Sarcoma Research: Latest Findings

Sarcoma Research: Latest Findings

Editor: Natalie Kasey

FOSTER ACADEMICS
www.fosteracademics.com

www.fosteracademics.com

FOSTER ACADEMICS

Cataloging-in-Publication Data

Sarcoma research : latest findings / edited by Natalie Kasey.
p. cm.
Includes bibliographical references and index.
ISBN 978-1-63242-914-8
1. Sarcoma. 2. Sarcoma--Research. 3. Sarcoma--Treatment. 4. Cancer. 5. Tumors. I. Kasey, Natalie.
RC270 .S273 2020
616.994--dc23

Foster Academics,
118-35 Queens Blvd., Suite 400,
Forest Hills, NY 11375, USA

ISBN 978-1-63242-914-8 (Hardback)

Contents

Contents

Preface

A sarcoma is a cancer which arises from the transformed cells of mesenchymal origin. Some types of sarcoma are chondrosarcoma, malignant hemangioendothelioma, chondrosarcoma, osteosarcoma, malignant schwannoma, soft tissue sarcomas, etc. Surgery is a recommended strategy for most cases of osteosarcoma. Amputation and limb-sparing surgery can be used for extremity tumor cases. Chemotherapy and radiation therapy can be administered before or after surgery. Prognosis is reasonably improved with chemotherapy, especially for bone sarcomas. Research in sarcoma explores ways to prevent, treat and manage sarcomas. New medications are being developed that are effective in the treatment of different subtypes of soft tissue sarcoma. Developing strategies for improved drug delivery and exploring new immune checkpoint inhibitors and targeted therapies are active areas of focus in sarcoma research. This book unravels the recent studies in sarcoma. The topics included herein are of utmost significance and bound to provide incredible insights to readers. Students, researchers, experts and oncologists will benefit alike from this book.

The information contained in this book is the result of intensive hard work done by researchers in this field. All due efforts have been made to make this book serve as a complete guiding source for students and researchers. The topics in this book have been comprehensively explained to help readers understand the growing trends in the field.

I would like to thank the entire group of writers who made sincere efforts in this book and my family who supported me in my efforts of working on this book. I take this opportunity to thank all those who have been a guiding force throughout my life.

Editor

1

Sarcopenia does not Affect Survival or Outcomes in Soft-Tissue Sarcoma

Robert J. Wilson,[1] Vignesh K. Alamanda,[2] Katherine G. Hartley,[3] Nathan W. Mesko,[4] Jennifer L. Halpern,[1] Herbert S. Schwartz,[1] and Ginger E. Holt[1]

[1]*Department of Orthopaedics and Rehabilitation, Vanderbilt University Medical Center, Nashville, TN 37232, USA*
[2]*Department of Orthopaedics, Carolinas Medical Center, Charlotte, NC 28203, USA*
[3]*Department of Radiology and Radiological Sciences, Vanderbilt University Medical Center, Nashville, TN 37232, USA*
[4]*Department of Orthopaedics, Cleveland Clinic, Cleveland, OH 44195, USA*

Correspondence should be addressed to Robert J. Wilson; robert.j.wilson@vanderbilt.edu

Academic Editor: C. Verhoef

Background and Objective. Sarcopenia is associated with decreased survival and increased complications in carcinoma patients. We hypothesized that sarcopenic soft-tissue sarcoma (STS) patients would have decreased survival, increased incidence of wound complications, and increased length of postresection hospital stay (LOS). *Methods.* A retrospective, single-center review of 137 patients treated surgically for STS was conducted. Sarcopenia was assessed by measuring the cross-sectional area of bilateral psoas muscles (total psoas muscle area, TPA) at the level of the third lumbar vertebrae on a pretreatment axial computed tomography scan. TPA was then adjusted for height (cm^2/m^2). The association between height-adjusted TPA and survival was assessed using Cox proportional hazard model. A logistical model was used to assess the association between height-adjusted TPA and wound complications. A linear model was used to assess the association between height-adjusted TPA and LOS. *Results.* Height-adjusted TPA was not an independent predictor of overall survival ($p = 0.746$). Patient age ($p = 0.02$) and tumor size ($p = 0.009$) and grade ($p = 0.001$) were independent predictors of overall survival. Height-adjusted TPA was not a predictor of increased hospital LOS ($p = 0.66$), greater incidence of postoperative infection ($p = 0.56$), or other wound complications ($p = 0.14$). *Conclusions.* Sarcopenia does not appear to impact overall survival, LOS, or wound complications in patients with STS.

1. Introduction

Sarcopenia, defined as the age-associated loss of skeletal muscle mass and function [1], has emerged as an important variable for predicting survival and complications for multiple malignancies. Sarcopenia has been shown to be an independent predictor of survival in patients with hepatocellular carcinoma [2], pancreatic adenocarcinoma [3], melanoma [4], and breast cancer [5]. Patients with sarcopenia have also been shown to be significantly more likely to have dose limiting toxicity from chemotherapeutic medications for renal cell carcinoma [6, 7], hepatocellular carcinoma [8], breast cancer [9], and thyroid cancer [10]. In addition, sarcopenia is associated with increased incidence of post-operative infection and length of hospital stay (LOS) in patients after colorectal cancer resections [11] and increased major complication rate and LOS in patients undergoing liver resection for colorectal cancer metastases [12].

The exact method of calculation of sarcopenia has been variable in the literature. However, calculating the area of skeletal muscle mass using computed tomography (CT) scans has become a commonly accepted modality for calculating sarcopenia and is considered by some to be the "gold standard" [13]. The use of the third or fourth lumbar vertebral level on an axial CT has become a common reference standard in multiple studies [3, 4, 11, 13] and a single cross-sectional slice for calculating muscle area has been shown to correlate strongly with whole body muscle mass [14, 15].

The numerical values for what constitutes sarcopenia are variable as well. Prado et al., in patients with gastrointestinal and pulmonary malignancies, established sex-specific cutoffs for sarcopenia: below 52.4 cm^2/m^2 for men and 38.5 cm^2/m^2

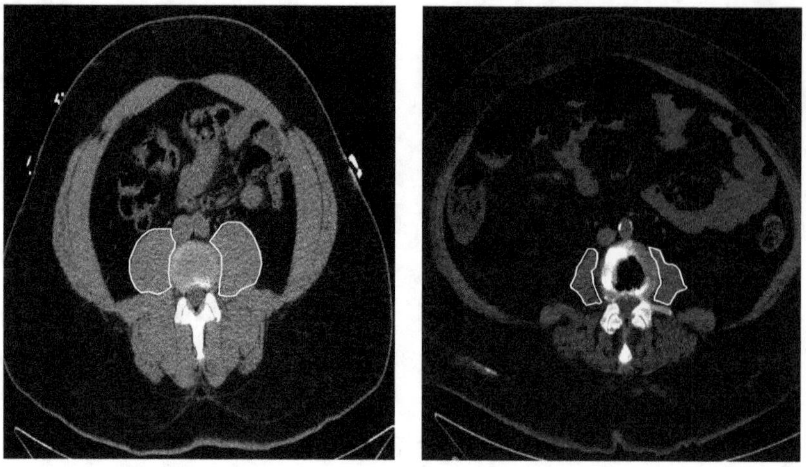

FIGURE 1: Example calculation method for TPA based on axial CT scan at L3 in two patients. Notice the difference in TPA between them.

for women, respectively, taken from mortality-based statistical stratification [16]. These values have since become reference standards for defining sarcopenia in multiple subsequent studies of carcinoma patients [8, 9, 11]. However, two other studies have used different cutoff values (43.75 cm^2/m^2 for men and 41.10 cm^2/m^2 for women) based on overall survival in patients undergoing resection of colorectal liver metastases [2, 17]. Yet another study defined sarcopenia as a total psoas area (TPA: combined surface area of bilateral psoas muscles) of less than 500 mm^2/m^2 based on optimum stratification [12].

To our knowledge, no prior studies exist that evaluate the relationship of sarcopenia to overall survival and treatment complications in patients with extremity soft-tissue sarcomas (STS) undergoing surgical resection. There are no established values for what constitutes sarcopenia in patients with soft-tissue sarcomas. We hypothesized that patients with STS and sarcopenia, as manifest by decreased height-adjusted TPA, would have decreased overall survival, increased incidence of postoperative wound complications including infection, and increased postresection LOS.

2. Materials and Methods

A retrospective, single-center review of 137 patients treated surgically for extremity STS between 2000 and 2008 was conducted. Relevant oncologic data and body mass index (weight (kg)/height (m^2)) were retrospectively extracted from our electronic medical record. Sarcopenia was assessed by manually measuring the cross-sectional area of the right and left psoas muscles (total psoas muscle area, TPA) on a single slice from a preoperative, staging CT scan at the level of the third lumbar vertebrae using Impax imaging software (version 6.3, Agfa Healthcare, Mortsel, Belgium), similar to the method outlined by Peng et al. [3]. TPA was then adjusted for height (cm^2/m^2). We chose this technique because it has been shown to be a valid method to calculate sarcopenia in the Peng et al. study and for the ease of manual measurement, given that only two muscle areas need to be traced out, as shown by the comparison scans of two patients in Figure 1.

In contrast, calculating the entire cross-sectional muscle area manually at the L3 level, unless aided by expensive computer software, is more time-consuming and potentially less reliable.

We used Wilcoxon rank sum test to compare continuous variables between two groups and Pearson chi-squared test to compare the categorical variables between groups. The association between height-adjusted TPA, age, gender, tumor grade, tumor depth, tumor size, surgical resection margin status, and overall survival was assessed using Cox proportional hazard model. A logistical model was used to assess the association between height-adjusted TPA and wound complications including infection with adjustment for age and gender. A wound infection was defined as requiring (1) oral or intravenous antibiotics, (2) in-clinic irrigation and debridement plus antibiotics, or (3) surgical irrigation and debridement plus antibiotics within 6 months of definitive sarcoma resection. Wound complications other than infection were defined as wound dehiscence requiring multiple gauze packing or negative pressure dressing changes or wound/flap necrosis requiring packing or debridement without need for antibiotics.

We applied a linear model with ordinary least squares to assess the association between height-adjusted TPA and length of stay with adjustment for age and gender. We did not establish gender-specific cutoffs to define sarcopenia as outlined elsewhere [16] as this is the first study to analyze sarcopenia in sarcoma patients. We instead linearly compared height-adjusted TPA with hospital LOS, wound infections, and wound complications as outlined above while controlling for gender. If sarcopenia, as manifested by decreased height-adjusted TPA, was found to be a significant predictor of poor outcomes on linear analysis, then risk stratification would be performed to establish appropriate cutoff values. A p

value < 0.05 was considered statistically significant. Statistical analyses were performed using open source R statistical software (version 3.0.2, Vienna, Austria) and SPSS (version 23, Armonk, NY). All statistical analyses were two-tailed. Our institution's internal review board gave approval for the study. No outside source of funding was used.

3. Results

Summary demographic, clinical, and outcome statistics are shown in Tables 1 and 2.

Height-adjusted TPA differed significantly between men and women ($p < 0.001$) (Table 2). Height-adjusted TPA was not an independent predictor of overall survival ($p = 0.746$), even after controlling for gender ($p = 0.712$), in Cox proportional hazard model as shown in Table 3. Similar to prior studies, both tumor size ($p = 0.009$) and grade ($p = 0.001$) were independent predictors of overall survival (Table 3). We also found increasing age ($p = 0.02$) to be an independent predictor of overall survival in Cox proportional hazard model. Tumor depth relative to investing fascia was not a significant predictor of survival ($p = 0.337$). Presence of a positive resection margin was not a significant predictor of survival as shown in Table 3 ($p = 0.422$).

Height-adjusted TPA was not a significant predictor of increased hospital LOS ($p = 0.66$), greater incidence of postoperative infection ($p = 0.56$), or incidence of other wound complications including dehiscence ($p = 0.14$), even after controlling for gender as shown in Table 4.

4. Discussion

This study is the first to analyze the influence of sarcopenia on survival and postoperative complications in patients with STS. Our study has several weaknesses. First, it is a single-center study with a relatively small number of patients and therefore the negative results could be due to the study being underpowered. However, multiple studies in the carcinoma literature have found sarcopenia to be a statistically significant predictor of outcomes, each with less patients enrolled than the 137 patients enrolled in this study [4, 7–9]. Second, the study is retrospective and does not contain any cancer-free control subjects. Third, our group of sarcomas was heterogeneous with regard to tumor grade, histologic subtype, and use of chemotherapy which may have influenced our results. Lastly, TPA was calculated based on manual measurements by authors Katherine G. Hartley and Vignesh K. Alamanda and may not be as precise as alternative methods such as using specially designed computer software.

We found no link between sarcopenia as manifest by height-adjusted TPA and overall survival, adverse events such as postoperative wound complications including infection, or increased hospital LOS. Using Cox proportional hazard model, we found that tumor grade and size were independent predictors of overall survival, similar to previous studies [18–20]. We also found that patient age was an independent predictor of overall survival, which has also been shown elsewhere [20].

The reasons our study did not find a link between sarcopenia, survival, LOS, and wound outcomes in STS are likely multifactorial. The average male and female height-adjusted TPA, shown in Table 2, were well above the 500 mm^2/m^2 TPA cutoff for sarcopenia used elsewhere [12]. Therefore the incidence, pathogenesis, and consequence of cancer cachexia and muscle wasting may be different in sarcomas than in carcinomas. However, we could find no studies in the literature looking at the clinical incidence or molecular and biochemical pathogenesis of muscle wasting and cachexia in soft-tissue sarcoma specifically. The predilection of most STS to metastasize to the lung hematogenously [21], in contradistinction to most carcinomas, is likely indicative of differential use of molecular signaling pathways and gene expression between the two cancer types [22].

In addition, 20% of the sarcomas in this study were superficial to the investing fascia, meaning direct structural influence on skeletal muscle was certainly limited and biochemical influence may be limited as well. The literature showing worse outcomes in carcinoma patients with sarcopenia includes multiple visceral abdominal tumors such as pancreatic, liver, and colorectal cancer which likely have a direct structural, as well as biochemical, effect on nutritional status that may be more significant than extremity sarcomas. For example, Lieffers et al. found that patients presenting with bowel obstruction from colorectal cancer were much more likely to have sarcopenia [11]. Our study also found no significant relationship between sarcopenia and postoperative wound complications, including infection. The principle study [11] to have shown a link between sarcopenia and "postoperative infections" also included postoperative pneumonia and urinary tract infections in addition to wound infections, which we did not.

The impact of sarcopenia on LOS has been variable with some carcinoma studies [11, 12] finding LOS increased in sarcopenic patients while another found no difference [3]. LOS on average in our study was 4 days, while the LOS in other studies with pancreaticoduodenectomies, liver resection, and bowel resections [3, 11, 12] varied from 10 to 15 days, likely indicative of a much larger physiologic insult than even large extremity STS resections. In addition, postoperative mobilization in our patient population is less likely to be limited by nausea, vomiting, ileus, and atelectasis thus possibly allowing for earlier discharges and less need for rehab or nursing facility placement.

We recommend performing further prospective clinical studies with larger sample sizes analyzing STS outcomes and correlating them with skeletal muscle mass and nutritional markers such as albumin and C-reactive protein. In addition, comparison of the molecular signaling pathways between sarcoma and carcinoma cachexia is needed to elucidate the likely differences between the two.

5. Conclusions

Sarcopenia, as manifested by decreased height-adjusted TPA, does not impact overall survival, hospital LOS, or wound complications including wound infection in patients with

TABLE 1: Demographic and clinical statistics.

		Range
Median age (years)	59	(42–70)
Median height (meters)	1.72	(1.6–1.8)
		Percentage
Gender	Male ($N = 69$)	50%
	Female ($N = 68$)	50%
Body mass index (BMI)	BMI < 30 ($N = 86$)	63%
	BMI 30–35 ($N = 30$)	22%
	BMI 35–40 ($N = 13$)	9%
	BMI 40–45 ($N = 4$)	3%
	BMI > 45 ($N = 4$)	3%
Surgery	Wide local excision ($N = 126$)	92%
	Amputation ($N = 11$)	8%
Surgical margins	Negative (R_0) ($N = 121$)	88%
	Positive (R_1) ($N = 16$)	12%
		Range
Median follow-up (years)	4.1	(1.7–5.6)
Median tumor size (cm)	9.0	(5.0–15.0)
Median time to death (months)	69	(40–89)
		Percentage
Tumor depth (relative to investing fascia)	Superficial ($N = 28$)	20%
	Deep ($N = 109$)	80%
Tumor grade	Low ($N = 25$)	18%
	Intermediate ($N = 15$)	11%
	High ($N = 97$)	71%
Histologic sarcoma type	Fibrosarcoma ($N = 5$)	4%
	Leiomyosarcoma ($N = 16$)	12%
	Liposarcoma ($N = 30$)	22%
	Malignant peripheral nerve sheath tumor ($N = 3$)	2%
	Undifferentiated pleiomorphic sarcoma ($N = 57$)	42%
	Synovial sarcoma ($N = 7$)	5%
	Vascular sarcoma ($N = 5$)	4%
	Rhabdomyosarcoma ($N = 1$)	1%
	Others ($N = 13$)	9%
AJCC stage at presentation	I ($N = 34$)	25%
	II ($N = 27$)	20%
	III ($N = 33$)	24%
	IV ($N = 42$)	31%
Preoperative radiation	Yes ($N = 32$)	23%
	No ($N = 105$)	77%
Postoperative radiation	Yes ($N = 84$)	61%
	No ($N = 53$)	39%
Chemotherapy	Yes ($N = 28$)	21%
	No ($N = 106$)	79%
Survival status at last follow-up	Alive ($N = 94$)	69%
	Died of disease ($N = 23$)	17%
	Died of other causes ($N = 10$)	7%
	Uncertain cause of death ($N = 5$)	4%

TABLE 2: Outcome variables by gender.

	Male (N = 69)	Female (N = 68)	p value
Average height-adjusted TPA (cm^2/m^2)	7.3	5.2	<0.001[2]
Median height-adjusted TPA (range, cm^2/m^2)	7.3 (6.1–8.2)	4.9 (4.4–5.9)	
Wound infection			0.12[1]
Yes (N = 23)	15	8	
No (N = 114)	54	60	
Wound complications			0.064[1]
Yes (N = 38)	24	14	
No (N = 99)	45	54	
Wound dehiscence			0.14[1]
Yes (N = 28)	15	13	
No (N = 10)	8	2	
Wound necrosis			0.8[1]
Yes (N = 11)	7	4	
No (N = 27)	16	11	
Average length of hospital stay (days)	3.9	4.3	0.7[2]
Median length of hospital stay (range in days)	3.0 (3.0–4.2)	3.0 (3.0–6.0)	
Postsurgical disposition			0.8[1]
Home (N = 116)	57	59	
Home with home health physical therapy (N = 5)	4	1	
Skilled nursing facility (N = 5)	2	3	
Inpatient rehab (N = 6)	3	3	
Transfer to another hospital (N = 3)	2	1	
Unknown disposition (N = 2)	1	1	

1 = Pearson test, 2 = Wilcoxon test.

TABLE 3: Results of Cox proportional hazard model for height-adjusted total psoas area (TPA) and overall survival.

Variable	X^2	d.f. (degrees of freedom)	p value
Height-adjusted TPA	0.105	1	0.746
Height-adjusted TPA controlling for gender	0.137	1	0.712
Patient age	5.403	1	0.02
Tumor size	6.796	1	0.009
Tumor grade	10.11	1	0.001
Tumor depth	0.920	1	0.337
R_1 resection margin (positive margin)	0.645	1	0.422

TABLE 4: Linear analysis of height-adjusted total psoas area (TPA) and hospital LOS, postoperative infection, and wound complications.

TPA category	Variable	X^2	d.f. (degrees of freedom)	p value
Height-adjusted TPA	Hospital LOS*		4	0.66
	Wound infection	1.16	2	0.56
	Wound complications	3.92	2	0.14
Height-adjusted TPA controlling for gender	Hospital LOS*		2	0.34
	Wound infection	1.02	1	0.31
	Wound complications	1.28	1	0.26

*Analysis of variance test performed instead of chi-squared analysis due to LOS being a noncategorical variable.

extremity STS. Biological, molecular, and pathological differences between patients with soft-tissue sarcomas and carcinomas may explain the differential effects of sarcopenia on patient outcomes.

References

[1] R. A. Fielding, B. Vellas, W. J. Evans et al., "Sarcopenia: an undiagnosed condition in older adults. Current consensus definition: prevalence, etiology, and consequences. International working group on sarcopeni," *Journal of the American Medical Directors Association*, vol. 12, no. 4, pp. 249–256, 2011.

[2] N. Harimoto, K. Shirabe, Y.-I. Yamashita et al., "Sarcopenia as a predictor of prognosis in patients following hepatectomy for hepatocellular carcinoma," *British Journal of Surgery*, vol. 100, no. 11, pp. 1523–1530, 2013.

[3] P. Peng, O. Hyder, A. Firoozmand et al., "Impact of sarcopenia on outcomes following resection of pancreatic adenocarcinoma," *Journal of Gastrointestinal Surgery*, vol. 16, no. 8, pp. 1478–1486, 2012.

[4] M. S. Sabel, J. Lee, S. Cai, M. J. Englesbe, S. Holcombe, and S. Wang, "Sarcopenia as a prognostic factor among patients with stage III melanoma," *Annals of Surgical Oncology*, vol. 18, no. 13, pp. 3579–3585, 2011.

[5] A. Villaseñor, R. Ballard-Barbash, K. Baumgartner et al., "Prevalence and prognostic effect of sarcopenia in breast cancer survivors: the HEAL Study," *Journal of Cancer Survivorship*, vol. 6, no. 4, pp. 398–406, 2012.

[6] S. Antoun, L. Birdsell, M. B. Sawyer, P. Venner, B. Escudier, and V. E. Baracos, "Association of skeletal muscle wasting with treatment with sorafenib in patients with advanced renal cell carcinoma: results from a placebo-controlled study," *Journal of Clinical Oncology*, vol. 28, no. 6, pp. 1054–1060, 2010.

[7] O. Huillard, O. Mir, M. Peyromaure et al., "Sarcopenia and body mass index predict sunitinib-induced early dose-limiting toxicities in renal cancer patients," *British Journal of Cancer*, vol. 108, no. 5, pp. 1034–1041, 2013.

[8] O. Mir, R. Coriat, B. Blanchet et al., "Sarcopenia predicts early dose-limiting toxicities and pharmacokinetics of sorafenib in patients with hepatocellular carcinoma," *PLoS ONE*, vol. 7, no. 5, Article ID e37563, 2012.

[9] C. M. M. Prado, V. E. Baracos, L. J. McCargar et al., "Sarcopenia as a determinant of chemotherapy toxicity and time to tumor progression in metastatic breast cancer patients receiving capecitabine treatment," *Clinical Cancer Research*, vol. 15, no. 8, pp. 2920–2926, 2009.

[10] M.-H. Massicotte, I. Borget, S. Broutin et al., "Body composition variation and impact of low skeletal muscle mass in patients with advanced medullary thyroid carcinoma treated with vandetanib: results from a placebo-controlled study," *Journal of Clinical Endocrinology and Metabolism*, vol. 98, no. 6, pp. 2401–2408, 2013.

[11] J. R. Lieffers, O. F. Bathe, K. Fassbender, M. Winget, and V. E. Baracos, "Sarcopenia is associated with postoperative infection and delayed recovery from colorectal cancer resection surgery," *British Journal of Cancer*, vol. 107, no. 6, pp. 931–936, 2012.

[12] P. D. Peng, M. G. van Vledder, S. Tsai et al., "Sarcopenia negatively impacts short-term outcomes in patients undergoing hepatic resection for colorectal liver metastasis," *HPB*, vol. 13, no. 7, pp. 439–446, 2011.

[13] C. M. M. Prado, L. A. Birdsell, and V. E. Baracos, "The emerging role of computerized tomography in assessing cancer cachexia," *Current Opinion in Supportive and Palliative Care*, vol. 3, no. 4, pp. 269–275, 2009.

[14] W. Shen, M. Punyanitya, Z. Wang et al., "Visceral adipose tissue: relations between single-slice areas and total volume," *American Journal of Clinical Nutrition*, vol. 80, no. 2, pp. 271–278, 2004.

[15] W. Shen, M. Punyanitya, Z. Wang et al., "Total body skeletal muscle and adipose tissue volumes: estimation from a single abdominal cross-sectional image," *Journal of Applied Physiology*, vol. 97, no. 6, pp. 2333–2338, 2004.

[16] C. M. Prado, J. R. Lieffers, L. J. McCargar et al., "Prevalence and clinical implications of sarcopenic obesity in patients with solid tumours of the respiratory and gastrointestinal tracts: a population-based study," *The Lancet Oncology*, vol. 9, no. 7, pp. 629–635, 2008.

[17] M. G. van Vledder, S. Levolger, N. Ayez, C. Verhoef, T. C. K. Tran, and J. N. M. Ijzermans, "Body composition and outcome in patients undergoing resection of colorectal liver metastases," *British Journal of Surgery*, vol. 99, no. 4, pp. 550–557, 2012.

[18] M. F. Brennan, C. R. Antonescu, N. Moraco, and S. Singer, "Lessons learned from the study of 10,000 patients with soft tissue sarcoma," *Annals of Surgery*, vol. 260, no. 3, pp. 416–422, 2014.

[19] I. Atean, Y. Pointreau, P. Rosset, P. Garaud, G. De-Pinieux, and G. Calais, "Prognostic factors of extremity soft tissue sarcoma in adults. A single institutional analysis," *Cancer/Radiothérapie*, vol. 16, no. 8, pp. 661–666, 2012.

[20] K. Maretty-Nielsen, N. Aggerholm-Pedersen, A. Safwat et al., "Prognostic factors for local recurrence and mortality in adult soft tissue sarcoma of the extremities and trunk wall," *Acta Orthopaedica*, vol. 85, no. 3, pp. 323–332, 2014.

[21] E. Pennacchioli, G. Tosti, M. Barberis et al., "Sarcoma spreads primarily through the vascular system: are there biomarkers associated with vascular spread?" *Clinical and Experimental Metastasis*, vol. 29, no. 7, pp. 757–773, 2012.

[22] K. Tschoep, A. Kohlmann, M. Schlemmer, T. Haferlach, and R.-D. Issels, "Gene expression profiling in sarcomas," *Critical Reviews in Oncology/Hematology*, vol. 63, no. 2, pp. 111–124, 2007.

2

Retinal Targets ALDH Positive Cancer Stem Cell and Alters the Phenotype of Highly Metastatic Osteosarcoma Cells

Xiaodong Mu,[1] Stuti Patel,[2] Damel Mektepbayeva,[3] Adel Mahjoub,[2] Johnny Huard,[1] and Kurt Weiss[2]

[1]*Department of Orthopaedic Surgery, University of Texas Health Science Center at Houston, Houston, TX 77030, USA*
[2]*Cancer Stem Cell Laboratory, Department of Orthopaedic Surgery, University of Pittsburgh, Pittsburgh, PA 15219, Kazakhstan*
[3]*Laboratory of Cellular Technology, Nazarbayev University, Astana, Akmola 010000, USA*

Correspondence should be addressed to Kurt Weiss; weiskr@upmc.edu

Academic Editor: Kanya Honoki

Aldehyde dehydrogenase (ALDH) is a cancer stem cell marker. Retinoic acid has antitumor properties, including the induction of apoptosis and inhibition of proliferation. Retinal, the precursor of retinoic acid, can be oxidized to retinoic acid by dehydrogenases, including ALDH. We hypothesized that retinal could potentially be transformed to retinoic acid with higher efficiency by cancer stem cells, due to the higher ALDH activity. We previously observed that ALDH activity is greater in highly metastatic K7M2 osteosarcoma (OS) cells than in nonmetastatic K12 OS cells. We also demonstrated that ALDH activity correlates with clinical metastases in bone sarcoma patients, suggesting that ALDH may be a therapeutic target specific to cells with high metastatic potential. Our current results demonstrated that retinal preferentially affected the phenotypes of ALDH-high K7M2 cells in contrast to ALDH-low K12 cells, which could be mediated by the more efficient transformation of retinal to retinoic acid by ALDH in K7M2 cells. Retinal treatment of highly metastatic K7M2 cells decreased their proliferation, invasion capacity, and resistance to oxidative stress. Retinal altered the expression of metastasis-related genes. These observations indicate that retinal may be used to specifically target metastatic cancer stem cells in OS.

1. Introduction

Retinoids are a class of compounds comprised of several signaling molecules, such as retinoic acid and retinaldehyde, that are structurally related to vitamin A (retinol) [1]. These molecules play a crucial role in the regulation of various cellular processes. Retinoids have been shown to exert a tumor-suppressive effect on cells based on their interaction with cyclins and cyclin-dependent kinases (CDKs) to prevent cell-cycle progression [1]. Additionally, they also influence cancer cell differentiation and apoptosis [2]. Many cancers have been shown to have abnormally low levels of various retinoids.

Retinoic acid, a derivative of retinol, has been shown to inhibit proliferation of malignant tumors and induce the apoptosis and differentiation in various types of cancer cells [1, 3–6]. Due to retinoic acid's antitumor properties, its role is being investigated in the treatment of various malignancies [3]. It is currently used in the treatment of acute promyelocytic leukemia and has been shown to result in complete remission [7]. Retinoic acid is derived from its precursor, all-trans-retinal (also called retinaldehyde or vitamin A aldehyde), by the action of dehydrogenases, including aldehyde dehydrogenase (ALDH) [8]. Previous studies have demonstrated that high ALDH activity predicted poor survival in various types of cancers [9, 10], such as breast cancer [11], epithelial cancer [12], and sarcoma [13]. ALDH activity is often specifically upregulated in cancer stem cells and has been recognized as a marker for cancer stem cells [10, 14–16]. Therefore, we believe it is reasonable to hypothesize that, because of the higher ALDH activity in cancer stem cells, retinal could be more efficiently transformed to retinoic acid by cancer stem cells, and thus preferentially induce the apoptosis and alteration of these cells.

Osteosarcoma (OS) is the most common primary tumor of the bone. It has a bimodal age distribution with a major peak during the second decade of life and a second smaller peak observed in patients over 50 years old. The lung is the most common site of metastatic spread, and survival is ultimately determined by the presence of absence of pulmonary metastatic disease. Deaths related to OS are thus the result of metastasis to the lung rather than the primary tumor itself. The prognosis of patients with OS has not improved in the past several decades due to the lack of treatment specifically targeting OS cell metastatic potential. Due to our limited understanding of the biology of sarcoma metastasis, this problem remains unsolved.

We have demonstrated the role of various cytokines and signaling pathways in OS metastasis using two related cell populations of a spontaneously occurring murine OS [17–20]. These cell lines, K12 and K7M2, differ in their metastatic potential, with K7M2 showing more features of cancer stem cells and a much greater metastatic rate to the lungs compared to K12 cells. The difference in their characteristics and metastatic potentials demonstrated that K7M2 and K12 feature different activation statuses of multiple biologic factors and signaling pathways: ALDH, Notchl, andmammalian target of rapamycin (mTOR). The inhibition of these signaling pathways alters OS cell behavior *in vitro* [17–20]. We observed that K7M2 cells demonstrated greater ALDH gene expression and activity than the less metastatic K12 cells. Additionally, ALDH activity was found to be greater in cultured cells from bone sarcoma patients who experienced clinical metastasis [21]. We thus hypothesized that ALDH might represent a means to specifically target sarcoma cells with high metastatic potential.

Our current research investigates the effect of novel treatment approaches to these metastasis-related genes. In the present study, we sought to take advantage of the increased level of ALDH activity in highly metastatic K7M2 OS cells to study the effects of retinal on cell growth and metastasis. Given the ability of retinal to be transformed into retinoic acid by ALDH and the high level of expression of ALDH in cancer stem cells, we hypothesized that treatment with retinal would selectively induce apoptosis and suppress tumor growth in K7M2 OS cells.

2. Materials and Methods

2.1. Cell Culture and Retinal Treatment. K12 and K7M2 cells were cultured in proliferation medium (10% FBS in DMEM). 5,000 cells were seeded in each well of a 12-well plastic plate. Cells were treated with either 1 μg/mL or 5 μg/mL of all-trans-retinal (Sigma) dissolved in 1 mL of proliferation medium. K7M2 cells treated with 1 μL of DMSO served as control. Cells were incubated for 2 days, before being fixed for observation or harvested for mRNA isolation.

2.2. Fluorescence-Activated Cell Sorting (FACS) Analysis of ALDH Activity and Sorting of Cells. ALDH enzymatic activity was determined using the Aldefluor Kit (STEMCELL Technologies). Cultured K7M2 cells from treatment as well as control groups were resuspended in Aldefluor buffer

TABLE 1: Primer sequences.

Gene	Primer sequence
GAPDH	Forward: TCCATGACAACTTTGGCATTG Reverse: TCACGCCACAGCTTTCCA
Notchl	Forward: GCCGCAAGAGGCTTGAGAT Reverse: GGAGTCCTGGCATCGTTGG
Hesl	Forward: CCAGCCAGTGTCAACACGA Reverse: AATGCCGGGAGCTATCTTTCT
BMP2	Forward: TCTTCCGGGAACAGATACAGG Reverse: TGGTGTCCAATAGTCTGGTCA
Aktl	Forward: ATGAACGACGTAGCCATTGTG Reverse: TTGTAGCCAATAAAGGTGCCAT
cMyc	Forward: TGACCTAACTCGAGGAGGAGCTGGAATC Reverse: AAGTTTGAGGCAGTTAAAATTATGGCTGAAGC
ALDHl	Forward: GACAGGCTTTCCAGATTGGCTC Reverse: AAGACTTTCCCACCATTGAGTGC
Klotho	Forward: CCCAAACCATCTATGAAAC Reverse: CTACCGTATTCTATGCCTTC

(1×10^6 cells/mL) and incubated at 37°C as per manufacturer's instructions. During the cell sorting process, cells were washed in Aldefluor buffer and maintained at 4°C. FL1 channel of a BD FACSAria Cell Sorting System and FACSDiva software (version 6.1.2; Becton, Dickinson and Company, San Jose, CA) was used to assess ALDH activity. Fluorescence-activated cell sorting (FACS) was utilized to collect cells according to their fluorescence intensity, which corresponds to cells' ALDH activity level. Cells with high and low ALDH levels were separately isolated and cultured.

2.3. Semiquantitative Reverse Transcription Polymerase Chain Reaction (RT-PCR). RNeasy plus mini kit (Qiagen) and the iScript cDNA Synthesis kit (Bio-Rad) were used to extract RNA from the cells and generate cDNA, respectively. RT-PCR was performed using a Bio-Rad MyiQ thermal cycler (Bio-Rad). Table 1 shows the sense and antisense primers for RT-PCR and their product. Following cycling parameters were used for all reactions: 94°C for 5 minutes; 30 cycles of the following: denature for 45 seconds at 95°C, anneal for 30 seconds (53°C–56°C), and extend for 45 seconds at 72°C. Expression of target genes was normalized to the expression of GAPDH, which served as a control gene. ImageJ software (version 1.32j, National Institutes of Health, Bethesda, MD) was used to perform RT-PCR analysis. The integrated density of bands was calculated based on product of the area and the mean gray value. All molecular bands were normalized to GAPDH.

2.4. Cell In Vitro Invasion Assay. In vitro invasion capacity of K7M2 cells treated with retinal was compared to control cells using a real-time cell invasion and migration (RT-CIM) assay system (ACEA Biosciences, Inc.), with a 16-well transwell plate (CIM-plate 16, Roche Diagnostics GmbH). The surface of the wells in the upper chamber was coated with Matrigel (BD BioSciences, Bedford, MA, USA) of different concentrations (2.5%, 5%, and 10%). Serum-containing medium (10% FBS) was added to the wells of the lower chamber. Cells (4×10^4 per well) in serum-free medium were seeded in the upper chamber. The migration of the cells through the Matrigel was monitored by the system every 15 minutes for 24 hours. Data analysis was carried out using RTCA Software 1.2 supplied with the instrument.

2.5. Actin Staining. Cells from each group were treated with phalloidin conjugated with Alexa Fluor 488 (Invitrogen) to observe actin organization. Treatment and control cells were grown overnight in proliferation medium in 12-well plates (50,000 cells/plate). The following day, the plates were washed twice with PBS, fixed in 3.7% formaldehyde solution for 10 minutes at room temperature, and washed two more times with PBS. The cells were then permeabilized in 0.1% Trition X-100 for 20 minutes and washed again with PBS. 5 μL of methanolic stock solution phalloidin, 200 μL PBS, and 1% BSA were added to each well and allowed to stand for 20 minutes, before being washed again with PBS. 300 μL of 300 nM DAPI was used for nuclear staining.

2.6. Statistical Analysis. Statistical analysis of all experiments for this study was carried out using data from at least three samples from each treatment group. Statistical significance was evaluated using Student's t-test. Difference between groups was considered significant for p value <0.05.

3. Results

3.1. Retinal Treatment of Highly Metastatic K7M2 Cells Decreased the Proliferation Capacity and Resistance to Oxidative Stress. K7M2 cells have been shown to feature much higher ALDH activity compared with K12 cells [17, 18]. K7M2 cells treated with all-trans-retinal (5 μg/mL) for 2 days were observed to have fewer cells on the culture dishes compared with the nontreated K7M2 cells (Figure 1(a)). Actually, compared to retinal-treated K12 cells, the proliferation of retinal-treated K7M2 cells was much more obviously decreased (Figure 1), indicating preferentially increased apoptosis in retinal-treated K7M2 cells. Furthermore, retinal-treated K7M2 cells also displayed higher levels of apoptosis induced by exposure to hydrogen peroxide (250 μM, 1 hr), as seen by propidium iodide (PI) staining (data not shown). Our previous results have shown that the sorted ALDH-high K7M2 cells are more resistant to oxidative stress-induced cell death, compared with the sorted ALDH-low cells [17]. Treatment of ALDH-high K7M2 cells with retinal (5 μg/mL) for 2 days significantly increased the ratio of apoptotic cells induced by exposure to hydrogen peroxide, compared to nontreated control ALDH-high K7M2 cells (Figure 2). The apoptotic effect was much more pronounced than in ALDH-low K7M2 cells. This observation indicates that the resistance to oxidative stress of K7M2 cells was preferentially decreased by retinal in cells with high ALDH activity.

3.2. Retinal Treatment of K7M2 Cells Resulted in Modified Gene Expression of Metastasis-Related Factors and Reduced ALDH Activity. Semiquantitative PCR analysis of K7M2 cells with and without retinal treatment was carried out to compare the expression levels of various signaling molecules involved in cell proliferation, apoptosis, and metastasis. Treatment with retinal resulted in the downregulation of Notch signaling as evidenced by decreased expression of Notchl and Hesl. Further, there was also a decrease in bone morphogenetic protein 2 (BMP2), cMyc, and ALDH levels while Klotho, a tumor suppressor, was up-egulated with retinal treatment (Figure 3(a)). Additionally, ALDH activity assay of K7M2 cells verified that retinal treatment (both 1 μg/mL and 5 μg/mL) was able to reduce the ALDH activity of K7M2 cells (Figure 3(b)).

3.3. Retinal Treatment of K7M2 Cells Altered Cell Morphological Characteristics and Decreased Invasion Capacity. Our previous results demonstrated that K7M2 cells feature different cell morphology than K12 cells and have significantly higher migration and invasion capacities *in vitro* [17, 18]. Here, actin staining by phalloidin demonstrated that K7M2 cells treated with retinal had undergone obvious alterations in migration-related cell morphological characteristics with reduced appearance of invadopodia, which play critical roles in cell migration/invasion (Figure 4(a)). Finally, *in vitro* invasion assays further displayed that treatment of K7M2 cells with retinal (5 μg/mL, 2 days) resulted in decreased cell invasion compared with untreated cells (Figure 4(b)).

4. Discussion

All-trans-retinal is a precursor of retinoic acid and can be transformed into retinoic acid by dehydrogenases, including ALDH. Retinoic acid has been shown to induce differentiation of hematopoietic and neural stem cells. Retinoic acid appears to induce apoptosis and differentiation in a number of cancers and has been successfully used to treat acute promyelocytic leukemia [1, 7]. However, the role of retinal as an antiproliferative agent in OS has not been studied. Based on the fact that retinal can be transformed to retinoic acid by ALDH, and ALDH activity is typically higher in cancer stem cells [9, 15, 18], we investigated the effect that retinal would have on highly metastatic OS cells.

Our study revealed that retinal was able to preferentially target the highly metastatic K7M2 cells which feature greater ALDH activity and other stem cell characteristics, by repressing their proliferation and inducing the apoptosis of these cells. The role of retinal in decreasing cell proliferation and cell survival was demonstrated by exposing cells to oxidative stress using hydrogen peroxide. ALDH-high K7M2 cells exhibited a greater increase in apoptosis compared to ALDH-low K7M2 cells. Additionally, our RT-PCR results also showed that retinal treatment results in the downregulation of various genes involved in cell-proliferation and cell survival. Namely, the expression level of Notchl, Hesl, cMyc, and BMP2 was decreased in a dose-dependent manner. Further, there was an upregulation of Klotho, a tumor suppressor gene.

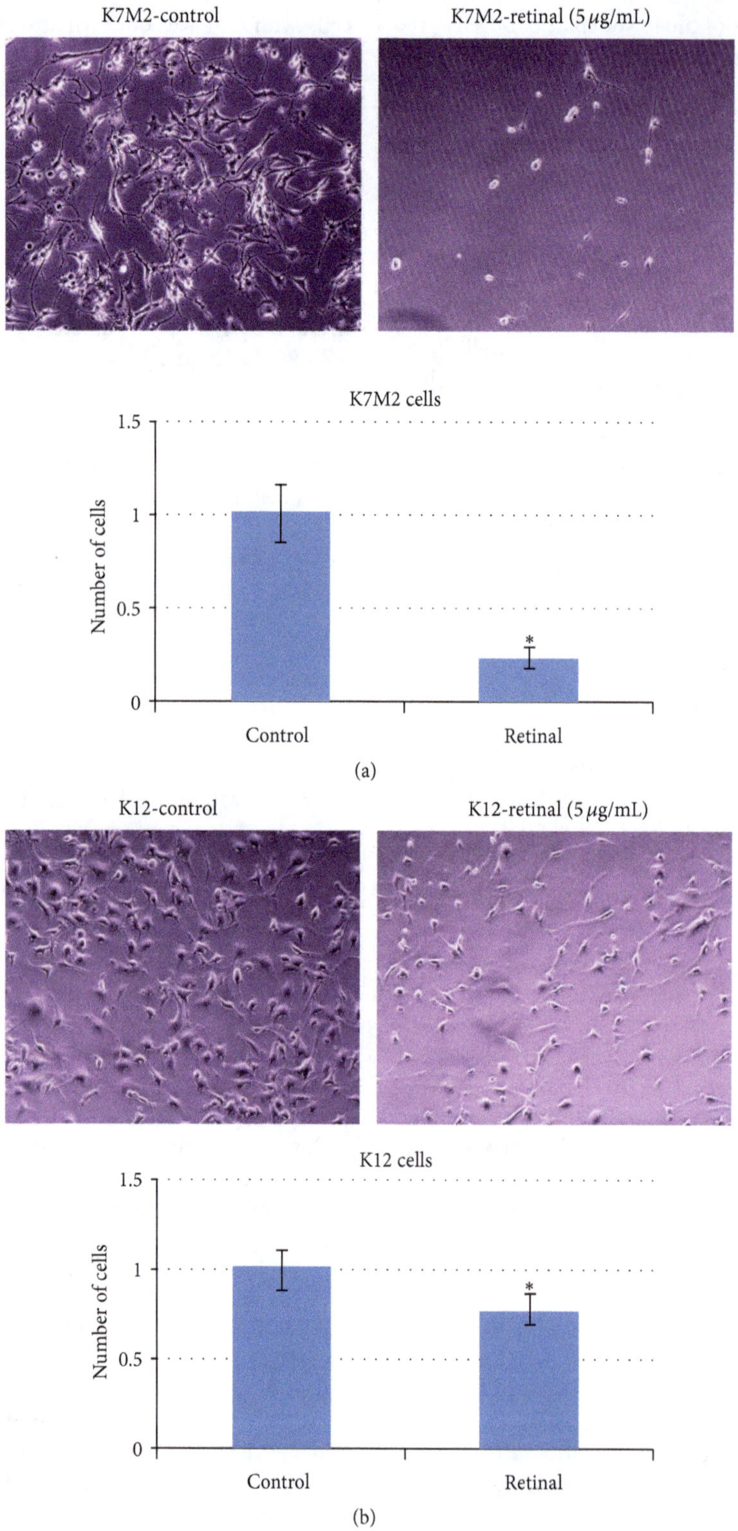

FIGURE 1: Retinal treatment of K7M2 cells decreased cell proliferation or survival. (a) and (b) The cell proliferation or survival capacity of K7M2 cells was more reduced with retinal treatment (5 μg/mL, 2 days), compared to K12 cells.

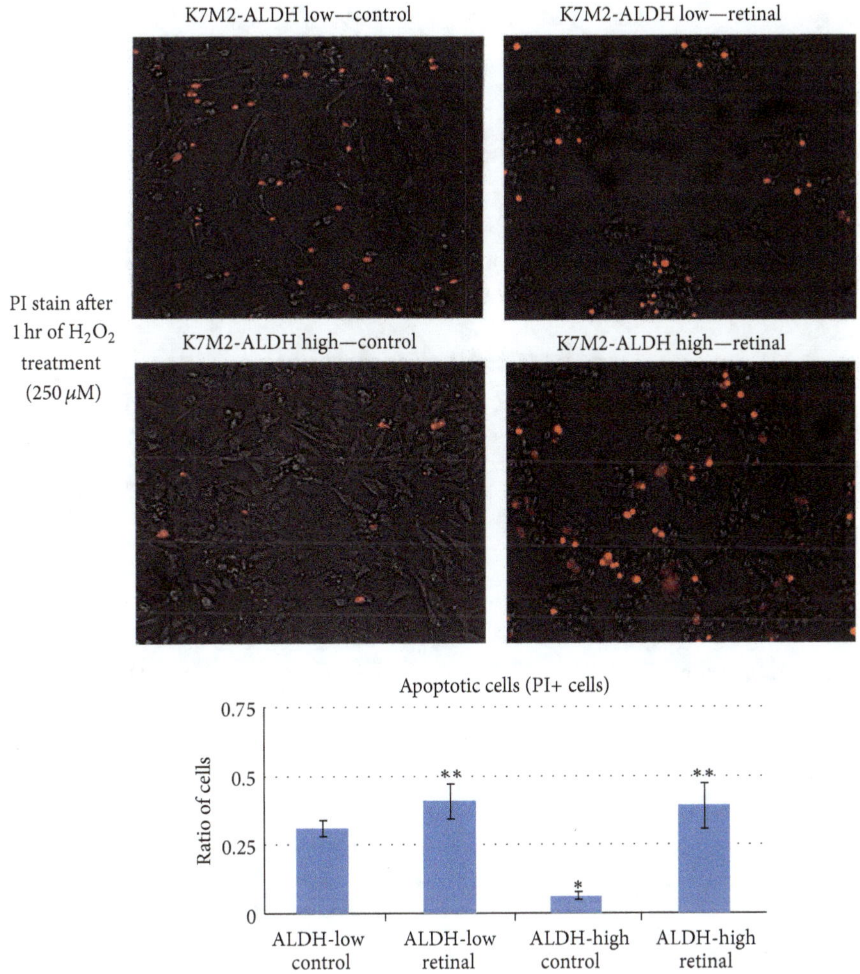

FIGURE 2: Retinal treatment of sorted ALDH-high K7M2 cells decreased antioxidative stress capacity. After cell sorting according to ALDH activity, it showed that the K7M2-ALDH high cells were more resistant to oxidative stress (H_2O_2, 250 μM for 1 hr) than the K7M2-ALDH low cells, while the retinal treatment of K7M2-ALDH high cells was able to greatly decrease their resistance to oxidative stress and resulted in more cell apoptosis. "*" indicates that ALDH-high control cells are significant different ($p < 0.05$) compared to ALDH-low control cells; "**" indicates retinal treated ALDH-high or ALDH-low cells are significant different ($p < 0.05$) compared to nontreated ALDH-high or ALDH-low control cells, respectively.

Additionally, use of retinal as a therapeutic agent not only employs the antiproliferative properties of retinoic acid but also takes advantage of certain factors produced by tumor stem cells specifically. The action of retinal on the cells is mediated by retinoic acid [2]. Given that the conversion of retinal to retinoic acid requires the action of dehydrogenases, it can be expected that the activity of retinal will be higher in tumor stem cells, which produce much higher quantities of ALDH, thereby making retinal therapy highly specific. Our results, therefore, indicate that retinal may be used as a cellular "Trojan Horse" of sorts to specifically target cancer stem cells.

Since pulmonary metastasis is the major cause of mortality in OS patients, it is crucial to devise therapeutic options that specifically target the metastatic potential of OS cells. Actin staining was performed to characterize the changes in cell morphology following treatment with retinal. We have previously demonstrated that changes in K7M2 cell shape and appearance of invadopodia relate to alteration in cells' migration/invasion potentials [17–21]. Our results demonstrate that in addition to acting as an antiproliferative agent, retinal also decreased cell invasiveness. Based on these results, we conclude that retinal therapy has the potential to specifically target metastatic OS cells and thus potentially decrease the incidence of pulmonary metastases, the ultimate cause of mortality in OS.

One of the limitations of this study is that the results are based on experiments carried out *in vitro*. While several studies have verified that the behavior of K7M2 cells parallels the growth of human OS cells, it is essential to conduct *in vivo* studies in order to validate these results.

5. Conclusion

Our current results demonstrate that retinal was capable of specifically acting on OS cells which express high levels of

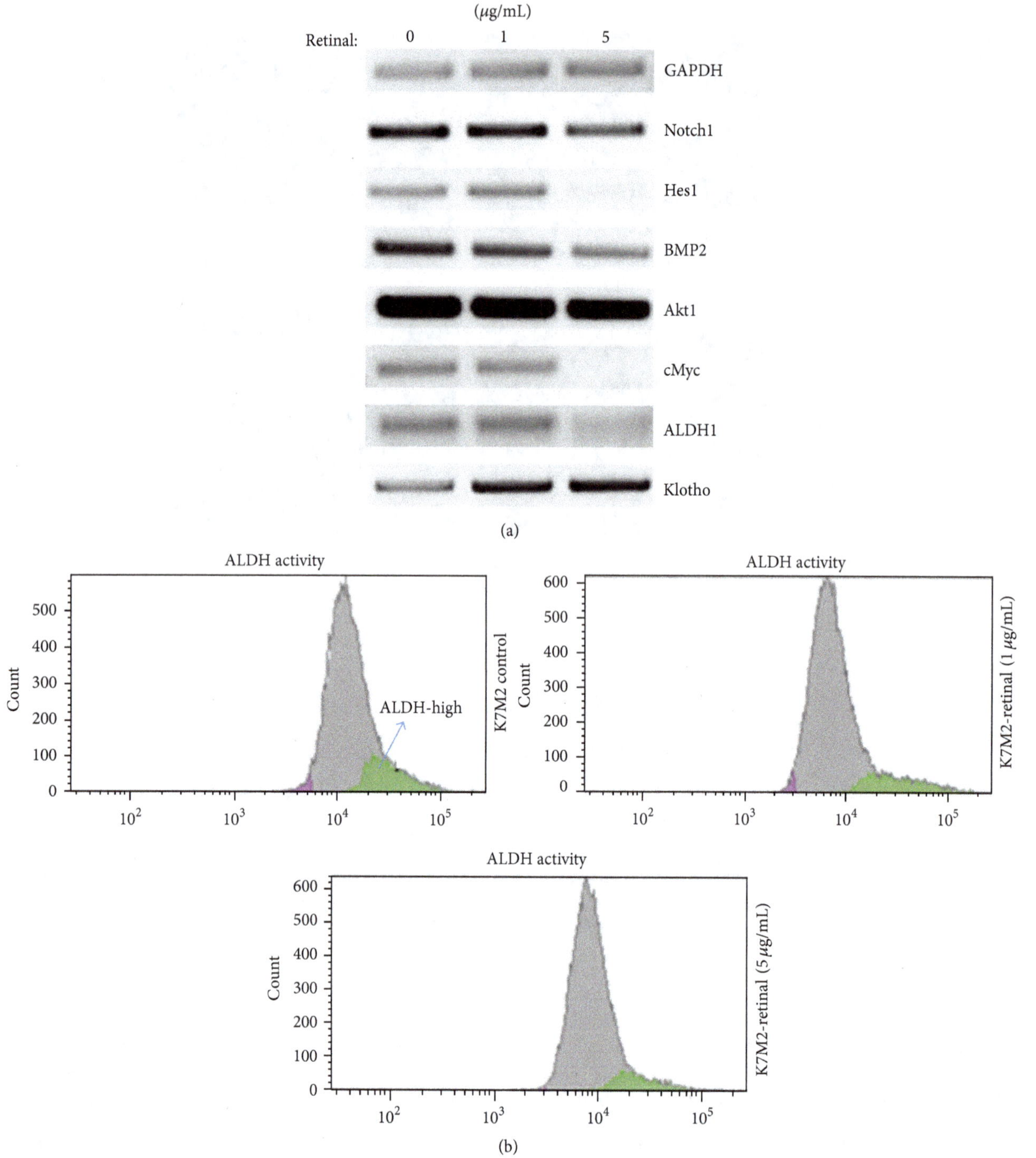

FIGURE 3: Retinal treatment of K7M2 cells modified the expression of metastasis-related genes and reduced ALDH activity. (a) RT-PCR results showed retinal treatment of K7M2 cells (1 or 5 μg/mL for 2 days) modified the expression of some key genes related with metastasis or tumorigenesis. (b) ALDH activity assay showed that retinal treatment of K7M2 cells reduced the aLDH activity of the cells.

ALDH and promoted these cells to undergo apoptosis. As cancer stem cells typically feature high ALDH activity, retinal could be used to specifically repress the growth of cancer stem cells with enhanced metastatic potential. Our study is the first to demonstrate the potential application of retinal for the treatment of tumorigenesis. We suggest that retinal could be potentially used to target OS cells with stem-like properties and ultimately decrease the ability of these cells to metastasize.

Abbreviations

ALDH: Aldehyde dehydrogenase
retinal: All-trans-retinal

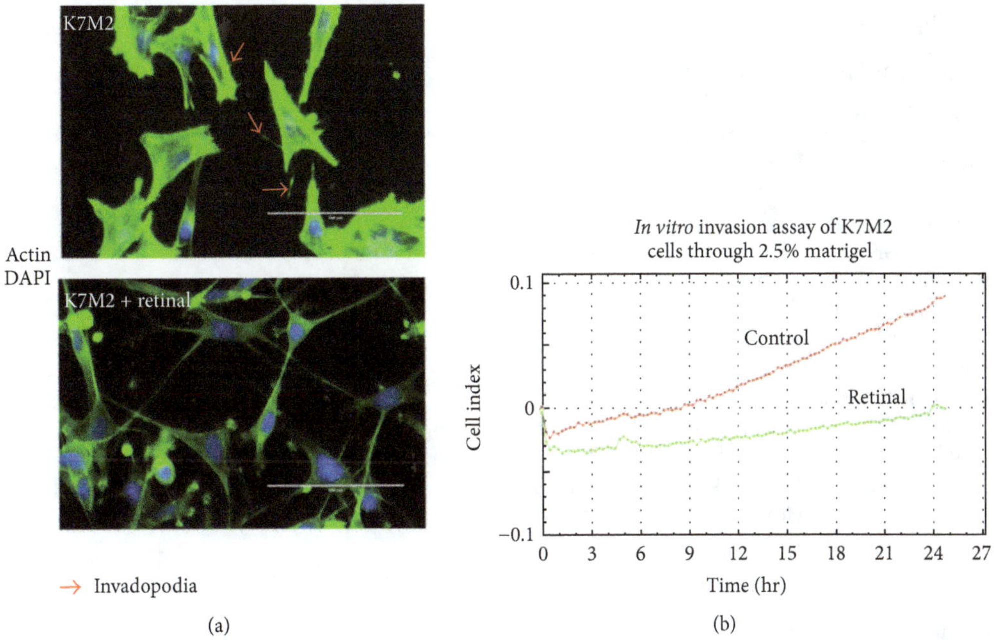

FIGURE 4: Retinal treatment of K7M2 cells changed migration-related cell morphological characteristics and decreased migration capacity. (a) Actin staining with phalloidin revealed that the cell morphology of K7M2 cells was modified with retinal treatment (5 μg/mL for 2 days), showing reduced presence of invadopodia. (b) *In vitro* invasion assay with 3D-matrigel (2.5%) revealed that K7M2 cells treated with retinal treatment (5 μg/mL for 2 days) migrated slower than nontreated K7M2 control cells.

FACS: Fluorescence-activated cell sorting
BMP: Bone morphogenetic protein
mTOR: Mammalian target of rapamycin.

Acknowledgments

The authors would acknowledge the funding support from NIH granted to Dr. Kurt Weiss (K08 CA177927), Sarcoma Foundation of America (SFA), University of Pittsburgh Cancer Institute, Pittsburgh Cure Sarcoma, and the Houy family in loving memory of Jon Houy.

References

[1] X.-H. Tang and L. J. Gudas, "Retinoids, retinoic acid receptors, and cancer," *Annual Review of Pathology*, vol. 6, pp. 345–364, 2011.

[2] N. Noy, "Between death and survival: retinoic acid in regulation of apoptosis," *Annual Review of Nutrition*, vol. 30, pp. 201–217, 2010.

[3] T. Schenk, S. Stengel, and A. Zelent, "Unlocking the potential of retinoic acid in anticancer therapy," *British Journal of Cancer*, vol. 111, pp. 2039–2045, 2014.

[4] M.-C. Chen, C.-Y. Huang, S.-L. Hsu et al., "Retinoic acid induces apoptosis of prostate cancer DU145 cells through Cdk5 overactivation," *Evidence-Based Complementary and Alternative Medicine*, vol. 2012, Article ID 580736, 11 pages, 2012.

[5] W. J. Huss, L. Lai, R. J. Barrios, K. K. Hirschi, and N. M. Greenberg, "Retinoic acid slows progression and promotes apoptosis of spontaneous prostate cancer," *The Prostate*, vol. 61, no. 2, pp. 142–152, 2004.

[6] C. Ginestier, J. Wicinski, N. Cervera et al., "Retinoid signaling regulates breast cancer stem cell differentiation," *Cell Cycle*, vol. 8, no. 20, pp. 3297–3302, 2009.

[7] M. E. Huang, Y. C. Ye, S. R. Chen et al., "Use of all-trans retinoic acid in the treatment of acute promyelocytic leukemia," *Blood*, vol. 72, no. 2, pp. 567–572, 1988.

[8] U. C. Dräger, E. Wagner, and P. McCaffery, "Aldehyde dehydrogenases in the generation of retinoic acid in the developing vertebrate: a central role of the eye," *The Journal of Nutrition*, vol. 128, supplement 2, pp. 463S–466S, 1998.

[9] D. Raha, T. R. Wilson, J. Peng et al., "The cancer stem cell marker aldehyde dehydrogenase is required to maintain a drug-tolerant tumor cell subpopulation," *Cancer Research*, vol. 74, no. 13, pp. 3579–3590, 2014.

[10] P. Marcato, C. A. Dean, C. A. Giacomantonio, and P. W. K. Lee, "Aldehyde dehydrogenase its role as a cancer stem cell marker comes down to the specific isoform," *Cell Cycle*, vol. 10, no. 9, pp. 1378–1384, 2011.

[11] E. Charafe-Jauffret, C. Ginestier, F. Iovino et al., "Aldehyde dehydrogenase 1-positive cancer stem cells mediate metastasis and poor clinical outcome in inflammatory breast cancer," *Clinical Cancer Research*, vol. 16, no. 1, pp. 45–55, 2010.

[12] S. Deng, X. Yang, H. Lassus et al., "Distinct expression levels and patterns of stem cell marker, aldehyde dehydrogenase isoform 1 (ALDH1), in human epithelial cancers," *PLoS ONE*, vol. 5, no. 4, Article ID e10277, 2010.

[13] K. Honoki, H. Fujii, A. Kubo et al., "Possible involvement of stem-like populations with elevated ALDH1 in sarcomas for chemotherapeutic drug resistance," *Oncology Reports*, vol. 24, no. 2, pp. 501–505, 2010.

[14] J. Feng, Q. Qi, A. Khanna et al., "Aldehyde dehydrogenase 1 is a tumor stem cell-associated marker in lung cancer," *Molecular Cancer Research*, vol. 7, no. 3, pp. 330–338, 2009.

[15] F. Zhou, Y.-D. Mu, J. Liang et al., "Aldehyde dehydrogenase 1: a specific cancer stem cell marker for human colorectal carcinoma," *Molecular Medicine Reports*, vol. 11, no. 5, pp. 3894–3899, 2015.

[16] H. Li, F. Ma, H. Wang et al., "Stem cell marker aldehyde dehydrogenase 1 (ALDH1)-expressing cells are enriched in triple-negative breast cancer," *The International Journal of Biological Markers*, vol. 28, no. 4, pp. e357–e364, 2013.

[17] X. Mu, C. Isaac, N. Greco, J. Huard, and K. Weiss, "Notch signaling is associated with ALDH activity and an aggressive metastatic phenotype in murine osteosarcoma cells," *Frontiers in Oncology*, vol. 3, article 143, 2013.

[18] X. Mu, C. Isaac, T. Schott, J. Huard, and K. Weiss, "Rapamycin inhibits ALDH activity, resistance to oxidative stress, and metastatic potential in murine osteosarcoma cells," *Sarcoma*, vol. 2013, Article ID 480713, 11 pages, 2013.

[19] X. Mu, D. Brynien, and K. R. Weiss, "The HDAC inhibitor vorinostat diminishes the *in vitro* metastatic behavior of osteosarcoma cells," *BioMed Research International*, vol. 2015, Article ID 290368, 6 pages, 2015.

[20] X. Mu, B. Sultankulov, R. Agarwal et al., "Chick embryo extract demethylates tumor suppressor genes in osteosarcoma cells," *Clinical Orthopaedics and Related Research*, vol. 472, no. 3, pp. 865–873, 2014.

[21] N. Greco, T. Schott, X. Mu et al., "ALDH activity correlates with metastatic potential in primary sarcomas of bone," *Journal of Cancer Therapy*, vol. 5, no. 4, pp. 331–338, 2014.

3

Clinical Outcomes of Surgical Treatments for Primary Malignant Bone Tumors Arising in the Acetabulum

Tomohiro Fujiwara, Koichi Ogura, Eisuke Kobayashi, Yoshikazu Tanzawa, Fumihiko Nakatani, Hirokazu Chuman, and Akira Kawai

Division of Musculoskeletal Oncology, National Cancer Center Hospital, 5-1-1 Tsukiji, Chuo-ku, Tokyo 104-0045, Japan

Correspondence should be addressed to Akira Kawai; akawai@ncc.go.jp

Academic Editor: Manish Agarwal

The functional and oncologic results of eighteen patients with primary malignant periacetabular tumors were reviewed to determine the impact of surgical treatment. The reconstruction procedures were endoprosthesis (11), hip transposition (4), iliofemoral arthrodesis (2), and frozen bone autograft (1). After a mean follow-up of 62 months, 13 patients were alive and 5 had died of their disease; the 5-year overall survival rate was 67.2%. The corresponding mean MSTS scores of patients with endoprosthesis (11) and other reconstructions (7) were 42% and 55% (49%, 68%, and 50%), respectively. Overall, postoperative complications including deep infection or dislocation markedly worsened the functional outcome. Iliofemoral arthrodesis provided better function than the other procedures, whereas endoprosthetic reconstruction demonstrated poor functional outcome except for patients who were reconstructed with the adequate soft tissue coverage. Avoiding postoperative complications is highly important for achieving better function, suggesting that surgical procedures with adequate soft tissue coverage or without the massive use of nonbiological materials are preferable. Appropriate selection of the reconstructive procedures for individual patients, considering the amount of remaining bone and soft tissues, would lead to better clinical outcomes.

1. Introduction

Although primary sarcomas arising in the pelvis are relatively rare, surgical treatment for these diseases remains difficult. Resections of pelvic bone are classified according to the system of Enneking and Dunham (Figure 1) [1, 2]. PII or periacetabular resections present a unique surgical challenge in that no specific form of reconstruction has proved superior [3]. There is still much debate about the best reconstructive option for these patients, and many such options exist. These include endoprosthetic reconstruction [4–6], hip transposition [7, 8], iliofemoral arthrodesis [9, 10], biologic reconstruction (using allografts or autografts from the tibia, fibula, iliac crest, or pelvis) [11, 12], or hip rotationplasty [13]. However, there is still no standard procedure for reconstruction after resection of malignant periacetabular tumors. Indeed, functional outcomes in patients who have undergone periacetabular resections also vary greatly depending on the type of reconstruction [14]. In several published series, musculoskeletal tumor society (MSTS) scores have been within the range of 40–60% [9, 15]. The major problem associated with these reconstructive procedures is their high rate of postoperative complications, such as delayed wound healing, infection, dislocation, aseptic loosening, or local recurrence [14–16]. Published series have reported complication rates of 18–65% depending on the reconstructive procedure employed [6]. The appropriateness of any reconstructive procedure needs to be decided on the basis of its functional results, as well as its rate of associated complications.

Over the past 10 years, a variety of reconstructive procedures have been employed at our institution. The purpose of the present study was to evaluate the surgical outcome, including complication rate and functional score, in patients after acetabular resection according to the surgical procedures employed, and to determine the clinical and functional outcome after resection of periacetabular tumors.

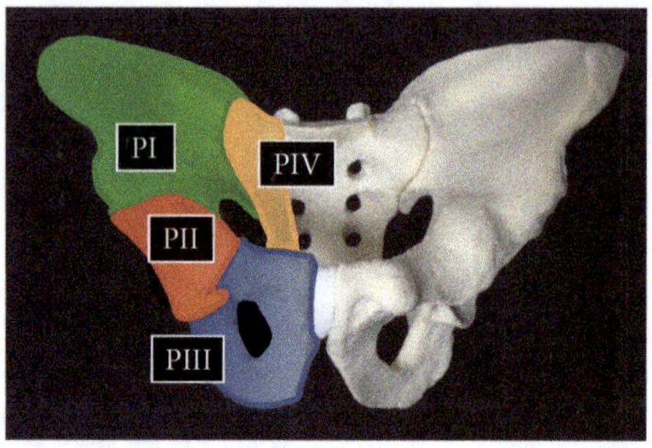

Figure 1: Diagram showing the resected area according to the classification system of Enneking and Dunham.

2. Patients and Methods

We retrospectively reviewed 18 patients with primary periacetabular bone tumors who underwent acetabular resection and reconstruction between June 1996 and December 2012. Their clinical data, treatment modalities, and treatment outcome were reviewed retrospectively by reference to the medical records. The following data were examined: demographic data (patient age at operation, gender, tumor size, and histologic diagnosis), surgical details (reconstructive procedures, lesion resected, and surgical margins), lesion resected, adjuvant therapy (chemotherapy and radiotherapy), postoperative complications (e.g., infection or dislocation), oncologic outcomes, and functional outcomes.

Acetabular lesions were resected using a variety of procedures according to the classification system of Enneking and Dunham (Figure 1). Surgical margins were evaluated on the basis of surgical and pathological reports according to the system described by Enneking [17]. Limb-sparing surgery was performed when the surgical margin would be comparable to that of external hemipelvectomy, as well as when adequate soft tissue and the sciatic nerve could be preserved during tumor resection. The reconstruction procedures after periacetabular tumor resection included endoprosthetic reconstruction (11), hip transposition (4), iliofemoral arthrodesis (2), and reconstruction using frozen bone autograft (1). The decision on the reconstruction procedure was made according to patient opinion based on the detailed informed consent obtained by the staff surgeon, including the characteristics of each procedure that had been reported [14, 15, 18–21]. For patients who underwent endoprosthetic reconstruction, we used an endoprosthetic system with a constrained hip mechanism (C-THA; Hip Reconstruction Cup; Japan Medical Materials) to obtain iliofemoral stability [6, 22], which was composed of a cup with a plate to anchor prosthesis into the remaining ilium. Hip transposition, iliofemoral arthrodesis, and reconstruction using frozen bone autograft were performed as previously reported [6–8, 10, 22–24].

Function was assessed at the final follow-up using the MSTS system developed by Enneking et al. [25]. The MSTS system is based on the analysis of factors pertinent to the patient as a whole (pain, restriction of activities and/or occupation, and emotional acceptance) and factors specific to the affected limb (the use of walking supports, walking distance, and gait). Each parameter is given a value ranging from 0 to 5, according to specific criteria, and the overall result is expressed as a summation of all the parameters, which then is converted to a percentage of the maximum possible score. We defined postoperative complications requiring surgical interventions within one year as major complications and all other complications as minor. Patient survivals were estimated by the Kaplan-Meier method calculated from the date of definitive surgery to the time of patient death or the last follow-up for survivors.

Ethical approval was obtained from the Institutional Review Boards of National Cancer Center Hospital.

Table 1: Patient characteristics for the entire study population and surgical/oncological outcome.

Description	Number
Patients	
Male 13, female 5	Total 18
Age (at diagnosis)	41 years (8–69)
Tumor size	11.7 cm (7–20)
Diagnosis	
Osteosarcoma	8
Chondrosarcoma	5
MFH of bone	2
Ewing sarcoma	2
Fibrosarcoma of bone	1
Neoadjuvant therapy	
Polychemotherapy	11
Radiotherapy	0
Adjuvant therapy	
Polychemotherapy	9
Radiotherapy	1
Follow-up	62 months (8–155)
Resected area (Enneking classification)	
PII	2
PI-II	4
PII-III	8
PI-II-III	4
Surgical outcome	
Wide margin	17
Marginal margin	0
Intralesional margin	1
Oncological outcome	
No evidence of disease (NED)	11
Alive with disease (AWD)	2
Dead of disease (DOD)	5
Prognosis	
Overall survival (five years)	67.2%

3. Results

3.1. Oncological Results for the Entire Group. Patient demographics and treatment data are summarized in Table 1. There were 13 males and 5 females with a mean age of 41 years

TABLE 2: Complications according to surgical treatment.

Surgical procedures	Number of patients	Number of patients with major complications	Complications (number)	Local recurrence (number)
Endoprosthesis	11	6 (55%)	Deep infection (2), superficial infection (2), dislocation (2), wound complication (3), abdominal hernia (1)	1
Other reconstructions	7	1 (14%)		0
Hip transposition	4	1 (25%)	Deep infection (1), superficial infection (1), leg-length discrepancy (4)	0
Iliofemoral arthrodesis	2	0	Implant breakage (1), leg-length discrepancy (2)	0
Frozen autograft	1	0	Osteoarthritis (1), wound complication (1)	0
Total	18	8 (44%)		1

(range, 8–69 years) at the time of surgical treatment. The mean tumor size was 11.7 cm (range, 7–20 cm). According to histological distribution, the primary tumor was recorded as osteosarcoma in 8 patients, chondrosarcoma in 5, malignant fibrous histiocytoma (MFH) of bone in 2, Ewing sarcoma in 2, and fibrosarcoma of bone in 1. The mean follow-up period was 62 months (range, 8–155 months). In this series, 11 patients received neoadjuvant chemotherapy and no patient received radiation therapy preoperatively. After surgery, 9 patients received adjuvant chemotherapy and 1 patient received radiation therapy.

The acetabular lesions were resected using a variety of procedures according to the classification system of Enneking and Dunham [1, 2]: type PII resection in 2 cases, type PI-II resection in 4 cases, type PII-III resection in 8 cases, and type PI-II-III resection in 4 cases (Table 1).

The surgical margins in this study group were classified as wide in 17 patients and intralesional in 1 patient (Table 1). One patient whose surgical margin was intralesional was reconstructed with endoprosthesis. This patient with dedifferentiated chondrosarcoma suffered local recurrence at 12 months after the operation, developed lung metastasis at 13 months, and died of the disease at 16 months after surgery.

After a mean overall follow-up of 62 months (range, 8–155 months), 11 patients (61%) had no evidence of disease (NED), 2 (11%) were alive with disease (AWD), and 5 (28%) had died of the disease (DOD) (Table 1). The 5-year overall survival rates were 67.2% (Figure 2).

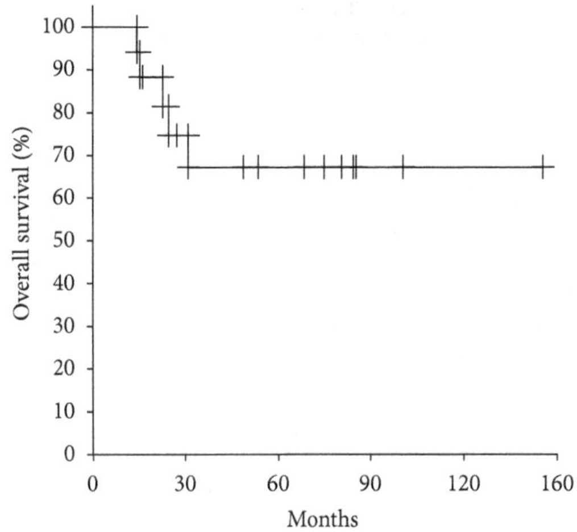

FIGURE 2: Cumulative overall survival curve for all patients estimated by the Kaplan-Meier method.

3.2. Complications according to Surgical Procedures. Postoperative complications are listed in Table 2.

After endoprosthesis replacement, most patients suffered postoperative complications. Among 11 patients who underwent endoprosthesis reconstruction, 6 (55%) had major complications, which required surgical interventions. The complications comprised superficial infection in 2 patients (18%), deep infection in 2 (18%), wound complication in 3 (27%), dislocation in 2 (18%), abdominal hernia in 1, and local recurrence in 1. Eight additional surgical procedures were performed in patients of this group, including 6 revisions for deep infection or wound complication and 2 for implant dislocation. No complications developed in 5 patients whose gluteus medius or gluteus maximus was preserved, or in those who underwent coverage of the large soft tissue defect with a rectus abdominis myocutaneous flap [26].

On the other hand, among those who performed other reconstructions than endoprosthesis, only one patient (14%) experienced major complication, which required surgical intervention. After hip transposition in 4 patients, one suffered postoperative infection, and all of the patients had leg-length discrepancy. One patient required additional surgical procedure for deep infection and wound problem. This patient underwent reconstruction with a Gore-Tex sheet around the iliac resection site, which was considered to have caused postoperative infection.

Of the 2 patients who underwent iliofemoral arthrodesis, both had leg-length discrepancy and one suffered implant complication. One patient suffered screw breakage at 2 years after surgery, which required an additional fixation. Later the patient underwent a limb-lengthening operation for leg-length discrepancy at another institution. The other patient died of metastatic disease at 2 years after surgery.

One patient who underwent reconstruction with a frozen bone autograft showed delayed postoperative wound healing.

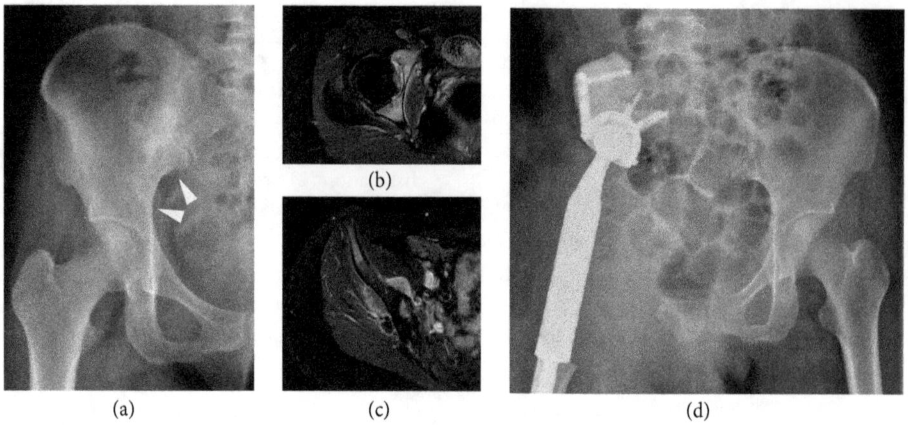

FIGURE 3: (a) Preoperative anteroposterior radiograph of the pelvis of a 28-year-old female who had osteosarcoma of the acetabulum and ilium. ((b) and (c)) Gadolinium-enhanced axial T1-weighted MRI showing the tumor arising in the acetabulum and ilium. After neoadjuvant chemotherapy, the patient underwent tumor wide resection and endoprosthetic reconstruction with no postoperative major complications. (d) Postoperative radiograph 3 years after endoprosthetic reconstruction.

TABLE 3: Functional outcomes according to surgical treatment.

Surgical procedure	Score according to musculoskeletal tumor society (MSTS score) system						
	Pain	Function	Acceptance	Support	Distance	Gait	Total
Endoprosthesis	64 (3.2)	42 (2.1)	46 (2.3)	6 (0.3)	44 (2.2)	42 (2.1)	42 (12.5)
Other reconstructions	82 (4.1)	54 (2.7)	57 (2.8)	17 (0.8)	57 (2.8)	60 (3)	55 (16.4)
Hip transposition	90 (4.5)	50 (2.5)	70 (3.5)	0 (0)	35 (1.75)	50 (2.5)	49 (14.7)
Iliofemoral arthrodesis	80 (4)	60 (3)	50 (2.5)	60 (3)	90 (4.5)	70 (3.5)	68 (20.5)
Frozen autograft	60 (3)	60 (3)	20 (1)	0 (0)	80 (4)	80 (4)	50 (15)
Mean scores	73 (3.6)	48 (2.4)	51 (2.5)	10 (0.5)	49 (2.5)	49 (2.5)	47 (14.2)

At 1 year after surgery, the patient presented with hip osteoarthritis, which has since shown gradual progression.

3.3. Functional Results according to the Surgical Procedures. The mean functional score in the present series, according to the MSTS system, was 14.2 points (47%) at the latest follow-up. The functional results according to the various surgical procedures employed are shown in Table 3.

The 11 patients who underwent endoprosthetic reconstruction had a mean functional score of 12.5 points (42%) out of a maximum of 30 points (range, 13–70%). All patients were unable to walk without walking aids; no patient had a score of >3 points (out of a possible 5 points). Eight patients required constant pain medication with nonnarcotic analgesics (four with moderate pain and four with mild pain). The mean emotional acceptance score was 46% (range, 0–60%). Notably, the mean MSTS score for the six patients without postoperative deep infection or dislocation was 55% (Figure 3), whereas that for the other five patients who suffered these complications was 28%.

The 4 patients who underwent reconstruction with hip transposition had a mean functional score of 49% (range, 33–67%). They complained of the least amount of pain. Only one patient required continuous use of analgesic medications. Notably, the mean emotional acceptance score was 70% (range, 40–100%), which was the highest among all the groups. All of these patients had limb-length discrepancy (Figure 4) and required a shoe lift. However, their walking ability was comparable to that of patients who underwent other surgical procedures.

Two patients who underwent iliofemoral arthrodesis had a mean functional score of 68%. One patient had no pain, and the other had mild pain. The mean emotional acceptance score was 50%. One patient required no support for walking (Figure 5), while the other was able to walk with one crutch. Both patients had limb-length discrepancy and required a shoe lift. One of them underwent additional limb-lengthening surgery after long-term survival and has maintained a high MSTS score.

The patient who was reconstructed with a frozen bone autograft had a functional score of 50%. He complained of moderate pain, which seemed to be caused by osteoarthritis, and used nonnarcotic analgesics (Figure 6). Two crutches were necessary for walking, and his emotional acceptance score was 20%.

Consequently, the mean functional score for patients with endoprosthesis (42%) was worse than that for patients with other reconstructions (55%), which seemed to be attributed to the high complication rate in the former group. The best results were obtained in patients who underwent iliofemoral arthrodesis, although the number of patients was small. Regardless of the surgical procedures, the functional scores

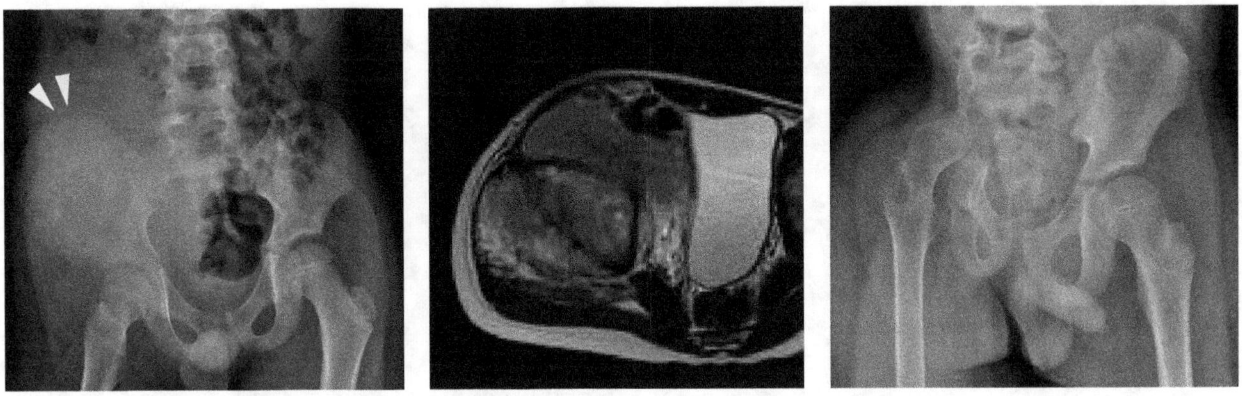

(a) (b) (c)

FIGURE 4: (a) Preoperative anteroposterior radiograph of the pelvis of an 8-year-old boy who had Ewing sarcoma in the ilium and acetabulum. (b) Axial T2-weighted MR image showing the tumor arising in the acetabulum. (c) Postoperative radiograph one year after hip transposition.

for patients with postoperative deep infections or dislocations were quite low; the mean MSTS scores for patients with these complications were less than 30%, whereas those for patients without these complications were more than 50%. Overall, the functional outcomes were similar between all the reconstructive options, except for those without postoperative major complications, indicating that avoiding these complications is highly important for achieving better functional outcome.

4. Discussion

Limb-sparing surgery for periacetabular tumors is one of the most challenging procedures for orthopaedic oncologists [6, 14, 15, 19]. While many surgical options after resection of periacetabular tumors have been reported [3, 27, 28] and several clinical studies have attempted its functional outcomes [14, 20, 21], no standard procedures have been determined. Usually, the technique selected for reconstruction is individualized for each patient. As the choice of the optimal technique for reconstruction after acetabular tumor resection depends on numerous parameters, surgeons need to understand the details of each case and the appropriate indications for each of the reconstructive procedures. In this study, we overviewed the clinical characteristics and postoperative functions in a series of patients who underwent various procedures in a single referral center and found that avoiding postoperative complications is highly important for achieving better function, suggesting that surgical procedures with adequate soft tissue coverage or without the massive use of nonbiological materials are preferable.

Pelvic reconstruction with an endoprosthesis has been a major challenge and in this series the functional results were not satisfactory. Postoperative function was markedly affected by major complications such as deep infection or implant dislocation. To date, various reports have demonstrated the high major complication rates by endoprosthetic replacement, ranging 18–65%; 40–65% in saddle prostheses [29–31], 28–41% in hemipelvic endoprosthesis [20, 21], 25–60% in custom-made hemipelvic endoprosthesis [4, 5, 32], and 18–58% in the other types of endoprosthesis such as ice cream cone endoprosthesis [33], modular hemipelvic endoprosthesis [18], PAR hemipelvic endoprosthesis [34], MUTARS hemipelvic endoprosthesis [35], and constrained hip reconstruction cup (C-THA) endoprosthesis [6]. The high rates of complications, and the associated poor functional results, have been considered to be related to the lack of soft tissue coverage, resection of muscles, and the creation of a large dead space [14]. In our series, patients with major complications also seemed to be attributable to the amount of remaining bone and soft tissues or a dead space. In two recent cases, relatively better function was achieved without postoperative complications using a rectus abdominis myocutaneous (RAM) flap, which is recommended for providing an adequate tissue mass to eliminate the dead space and for covering any exposed bone or implants with well vascularized tissue [26]. Therefore, reconstruction with adequate soft tissue coverage could avoid postoperative complications and improve clinical outcomes of endoprosthetic reconstruction. Recently, an extended application of computer navigation-assisted resection in pelvic tumors has been described [36–38]. Successful case reports have indicated that incorporating computer navigation may aid in accurate intraoperative identification of tumor extent and facilitate bone resections with clear surgical margins in musculoskeletal tumor surgery. Furthermore, CT and MRI fusion images when combined with surgical navigation help surgeons produce a reliable preoperative plan and may improve identification of margins on planned resections, thus avoiding unnecessary resection in musculoskeletal tumor surgery [38, 39]. Therefore, these novel techniques or carefully considered selection criteria, including patients with adequate normal bone and soft tissue after resection or who are suitable for RAM flap, could probably improve the outcome of endoprosthetic reconstruction. Alternately, surgical procedures other than endoprosthetic reconstruction appear to be reasonable options for many of these patients, considering the high complication rate and modest functional scores associated with periacetabular reconstructions as shown in previous reports and our current data.

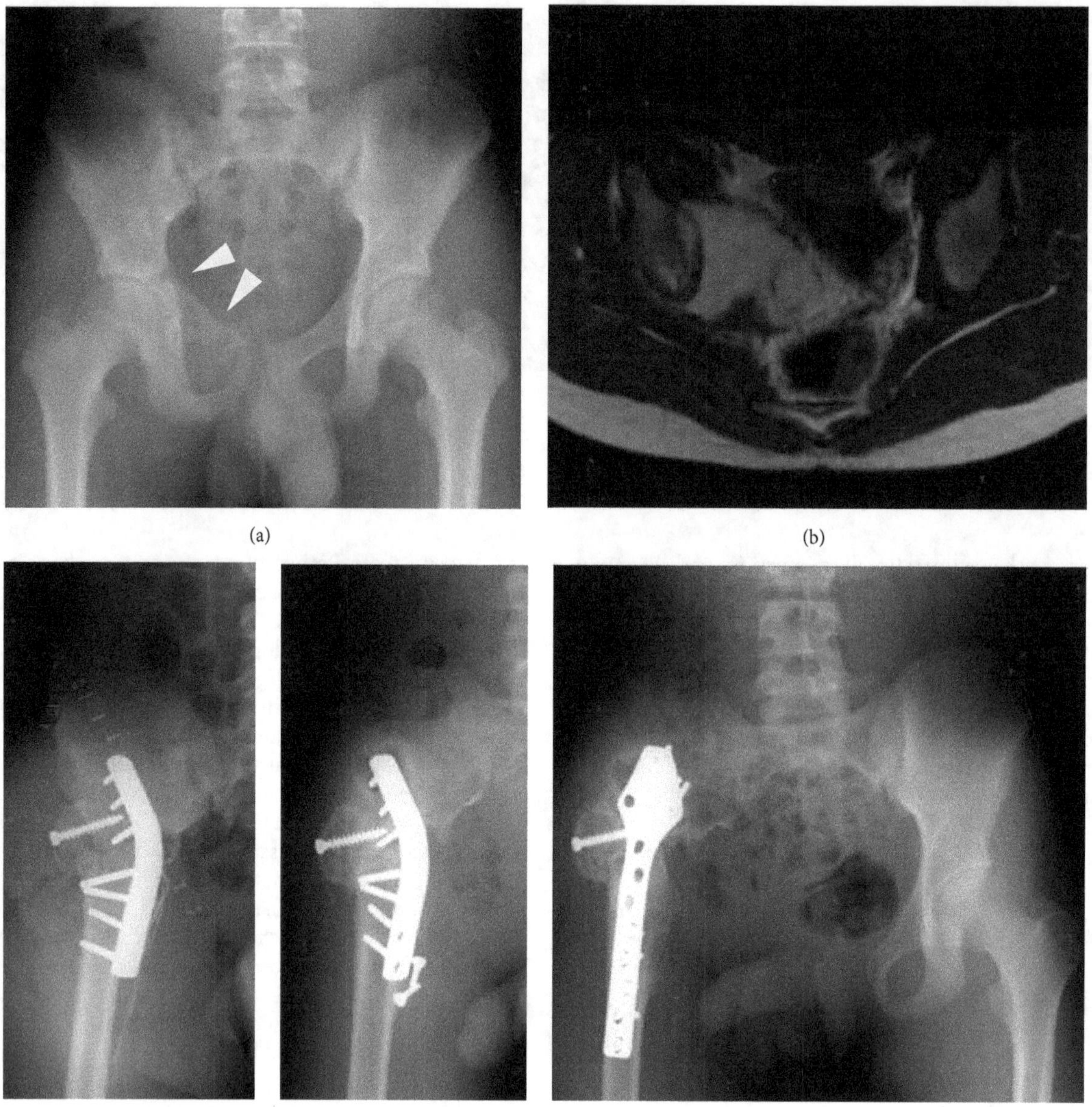

(a) (b) (c) (d) (e)

FIGURE 5: (a) Preoperative anteroposterior radiograph of the pelvis of a 14-year-old boy who had Ewing sarcoma of the acetabulum and pubis. (b) Axial T2-weighted MRI showing the tumor arising in the acetabulum. (c) Postoperative radiograph showing plate fixation of the proximal femur to the remaining ilium after PII-III resection. (d) Plain radiograph showing screw breakage 2 years after first iliofemoral arthrodesis. (e) Plain radiograph 11 years after refixation.

Patients in this series who underwent hip transposition achieved relatively good function. Hip transposition, reported in 1988 by Winkelmann at the University Hospital of Münster, is characterized by a lower incidence of complications and revision surgery in comparison with other reconstructive procedures [7, 8, 14, 40]. The lower complication rate associated with this procedure is attributed to the smaller dead space resulting from a shift of the hip proximally to the pelvis [40]. Postoperative deep infection in one of the patients in this series might have been caused by the use of a Gore-Tex sheet, which is a nonbiological material. A better functional prognosis would have been expected in this patient if simple reconstruction without nonbiological materials had been possible. In general, patients with pelvic sarcoma have a poor prognosis [41, 42]. Therefore, safer procedures with higher success rates and lower complication rates are desirable. Leg-length discrepancy after surgery is the major problem of this procedure [7, 8]. However, Rödl et al. reported that such leg-length discrepancy could be corrected using distraction osteogenesis [40]. They demonstrated that four patients who underwent limb lengthening after long-term survival achieved good average MSTS scores of 73%. Recent report from Okayama University [43] has also demonstrated good to excellent MSTS scores of 60–93% by using postoperative

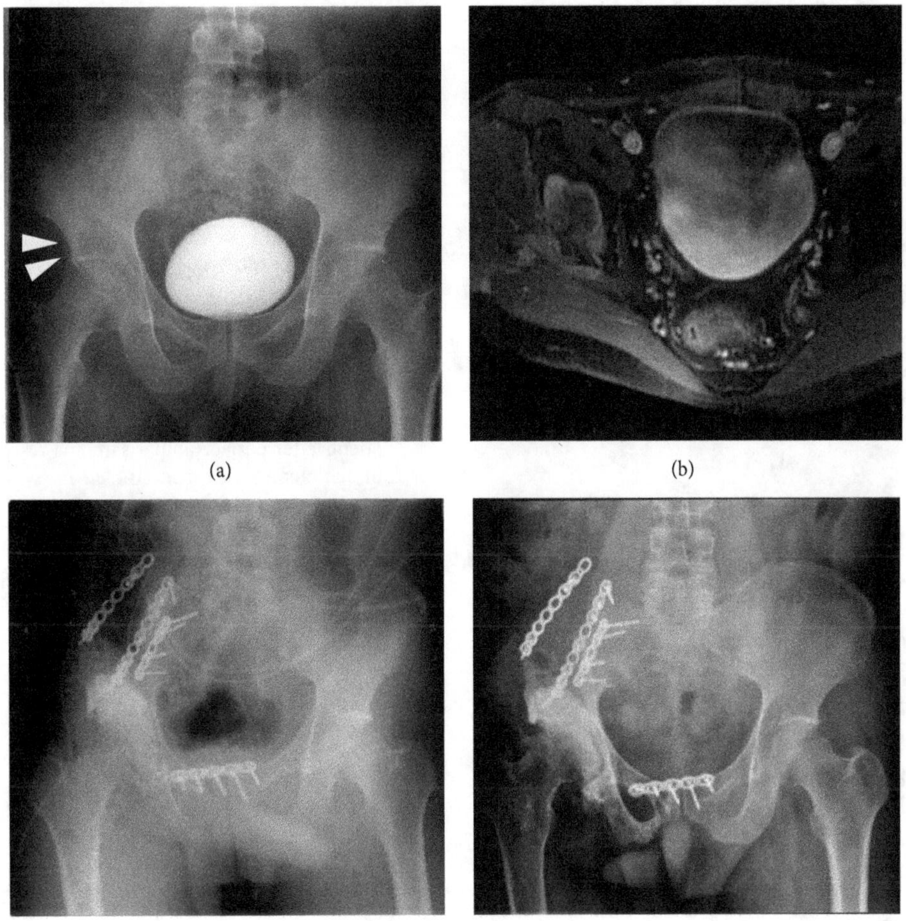

(a) (b) (c) (d)

Figure 6: (a) Preoperative anteroposterior radiograph of the pelvis of a 38-year-old man who had MFH of bone in the acetabulum. (b) Gadolinium-enhanced axial T1-weighted MRI showing the tumor arising in the acetabulum. (c) Postoperative radiograph after reconstruction using a frozen bone autograft. (d) Follow-up radiograph 1.5 years after surgery showing osteoarthritis of the hip joint.

external fixation instead of pelvic cast which was described as the original method [7]. Collectively, hip transposition is a reasonable reconstruction method with lower complication rates for patients with periacetabular tumors.

Iliofemoral arthrodesis achieved the best functional scores in this series, attributable to a good gait performance with a stiff hip. Previous studies have also mentioned the advantage of a durable, pain-free, but stiff hip and less leg-length discrepancy [10, 28]. We consider that iliofemoral arthrodesis is suitable for patients with strenuous activity requirements. One major problem of iliofemoral arthrodesis is a high rate of nonunion (60%) after primary fusion [44]. However, no patients in this series suffered nonunion, and a recent report has indicated a relatively lower nonunion rate of 14% [10]. One of the suggested reasons for nonunion is that a solid iliofemoral fusion is difficult to achieve, since the surface for bone contact is usually small [10]. Therefore, this reconstruction procedure would be most suitable when the proximal osteotomy is at the lower part of the ilium, as shown in Figure 5. One patient in the present series achieved bone union using a vascularized fibular graft. Appropriate indications and use of a vascularized iliac bone block or fibular graft might improve the union rate.

Although the small number of patients who underwent reconstruction with a frozen bone autograft limits the interpretation of our results, we achieved relatively good functional results. However, the patient developed hip osteoarthritis and has complained of continuous pain. Resurfacing total hip arthroplasty may therefore be necessary in the future. As a previous report has indicated, the advantages of this procedure include a perfect fit, the lack of any need for a bone bank, easy attachment of tendons and ligaments, and a related desirable bone stock [24]. However, this procedure has certain disadvantages, such as a high rate of postoperative infection, degeneration of cartilage over time, and therefore late osteoarthritis. Accordingly, the long-term outcome of reconstruction using a frozen bone autograft remains unknown.

We found that patients with major complications had markedly reduced functional scores. Thus, reduction of the postoperative complication rate is highly important to obtain better function. In general, since the patients with pelvic sarcoma have a poor prognosis, complete resection of the tumor as well as reconstruction without postoperative complications is desirable for them. From this viewpoint, we consider that the surgical procedures without massive use of nonbiological materials, including endoprosthesis, are preferable to achieve better function and fewer complications, although the rarity and variability of these tumors preclude a statistical comparison of outcomes. Alternately, appropriate selection of reconstruction procedures for individual patients, considering the amount of remaining bone and soft tissues and novel techniques such as tissue transfer or computer-assisted surgery, would lead to fewer complications and better function.

5. Conclusions

This study summarized the clinical outcomes of major reconstructive procedures after resection of periacetabular tumors. Postoperative major complications, including deep infection or hip dislocation, remarkably worsened functional outcome. Endoprosthetic reconstruction failed without adequate soft tissue coverage. Therefore, avoiding postoperative complications is highly important for achieving better function, suggesting that surgical procedures with adequate soft tissue coverage or without the massive use of nonbiological materials are preferable. Appropriate selection of reconstruction procedures for individual patients, considering the amount of resection and remaining bone and soft tissues, would lead to fewer complications and better function.

Acknowledgments

The authors would like to thank all participating patients, as well as the study nurses, coinvestigators, and colleagues who made this trial possible.

References

[1] W. F. Enneking, "Local resection of malignant lesions of the hip and pelvis," *The Journal of Bone & Joint Surgery—American Volume*, vol. 48, no. 5, pp. 991–1007, 1966.

[2] W. F. Enneking and W. K. Dunham, "Resection and reconstruction for primary neoplasms involving the innominate bone," *The Journal of Bone & Joint Surgery—American Volume*, vol. 60, no. 6, pp. 731–746, 1978.

[3] R. Hugate Jr. and F. H. Sim, "Pelvic reconstruction techniques," *Orthopedic Clinics of North America*, vol. 37, no. 1, pp. 85–97, 2006.

[4] A. Abudu, R. J. Grimer, S. R. Cannon, S. R. Carter, and R. S. Sneath, "Reconstruction of the hemipelvis after the excision of malignant tumours," *The Journal of Bone & Joint Surgery—British Volume*, vol. 79, no. 5, pp. 773–779, 1997.

[5] P. K. Jaiswal, W. J. S. Aston, R. J. Grimer et al., "Peri-acetabular resection and endoprosthetic reconstruction for tumours of the acetabulum," *Journal of Bone & Joint Surgery—British Volume*, vol. 90, no. 9, pp. 1222–1227, 2008.

[6] T. Ueda, S. Kakunaga, S. Takenaka, N. Araki, and H. Yoshikawa, "Constrained total hip megaprosthesis for primary periacetabular tumors," *Clinical Orthopaedics and Related Research*, vol. 471, no. 3, pp. 741–749, 2013.

[7] C. Gebert, G. Gosheger, and W. Winkelmann, "Hip transposition as a universal surgical procedure for periacetabular tumors of the pelvis," *Journal of Surgical Oncology*, vol. 99, no. 3, pp. 169–172, 2009.

[8] C. Gebert, M. Wessling, C. Hoffmann et al., "Hip transposition as a limb salvage procedure following the resection of periacetabular tumors," *Journal of Surgical Oncology*, vol. 103, no. 3, pp. 269–275, 2011.

[9] E. E. Carmody Soni, B. J. Miller, M. T. Scarborough, and C. Parker Gibbs, "Functional outcomes and gait analysis of patients after periacetabular sarcoma resection with and without ischiofemoral arthrodesis," *Journal of Surgical Oncology*, vol. 106, no. 7, pp. 844–849, 2012.

[10] B. Fuchs, M. I. O'Connor, K. R. Kaufman, D. J. Padgett, and F. H. Sim, "Iliofemoral arthrodesis and pseudarthrosis: a long-term functional outcome evaluation," *Clinical Orthopaedics and Related Research*, vol. 397, pp. 29–35, 2002.

[11] D. Campanacci, S. Chacon, N. Mondanelli et al., "Pelvic massive allograft reconstruction after bone tumour resection," *International Orthopaedics*, vol. 36, no. 12, pp. 2529–2536, 2012.

[12] J.-M. Laffosse, A. Pourcel, N. Reina et al., "Primary tumor of the periacetabular region: resection and reconstruction using a segmental ipsilateral femur autograft," *Orthopaedics & Traumatology: Surgery & Research*, vol. 98, no. 3, pp. 309–318, 2012.

[13] W. W. Winkelman, "Hip rotationplasty for malignant tumors of the proximal part of the femur," *The Journal of Bone & Joint Surgery—American Volume*, vol. 68, no. 3, pp. 362–369, 1986.

[14] C. Hoffmann, G. Gosheger, C. Gebert, H. Jürgens, and W. Winkelmann, "Functional results and quality of life after treatment of pelvic sarcomas involving the acetabulum," *Journal of Bone and Joint Surgery A*, vol. 88, no. 3, pp. 575–582, 2006.

[15] A. Hillmann, C. Hoffman, G. Gosheger, R. Rödl, W. Winkelmann, and T. Ozaki, "Tumors of the pelvis: complications after reconstruction," *Archives of Orthopaedic and Trauma Surgery*, vol. 123, no. 7, pp. 340–344, 2003.

[16] T. Ozaki, A. Hillmann, D. Bettin, P. Wuisman, and W. Winkelmann, "High complication rates with pelvic allografts: experience of 22 sarcoma resections," *Acta Orthopaedica Scandinavica*, vol. 67, no. 4, pp. 333–338, 1996.

[17] W. F. Enneking, "A system of staging musculoskeletal neoplasms," *Clinical Orthopaedics and Related Research*, vol. 204, pp. 9–24, 1986.

[18] Z. Guo, J. Li, G.-X. Pei, X.-D. Li, and Z. Wang, "Pelvic reconstruction with a combined hemipelvic prostheses after resection of primary malignant tumor," *Surgical Oncology*, vol. 19, no. 2, pp. 95–105, 2010.

[19] E. Schwameis, M. Dominkus, P. Krepler et al., "Reconstruction of the pelvis after tumor resection in children and adolescents," *Clinical Orthopaedics and Related Research*, vol. 402, pp. 220–235, 2002.

[20] R. Windhager, J. Karner, H.-P. Kutschera, P. Polterauer, M. Salzer-Kuntschik, and R. Kotz, "Limb salvage in periacetabular sarcomas: review of 21 consecutive cases," *Clinical Orthopaedics and Related Research*, vol. 331, pp. 265–276, 1996.

[21] R. J. Wirbel, M. Schulte, and W. E. Mutschler, "Surgical treatment of pelvic sarcomas: oncologic and functional outcome," *Clinical Orthopaedics and Related Research*, vol. 390, pp. 190–205, 2001.

[22] A. Uchida, A. Myoui, N. Araki, H. Yoshikawa, T. Ueda, and Y. Aoki, "Prosthetic reconstruction for periacetabular malignant tumors," *Clinical Orthopaedics and Related Research*, no. 326, pp. 238–245, 1996.

[23] S. Nagoya, T. Wada, S. Kawaguchi, M. Kaya, T. Takebayashi, and T. Yamashita, "Functional results of reconstructive hip arthrodesis for periacetabular malignant tumor," *European Orthopaedics and Traumatology*, vol. 3, no. 2, pp. 121–125, 2012.

[24] H. Tsuchiya, S. L. Wan, K. Sakayama, N. Yamamoto, H. Nishida, and K. Tomita, "Reconstruction using an autograft containing tumour treated by liquid nitrogen," *The Journal of Bone & Joint Surgery—British Volume*, vol. 87, no. 2, pp. 218–225, 2005.

[25] W. F. Enneking, W. Dunham, M. C. Gebhardt, M. Malawar, and D. J. Pritchard, "A system for the functional evaluation of reconstructive procedures after surgical treatment of tumors of the musculoskeletal system," *Clinical Orthopaedics and Related Research*, vol. 286, pp. 241–246, 1993.

[26] K. Ogura, S. Miyamoto, M. Sakuraba, H. Chuman, T. Fujiwara, and A. Kawai, "Immediate soft-tissue reconstruction using a rectus abdominis myocutaneous flap following wide resection of malignant bone tumours of the pelvis," *Bone & Joint Journal*, vol. 96, no. 2, pp. 270–273, 2014.

[27] R. J. Grimer, S. R. Carter, R. M. Tillman, D. Spooner, D. C. Mangham, and Y. Kabukcuoglu, "Osteosarcoma of the pelvis," *Journal of Bone and Joint Surgery B*, vol. 81, no. 5, pp. 796–802, 1999.

[28] M. I. O'Connor, "Malignant pelvic tumors: limb-sparing resection and reconstruction," *Seminars in Surgical Oncology*, vol. 13, no. 1, pp. 49–54, 1997.

[29] P. Cottias, C. Jeanrot, T. S. Vinh, B. Tomeno, and P. Anract, "Complications and functional evaluation of 17 saddle prostheses for resection of periacetabular tumors," *Journal of Surgical Oncology*, vol. 78, no. 2, pp. 90–100, 2001.

[30] Y. Kitagawa, E. T. Ek, and P. F. Choong, "Pelvic reconstruction using saddle prosthesis following limb salvage operation for periacetabular tumour.," *Journal of Orthopaedic Surgery*, vol. 14, no. 2, pp. 155–162, 2006.

[31] A. J. S. Renard, R. P. H. Veth, H. W. B. Schreuder et al., "The saddle prosthesis in pelvic primary and secondary musculoskeletal tumors: functional results at several postoperative intervals," *Archives of Orthopaedic and Trauma Surgery*, vol. 120, no. 3-4, pp. 188–194, 2000.

[32] T. Ozaki, C. Hoffmann, A. Hillmann, G. Gosheger, N. Lindner, and W. Winkelmann, "Implantation of hemipelvic prosthesis after resection of sarcoma," *Clinical Orthopaedics and Related Research*, vol. 396, pp. 197–205, 2002.

[33] N. E. Fisher, J. T. Patton, R. J. Grimer et al., "Ice-cream cone reconstruction of the pelvis: a new type of pelvic replacement EARLY RESULTS," *The Journal of Bone & Joint Surgery—British Volume*, vol. 93, no. 5, pp. 684–688, 2011.

[34] L. R. Menendez, E. R. Ahlmann, Y. Falkinstein, and D. C. Allison, "Periacetabular reconstruction with a new endoprosthesis," *Clinical Orthopaedics and Related Research*, vol. 467, no. 11, pp. 2831–2837, 2009.

[35] D. Witte, L. Bernd, J. Bruns et al., "Limb-salvage reconstruction with MUTARS hemipelvic endoprosthesis: a prospective multicenter study," *European Journal of Surgical Oncology*, vol. 35, no. 12, pp. 1318–1325, 2009.

[36] T. Hüfner, M. Kfuri Jr., M. Galanski et al., "New indications for computer-assisted surgery: tumor resection in the pelvis," *Clinical Orthopaedics and Related Research*, no. 426, pp. 219–225, 2004.

[37] C. Krettek, J. Geerling, L. Bastian et al., "Computer aided tumor resection in the pelvis," *Injury*, vol. 35, no. 1, pp. 79–83, 2004.

[38] K. C. Wong and S. M. Kumta, "Computer-assisted tumor surgery in malignant bone tumors," *Clinical Orthopaedics and Related Research*, vol. 471, no. 3, pp. 750–761, 2013.

[39] K. C. Wong, S. M. Kumta, G. E. Antonio, and L. F. Tse, "Image fusion for computer-assisted bone tumor surgery," *Clinical Orthopaedics and Related Research*, vol. 466, no. 10, pp. 2533–2541, 2008.

[40] R. Rödl, G. Gosheger, B. Leidinger, N. Lindner, W. Winkelmann, and T. Ozaki, "Correction of leg-length discrepancy after hip transposition," *Clinical Orthopaedics and Related Research*, no. 416, pp. 271–277, 2003.

[41] A. Kawai, J. H. Healey, P. J. Boland, P. P. Lin, A. G. Huvos, and P. A. Meyers, "Prognostic factors for patients with sarcomas of the pelvic bones," *Cancer*, vol. 82, no. 5, pp. 851–859, 1998.

[42] T. Ozaki, S. Flege, M. Kevric et al., "Osteosarcoma of the pelvis: experience of the cooperative osteosarcoma study group," *Journal of Clinical Oncology*, vol. 21, no. 2, pp. 334–341, 2003.

[43] T. Fujiwara, T. Kunisada, S. Itani, Y. Morimoto, T. Sasaki, and T. Ozaki, "Short-term follow-up of hip transposition using external fixator after resection of pelvic tumor," *Central Japan Journal of Orthopaedic Surgery and Traumatology*, vol. 53, pp. 937–938, 2010 (Japanese).

[44] M. Campanacci and R. Capanna, "Pelvic resections: the Rizzoli Institute experience," *The Orthopedic Clinics of North America*, vol. 22, no. 1, pp. 65–86, 1991.

4

Whole Lung Irradiation in Adults with Metastatic Ewing Sarcoma: Practice Patterns and Implications for Treatment

Shyam K. Tanguturi,[1] Suzanne George,[2,3] Karen J. Marcus,[2,4,5,6] George D. Demetri,[2,3] and Elizabeth H. Baldini[2,4,5,6]

[1]*Harvard Radiation Oncology Program, Boston, MA 02115, USA*
[2]*Center for Sarcoma and Bone Oncology, Dana-Farber Cancer Institute, Boston, MA 02115, USA*
[3]*Department of Medical Oncology, Dana-Farber Cancer Institute, Boston, MA 02115, USA*
[4]*Department of Radiation Oncology, Dana-Farber Cancer Institute, Boston, MA 02115, USA*
[5]*Department of Radiation Oncology, Brigham and Women's Hospital, Boston, MA 02115, USA*
[6]*Department of Radiation Oncology, Boston's Children's Hospital, Boston, MA 02115, USA*

Correspondence should be addressed to Elizabeth H. Baldini; ebaldini@partners.org

Academic Editor: Uta Dirksen

Background. Whole lung irradiation (WLI) is a standard treatment component for children with metastatic Ewing Sarcoma (ES), but data on WLI for adults are sparse. *Design*. An email survey was sent to expert sarcoma-dedicated oncologists worldwide: *An adult with excellent performance status presents with primary ES in the leg and multiple pulmonary metastases. The patient achieves complete radiographic response after chemotherapy and resection of the primary. Would you give bilateral WLI to (1) this adult patient?, (2) this patient if 20 years old (yo)?, (3) this patient if 45 yo?, or (4) this patient if 60 yo? Results*. 38 experts responded, including 24 adult, 1 adolescent young adult, and 13 pediatric oncologists. 63%, 63%, 62%, and 50% of respondents offered WLI to the adult, 20-year-old, 45-year-old, and 60-year-old, respectively. Pediatric oncologists more likely endorsed WLI across all ages including the adult ($P = 0.01$), 20-year-old ($P = 0.005$), 45-year-old ($P = 0.01$), and 60-year-old ($P = 0.08$). There were no significant differences between medical and radiation oncologists or between European/Australian and American providers. *Conclusions*. Almost two-thirds of experts surveyed supported WLI for adults with metastatic ES up to age 45 and half supported WLI for a 60-year-old. Continued collaboration across adult and pediatric oncology is needed to define evidence-based strategies across the age spectrum.

1. Introduction

Ewing Sarcoma (ES) is a mesenchymal malignancy of unclear histogenetic derivation characterized by distinct chromosomal translocations at the EWSR1 gene [1]; this disease occurs primarily in children and young adults and less commonly in older adults. Although 20–25% of patients with ES present with distant metastatic disease at diagnosis [2], some patients, such as those with limited pulmonary metastases (PM), may be cured with aggressive multimodality therapy. Whole lung irradiation (WLI) is one such treatment designed with curative-intent for patients with PM. In the Intergroup Ewing's Sarcoma Study (IESS-I) of primarily pediatric patients with localized disease, prophylactic WLI with VAC chemotherapy (vincristine, doxorubicin, and cyclophosphamide) was associated with improved survival and fewer PM relative to those treated with VAC alone [3]. Similarly, other retrospective studies have suggested benefits in disease control and survival with the use of WLI for patients with metastatic ES and clinically evident PM [4–8]. Fractionated WLI at doses between 12 and 21 Gy appears to be well tolerated with acceptable rates of toxicity [3–7, 9–11], although data across all age ranges are lacking. Despite the lack of prospective randomized studies, the available data have supported use of WLI as a component of curative therapy for the majority of pediatric ES patients with PM, and this practice is strongly supported by the U.S. National Cancer Institute (NCI) [12].

TABLE 1: Surveyed expert oncologists' recommendations for whole lung irradiation for Ewing Sarcoma patients with pulmonary metastases in complete response following chemotherapy.

Whole lung irradiation recommendation	*N*	Adult*	*P*	20-year-old	*P*	45-year-old	*P*	60-year-old	*P*
All oncologists surveyed	38	63%		63%		62%		50%	
Oncologist discipline									
Medical oncologist	26	58%	NS	58%	NS	60%	NS	46%	NS
Radiation oncologist	12	73%		75%		67%		58%	
AYA/pediatric oncologist	14	92%	0.01	93%	0.005	92%	0.01	75%	0.08
Adult oncologist	24	48%		46%		46%		38%	
Oncologist country									
Europe/Australia	15	57%	NS	60%	NS	53%	NS	40%	NS
United States	23	67%		65%		68%		57%	

*Adult age not specified.
P = 2-tail Fisher Exact Test *P* value; NS = not significant; AYA = adolescent and young adult.

However, given the limited efficacy and toxicity data pertaining to WLI for adults, the use of WLI in adult ES patients is appropriately more controversial. Like other sarcomas that impact both adult and pediatric patients, ES presents distinct challenges with respect to forming consensus on best practice treatment strategies across the age spectrum. Clinical studies are ongoing, such as the Euro-Ewing-Intergroup EE99 (COG-AEWSO331) trial, which randomizes patients with pulmonary metastatic disease alone to standard consolidation chemotherapy with WLI or to high dose chemotherapy plus peripheral blood stem cell (PBSC) rescue in patients up to 50 years old. In the absence of robust data regarding efficacy and toxicity, there is no clear consensus on the use of WLI for adult ES patients with PM. In this context, we conducted a survey of expert sarcoma-dedicated oncologists to ascertain practice patterns regarding WLI for adults with ES and PM.

2. Methods

We developed a brief survey, in which we described the following clinical scenario: *An adult with excellent performance status presents with a primary ES in the leg and multiple PM. The patient achieves a complete radiographic response after chemotherapy and resection of the primary.* Participants were asked: *Would you give bilateral WLI to (1) this adult patient?, (2) this patient if 20 years old?, (3) this patient if 45 years old?, or (4) this patient if 60 years old?* The survey was emailed to 54 expert sarcoma-dedicated medical and radiation oncologists from adult and pediatric practices located in the US, Europe, and Australia. Experts were identified on the basis of their active involvement in sarcoma clinical trial groups such as EORTC, Children's Oncology Group (COG), NCI Canada Clinical Trials Group, Sarcoma Alliance for Research through Collaboration (SARC), and NRG Oncology. This study was approved by the Dana-Farber/Harvard Cancer Center Institutional Review Board.

Basic demographic information about survey participants was collected including practice discipline, country of practice, adult versus pediatric specialty, and institution. Responses among participant groups were compared using Fisher's Exact Test.

3. Results

Thirty-eight of the 54 (70%) emailed participants responded to our survey, including 26 medical and 12 radiation oncologists; 24 adult, 1 adolescent and young adult (AYA), and 13 pediatric oncologists; and 1 from Australia, 14 from Europe, and 23 from the US. Overall, 63% of participants opted to offer WLI to the adult patient, 63% to the 20-year-old, 62% to the 45-year-old, and 50% to the 60-year-old (Table 1).

Table 1 also shows rates of WLI recommendation according to type of oncologist and geographic region. Pediatric oncologists were significantly more likely than adult oncologists to endorse WLI for the adult with no age specified (92% versus 48%, $P = 0.01$), for the 20-year-old (93% versus 46%, $P = 0.005$), and for the 45-year-old (92% versus 46%, $P = 0.01$); the trend was similar for the 60-year-old, but the results were not statistically different (75% versus 38%, $P = 0.08$). No statistically significant differences were seen between responses for medical and radiation oncologists or between oncologists in Europe or Australia versus in the US. Among all categories, WLI was recommended the least for the 60-year-old, but still approximately 50% of the time.

4. Discussion

Despite a relatively poor prognosis among patients with metastatic ES, some of these patients are potentially curable, and as such, aggressive multimodal therapy is a standard approach for metastatic ES. Since the 1970s, WLI has been a component of this aggressive therapy [13] although clear data supporting the necessity of its use, particularly for adults, are lacking.

To illustrate practice patterns and to gather expert opinions on this topic, we surveyed a global sample of oncologists with dedicated expertise in sarcoma management on the use of WLI in adults with ES. Almost two-thirds of sarcoma experts in our survey supported WLI for adults with ES and PM up to age 45, and half supported it up to age 60. Although there were no significant differences in recommendations between medical and radiation oncologists, or by practice location, we found that pediatric oncologists were the most likely to recommend WLI for adults at nearly double the rate across all age groups.

In the pediatric literature, there is substantial evidence to support WLI among ES patients with localized disease [3] as well as for those with metastatic disease limited to the lungs in combination with older chemotherapy regimens [4–6, 8]. Data addressing the potential benefits of WLI in combination with more modern dose- and schedule-intensive chemotherapy regimens are lacking, although the ongoing Euro-Ewing-Intergroup EE99 (COG-AEWSO331) trial is asking this important question. Moreover, although many of these early landmark studies did include adult patients, the vast majority of studied patients were young with median ages of 13 (Nesbit et al. [3]), 13.8 (range: 4.6–21.3; Spunt et al. [6]), and 15 (range: 2–45; Paulussen et al. [4]) further highlighting the limited evidence to support or refute the use of WLI in older age groups. Lastly, the appropriate clinical setting in which to employ WLI has never been defined. WLI could be considered (1) as prophylaxis in the setting of local disease, (2) as treatment in the setting of isolated PM either in complete response or present as residual disease following chemotherapy, and (3) as treatment in the setting of PM and extrapulmonary metastases with PM either in complete response or present as residual disease following chemotherapy. At present, the use of WLI is an integral component of many treatment regimens for pediatric patients with ES and PM, but this practice is less standardized for adults in similar clinical situations.

Broad recommendations for the use of WLI in all age ranges of patients with PM are further complicated by the unique side effect profile and comorbidities relevant to each age group. Toxicity concerns in the pediatric population center on the risks of late pulmonary fibrosis, impaired pulmonary function, chest wall hypoplasia/deformity, and secondary malignancy [14]. The latter two are less relevant for adult patients who may be inherently less susceptible to these events, although second malignancies remain an important concern for young adults [15]. Older adults may be more at risk for acute toxicities like pneumonitis or another pulmonary toxicity which is additive to coexisting health conditions and habits such as lung disease and smoking. Significant cardiac toxicity from WLI *per se* has not been described for any age group, but there is a preponderance of evidence associating RT with the heart with subsequent adverse cardiac events for both pediatric and adult cohorts [16–20]. For this reason, potential cardiac toxicity from WLI must be acknowledged, along with consideration of research and efforts to minimize cardiac dose such as the cardiac-sparing IMRT technique for WLI [21].

To help fill the data void relating to WLI for adults, investigators from Memorial Sloan Kettering Cancer Center studied a series of 26 adult patients with ES and PM who were treated with WLI [11]. In this cohort, the median age was 26 years old, and the range was 18–40 years old. Reported 3-year freedom from pulmonary relapse, event-free survival, and overall survival rates were 45%, 38%, and 45%, respectively, and there was excellent treatment tolerability. Acute toxicity was limited to 12 of 26 patients (46%) who experienced Grade 1 toxicities and three patients (12%) who experienced Grade 2 toxicities including esophagitis, fatigue, and nausea. Two patients (8%) developed herpes zoster in a dermatome corresponding to the RT field within three months of RT. There were no observed cases of late pneumonitis, cardiac toxicities, radiographic sequelae, or other toxicities ≥grade 2. Compared with pulmonary metastases only, the presence of extrapulmonary metastases at diagnosis was associated with inferior 3-year PM-free survival (24%), event-free survival (14%), and overall survival (13%); the authors suggested that WLI may not be sufficiently beneficial to justify its use in patients with extrapulmonary metastases. Lower WLI doses of <15 Gy versus ≥15 Gy ($P = 0.05$) predicted for inferior overall survival, whereas a history of smoking predicted for poorer event-free survival ($P = 0.04$) and showed a trend for inferior overall survival ($P = 0.06$). Smokers and former smokers also appeared to have higher rates of acute toxicity (73% versus 36%), but this did not reach significance ($P = 0.11$). No significant differences in outcomes were seen according to response of PM to chemotherapy. This study is an important step towards understanding outcomes of WLI in adult patients with ES but is limited by the relatively young age of patients included and likely selection bias acknowledged by the authors related to the retrospective design, high rate of patients with isolated pulmonary metastases (65%), and high proportion of adults who did not receive WLI at their institution (35%).

In our survey, we identified significant differences in recommendations for WLI between pediatric and adults oncologists. These divergent practice patterns illustrate not only the challenges in the interpretation of limited data sets in rare tumors but also some of the inherent biases that may arise through a practice devoted to either adult or pediatric patients. Practice variation across adult and pediatric providers has been reported in other soft tissue cancers as well. For example, a survey of adult and pediatric oncologists on the treatment of adult medulloblastoma patients similarly demonstrated substantial variation in practice, particularly with the choice of chemotherapeutic agents, likely reflecting the limited data available relevant to older adult population [22]. Likewise, population studies have demonstrated less aggressive protocols for diagnosis, staging, and treatment for adults with Wilms' Tumor relative to their pediatric counterparts and cited this less aggressive approach as an explanation for inferior survival outcomes among adults [23].

Together, these data call for renewed and continued collaboration across the artifactual divides of adult and pediatric oncology to define evidence-based treatment strategies and appropriate prospective trials across the age spectrum. A vibrant form of this collaboration is seen in the emergence of interest in adolescent and young adult (AYA) oncology as a resource-dedicated discipline dedicated to bridging service and survival gaps in the young adult population and in cancers affecting many age groups which span the traditional "lines" demarcating pediatric and adult oncology [24–26]. Efforts of the AYA Oncology Progress Review Group and others have produced an increased understanding of the distinct survival outcomes, survivorship concerns, barriers to care, and challenges to clinical trial enrollment relevant to these patients [26–28]. Increased participation by AYA providers in both patient care and in clinical trial development will undoubtedly expand our understanding of these understudied populations and encourage inclusion of these patients in forthcoming clinical studies.

The ongoing Euro-Ewing-Intergroup EE99 (COG-AEWSO331) trial comparing standard consolidation chemotherapy with WLI to high dose chemotherapy plus peripheral blood stem cell (PBSC) rescue in patients up to 50 years old with EW and PM is one example of such interdisciplinary collaboration, which promises to help elucidate the role of WLI across a broad range of ages. As we await those results, our survey suggests that the majority of expert oncologists would offer WLI for most adults with ES and PM in complete response, particularly for younger patients up to the age of 45. While it may be reasonable to treat younger adults with WLI, outside of a clinical trial, we would recommend caution in older adults with comorbidities due to limited safety data in this patient population. For clinical scenarios of localized disease, PM that do not completely respond to induction therapy, or PM in combination with extrapulmonary disease, we agree with others that the potential benefits of WLI are limited and we would not endorse the use of WLI in these scenarios.

5. Conclusion

In this survey of worldwide expert sarcoma-oncologists, approximately two-thirds of respondents supported WLI for adult patients with metastatic ES up to 45 years old, and half supported WLI for patients 60 years old. Pediatric oncologists were most likely to recommend WLI at nearly double the rate across all age groups. These data call for continued collaboration across adult and pediatric oncology to define evidence-based treatment strategies and appropriate prospective trials across the age spectrum. As we await the results of the ongoing Euro-Ewing-Intergroup EE99 study investigating the role of WLI, these data suggest that the majority of expert oncologists would offer WLI for most adults with ES and PM, particularly for younger patients up to the age of 45.

Acknowledgment

The authors acknowledge Ewing's Practice Pattern Survey respondents for their responses and contributions to this study.

References

[1] O. Delattre, J. Zucman, T. Melot et al., "The Ewing family of tumors—a subgroup of small-round-cell tumors defined by specific chimeric transcripts," *The New England Journal of Medicine*, vol. 331, no. 5, pp. 294–299, 1994.

[2] S. J. Cotterill, S. Ahrens, M. Paulussen et al., "Prognostic factors in Ewing's tumor of bone: analysis of 975 patients from the European Intergroup Cooperative Ewing's Sarcoma Study Group," *Journal of Clinical Oncology*, vol. 18, no. 17, pp. 3108–3114, 2000.

[3] M. E. Nesbit, E. A. Gehan, E. O. Burgert et al., "Multimodal therapy for the management of primary, nonmetastatic Ewing's Sarcoma of bone: a long-term follow-up of the first intergroup study," *Journal of Clinical Oncology*, vol. 8, no. 10, pp. 1664–1674, 1990.

[4] M. Paulussen, S. Ahrens, A. W. Craft et al., "Ewing's tumors with primary lung metastases: survival analysis of 114 (European intergroup) cooperative Ewing's sarcoma studies patients," *Journal of Clinical Oncology*, vol. 16, no. 9, pp. 3044–3052, 1998.

[5] J. Dunst, M. Paulussen, and H. Jürgens, "Lung irradiation for Ewing's sarcoma with pulmonary metastases at diagnosis: results of the CESS-studies," *Strahlentherapie und Onkologie*, vol. 169, no. 10, pp. 621–623, 1993.

[6] S. L. Spunt, M. B. McCarville, L. E. Kun et al., "Selective use of whole-lung irradiation for patients with Ewing sarcoma family tumors and pulmonary metastases at the time of diagnosis," *Journal of Pediatric Hematology/Oncology*, vol. 23, no. 2, pp. 93–98, 2001.

[7] T. Bölling, A. Schuck, M. Paulussen et al., "Whole lung irradiation in patients with exclusively pulmonary metastases of Ewing tumors: toxicity analysis and treatment results of the EICESS-92 trial," *Strahlentherapie und Onkologie*, vol. 184, no. 4, pp. 193–197, 2008.

[8] J. S. Whelan, R. J. Burcombe, J. Janinis, A. M. Baldelli, and A. M. Cassoni, "A systematic review of the role of pulmonary irradiation in the management of primary bone tumours," *Annals of Oncology*, vol. 13, no. 1, pp. 23–30, 2002.

[9] L. B. Marks, S. M. Bentzen, J. O. Deasy et al., "Radiation dose-volume effects in the lung," *International Journal of Radiation Oncology Biology Physics*, vol. 76, no. 3, pp. S70–S76, 2010.

[10] C. J. H. Fryer, P. J. Fitzpatrick, W. D. Rider, and P. Pooh, "Radiation pneumonitis: experience following a large single dose of radiation," *International Journal of Radiation Oncology, Biology, Physics*, vol. 4, no. 11-12, pp. 931–936, 1978.

[11] D. L. Casey, K. M. Alektiar, N. K. Gerber, and S. L. Wolden, "Whole lung irradiation for adults with pulmonary metastases from Ewing sarcoma," *International Journal of Radiation Oncology Biology Physics*, vol. 89, no. 5, pp. 1069–1075, 2014.

[12] National Cancer Institute, Ewing Sarcoma Treatment (PDQ), http://www.cancer.gov/cancertopics/pdq/treatment/ewings/HealthProfessional/page6.

[13] N. Jaffe, D. Paed, D. Traggis, S. Salian, and J. R. Cassady, "Improved outlook for Ewing's sarcoma with combination chemotherapy (vincristine, actinomycin D and cyclophosphamide) and radiation therapy," *Cancer*, vol. 38, no. 5, table 1, pp. 1925–1930, 1976.

[14] T. Bölling, S. Könemann, I. Ernst, and N. Willich, "Late effects of thoracic irradiation in children," *Strahlentherapie und Onkologie*, vol. 184, no. 6, pp. 289–295, 2008.

[15] S. L. Hancock, M. A. Tucker, and R. T. Hoppe, "Breast cancer after treatment of Hodgkin's disease," *Journal of the National Cancer Institute*, vol. 85, no. 1, pp. 25–31, 1993.

[16] V. King, L. S. Constine, D. Clark et al., "Symptomatic coronary artery disease after mantle irradiation for Hodgkin's disease," *International Journal of Radiation Oncology Biology Physics*, vol. 36, no. 4, pp. 881–889, 1996.

[17] M. Tukenova, C. Guibout, O. Oberlin et al., "Role of cancer treatment in long-term overall and cardiovascular mortality after childhood cancer," *Journal of Clinical Oncology*, vol. 28, no. 8, pp. 1308–1315, 2010.

[18] E. J. Chow, Y. Chen, L. C. Kremer et al., "Individual prediction of heart failure among childhood cancer survivors," *Journal of Clinical Oncology*, vol. 33, no. 5, pp. 394–402, 2014.

[19] D. A. Mulrooney, M. W. Yeazel, T. Kawashima et al., "Cardiac outcomes in a cohort of adult survivors of childhood and adolescent cancer: retrospective analysis of the Childhood Cancer Survivor Study cohort," *British Medical Journal*, vol. 339, no. 7736, Article ID b4606, 2009.

[20] S. C. Darby, M. Ewertz, P. McGale et al., "Risk of ischemic heart disease in women after radiotherapy for breast cancer," *The New England Journal of Medicine*, vol. 368, no. 11, pp. 987–998, 2013.

[21] J. A. Kalapurakal, Y. Zhang, A. Kepka et al., "Cardiac-sparing whole lung IMRT in children with lung metastasis," *International Journal of Radiation Oncology, Biology, Physics*, vol. 85, no. 3, pp. 761–767, 2013.

[22] R. Cosman, C. S. B. Brown, K. C. DeBraganca, and M. Khasraw, "Patterns of care in adult medulloblastoma: results of an international online survey," *Journal of Neuro-Oncology*, vol. 120, no. 1, pp. 125–129, 2014.

[23] A. N. Ali, R. Diaz, H.-K. Shu, A. C. Paulino, and N. Esiashvili, "A Surveillance, Epidemiology and End Results (SEER) program comparison of adult and pediatric Wilms' tumor," *Cancer*, vol. 118, no. 9, pp. 2541–2551, 2012.

[24] National Cancer Institute and Lance Armstrong Foundation, "Closing the gap: research and care imperatives for adolescents and young adults with cancer," Report of the Adolescent and Young Adult Oncology Progress Review Group, 2006.

[25] B. Hayes-Lattin, B. Mathews-Bradshaw, and S. Siegel, "Adolescent and young adult oncology training for health professionals: a position statement," *Journal of Clinical Oncology*, vol. 28, no. 32, pp. 4858–4861, 2010.

[26] P. H. Shaw, D. R. Reed, N. Yeager, B. Zebrack, S. M. Castellino, and A. Bleyer, "Adolescent and young adult (AYA) oncology in the United States: a specialty in its late adolescence," *Journal of Pediatric Hematology/Oncology*, vol. 37, no. 3, pp. 161–169, 2015.

[27] H. Soliman and S. V. Agresta, "Current issues in adolescent and young adult cancer survivorship," *Cancer Control*, vol. 15, no. 1, pp. 55–62, 2008.

[28] M. E. Burke, K. Albritton, and N. Marina, "Challenges in the recruitment of adolescents and young adults to cancer clinical trials," *Cancer*, vol. 110, no. 11, pp. 2385–2393, 2007.

5

The Identification of Prognostic Factors and Survival Statistics of Conventional Central Chondrosarcoma

Sjoerd P. F. T. Nota,[1] Yvonne Braun,[1] Joseph H. Schwab,[1] C. Niek van Dijk,[2] and Jos A. M. Bramer[2]

[1] *Orthopaedic Oncology Service, Massachusetts General Hospital, Harvard Medical School, Boston, MA 02114, USA*
[2] *Department of Orthopaedic Surgery, Academic Medical Center, 1105 AZ Amsterdam, Netherlands*

Correspondence should be addressed to Sjoerd P. F. T. Nota; snota@mgh.harvard.edu

Academic Editor: Manish Agarwal

Introduction. Chondrosarcomas are malignant bone tumors that are characterized by the production of chondroid tissue. Since radiation therapy and chemotherapy have limited effect on chondrosarcoma, treatment of most patients depends on surgical resection. We conducted this study to identify independent predictive factors and survival characteristics for conventional central chondrosarcoma and dedifferentiated central chondrosarcoma. *Methods.* A systematic literature review was performed in September 2014 using the Pubmed, Embase, and Cochrane databases. Subsequent to a beforehand-composed selection procedure we included 13 studies, comprising a total of 1114 patients. *Results.* The prognosis of central chondrosarcoma is generally good for the histologically low-grade tumors. Prognosis for the high-grade chondrosarcoma and the dedifferentiated chondrosarcoma is poor with lower survival rates. Poor prognostic factors in conventional chondrosarcoma for overall survival are high-grade tumors and axial/pelvic tumor location. In dedifferentiated chondrosarcoma the percentage of dedifferentiated component has significant influence on disease-free survival. *Conclusion.* Despite the fact that there are multiple prognostic factors identified, as shown in this study, there is a need for prospective and comparative studies. The resulting knowledge about prognostic factors and survival can give direction in the development of better therapies. This could eventually lead to an evidence-based foundation for treating chondrosarcoma patients.

1. Introduction

Chondrosarcomas are malignant bone tumors that can be characterized by the production of chondroid tissue [1]. This heterogeneous group of tumors occupy about a quarter of all the primary malignant osseous neoplasms of the bone [2]. Chondrosarcomas are the most common occurring primary sarcoma of the bone after osteosarcoma [2, 3]. The clinical behavior and prognosis of these tumors depend on many variables of which tumor grade is one of the most important; high-grade tumors have a worse prognosis compared to low-grade tumors [4, 5]. This poor prognosis can partially be explained by the high tendency to metastasize. About three-quarters of all chondrosarcomas consist of conventional central chondrosarcoma. These central chondrosarcomas have the outgrowth of the sarcomatous tumor in the intramedullary cavity in common. The central chondrosarcoma's anatomical counterpart is the peripheral chondrosarcoma. These specific chondrosarcomas develop from a preexisting osteochondroma and are situated on the outside of the cortex of the bone. The peripheral chondrosarcoma tumors have a better prognosis when compared to the central chondrosarcoma and tend to affect younger patients [6].

Radiation therapy and chemotherapy have limited to arguably no effect on conventional chondrosarcoma [7, 8]. There are rarer chondrosarcoma subtypes that are more responsive to chemotherapy and/or radiation therapy [9]. The vast majority of chondrosarcoma patients solely depended on the surgical treatment by tumor resection. Chemotherapy might have a role in dedifferentiated chondrosarcoma [10, 11] although the positive effect is not consistently reported in literature [11–13].

Identification of prognostic factors and knowledge about survival are important. For patients this knowledge can provide insight into their future perspective and it may provide guidance in the decision-making concerning treatment. Physicians can use the prognostic and survival information as a tool to select the optimal treatment strategy and inform patients. To direct efforts in the development of new therapeutic strategies the identification of proven prognostic factors of central chondrosarcoma is important, especially since the treatment options are limited. We conducted this systematic review with the aim of identifying independent predictive factors and survival characteristics for both conventional central chondrosarcoma and dedifferentiated central chondrosarcoma.

2. Materials and Methods

This systematic review was registered on PROSPERO prior to data extraction (registration number: CRD42014008961). The MOOSE checklist for meta-analysis of observational studies in epidemiology study was applied for the evaluation of meta-analysis and observational studies [14].

2.1. Search Strategy. We searched Pubmed, Embase, and the Cochrane database for title and abstract, without any limits on September 9, 2014, using the following search terms: ((“chondrosarcoma*” OR “chondroid sarcoma” OR “chondroid sarcomas”) AND “prognos*”) OR ((“chondrosarcoma*” OR “chondroid sarcoma” OR “chondroid sarcomas”) AND “surviv*”) resulting in a total of 2253 publications.

2.2. Study Selection, Data Extraction, and Critical Appraisal. Two reviewers (Sjoerd P. F. T. Nota, Yvonne Braun) independently screened all the studies’ titles and abstracts and retrieved the full-text manuscripts for the articles that met our inclusion criteria. If consensus was not reached between the two reviewers, a third reviewer (Jos A. M. Bramer) was consulted. We included all articles focusing on any prognostic factors and/or survival statistics on all grades (including dedifferentiated chondrosarcoma) of primary central chondrosarcoma of the bone.

We excluded congress proceedings, letter to the editors, cohorts that were not independently identifiable, all studies published in a different language than English, and studies published before 1980. In addition we excluded case-reports and case-series with less than 10 patients. Furthermore we excluded papers reporting on surgical procedures and studies focusing solely on metastasis. Finally we excluded all papers that did not clearly distinguish between central and peripheral chondrosarcoma and reviews were excluded as well.

After applying our exclusion criteria on the title and abstract 274 papers remained for full-text screening.

The quality of the data was assessed by application of predetermined critical appraisal criteria by two independent researchers. Lack of consensus was solved again as described above. The criteria assessed were as follows: study participation, study attrition, prognostic factor measurement, outcome measurement, confounding measurement, analysis performed, population included, the time of follow-up, the level of evidence, the presence of a disclosure statement, and the presence of a baseline characteristics table (Appendix).

2.3. Outcome Measurements. We extracted the data of the following variables from the selected studies: author/year, type of study, mean age, sex distribution, mean duration of follow-up, primary tumors only, metastasis at presentation, grading method, tumor grade, anatomical location, overall survival, and 5- and 10-year survival per grade. In addition we registered the disease-free survival, the percentage of patients with no evidence of disease, and the percentage of patients with no evidence of disease after tumor relapse. Furthermore we looked at the percentage of patients alive with disease and dead of disease and the percentage of patients that died of a different cause. We also looked at the local recurrence rate, the time to local recurrence, metastasis rate and time to metastasis, and the use of chemo- and radiation therapy. Finally to account for the homogeneity of the treatment of the patients in the studies we also reported the status of the surgical margins of the included subjects.

2.4. Analysis. To prevent reporting biased results due to the high quantity of cohort studies and case-series and potential overlap of patients’ population we choose to only report our results narratively and did not attempt to merge results and do additional analyses.

2.5. Prognostic Factors and Survival Statistics. In this review we will narratively summarize the prognostic factors and survival statistics reported in our selected studies.

2.6. Study Characteristic. After screening the full-text articles we included 13 studies that met our inclusion criteria for this review [10, 15–26]. The 13 studies included were based on retrospective evidence. All studies reported clearly the dates of researched period, the patient sample, and the point of the course of the disease. Nine out of the 13 studies (69%) reported a sufficient long follow-up (more than 1 year) and explained the reason of patients being lost to follow-up. Four studies (31%) did not report these factors and may therefore be subject to more selection bias (see the appendix).

2.7. Study Population. The 13 included studies comprised the data of 1114 patients, although population overlap is likely since multiple studies are performed in the same institution. In the studies where we could determine the age the average age of the patients ranged from 35 to 59 years and the percentage of males ranged from 42% to 79% with only 1 study reporting more females in the cohort. The mean follow-up ranged from at least more than 2 years to 13 years. The individual follow-up ranged from a minimum of 0 years to a maximum of 26 years (Table 1).

Not all studies mentioned the fact if only primary tumors and if recurrences were excluded or did included patient with such tumors (Table 2). There were a wide variety of tumor grades in the included studies. Three studies focused on central dedifferentiated chondrosarcoma and 1 study focused on grade 2 chondrosarcoma only; all other studies

TABLE 1: Demographic patient and study characteristics of the included studies.

Study	Study design	Patients (number)	Mean age (range) (years)	Male (%)	Follow-up (range) (years)
Andreou et al., 2011 [15]	R	115	47 (14–79)	61%	12 (5–24)
Angelini et al., 2012 [16]	R	296	50 (13–88)	57%	7 (1.6–20)
Briccoli et al., 2002 [17]	R	14	·	·	5.8 (0–19)
Cho et al., 2011 [18]	R	32	·	72%	9.2 (2.6–19)
de Camargo et al., 2010 [19]	R	46	43 (17–79)	54%	8.3 (2.7–26)
Donati et al., 2010 [20]	R	31	35 (13–67)	42%	13 (5.5–25)
Donati et al., 2005 [21]	R	63	·	·	·
Gitelis et al., 1981 [22]	R	69	44 (14–78)	68%	>5 year
Mavrogenis et al., 2013 [23]	R	119	·	·	>2 year
Mitchell et al., 2000 [10]	R	14	57 (37–79)	79%	4.7 (1.7–7.5)$^{+}$
Ozaki et al., 1996 [24]	R	21	51 (25–71)	67%	12 (5–22)
Staals et al., 2006 [25]	R	123*	59 (24–83)	54%	2.8 (0–17)
van Maldegem et al., 2014 [26]	R	171	53 (17–90)	63%	·

*110 patients with actual follow-up data, R = retrospective, and $^{+}$surviving patients.

included patients with a variety of different tumor grades. The localizations of the tumors comprise the entire skeleton throughout the different studies (Table 2).

In 10 out of the 13 studies the surgical margin status was determined showing a wide range in the percentages of patients having wide and radical resection (Table 6).

The additional use of chemotherapy and radiotherapy is only registered in, respectively, 9 out of 13 (69%) and 6 out of 13 (46%) studies. Chemotherapy is used in 6 out of the 9 (67%) studies where chemotherapy is mentioned. Radiotherapy is used in 4 out of the 6 (67%) studies where its use is mentioned (Table 5).

3. Results

3.1. Survival: General. Overall survival ranged from 21% to 100% at the time of follow-up depending on the specific study. Five- and 10-year survival ranged from 2% to 100% and 32% to 85%, respectively (Table 3). Disease-free survival ranged from 30% to 89% and the local recurrence rate ranged from 6.2% to 35%. In the 5 studies reporting the metastasis rate the rate ranges from 0% to 38% (Table 4).

3.2. Survival: Grades 1, 2, and 3 and Dedifferentiated Chondrosarcoma. The reported 5-year survival for grade 1 chondrosarcoma ranged from 82% to 99%. The 10-year survival ranged from 89% to 95%. The 5-year survival for grade 2 chondrosarcoma ranged from 63% to 92%. The 10-year survival ranged from 58% to 86%. The 5-year survival for grade 3 chondrosarcoma ranged from 0% to 77%. The lowest (0%) survival was displayed in a study looking at a very small subgroup of patients treated with an intralesional resection. The 10-year survival ranged from 0% to 55%. The 5-year survival for dedifferentiated chondrosarcoma was 24% as reported in 1 study (Table 3).

3.3. Prognostic Factors. In 7 of the included studies prognostic factors for overall survival were reported. Cho et al. found no difference in event-free survival between curettage in combination with subsequent treatment versus standard treatment of wide excision ($p = 0.16$) in their cohort of grade 2 chondrosarcoma of the extremities [18]. Donati et al. compared survival of central with peripheral chondrosarcoma and found a difference in survival in their cohort of pelvis tumors ($p = 0.00093$) as did Gitelis et al. at 5-year ($p < 0.001$) and 10-year ($p < 0.001$) as well as in total disease-free survival ($p < 0.005$) between central and peripheral chondrosarcoma [21, 22].

Andreou et al., Angelini et al., and Staals et al. investigated multiple potential prognostic factors [15, 16, 25] as summarized in Table 7. The main significant poor prognostic factors Andreou et al. and/or Angelini et al. reported were larger tumor volume, higher grade and distant metastasis, and a worse prognosis for axial located tumors (including the pelvis) compared to in the extremity located tumors. Worst prognosis for a pathologic fracture and supportive care in comparison with multidisciplinary treatment (chemotherapy, radiotherapy, and further surgery) were reported as well. Staals et al. most prominent findings were the significant impact of Stage 3 lesions versus, respectively, Stages 2a and 2b lesions and the poor prognostic value of a higher percentage of dedifferentiated component within the tumor [25]. van Maldegem et al. show in unresectable chondrosarcoma a survival benefit for the use of chemotherapy compared to not using systemic treatment. When interpreting these results, the large heterogeneity in the treatment groups should be accounted for. In addition they show significant impact of solely unresectable disease compared to unresectable disease in combination with the presence of metastasis. Finally they showed that an age younger than 40 and grade 2 tumors have a better survival [26] (Table 7).

Table 2: Oncologic patient and study characteristics of the included studies.

Study	Primary tumors only	Metastasis at presentation	Grading	Grade 1	Grade 2	Grade 3	Dediff.
Andreou et al., 2011 [15]	Yes	No	Evans et al.	56 (49%)	41 (36%)	18 (15%)	0
Angelini et al., 2012 [16]	·	·	Lichtenstein and Jaffe	87 (29%)	162 (55%)	47 (16%)	0
Briccoli et al., 2002 [17]	No	Yes	·	0	9 (64%)	4 (29%)	1 (7.1%)
Cho et al., 2011 [18]	No	No	Evans et al.	0	32 (100%)	0	0
de Camargo et al., 2010 [19]	Yes	Yes	Lichtenstein and Jaffe	23 (50%)	23 (50%)	0	0
Donati et al., 2010 [20]	No	No	Mirra et al. + Schiller et al.	31 (100%)	0	0	0
Donati et al., 2005 [21]	No	·	·	1 (1.6%)	44 (70%)	18 (29%)	0
Gitelis et al., 1981 [22]	·	·	·	9 (13%)	46 (67%)	14 (20%)	0
Mavrogenis et al., 2013 [23]	·	·	·	·	·	·	22 (18%)
Mitchell et al., 2000 [10]	·	·	·	0	0	0	14 (100%)
Ozaki et al., 1996 [24]	No	·	Evans et al.	11 (52%)	6 (29%)	4 (19%)	0
Staals et al., 2006 [25]	·	·	·	0	0	0	123 (100%)
van Maldegem et al., 2014 [26]	No	Yes	·	9	118	44	0

Study	Lower extremity	Upper extremity (incl. shoulder girdle)	Hand*	Pelvis girdle (incl. sacrum)	Axial skeleton	Thorax	Other
Andreou et al., 2011 [15]	48 (42%)	20 (17%)	0	42 (37%)	5 (4.3%)	0	0
Angelini et al., 2012 [16]	134 (45%)	50 (17%)	4 (1.4%)	82 (28%)	10 (3.4%)	16 (5.4%)	0
Briccoli et al., 2002 [17]	0	0	0	0	0	14 (100%)	0
Cho et al., 2011 [18]	22 (69%)	7 (22%)	0	0	0	0	3 (9.4%)
de Camargo et al., 2010 [19]	25 (54%)	10 (22%)	4 (8.7%)	6 (13%)	1 (2.2%)	0	0
Donati et al., 2010 [20]	24 (77%)	7 (23%)	0	0	0	0	0
Donati et al., 2005 [21]	0	0	0	63 (100%)	0	0	0
Gitelis et al., 1981 [22]	·	·	·	·	·	·	·
Mavrogenis et al., 2013 [23]	0	0	0	119 (100%)	0	0	0
Mitchell et al., 2000 [10]	8 (57%)	2 (14%)	0	4 (29%)	0	0	0
Ozaki et al., 1996 [24]	6 (29%)	2 (9.5%)	0	13 (62%)	0	0	0
Staals et al., 2006 [25]	67 (54%)	27 (22%)	0	28 (23%)	0	0	0
van Maldegem et al., 2014 [26]	^	^	^	63 (37%)	9 (5.3%)	15 (8.8%)	^

*If specifically mentioned; ^no differentiation possible.

TABLE 3: Oncologic outcome, survival.

Study	Overall survival	5 y survival	10 y survival	Grade 1 5 y survival	Grade 1 10 y survival
Andreou et al., 2011 [15]	63%	72%	69%	89%	89%
Angelini et al., 2012 [16]	84%	92%	84%	99%	95%
Briccoli et al., 2002 [17]	86%	·	·	·	·
Cho et al., 2011 [18]	84%	·	85%^	·	·
de Camargo et al., 2010 [19]	94%^^	·	·	·	·
Donati et al., 2010 [20]	100%	100%	·	·	·
Donati et al., 2005 [21]	73%	·	·	·	·
Gitelis et al., 1981 [22]	·	49%	32%	·	·
Mavrogenis et al., 2013 [23]	·	80%*	65%*	·	·
Mitchell et al., 2000 [10]	21%	·	·	·	·
Ozaki et al., 1996 [24]	57%	·	·	82%	·
Staals et al., 2006 [25]	24%	24%	·	·	·
van Maldegem et al., 2014 [26]	·	2%	·	·	·
Study	**Grade 2 5 y survival**	**Grade 2 10 y survival**	**Grade 3 5 y survival**	**Grade 3 10 y survival**	**Dedifferentiated 5 y survival**
Andreou et al., 2011 [15]	63%	58%	39%	33%	·
Angelini et al., 2012 [16]	92%	86%	77%	55%	·
Briccoli et al., 2002 [17]	·	·	50%	·	·
Cho et al., 2011 [18]	·	85%^	·	·	·
de Camargo et al., 2010 [19]	·	·	·	·	·
Donati et al., 2010 [20]	·	·	·	·	·
Donati et al., 2005 [21]	·	·	·	·	·
Gitelis et al., 1981 [22]	·	·	·	·	·
Mavrogenis et al., 2013 [23]	·	·	·	·	·
Mitchell et al., 2000 [10]	·	·	·	·	·
Ozaki et al., 1996 [24]	67%	·	0%	·	·
Staals et al., 2006 [25]	·	·	·	·	24%
van Maldegem et al., 2014 [26]	·	·	·	·	·

*Extracted from Kaplan Meier curve, ^^43/46 = 93%, and ^discrepancy calculation and manuscript.

TABLE 4: Oncologic outcome, survival.

Study	Disease-free survival	No evidence of disease	No evidence of disease after tumor relapse	Alive with disease	Dead of disease	Dead of other causes
Andreou et al., 2011 [15]	63%	73 (63%)	0	0	38* (33%)	4 (3.5%)
Angelini et al., 2012 [16]	79%	201 (68%)	33 (11%)	15 (5.1%)	35 (12%)	12 (4.1%)
Briccoli et al., 2002 [17]	71%	10 (71%)	·	2 (14%)	1 (7.1%)	1 (7.1%)
Cho et al., 2011 [18]	75%	24 (75%)	2 (6.3%)	3 (9.4%)	5 (16%)	0
de Camargo et al., 2010 [19]	89%	·	·	6 (13%)	3 (7%)	0
Donati et al., 2010 [20]	·	29 (94%)	2 (6.5%)	0	0	0
Donati et al., 2005 [21]	·	·	·	·	·	·
Gitelis et al., 1981 [22]	30%	·	·	·	·	·
Mavrogenis et al., 2013 [23]	·	·	·	·	·	·
Mitchell et al., 2000 [10]	·	·	·	·	·	·
Ozaki et al., 1996 [24]	62%	4 (19%)	9 (43%)	0	7 (33%)	1 (4.8%)
Staals et al., 2006 [25]	·	·	·	·	84 (76%)	·
van Maldegem et al., 2014 [26]	·	·	·	·	·	·

*Including 6 treatment related deaths.

Table 5

Study	Local recurrence	Time to local recurrence (months)	Metastasis	Time to metastasis (months)	Chemotherapy	Radiation
Andreou et al., 2011 [15]	38 (33%)	21 (2–96)	30 (26%)	27 (2–141)	Used	Used
Angelini et al., 2012 [16]	50 (17%)	.	41 (14%)	.	Not used	Not used
Briccoli et al., 2002 [17]	6 (43%)	.	.	.	Used	.
Cho et al., 2011 [18]	2 (6.2%)	.	10 (31%)	49 (7–181)*	.	.
de Camargo et al., 2010 [19]	16 (35%)	24 (9–46)	.	.	Not used	Not used
Donati et al., 2010 [20]	2 (6.5%)	31 (31–31)	0	.	.	.
Donati et al., 2005 [21]	15 (24%)	.	.	.	.	.
Gitelis et al., 1981 [22]	22 (32%)	.	26 (38%)	.	.	.
Mavrogenis et al., 2013 [23]	.	.	.	.	Used	.
Mitchell et al., 2000 [10]	.	.	.	.	Used	Used
Ozaki et al., 1996 [24]	.	.	.	.	Not used	Used
Staals et al., 2006 [25]	.	.	.	.	Used	.
van Maldegem et al., 2014 [26]	.	.	.	.	Used	Used

*Different numbers calculable in paper.

Table 6

Study	Inadequate surgical margins Enneking: intralesional or marginal	Wide and radical margin
Andreou et al., 2011 [15]	21 (18%)	94 (82%)
Angelini et al., 2012 [16]	74 (25%)	222 (75%)
Briccoli et al., 2002 [17]	3 (21%)	11 (79%)
Cho et al., 2011 [18]	7 (22%)	25 (78%)
de Camargo et al., 2010 [19]	25 (54%)	18 (39%)
Donati et al., 2010 [20]	17 (55%)	14 (45%)
Donati et al., 2005 [21]	17 (27%)	46 (73%)
Gitelis et al., 1981 [22]	37 (54%)	32 (46%)
Mavrogenis et al., 2013 [23]	.	.
Mitchell et al., 2000 [10]	.	.
Ozaki et al., 1996 [24]	21 (100%)	0
Staals et al., 2006 [25]	.	.
van Maldegem et al., 2014 [26]	52 (30%)*	87 (51%)*

*Initial surgery.

4. Discussion and Conclusions

The results of our study show that the prognosis of central chondrosarcoma is fairly good for the low histological grade tumors with a 5- and 10-year survival of over 80%. High-grade chondrosarcoma and the highly lethal dedifferentiated chondrosarcoma have a poor prognosis with lower survival rates. The main negative prognostic factors for overall survival displayed in this review are a higher tumor grade and an axial/pelvis location of the tumor for the conventional chondrosarcoma. The percentage of dedifferentiated component within dedifferentiated chondrosarcoma has significant influence on disease-free survival of these tumors.

This review should be interpreted with its limitations in mind. First of all there are only limited studies in literature that describe solely central chondrosarcoma (or where the central chondrosarcomas are identifiable). The included studies are all retrospective and, even though we used strict inclusion criteria, have a large heterogeneity between patients and treatments. The heterogeneity in histologic type of grading used to evaluate the tumors, the variability in the use of chemo- and radiotherapy, and the differences in the presence of inadequate surgical margins might all have influenced our study's main outcomes. Second limitation is the likely overlap in patient population that can be explained by the centralization of care in large institutions due to the low incidence of primary orthopaedic tumors in general populations. This might introduce a bias and might amplify the experience of a single (experienced) center. Finally there is a large heterogeneity in the outcome measures, partially explained by differences in follow-up time, which makes the direct comparison and getting a general overview of the

TABLE 7: Prognostic factors.

Andreou et al. [15] Overall survival	
Variable (bivariate analysis)	*p value*
Sex	$p = 0.6$
Age (higher)	$p = 0.04$
Extremity versus axial + pelvis	$p = 0.002$
Tumor volume (0–100 cc vs. >100 cc)	$p < 0.001$
Grade tumor	$p < 0.001$
Local recurrences	$p < 0.001$
Distant metastasis	$p < 0.001$
Surgical margins	$p = 0.9$
Type of surgery	
Low grade: ablative versus limb-sparing	$p = 0.7$
High grade: ablative versus limb-sparing	$p = 0.1$
Pathologic fracture	$p = 0.002$
ACJCC	$p < 0.001$
Multi disc. versus support. care	$p = 0.001$
Variable (multivariate analysis)	
High grade: RR = 5	$p < 0.001$
Axial + pelvis: RR = 2	$p = 0.04$
Staals et al. [25] Disease-free survival	
Variable (bivariate analysis)	*p value*
Gender	NS
Age	NS
Duration of symptoms	NS
Lesion size	NS
Anatomic location	NS
Stage 3 versus Stage 2a	$p = 0.003$
Stage 3 versus Stage 2b	$p < 0.00005$
Stage 2a versus Stage 2b	$p = 0.27$
Histologic subtype, MFH versus OS	$p = 0.046$
Histologic subtype, MFH versus fibr. sarc.	$p = 0.08$
Histologic subtype, OS versus fibr. sarc.	$p = 0.96$
Grade 3DD versus grade 4DD	$p = 0.10$
Percentage of DD component	$p = 0.0102$
Percentage of DD component, >50% versus <50%	$p < 0.00005$
Limb-sparing versus resection	$p = 0.08$
Surgery versus surgery + chemotherapy	$p = 0.88$
Variable (multivariate analysis, overall survival)	
Percentage of DD component	$p = 0.0102$
Angelini et al. [16] Overall survival	
Variable (bivariate analysis)	*p value*
G1: wide versus intralesional	$p = 0.495$
G1: extremity versus trunk	$p = 0.595$
G2: wide versus intralesional	$p = 0.948$
G2: extremity versus trunk	$p = 0.589$
G2: resect. versus amputation	$p = 0.496$
G3: extremity versus trunk	$p = 0.039$
G3: resect. versus amputation	$p = 0.051$
Variable (multivariate analysis)	
G3: resect. versus amputation	$p = 0.0943$
G3: extr. versus trunk	$p = 0.0889$
van Maldegem et al. [26] Overall survival from the day of unresectability	
Variable (bivariate analysis)	*p value*
Only local unresectable disease versus local unresectable disease + metastasis	$p = 0.0014$
Age (<40 years)	$p = 0.001$
Grade II tumors	$p = 0.022$
Sex	NS
Site	NS
Resectable versus nonresectable disease at primary diagnosis	NS
Systemic treatment	$p < 0.0487$

RR = Relative Risk, G = grade, MFH = malignant fibrohistocytoma, OS = osteosarcoma, and DD = dedifferentiated.

included studies challenging. This is, for example, displayed in the wide ranges in survival statistics. The grade 3 tumors have a range of 0–77% 5-year survival. Most likely this difference is caused by comparing a small subgroup of intralesional treated tumors with the results from a highly specialized center. Also significant interobserver variability in pathologists' histologic grading is known to be present in these types of tumors [27]. This might also directly influence the reported outcomes.

Remarkably in contrast to reports in literature on chondrosarcoma [28, 29], surgical margins were not identified as independent predictor of survival in this review. However, as stated by Andreou et al. as well, in multivariable analysis Lee et al. showed only a small effect of surgical margin status on survival and Fiorenza et al. were not able to determine the effect when accounting for confounders factors [15]. Caution is needed when interpreting these conclusions and their potential consequences in practice. Relative small retrospective studies with a large heterogeneity of patients might be the cause of the inability to identify, in oncology commonly accepted, prognostic factors such as wide surgical margins.

Our study points out that there is a need for prospective and comparative studies identifying factors and treatments influencing the survival of patients suffering from central chondrosarcoma. More evidence from high quality research might eventually lead to a more evidence-based foundation of treatments while preventing abundant exposure of patients to potentially harmful therapies such as radiation and chemotherapy. Further centralization of care for patients with relatively rare diseases would be desirable from a patient's point of view but might also generate opportunities for researchers to set up prospective and comparative studies. To improve survival in central chondrosarcoma patients,

TABLE 8

(a)

Author, year	Study participation: Dates of researched period stated Clearly defined patient sample, assembled at a common point in course of the disease	Study attrition: Sufficiently long and complete follow-up (≥2 years and ≥80%) Explaining reasons for patients being lost to follow-up	Confounding measurement: Defined and comparable treatment for patients
Andreou et al., 2011 [15]	1	1	1, types of surgery mentioned
Angelini et al., 2012 [16]	1	1	1, types of surgery mentioned
Briccoli et al., 2002 [17]	1	0	1, types of surgery mentioned
Cho et al., 2011 [18]	1	1	1, types of surgery mentioned
de Camargo et al., 2010 [19]	1	1	1, types of surgery mentioned
Donati et al., 2010 [20]	1	1	1, types of surgery mentioned
Donati et al., 2005 [21]	1	1	1, types of surgery mentioned
Gitelis et al., 1981 [22]	1	1	1, types of surgery mentioned
Mavrogenis et al., 2013 [23]	1	1	1, types of surgery mentioned
Mitchell et al., 2000 [10]	1	0	1, types of surgery mentioned
Ozaki et al., 1996 [24]	1	1	1, types of surgery mentioned
Staals et al., 2006 [25]	1	0	1, types of surgery mentioned
van Maldegem et al., 2014 [26]	1	0	1, types of surgery mentioned

(b)

Author, year	Analysis: Valid statistical analysis is done Multivariable analysis is done	Population: (no overlap)	Disclosure
Andreou et al., 2011 [15]	1	1	1
Angelini et al., 2012 [16]	1	0	1
Briccoli et al., 2002 [17]	0	0	0
Cho et al., 2011 [18]	0	1	1
de Camargo et al., 2010 [19]	0	1	1
Donati et al., 2010 [20]	0	0	1
Donati et al., 2005 [21]	1, but not on central survival	0	1
Gitelis et al., 1981 [22]	0	0	0
Mavrogenis et al., 2013 [23]	1	0	1
Mitchell et al., 2000 [10]	0	1	1
Ozaki et al., 1996 [24]	0	1	0
Staals et al., 2006 [25]	0	0	0
van Maldegem et al., 2014 [26]	0	0	1

(c)

Author, year	Prognostic factor measurement: Clear definition and valid assessment of prognostic factors	Outcome measurement: Well defined outcome parameters (survival: overall, metastatic-free, event-free)
Andreou et al., 2011 [15]	1	1
Angelini et al., 2012 [16]	1	1
Briccoli et al., 2002 [17]	0	0
Cho et al., 2011 [18]	1	1
de Camargo et al., 2010 [19]	1	1
Donati et al., 2010 [20]	1	0
Donati et al., 2005 [21]	1	0
Gitelis et al., 1981 [22]	1	1
Mavrogenis et al., 2013 [23]	1	1
Mitchell et al., 2000 [10]	1	0
Ozaki et al., 1996 [24]	1	1
Staals et al., 2006 [25]	1	1
van Maldegem et al., 2014 [26]	1	1

(d)

Author, year	FU >1 year	Level of evidence I–IV
Andreou et al., 2011 [15]	1	4, prognostic
Angelini et al., 2012 [16]	1	4, prognostic
Briccoli et al., 2002 [17]	0	4, prognostic
Cho et al., 2011 [18]	1	3, therapeutic
de Camargo et al., 2010 [19]	1	4, prognostic
Donati et al., 2010 [20]	1	2, prognostic
Donati et al., 2005 [21]	1	4, prognostic
Gitelis et al., 1981 [22]	1	4, prognostic
Mavrogenis et al., 2013 [23]	1	4, prognostic
Mitchell et al., 2000 [10]	1	4, prognostic
Ozaki et al., 1996 [24]	1	4, prognostic
Staals et al., 2006 [25]	0	4, prognostic
van Maldegem et al., 2014 [26]	1	4, prognostic

(e)

Author, year	Confounding measurement Defined and comparable treatment for patients	Baseline
Andreou et al., 2011 [15]	1, types of surgery mentioned	0
Angelini et al., 2012 [16]	1, types of surgery mentioned	0
Briccoli et al., 2002 [17]	1, types of surgery mentioned	1
Cho et al., 2011 [18]	1, types of surgery mentioned	0
de Camargo et al., 2010 [19]	1, types of surgery mentioned	0
Donati et al., 2010 [20]	1, types of surgery mentioned	1
Donati et al., 2005 [21]	1, types of surgery mentioned	0
Gitelis et al., 1981 [22]	1, types of surgery mentioned	1
Mavrogenis et al., 2013 [23]	1, types of surgery mentioned	0
Mitchell et al., 2000 [10]	1, types of surgery mentioned	1
Ozaki et al., 1996 [24]	1, types of surgery mentioned	1
Staals et al., 2006 [25]	1, types of surgery mentioned	0
van Maldegem et al., 2014 [26]	1, types of surgery mentioned	1

(f)

Author, year	Disclosure
Andreou et al., 2011 [15]	1
Angelini et al., 2012 [16]	1
Briccoli et al., 2002 [17]	0
Cho et al., 2011 [18]	1
de Camargo et al., 2010 [19]	1
Donati et al., 2010 [20]	1
Donati et al., 2005 [21]	1
Gitelis et al., 1981 [22]	0
Mavrogenis et al., 2013 [23]	1
Mitchell et al., 2000 [10]	1
Ozaki et al., 1996 [24]	0
Staals et al., 2006 [25]	0
van Maldegem et al., 2014 [26]	1

the high-grade chondrosarcoma and the dedifferentiated chondrosarcoma seem to be good candidates for future studies exploring better treatments options due to their poor prognosis.

Appendix

See Table 8.

Authors' Contribution

All authors have made substantial contributions to all of the following: (1) the conception and design of the study, or acquisition of data, or analysis and interpretation of data, (2) drafting the paper or revising it critically for important intellectual content, and (3) final approval of the version to be submitted.

References

[1] P. B. Hogendoorn, J. M. Bovee, and G. P. Nielsen, "Chondrosarcoma (grades I-III), including primary and secondary variants and periosteal chondrosarcoma," in *World Health Organization Classification of Tumours of Soft Tissue and Bone*, C. D. M. Fletcher, J. A. Bridge, P. C. W. Hogendoorn, and F. Mertens, Eds., vol. 5, p. 264, IARC, Lyon, France, 2013.

[2] H. D. Dorfman and B. Czerniak, "Bone cancers," *Cancer*, vol. 75, no. 1, supplement, pp. 203–210, 1995.

[3] T. A. Damron, W. G. Ward, and A. Stewart, "Osteosarcoma, chondrosarcoma, and Ewing's sarcoma: national cancer data base report," *Clinical Orthopaedics and Related Research*, vol. 459, pp. 40–47, 2007.

[4] H. L. Evans, A. G. Ayala, and M. M. Romsdahl, "Prognostic factors in chondrosarcoma of bone: a clinicopathologic analysis with emphasis on histologic grading," *Cancer*, vol. 40, no. 2, pp. 818–831, 1977.

[5] A. Y. Giuffrida, J. E. Burgueno, L. G. Koniaris, J. C. Gutierrez, R. Duncan, and S. P. Scully, "Chondrosarcoma in the United States (1973 to 2003): an analysis of 2890 cases from the SEER database," *The Journal of Bone & Joint Surgery—American Volume*, vol. 91, no. 5, pp. 1063–1072, 2009.

[6] A. R. Ahmed, T.-S. Tan, K. K. Unni, M. S. Collins, D. E. Wenger, and F. H. Sim, "Secondary chondrosarcoma in osteochondroma: report of 107 patients," *Clinical Orthopaedics and Related Research*, no. 411, pp. 193–206, 2003.

[7] A. Italiano, O. Mir, A. Cioffi et al., "Advanced chondrosarcomas: role of chemotherapy and survival," *Annals of Oncology*, vol. 24, no. 11, Article ID mdt374, pp. 2916–2922, 2013.

[8] F. Moussavi-Harami, A. Mollano, J. A. Martin et al., "Intrinsic radiation resistance in human chondrosarcoma cells," *Biochemical and Biophysical Research Communications*, vol. 346, no. 2, pp. 379–385, 2006.

[9] S. Kawaguchi, I. Weiss, P. P. Lin, W. W. Huh, and V. O. Lewis, "Radiation therapy is associated with fewer recurrences in mesenchymal chondrosarcoma," *Clinical Orthopaedics and Related Research*, vol. 472, no. 3, pp. 856–864, 2014.

[10] A. D. Mitchell, K. Ayoub, D. C. Mangham, R. J. Grimer, S. R. Carter, and R. M. Tillman, "Experience in the treatment of dedifferentiated chondrosarcoma," *The Journal of Bone and Joint Surgery—British Volume*, vol. 82, no. 1, pp. 55–61, 2000.

[11] E. L. Staals, P. Bacchini, M. Mercuri, and F. Bertoni, "Dedifferentiated chondrosarcomas arising in preexisting osteochondromas," *The Journal of Bone & Joint Surgery—American Volume*, vol. 89, no. 5, pp. 987–993, 2007.

[12] I. D. Dickey, P. S. Rose, B. Fuchs et al., "Dedifferentiated chondrosarcoma: the role of chemotherapy with updated outcomes," *The Journal of Bone & Joint Surgery—American Volume*, vol. 86, no. 11, pp. 2412–2418, 2004.

[13] R. J. Grimer, G. Gosheger, A. Taminiau et al., "Dedifferentiated chondrosarcoma: prognostic factors and outcome from a European group," *European Journal of Cancer*, vol. 43, no. 14, pp. 2060–2065, 2007.

[14] D. F. Stroup, J. A. Berlin, S. C. Morton et al., "Meta-analysis of observational studies in epidemiology: a proposal for reporting," *Journal of the American Medical Association*, vol. 283, no. 15, pp. 2008–2012, 2000.

[15] D. Andreou, S. Ruppin, S. Fehlberg, D. Pink, M. Werner, and P.-U. Tunn, "Survival and prognostic factors in chondrosarcoma: results in 115 patients with long-term follow-up," *Acta Orthopaedica*, vol. 82, no. 6, pp. 749–755, 2011.

[16] A. Angelini, G. Guerra, A. F. Mavrogenis, E. Pala, P. Picci, and P. Ruggieri, "Clinical outcome of central conventional chondrosarcoma," *Journal of Surgical Oncology*, vol. 106, no. 8, pp. 929–937, 2012.

[17] A. Briccoli, M. De Paolis, L. Campanacci et al., "Chondrosarcoma of the chest wall: a clinical analysis," *Surgery Today*, vol. 32, no. 4, pp. 291–296, 2002.

[18] W. H. Cho, W. S. Song, D.-G. Jeon et al., "Oncologic impact of the curettage of grade 2 central chondrosarcoma of the extremity," *Annals of Surgical Oncology*, vol. 18, no. 13, pp. 3755–3761, 2011.

[19] O. P. de Camargo, A. M. Baptista, M. J. Atanásio, and D. R. Waisberg, "Chondrosarcoma of bone: lessons from 46 operated cases in a single institution," *Clinical Orthopaedics and Related Research*, vol. 468, no. 11, pp. 2969–2975, 2010.

[20] D. Donati, S. Colangeli, M. Colangeli, C. Di Bella, and F. Bertoni, "Surgical treatment of grade I central chondrosarcoma," *Clinical Orthopaedics and Related Research*, vol. 468, no. 2, pp. 581–589, 2010.

[21] D. Donati, A. El Ghoneimy, F. Bertoni, C. Di Bella, and M. Mercuri, "Surgical treatment and outcome of conventional pelvic chondrosarcoma," *The Journal of Bone & Joint Surgery—British Volume*, vol. 87, no. 11, pp. 1527–1530, 2005.

[22] S. Gitelis, F. Bertoni, P. Picci, and M. Campanacci, "Chondrosarcoma of bone. The experience at the Istituto Ortopedico Rizzoli," *The Journal of Bone and Joint Surgery—American Volume*, vol. 63, no. 8, pp. 1248–1257, 1981.

[23] A. F. Mavrogenis, A. Angelini, G. Drago, B. Merlino, and P. Ruggieri, "Survival analysis of patients with chondrosarcomas of the pelvis," *Journal of Surgical Oncology*, vol. 108, no. 1, pp. 19–27, 2013.

[24] T. Ozaki, N. Lindner, A. Hillmann, R. Rödl, S. Blasius, and W. Winkelmann, "Influence of intralesional surgery on treatment outcome of chondrosarcoma," *Cancer*, vol. 77, no. 7, pp. 1292–1297, 1996.

[25] E. L. Staals, P. Bacchini, and F. Bertoni, "Dedifferentiated central chondrosarcoma," *Cancer*, vol. 106, no. 12, pp. 2682–2691, 2006.

[26] A. M. van Maldegem, H. Gelderblom, E. Palmerini et al., "Outcome of advanced, unresectable conventional central chondrosarcoma," *Cancer*, vol. 120, no. 20, pp. 3159–3164, 2014.

[27] D. Eefting, Y. M. Schrage, M. J. A. Geirnaerdt et al., "Assessment of interobserver variability and histologic parameters to improve reliability in classification and grading of central cartilaginous tumors," *American Journal of Surgical Pathology*, vol. 33, no. 1, pp. 50–57, 2009.

[28] F. Fiorenza, A. Abudu, R. J. Grimer et al., "Risk factors for survival and local control in chondrosarcoma of bone," *Journal of Bone and Joint Surgery—British Volume*, vol. 84, no. 1, pp. 93–99, 2002.

[29] F. Y. Lee, H. J. Mankin, G. Fondren et al., "Chondrosarcoma of bone: an assessment of outcome," *The Journal of Bone & Joint Surgery—American Volume*, vol. 81, no. 3, pp. 326–338, 1999.

6

Aberrant Hedgehog Signaling and Clinical Outcome in Osteosarcoma

Winnie W. Lo,[1,2] Dushanthi Pinnaduwage,[2] Nalan Gokgoz,[2] Jay S. Wunder,[2,3,4] and Irene L. Andrulis[1,2]

[1] *Department of Molecular Genetics, University of Toronto, ON, Canada M5S 1A8*
[2] *Lunenfeld-Tanenbaum Research Institute, Mount Sinai Hospital, 600 University Avenue, Toronto, ON, Canada M5G 1X5*
[3] *University Musculoskeletal Oncology Unit, Mount Sinai Hospital, Toronto, ON, Canada M5G 1X5*
[4] *Department of Surgery, University of Toronto, ON, Canada M5G 1L5*

Correspondence should be addressed to Irene L. Andrulis; andrulis@lunenfeld.ca

Academic Editor: Akira Kawai

Despite the importance of Hedgehog signaling in bone development, the relationship between Hedgehog pathway expression and osteosarcoma clinical characteristics and outcome has not been investigated. In this study of 43 high-grade human osteosarcoma samples, we detected high expression levels of the Hedgehog ligand gene, *IHH*, and target genes, *PTCH1* and *GLI1*, in most samples. Further analysis in tumors of patients with localized disease at diagnosis identified coexpression of *IHH* and *PTCH1* exclusively in large tumors. Higher levels of *IHH* were observed more frequently in males and patients with higher levels of *GLI1* were more responsive to chemotherapy. Subgroup analysis by tumor size and *IHH* expression indicated that the well-known association between survival and tumor size was further refined when *IHH* levels were taken into consideration.

1. Introduction

Osteosarcoma is the most common primary bone cancer and typically affects children and young adults. Although osteosarcoma is relatively rare, the disease afflicts individuals in the prime of their productive life and the clinical behaviour is highly aggressive [1]. Almost all osteosarcomas are high grade and have a poor prognosis, with 10–20% of patients having detectable metastases to the lungs at diagnosis. With the combination of surgery and chemotherapy, 50–60% of patients with a localized osteosarcoma will achieve long term disease-free survival, while the long term survival for patients with metastasis at diagnosis is only 20–30% [2–4].

The Hedgehog (Hh) signaling pathway is crucial for the regulation of proliferation and differentiation during embryonic development (for reviews, see [5, 6]), and its complexity is reflected from the involvement of multiple regulatory proteins at different cellular levels. In the absence of Hh ligands, patched homologue (PTCH1), a twelve-transmembrane protein, inhibits the localization of smoothened homologue (SMO), a seven-transmembrane protein, to cilia, thus preventing the activation of downstream signaling. Binding of the Hedgehog ligand to PTCH1 prevents PTCH1-mediated inhibition of SMO, thereby allowing SMO to localize to cilia and promote downstream activation of transcription factors encoded by the GLI zinc-finger family. In vertebrates, there are three Hedgehog-family ligands, sonic (SHH), Indian (IHH), and desert (DHH), and three GLI proteins. GLI1 and GLI2 act mainly as transcriptional activators, while GLI3 functions mainly as a repressor. Expression of GLI activators results in the induction of Hh target genes, including *GLI1* and *PTCH1*, that participate in positive and negative feedback mechanisms.

The Hh pathway is dormant in most adult tissues but becomes aberrantly activated in many cancers in a ligand-dependent or ligand-independent manner [6–12]. Both mechanisms are accompanied by overexpression of downstream Hh pathway targets, such as *PTCH1* and *GLI1*. Ligand-dependent Hh activation is caused by overproduction of the Hh ligand. Inactivating mutations of *PTCH1* are the most common causes of ligand-independent activation and are frequently found in basal cell carcinomas and medulloblastomas [13–16].

The origin of osteosarcoma is unknown, although these tumors tend to form in areas of rapid bone growth or turnover, such as in the long bones of developing adolescents. The long bones of the limbs and ribs develop by a process known as endochondral ossification. The Hedgehog pathway, more specifically the Indian Hedgehog (Ihh) ligand, regulates endochondral ossification by coordinating chondrocyte proliferation and differentiation and osteoblast differentiation [17]. Bone formation has been demonstrated to be reduced in $Ihh^{-/-}$ mice [18]. In addition, the IHH pathway has been found to be constitutively active in chondrosarcoma [19–22]; however, the role of Hedgehog signaling in osteosarcoma has not been investigated extensively. We previously identified Hedgehog dysregulation and signaling crosstalk between the tumor and the stroma in osteosarcoma cell lines and patient-derived xenograft models and demonstrated specific blockage of signaling exerted by Hedgehog inhibitors [23]. In the current study, we determined the levels of expression of Hedgehog pathway components (*IHH, SMO, PTCH1,* and *GLI1*) in primary human osteosarcoma specimens and examined the association with clinical characteristics and patient outcome.

2. Materials and Methods

2.1. Tumor Specimen. Tumors from forty-three patients with high-grade osteosarcoma of the extremity were evaluated in this study. Eleven were obtained from patients who had metastases at diagnosis, and the remaining thirty-two were from patients who had no metastasis at diagnosis. Of these thirty-two samples, twenty were from patients who remained free of systemic disease, and twelve were from those who developed metastasis after diagnosis. Patients were treated at 1 of 5 tertiary care medical institutions: Mount Sinai Hospital, Toronto, Canada; Vancouver Hospital and Health Sciences Center, Vancouver, Canada; Royal Orthopaedic Hospital, Birmingham, UK; Memorial Sloan Kettering Cancer Center, New York, NY, USA; and Mayo Clinic, Rochester, MN. Patients were seen in regular follow-up for at least 4 years from the time of diagnosis or until systemic recurrence, except for patients who presented with metastases at the time of diagnosis.

Patients were selected from a larger tumor bank cohort on the basis of availability of tumor material. Each eligible patient provided a signed consent form before study entry, as approved by each participating institution's Research Ethics Board. Tumor specimens were obtained at the time of surgical biopsy and were chosen by a pathologist with the aid of frozen histological analysis to ensure the presence of viable tumor without normal tissue contamination. Tumor samples were collected immediately after surgery, snap-frozen in liquid nitrogen, and stored at −70°C.

2.2. Differentiation of Human Osteoblastic Cells. Human bone marrow from two cancer-free individuals was obtained directly from surgical specimens. Bone marrow specimens were washed with Minimum Essential Medium Alpha with 300 U of Penicillin-Streptomycin for 15 to 20 minutes and repeated 2 times with fresh media with antibiotics. To differentiate cells of the osteoblastic lineage, tissues were cut into small pieces, placed in 10 cm plates, and cultured in fully supplemented media (α-MEM with 15% FBS, 100 U Penicillin-Streptomycin, 50 μg ascorbic acid/mL, 10 mM Na β-glycerophosphate, and 10^{-8} M dexamethasone) at 37°C undisturbed for 3 days. Fresh media were replaced every 3 to 4 days with regular monitoring under the microscope. Tissues were removed once spindle-shaped cells became visible for 1 week or more. Cells were cultured until confluent, at which time the cells were collected for RNA and DNA extraction or trypsinized and replated in 96-well plates. Differentiated cells were fixed and evaluated for the presence of alkaline phosphatase, using Naphthol AS phosphate (Sigma) coupled with Fast Blue BB Salt (Sigma), and for mineralization, using 0.2% Alizarin Red S solution (Sigma).

2.3. Quantitative Assessment of IHH, SMO, PTCH1, and GLI1 mRNA Expression by Real-Time RT-PCR. Frozen tumor samples were crushed in a Brinkman Retch crusher. Total RNA was extracted using TRIzol (Invitrogen). Total RNA was reverse transcribed to cDNA using M-MLV Reverse Transcriptase (Invitrogen). Gene-specific TaqMan Assay-on-Demand (Applied Biosystems) was used to quantify the transcript levels of *IHH, SMO, GLI1,* and *PTCH1* in the samples. The absolute standard curve method was used to determine the levels of expression by relating the PCR signal to a standard curve that was first constructed from RNA of known concentration. This curve was then used as a reference standard for extrapolating quantitative information for mRNA targets of unknown concentrations. cDNA from colon cancer cell lines SW1417 and RW948 was used as reference standards for *IHH* and *PTCH1*, respectively, because of the known high levels of expression found in these cells. cDNA from a pool of 11 tumor cell lines was used as a reference standard for *SMO* and *GLI1*. Asparagine synthetase (*AS*) was used as an endogenous control for expression normalization of *IHH*, while glyceraldehyde-3-phosphate dehydrogenase (*GAPDH*) was used for *SMO, GLI1,* and *PTCH1*. The housekeeping genes *AS* and *GAPDH* were chosen based on their similarity in the dynamic quantification range to the genes of interest.

2.4. Data Analysis and Statistical Tests. The expression values of *IHH, SMO, PTCH1,* and *GLI1* were log2 transformed to achieve approximate normality of the error distribution. Histograms showed that the log2 transformed expression data were still skewed to the left, with the exception of *GLI1* data. Therefore, the median was taken as a measure of center, and samples were assigned to the "High" or "Low" expression group, using the median as a cutoff. Descriptive baseline analyses by Chi-square test or Fisher's exact test or t-test compared frequency distribution of selected clinical and demographic variables among groups defined by expression status (high versus low expression, using the median as cutoff). Categoric or continuous coding schemes

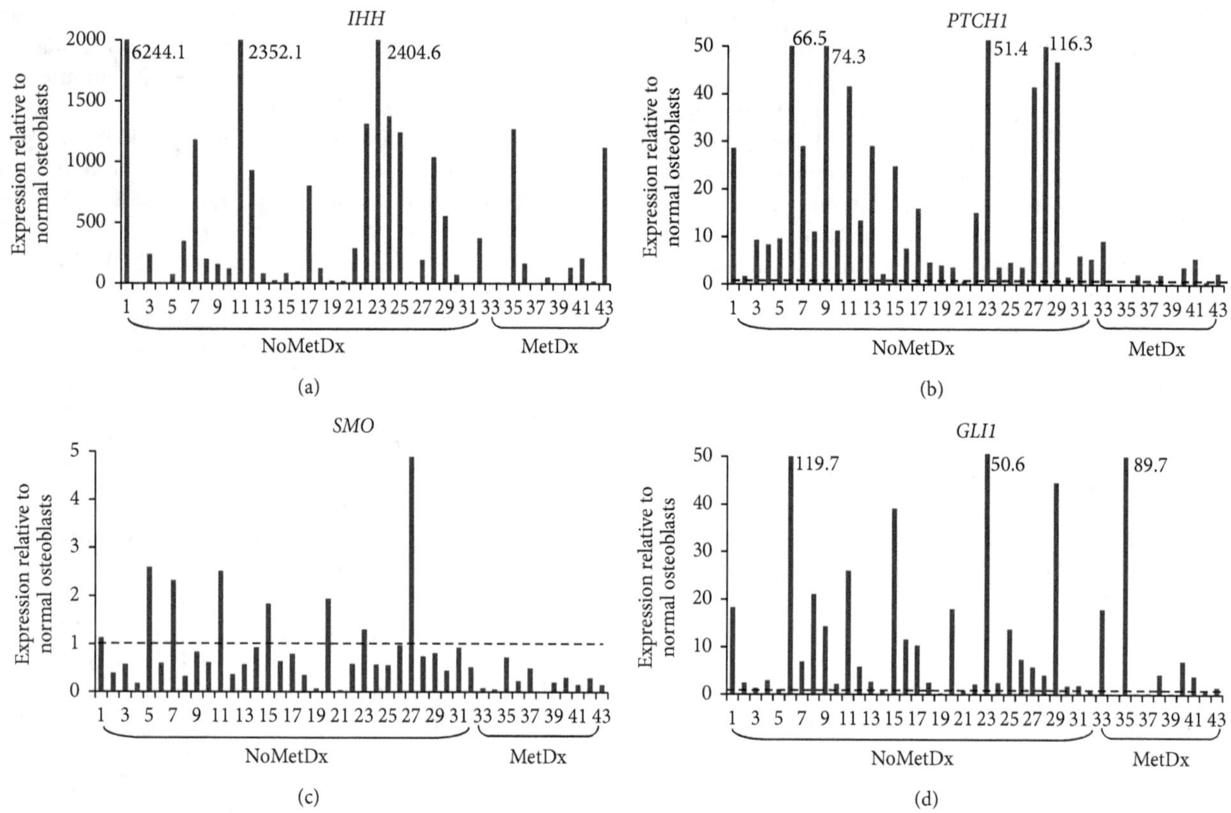

FIGURE 1: Expression levels of *IHH*, *PTCH1*, *SMO*, and *GLI1* in 43 osteosarcoma tumors relative to normal osteoblasts. Expression levels in tumors were normalized to the average level of 2 normal osteoblast samples and presented as fold change. Fold changes greater than the y-axis are labelled next to the representing bars (NoMetDx = no metastasis at diagnosis; MetDx = metastasis at diagnosis).

for the variables were selected before the analysis, on the basis of previous study or clinical convention. The selected clinical and demographic variables included were tumor size (>9 cm versus ≤9 cm), chemotherapy-induced necrosis (>90% versus ≤90%), gender (female versus male), and age at diagnosis (continuous). Univariate disease-free survival (metastasis-free, DFS) analysis according to subgroups of expression status was assessed by the Log-Rank test with Kaplan-Meier survival curves and by the Cox Proportional Hazards model. The Cox Proportional Hazards model was used for multivariate DFS analysis to assess the contribution of each gene in addition to traditional prognostic factors. Prognostic factors included in the analysis were clinical and demographic variables mentioned above. Relative risks (RR) for each gene and each factor were estimated by the hazard ratio in the Cox Proportional Hazards model [24, 25]. To further assess the contribution of each gene status in combination with tumor size (dichotomous), univariate and multivariate survival analyses were repeated considering the four groups of gene status and tumor size (high/>9 cm, low/>9 cm, high/≤9 cm, and low/≤9 cm) as the main variable in each model. Firth's correction was applied to the Cox modeling with sparse data [26].

All tests were two sided. Disease-free survival (DFS) was taken as the time between diagnosis and the confirmation of metastasis. Patient status on October 26, 2012, determined DFS times and censoring status using clinical follow-up data. We observed that 15 patients developed metastases out of 32. There were no lost to follow-ups. Excluding the patients with metastases, the minimum follow-up time was 60 months and the median follow-up time was 108 months. Patients with disease-free status were censored at the last follow-up date. A test with a P value <0.05 was considered statistically significant. All statistical analyses were performed using SAS 9.2 software (SAS Inc., Cary, NC, USA) with P values unadjusted for multiple testing and Kaplan-Meier plots generated using R statistical software version 2.3.0 (http://www.r-project.org/).

3. Results

3.1. High Levels of Expression of Indian Hedgehog Genes in Osteosarcoma Samples. Since there are currently no specific antibodies for endogenous human Hedgehog pathway genes that work reliably in immunohistochemistry assays [27], the transcript levels of *IHH*, *SMO*, *PTCH1*, and *GLI1* were determined using real-time RT-PCR in 43 human primary high-grade osteosarcoma samples and normalized to the levels detected in normal osteoblasts (Figure 1). Variable levels of *IHH*, *SMO*, *PTCH1*, and *GLI1* expression were observed in the osteosarcoma samples. The expression levels of *IHH* were low in the normal osteoblasts and most tumors exhibited higher *IHH* levels relative to the normal osteoblasts. Likewise,

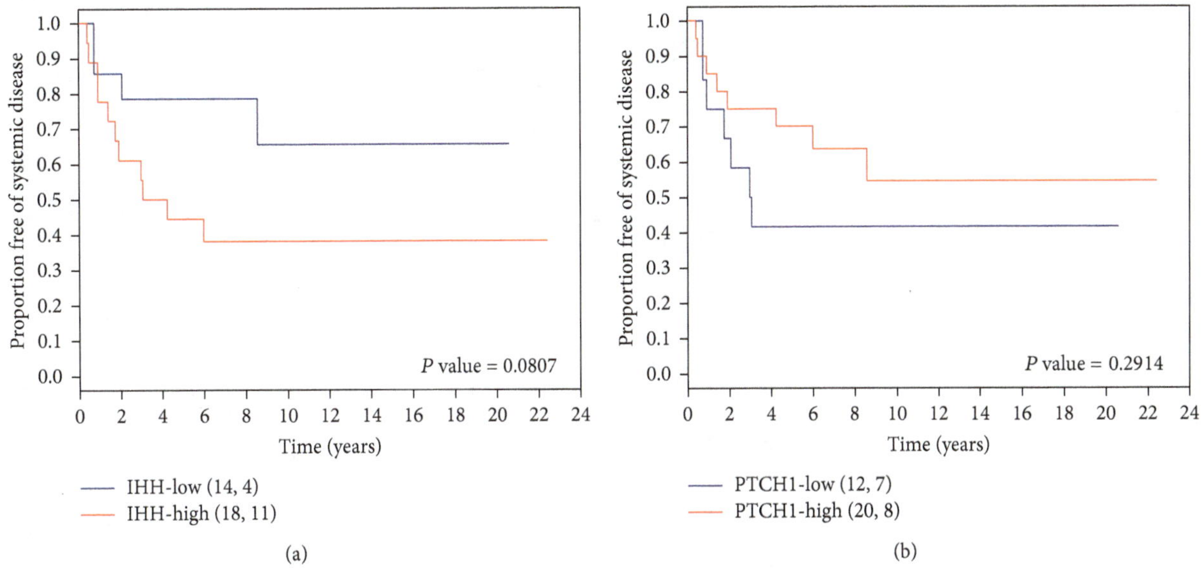

FIGURE 2: Kaplan-Meier survival curves of systemic disease-free survival for patients without metastasis at diagnosis with high and low levels of (a) *IHH* and (b) *PTCH1* gene expression. *P* value = Log-Rank *P* value.

the majority of the samples exhibited higher than normal levels of *PTCH1* and *GLI1*, with some exhibiting very high levels of expression. With the exception of a few specimens, *SMO* was not highly expressed in the tumors.

3.2. Coexpression of Indian Hedgehog Pathway Genes in Tumors from Subjects Presenting without Metastasis at Diagnosis. Thirty to forty percent of osteosarcoma patients who have localized disease at diagnosis will eventually develop metastasis. To determine whether expression of the Hh pathway genes is associated with patient clinical characteristics and outcome, expression was further analyzed in the subgroup ($n = 32$) presenting without metastasis at diagnosis (NoMetDx). In this subgroup, the mean age was 26.5 years (SD = 17.3, minimum = 7, and maximum = 73); 68.8% were male; 46.9% had small tumors; 46.9% had large tumors; 6.2% (2 tumors) had no tumor size data; 50% of tumors had low necrosis; 28.1% had high necrosis; 21.9% (7 tumors) had no necrosis data. Furthermore, as shown in Table 1, with the exception of the *IHH* and *SMO* pair, the levels of *IHH*, *PTCH1*, *SMO*, and *GLI1* are positively correlated with each other in tumors from patients presenting without metastasis at diagnosis. Interestingly, a strong coexpression of *IHH* with *PTCH1* was observed only in the subgroup of large tumors ($n = 15$), whereas expression of *PTCH1*, *SMO*, and *GLI1* was coexpressed in small tumors ($n = 15$) (Table 1).

3.3. Associations between Levels of Hedgehog Pathway Components with Clinical Characteristics in Tumors from Subjects Presenting without Metastasis at Diagnosis. Gene expression levels were not related to clinical characteristics (data not shown) with the exception of an association of *IHH* expression with gender and *GLI1* expression with chemotherapy-induced necrosis. Higher levels of *IHH* were observed more frequently in males than in females (72.7% versus 20.0%; $P = 0.0084$). Patients with higher levels of *GLI1* were more responsive to chemotherapy as demonstrated by higher percentage of chemotherapy-induced necrosis compared to patients with lower *GLI1* levels (53.3% versus 10.0%; $P = 0.0405$).

3.4. Effects of IHH and PTCH1 Levels on Survival. Log-Rank tests suggested a borderline significant survival difference for high versus low expression of *IHH* (P value = 0.0807). A trend toward a worse disease-free survival was observed for patients in the high *IHH* expression group compared to patients in the low *IHH* expression group from the univariate Cox Proportional Hazards model ($n = 32$) ($P = 0.0948$, hazard ratio (HR) = 2.66; confidence interval (CI): (0.84, 8.40)) (Table 2; Figure 2(a)). In contrast, a trend towards better survival was found in patients in the high *PTCH1* group ($P = 0.2927$; HR = 1.73; CI: (0.62, 4.79)) (Figure 2(b)). No survival differences were identified in the high and low expression groups of *GLI1* and *SMO* (data not shown).

In the multivariate Cox Proportional Hazards model ($n = 23$) (Table 2), to assess whether tumor size in combination with the expression of *IHH* correlates with poor survival, borderline significance ($P = 0.0970$; HR = 6.4; CI: (0.7, 57.9)) was achieved for high *IHH* expression group. No statistically significant difference for *PTCH1* was detected in the multivariate model (data not shown).

3.5. Ability of IHH Levels to Better Predict Outcome Groups in Patients with Different Tumor Sizes. Disease-free survival was compared among patients with tumors exhibiting different combinations of size (>9 cm or ≤9 cm) and gene expression status (high or low). Interestingly, we found that the group with both low *IHH* expression and smaller tumors remained disease-free and thus had the best disease-free survival compared to the other three groups (Log-Rank P value = 0.0496

Table 1: Pairwise Pearson correlation coefficients between log-transformed *IHH*, *PTCH1*, *GLI1*, and *SMO* expression in osteosarcoma samples and *P* value for test of the null hypothesis that correlation is zero.

	NoMetDx ($n = 32$)				Large tumors ($n = 15$)				Small tumors ($n = 15$)			
	log IHH	log PTCH1	log SMO	log GLI1	log IHH	log PTCH1	log SMO	log GLI1	log IHH	log PTCH1	log SMO	log GLI1
log IHH	1.00	**0.44 (P = 0.011)**	0.20 ($P = 0.27$)	**0.34 (P = 0.056)**	1.00	**0.56 (P = 0.029)**	0.05 ($P = 0.86$)	0.39 ($P = 0.15$)	1.00	0.37 ($P = 0.18$)	0.28 ($P = 0.31$)	0.34 ($P = 0.21$)
log PTCH1		1.00	**0.52 (P = 0.002)**	**0.61 (P = 0.0002)**		1.00	0.43 ($P = 0.11$)	0.44 ($P = 0.10$)		1.00	**0.53 (P = 0.04)**	**0.70 (P = 0.004)**
log SMO			1.00	**0.45 (P = 0.009)**			1.00	0.24 ($P = 0.40$)			1.00	**0.56 (P = 0.03)**
log GLI1				1.00				1.00				1.00

Bold text indicates statistically significant positive correlations.
Two patients have missing tumor size information.

TABLE 2: Results of DFS analysis by Cox Proportional Hazards model in no metastasis at diagnosis group (n = 32) for IHH.

Prognostic factor	Univariate				Multivariate*			
	HR	95% CI		P value	HR	95% CI		P value
IHH								
High versus low	2.66	0.84	8.40	0.0948	6.43	0.71	57.97	0.0970
Size								
>9 cm versus ≤9 cm	3.52	1.06	11.67	0.0394	22.81	2.22	234.02	0.0085
Necrosis								
>90% versus ≤90%	0.71	0.21	2.35	0.5716	0.53	0.13	2.14	0.3733
Gender								
Male versus female	1.39	0.44	4.36	0.5795	0.22	0.02	2.25	0.1998
Age (years)	1.02	0.99	1.05	0.1676	1.03	0.99	1.07	0.0965

*Firth correction to handle small sample sizes.

(for 4-group comparison)) (Figure 3(a)). Moreover, in the small tumor subgroup, patients with low *IHH* expression had better disease-free survival than those with high *IHH* expression (P value = 0.0163; HR = 3.19; CI: (0.58, 17.44)). These results suggest that *IHH* levels can better predict outcome in patients with small tumors. We also found that the group with both low *PTCH1* expression and larger tumors tended to have poorer disease-free survival compared to the other three groups (Log-Rank P value = 0.0649 (for 4-group comparison)) (Figure 3(b)).

Furthermore, a multivariate model for *IHH* in combination with size (Table 3) shows that *IHH* in combination with size can identify a higher risk group than *IHH* or size alone. Patients in the large tumor and high *IHH* group are at much higher risk compared to those in the smaller tumor and low *IHH* group (low risk group) (P = 0.0378; HR = 52.30; CI: 3.27, 10906.34). We also noticed that when compared to the low risk group, patients in the large tumor and low *IHH* group are at a trend of lower risk than those in the large tumor and high *IHH* group (HR: 17.62 versus 52.3) (Table 3). Furthermore, patients in the small tumor and high *IHH* group are at a trend of higher risk than those in the small tumor and low *IHH* group (low risk group) (P = 0.2831; HR = 6.31; CI: 0.47, 934.10).

4. Discussion

While previous expression studies have suggested the involvement of dysregulated Hedgehog signaling in osteosarcoma, most of them were carried out in osteosarcoma cell lines with the inclusion of limited numbers of clinical samples [28–32]. The transcript levels of Hedgehog pathway genes have been associated with outcome in many cancer types [33, 34], but this is the first report to show the relationship between Hedgehog pathway gene expression and osteosarcoma outcome.

In this study of 43 osteosarcoma samples, we detected high expression levels of the Hedgehog ligand gene, *IHH*, and IHH target genes, *PTCH1* and *GLI1*, in most osteosarcoma samples. We found that tumors from patients presenting without metastasis at diagnosis exhibited pairwise coexpression of *IHH*, *PTCH1*, *SMO*, and *GLI1* with the exception of the pair of *IHH* and *SMO*. In addition, a correlation of expression of the ligand gene, *IHH*, and the target gene, *PTCH1*, found exclusively in large tumors, is indicative of ligand-dependent activation. In contrast, levels of *SMO*, *PTCH1*, and *GLI1* were found to be positively correlated with each other in small tumors, suggesting ligand-independent activation. These data suggest that both ligand-dependent and ligand-independent mechanisms may lead to Hedgehog activation in osteosarcoma but having ligand-dependent activation due to high levels of *IHH* may lead to larger tumor size, which is a well-known prognostic factor for osteosarcoma. Indeed, we found that patients with higher levels of *IHH* tended to exhibit a worse outcome compared to those with lower levels of expression (HR = 2.66; CI: (0.84, 8.40)). Interestingly, even though the levels of *IHH* and *PTCH1* are coexpressed, patients with higher levels of *PTCH1* (HR = 1.73; CI: (0.62, 4.79)) tended to have a better outcome.

In this exploratory study, we did not detect statistically significant differences with our limited sample size; however, HR values as large as 8.4 and 4.8 cannot be ignored. Furthermore, the opposite effects of high levels of *IHH* and *PTCH1* on survival are in line with the biological roles of IHH and PTCH1 in the pathway. The PTCH1 receptor negatively regulates signaling in the absence of Hh ligands by preventing the SMO receptor from activating downstream signaling. The Hh ligands positively regulate signaling by binding to PTCH1 and relieving its inhibition of SMO, thereby allowing SMO to induce downstream signaling.

Nonetheless, even with our limited sample size, we found that the well-known association between survival and tumor size was further refined when *IHH* levels were taken into consideration. Patients with lower *IHH* expression and small tumors remained disease-free and had better survival compared to patients with higher *IHH* expression and small tumors which demonstrated similar survival to those with large tumors. Similarly in the large tumor group, patients with lower *IHH* tumors had better survival than those with higher *IHH* expression. Since the Hedgehog pathway controls the proliferation of chondrocytes during bone development [17], an interaction between IHH and proliferation, which presumably contribute to tumor size, likely exists. However, the available sample size limits the precision of the results

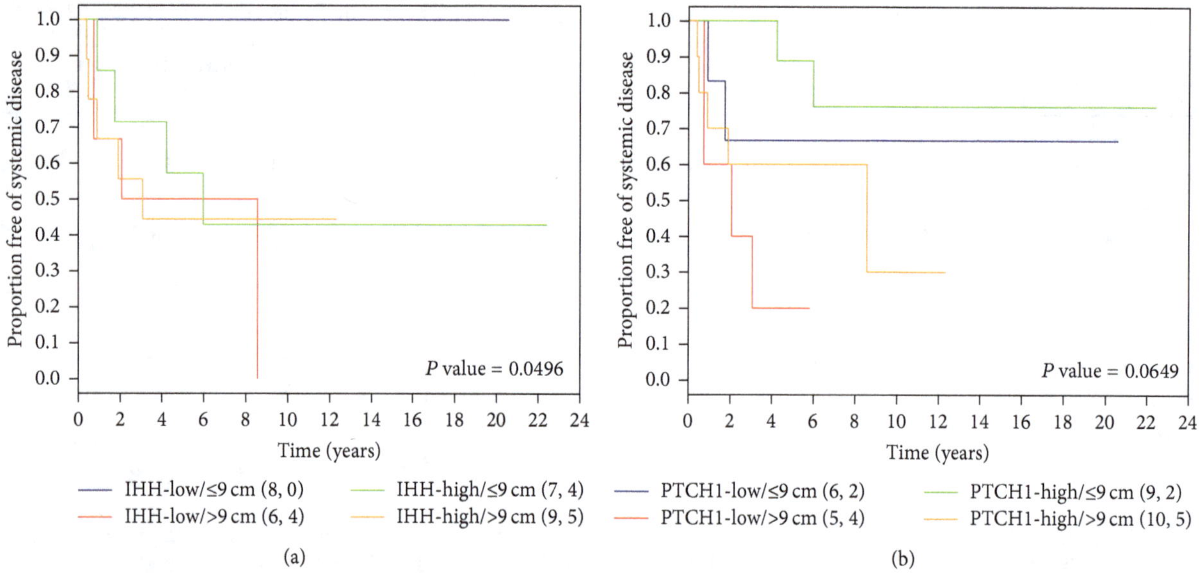

FIGURE 3: Kaplan-Meier survival curves of systemic disease-free survival for patients without metastasis at diagnosis in combination with tumor size and (a) *IHH* or (b) *PTCH1* expression status. *P* value = Log-Rank *P* value.

TABLE 3: Results of DFS analysis by Cox Proportional Hazards model in no metastasis at diagnosis group ($n = 32$) for IHH in combination with size.

Prognostic factor	Univariate HR	Univariate 95% CI		Univariate *P* value	Multivariate* HR	Multivariate* 95% CI		Multivariate* *P* value
IHH/size								
IHH+/≤9 cm versus IHH−/≤9 cm	12.78	1.36	1694.88	0.1128*	6.31	0.47	934.10	0.2831
IHH+/>9 cm versus IHH−/≤9 cm	17.10	1.91	2253.96	0.0754*	52.30	3.27	10906.34	0.0378
IHH−/>9 cm versus IHH−/≤9 cm	20.48	2.14	2727.27	0.0611*	17.62	1.48	2614.55	0.0907
Necrosis								
>90% versus ≤90%	0.71	0.21	2.35	0.5716	0.62	0.16	2.39	0.5027
Gender								
Male versus female	1.39	0.44	4.36	0.5795	0.33	0.03	2.10	0.2700
Age (years)	1.02	0.99	1.05	0.1676	1.03	0.99	1.07	0.2034

*Firth correction to handle small sample sizes.
IHH+: high IHH levels.
IHH−: low IHH levels.

obtained (see wide confidence intervals in Table 3); therefore, it will be important to replicate the results in a larger study.

Our descriptive analyses demonstrated that higher levels of *IHH* were more frequently observed in males than in females. The incidence of osteosarcoma is more frequent in males than females [35], which is also found in our cohort (68.8% male versus 31.2% female). In addition, in our cohorts, males tend to have larger tumors than females (80% versus 20%; $P = 0.12$). High levels of *IHH* found in males may suggest that ligand-dependent Hedgehog activation may contribute to abnormal cell proliferation and thus larger tumors and higher incidence of osteosarcoma in males. A positive correlation was identified between *GLI1* expression and chemotherapy-induced necrosis. This could suggest that although GLI1 is a positive regulator of the pathway, tumors with higher levels of *GLI1* may be more responsive to therapy. Future studies that include larger number of osteosarcoma cases will be required to further examine the relationship between the Hedgehog pathway genes and clinical characteristics and outcome.

The observation that *IHH* expression is predictive of outcome in combination with tumor size suggests that *IHH* expression may be used to improve the prognostic value of tumor size and possibly improve the stratification of patients prior to starting chemotherapy. For instance, patients determined to be at lower risk of developing metastasis due to both small tumor size and low *IHH* expression may require less prolonged or less intensive chemotherapy treatment to prevent development of metastatic disease. In addition, with the development of inhibitors that target aberrant Hh signaling, it will be important to determine whether our findings can be replicated in larger study cohorts to identify patients with tumors exhibiting constitutive ligand-dependent signaling that may also be responsive to Hedgehog inhibitors.

Acknowledgments

The authors thank their colleagues in the Department of Pathology and Laboratory Medicine, Mount Sinai Hospital, and Drs. Beauchamp (Vancouver General Hospital, Vancouver, BC, Canada), Grimer (Royal Orthopaedic Hospital, Birmingham, England), Healey (Memorial Sloan Kettering Cancer Center, New York, NY, USA), and Rock (Mayo Clinic, Rochester, MN, USA) for providing osteosarcoma specimens. They also thank Robert Parkes for statistical assistance, Dr. Sukhu, Mount Sinai Hospital, for technical and reagent support, and Dr. Bull, Lunenfeld-Tanenbaum Research Institute and Prosserman Centre for Health Research, for the comments on the paper. This work was supported by grants to Irene L. Andrulis and Jay S. Wunder from Ontario Cancer Research Network, the Canadian Institutes of Health Research, Ontario Research Fund, and the Canadian Foundation for Innovation and funding from Sydney Cooper Program for the Prevention of Cancer Progression. Winnie W. Lo received support from the Canadian Institutes of Health Research Collaborative Training Program in Molecular Medicine.

References

[1] J. Levesque, R. Marx, R. S. Bell, J. S. Winder, R. A. Kandel, and L. M. White, *A Clinical Guide to Primary Bone Tumors*, Williams & Wilkins, Philadelphia, Pa, USA, 1998.

[2] M. P. Link, A. M. Goorin, and A. W. Miser, "The effect of adjuvant chemotherapy on relapse-free survival in patients with osteosarcoma of the extremity," *The New England Journal of Medicine*, vol. 314, no. 25, pp. 1600–1606, 1986.

[3] F. Eilber, A. Giuliano, and J. Eckhardt, "Adjuvant chemotherapy for osteosarcoma: a randomized prospective trial," *Journal of Clinical Oncology*, vol. 5, no. 1, pp. 21–26, 1987.

[4] S. S. Bielack, B. Kempf-Bielack, G. Delling et al., "Prognostic factors in high-grade osteosarcoma of the extremities or trunk: an analysis of 1,702 patients treated on neoadjuvant cooperative osteosarcoma study group protocols," *Journal of Clinical Oncology*, vol. 20, no. 3, pp. 776–790, 2002.

[5] L. L. Rubin and F. J. de Sauvage, "Targeting the Hedgehog pathway in cancer," *Nature Reviews Drug Discovery*, vol. 5, no. 12, pp. 1026–1033, 2006.

[6] J. Jiang and C. C. Hui, "Hedgehog signaling in development and cancer," *Developmental Cell*, vol. 15, no. 6, pp. 801–812, 2008.

[7] D. M. Berman, S. S. Karhadkar, A. Maitra et al., "Widespread requirement for Hedgehog ligand stimulation in growth of digestive tract tumours," *Nature*, vol. 425, no. 6960, pp. 846–851, 2003.

[8] C. Dierks, J. Grbic, K. Zirlik et al., "Essential role of stromally induced Hedgehog signaling in B-cell malignancies," *Nature Medicine*, vol. 13, no. 8, pp. 944–951, 2007.

[9] G. V. Hegde, K. J. Peterson, K. Emanuel et al., "Hedgehog-induced survival of B-cell chronic lymphocytic leukemia cells in a stromal cell microenvironment: a potential new therapeutic target," *Molecular Cancer Research*, vol. 6, no. 12, pp. 1928–1936, 2008.

[10] S. S. Karhadkar, G. S. Bova, N. Abdallah et al., "Hedgehog signalling in prostate regeneration, neoplasia and metastasis," *Nature*, vol. 431, no. 7009, pp. 707–712, 2004.

[11] S. P. Thayer, M. P. Di Magliano, P. W. Heiser et al., "Hedgehog is an early and late mediator of pancreatic cancer tumorigenesis," *Nature*, vol. 425, no. 6960, pp. 851–856, 2003.

[12] R. L. Yauch, S. E. Gould, S. J. Scales et al., "A paracrine requirement for Hedgehog signalling in cancer," *Nature*, vol. 455, no. 7211, pp. 406–410, 2008.

[13] N. Dahmane, J. Lee, P. Robins, P. Heller, and A. R. Altaba, "Activation of the transcription factor Gli1 and the sonic Hedgehog signalling pathway in skin tumours," *Nature*, vol. 389, no. 6653, pp. 876–881, 1997.

[14] A. B. Undén, P. G. Zaphiropoulos, K. Bruce, R. Toftgård, and M. Ståhle-Bäckdahl, "Human patched (PTCH) mRNA is overexpressed consistently in tumor cells of both familial and sporadic basal cell carcinoma," *Cancer Research*, vol. 57, no. 12, pp. 2336–2340, 1997.

[15] Y. Lee, H. L. Miller, P. Jensen et al., "A molecular fingerprint for medulloblastoma," *Cancer Research*, vol. 63, no. 17, pp. 5428–5437, 2003.

[16] C. Raffel, R. B. Jenkins, L. Frederick et al., "Sporadic medulloblastomas contain PTCH mutations," *Cancer Research*, vol. 57, no. 5, pp. 842–845, 1997.

[17] H. M. Kronenberg, "Developmental regulation of the growth plate," *Nature*, vol. 423, no. 6937, pp. 332–336, 2003.

[18] B. St-Jacques, M. Hammerschmidt, and A. P. McMahon, "Indian Hedgehog signaling regulates proliferation and differentiation of chondrocytes and is essential for bone formation," *Genes and Development*, vol. 13, no. 16, pp. 2072–2086, 1999.

[19] L. Ho, A. Stojanovski, H. Whetstone et al., "Gli2 and p53 cooperate to regulate IGFBP-3-mediated chondrocyte apoptosis in the progression from benign to malignant cartilage tumors," *Cancer Cell*, vol. 16, no. 2, pp. 126–136, 2009.

[20] S. Hopyan, N. Gokgoz, R. Poon et al., "A mutant PTH/PTHrP type I receptor in enchondromatosis," *Nature Genetics*, vol. 30, no. 3, pp. 306–310, 2002.

[21] T. D. Tiet and B. A. Alman, "Developmental pathways in musculoskeletal neoplasia: involvement of the Indian Hedgehog-parathyroid hormone-related protein pathway," *Pediatric Research*, vol. 53, no. 4, pp. 539–543, 2003.

[22] T. D. Tiet, S. Hopyan, P. Nadesan et al., "Constitutive Hedgehog signaling in chondrosarcoma up-regulates tumor cell proliferation," *The American Journal of Pathology*, vol. 168, no. 1, pp. 321–330, 2006.

[23] W. W. Lo, J. S. Wunder, B. C. Dickson et al., "Involvement and targeted intervention of dysregulated Hedgehog signaling in osteosarcoma," *Cancer*, vol. 120, no. 4, pp. 537–547, 2014.

[24] D. R. Cox and D. Oakes, *Analysis of Survival Data*, Chapman & Hall/CRC, New York, NY, USA, 1984.

[25] D. R. Cox, "Regression models and life-tables," *Journal of the Royal Statistical Society B: Methodological*, vol. 34, no. 2, pp. 187–220, 1972.

[26] G. Heinze and M. Schemper, "A solution to the problem of monotone likelihood in Cox regression," *Biometrics*, vol. 57, no. 1, pp. 114–119, 2001.

[27] J. M. Y. Ng and T. Curran, "The Hedgehog's tale: developing strategies for targeting cancer," *Nature Reviews Cancer*, vol. 11, no. 7, pp. 493–501, 2011.

[28] J. Warzecha, S. Göttig, K. U. Chow et al., "Inhibition of osteosarcoma cell proliferation by the Hedgehog-inhibitor cyclopamine," *Journal of Chemotherapy*, vol. 19, no. 5, pp. 554–561, 2007.

[29] M. Hirotsu, T. Setoguchi, H. Sasaki et al., "Smoothened as a new therapeutic target for human osteosarcoma," *Molecular Cancer*, vol. 9, article 5, 2010.

[30] H. Nagao, K. Ijiri, M. Hirotsu et al., "Role of GLI2 in the growth of human osteosarcoma," *Journal of Pathology*, vol. 224, no. 2, pp. 169–179, 2011.

[31] W. Yang, X. Liu, E. Choy, H. Mankin, F. J. Hornicek, and Z. Duan, "Targeting Hedgehog-GLI-2 pathway in osteosarcoma," *Journal of Orthopaedic Research*, vol. 31, no. 3, pp. 502–509, 2013.

[32] A. B. Mohseny, Y. Cai, M. Kuijjer et al., "The activities of Smad and Gli mediated signalling pathways in high-grade conventional osteosarcoma," *European Journal of Cancer*, vol. 48, no. 18, pp. 3429–3438, 2012.

[33] Y. Mori, T. Okumura, S. Tsunoda, Y. Sakai, and Y. Shimada, "Gli-1 expression is associated with lymph node metastasis and tumor progression in esophageal squamous cell carcinoma," *Oncology*, vol. 70, no. 5, pp. 378–389, 2007.

[34] S. You, J. Zhou, S. Chen et al., "PTCH1, a receptor of Hedgehog signaling pathway, is correlated with metastatic potential of colorectal cancer," *Upsala Journal of Medical Sciences*, vol. 115, no. 3, pp. 169–175, 2010.

[35] C. D. M. Fletcher, K. K. Unni, and F. Mertens, *Pathology and Genetics of Tumours of Soft Tissue and Bone*, vol. 4, World Health Organization, Lyon, France, 2002.

7

Intercalary Reconstruction after Wide Resection of Malignant Bone Tumors of the Lower Extremity using a Composite Graft with a Devitalized Autograft and a Vascularized Fibula

Koichi Ogura,[1] Shimpei Miyamoto,[2] Minoru Sakuraba,[2] Tomohiro Fujiwara,[1] Hirokazu Chuman,[1] and Akira Kawai[1]

[1] *Department of Musculoskeletal Oncology, National Cancer Center Hospital, 5-1-1 Tsukiji, Chuo-ku, Tokyo 104-0045, Japan*
[2] *Department of Plastic and Reconstruction Surgery, National Cancer Center Hospital, 5-1-1 Tsukiji, Chuo-ku, Tokyo 104-0045, Japan*

Correspondence should be addressed to Akira Kawai; akawai@ncc.go.jp

Academic Editor: Valerae O. Lewis

Introduction. Although several intercalary reconstructions after resection of a lower extremity malignant bone tumor are reported, there are no optimal methods which can provide a long-term reconstruction with fewest complications. We present the outcome of reconstruction using a devitalized autograft and a vascularized fibula graft composite. *Materials and Methods.* We conducted a retrospective review of 11 patients (7 males, 4 females; median age 27 years) undergoing reconstruction using a devitalized autograft (pasteurization (n = 6), deep freezing (n = 5)) and a vascularized fibula graft composite for lower extremity malignant bone tumors (femur (n = 10), tibia (n = 1)). *Results.* The mean period required for callus formation and bone union was 4.4 months and 9.9 months, respectively. Four postoperative complications occurred in 3 patients: 2 infections (1 pasteurized autograft, 1 frozen autograft) and 1 fracture and 1 implant failure (both in pasteurized autografts). Graft removal was required in 2 patients with infections. The mean MSTS score was 81% at last follow-up. *Conclusions.* Although some complications were noted in early cases involving a pasteurized autograft, our novel method involving a combination of a frozen autograft with a vascularized fibula graft and rigid fixation with a locking plate may offer better outcomes than previously reported allografts or devitalized autografts.

1. Introduction

Limb salvage surgery has replaced amputation for malignant musculoskeletal tumors. Most bone sarcomas occur in the metaphyseal portion of the bone and typical resection involves the whole proximal or distal part of the bone. Therefore, in most cases, the resected segment of bone is replaced by a prosthesis, which provides satisfactory results quickly after surgery. However, when the tumor involves the diaphyseal portion of the bone, an intercalary reconstruction method is required, and this has not been standardized. Intercalary allografts, which is the most widely accepted reconstruction method, are associated with high incidences of nonunion (12–57%), fracture (17–30%), and infection (10–15%). [1–6]. In addition, single use of devitalized autograft such as frozen autograft or pasteurized autograft was also associated with nonunion (20% and 7%, resp.) [7, 8]. Although a segmental prosthesis can provide immediate stability and good short-term postoperative function, it is associated with long-term problems including implant wear, breakage, and loosening with the 10-year implant survival of 63% [9]. Therefore there is an urgent need to develop an optimal reconstruction method for this type of condition.

Vascularized fibula grafts have been reported to yield favorable outcomes in terms of bone union in cases of trauma, infection, or musculoskeletal tumors [10–15]. Recently, several investigators have reported an intercalary reconstruction technique using a composite graft comprising a free vascularized fibula graft with an allograft, or an extracorporeally irradiated or pasteurized autograft, in order to overcome shortcomings such as nonunion, infection, and fracture resulting from deterioration of mechanical strength [10, 16–18].

The aim of the present study was to analyze the clinical and functional outcomes of intercalary reconstruction using a composite graft comprising a devitalized autograft and a vascularized fibula graft after wide resection of malignant bone tumor of the lower extremity and compare the results with those reported previously for other reconstruction methods. In addition, we investigated the applicability of a novel surgical technique using a frozen autograft and a vascularized fibula graft composite and compared it with pasteurized autograft group.

2. Patients and Methods

We conducted a retrospective review of 11 consecutive patients who underwent intercalary bone defect reconstruction using a devitalized autograft combined with a vascularized fibula graft composite between 2007 and 2011. Their clinical data, treatment modalities, and outcome were reviewed retrospectively with reference to the medical records. The mean follow-up period was 68 months (range, 25–131 months).

The following data were examined: demographic data (patient age at operation, gender, tumor site, and histologic diagnosis), surgical details (length of bone defect, methods of devitalization, operation time, total blood loss, and reconstruction details), adjuvant therapy (chemotherapy and radiotherapy), postoperative complications (nonunion, fracture, implant failure, or infection), the time required for bone union, the findings of bone scintigraphy, oncologic outcomes, and functional outcomes.

Wide resection of the tumor was performed in all cases, and the bone defect was reconstructed with a devitalized autograft and a vascularized fibula graft placed into the medullary canal of the autograft. The composite graft was rigidly fixed with a plate and screws (Figure 1). The pasteurized or frozen autografts were prepared as described previously [7, 19, 20]. Bone union was defined as the presence of fusion between the host bone and the devitalized autograft at both ends and full weight-bearing without pain. Bone scintigraphy was performed soon after surgery (within 2 months) and late after surgery (more than 6 months) in selected cases. Functional outcome of the reconstructed limb was assessed using the Musculoskeletal Tumor Society (MSTS) scoring system [21], which included pain, function, emotional acceptance, use of any external support, walking ability, and gait alteration.

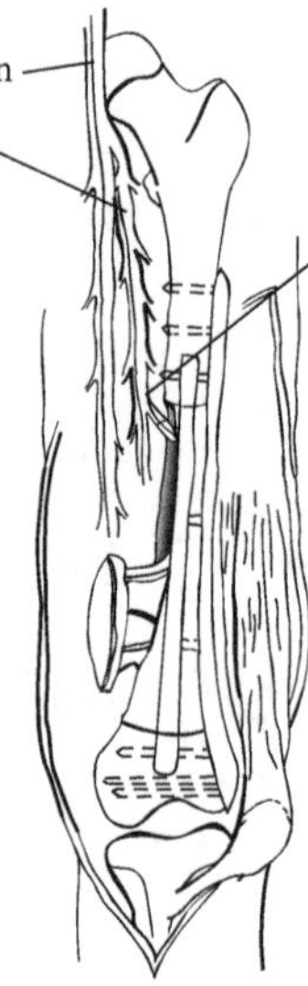

FIGURE 1: Illustration showing reconstruction of a femur diaphysis using a composite graft with a devitalized autograft and a vascularized fibula graft.

3. Results

Patient demographics and treatment data are summarized in Tables 1 and 2. There were 7 males and 4 females with a mean age of 29 years (range, 11–63 years). No patients had preoperative comorbidities that might have influenced the bone healing time. The histological diagnoses were osteosarcoma ($n = 6$), bone involving soft tissue sarcoma ($n = 3$), Ewing's sarcoma ($n = 1$), and chondrosarcoma ($n = 1$). The locations of the resected bone were the femur ($n = 10$) and tibia ($n = 1$). Adjuvant chemotherapy and radiotherapy were performed in 8 and 1 patients, respectively. The mean length of the bone defect was 19 cm (range, 10–22 cm). The methods of devitalization included pasteurization ($n = 6$) and deep freezing ($n = 5$). Free bone grafting from iliac crest at the junction was performed in 8 patients. The fixation method included a plate in 5 patients, a locking plate in 5 patients, and only screws in 1 patient. The total operation time ranged from 430 to 910 minutes (mean, 698 minutes) and mean blood loss was 1,086 mL (range, 354–2,162 mL). Although the mean operation time was shorter and mean blood loss was less in the frozen autograft group (645 minutes, 841 mL) than in the pasteurized autograft group (710 minutes, 1,291 mL), the differences were not statistically significant ($P = 0.511$ and 0.319, resp.).

Treatment results are summarized in Table 3. Bone union was achieved in 10 patients (91%). In case 5, deep infection occurred and resulted in graft removal to cure the infection at 2 months after surgery. Therefore, bone union was not evaluable. The mean period required for callus formation and bone union was 4.4 months (range, 3–11 months) and 9.9 months (range, 4–14 months), respectively. Time required for bone union was significantly shorter in the frozen autograft group (7.0 months) than in the pasteurized autograft group (11.2 months) (Student's t-test, $P = 0.042$). Although no statistical significance was noted, the mean period until bone union in patients who underwent free bone grafting was shorter than in those who did not (8.9 months versus 11.0 months; Student's t-test, $P = 0.320$). Hypertrophy of the vascularized fibula and subsequent bone integration into the devitalized autograft was seen in only 2 patients at 21 months (Patient 4) and 39 months (Patient 7) after surgery, respectively. Bone scintigraphy in the early phase was performed in 7 patients and all of them showed increased uptake in the fibula graft and no uptake in the devitalized autograft. Among these patients, 3 underwent bone scintigraphy in the late phase; 2 patients showed increased uptake in both the fibula graft and the devitalized autograft, and 1 patient showed increased

TABLE 1: Patient demographics and adjuvant therapy data.

Number	Age	Gender	Histologic diagnosis	Tumor site	Tumor size (cm)	Chemotherapy	Radiotherapy
1	20	M	Osteosarcoma	Femur	16	Preoperative/postoperative	None
2	11	F	Osteosarcoma	Femur	16	Preoperative/postoperative	None
3	49	M	Bone involving recurrent myxoid liposarcoma	Femur	14	Preoperative/postoperative	Preoperative
4	27	M	Fibrosarcoma (grade 2)	Femur	13	None	None
5	37	M	Ewing's sarcoma	Femur	13	Preoperative/postoperative	None
6	29	F	Parosteal osteosarcoma	Femur	6	None	None
7	16	F	Osteosarcoma	Femur	14	Preoperative/postoperative	None
8	36	M	Osteosarcoma	Tibia	10	Preoperative/postoperative	None
9	11	F	Osteosarcoma	Femur	16	Preoperative/postoperative	None
10	63	M	Bone involving myxofibrosarcoma	Femur	12	Preoperative	None
11	19	M	Chondrosarcoma (grade 2)	Femur	16	None	None

TABLE 2: Surgical details of the patients.

Number	Length of bone defect (cm)	Method of devitalization	Free bone graft at the junction	Fixation	Operation time (min)	Blood loss (mL)
1	22	Pasteurization	Yes	Plate	630	1615
2	22	Pasteurization	Yes	Plate	540	574
3	20	Pasteurization	Yes	Plate	670	713
4	18	Pasteurization	No	Plate	910	1900
5	20	Pasteurization	No	Plate	660	823
6	10	Pasteurization	No	Screw	848	2121
7	20	Deep freezing	Yes	Locking plate	430	634
8	16	Deep freezing	Yes	Locking plate	854	604
9	22	Deep freezing	Yes	Locking plate	684	354
10	18	Deep freezing	Yes	Locking plate	750	450
11	22	Deep freezing	Yes	Locking plate	506	2162

uptake in the fibula graft and no uptake in the devitalized autograft.

Four postoperative complications occurred in 3 patients: 2 infections (1 pasteurized autograft, 1 frozen autograft) and 1 fracture at the proximal host-graft junction and 1 implant failure (screw breakage) (both in pasteurized autografts). No significant difference in the postoperative complication rate was seen between the pasteurized and frozen autograft groups (Fisher's exact test, $P = 0.621$). Graft removal was required in 2 patients with infections. Two patients suffered from local recurrence out of the pasteurized autograft, which necessitated amputation. Oncological outcomes for the patients overall were CDF in 5, NED in 1, AWD in 3, and DOD in 2 patients at the time of last follow-up. The mean MSTS score was 81% (range, 43–100%). The mean MSTS score was relatively higher in the frozen autograft group (85%) than in the pasteurized autograft group (70%), but the difference was not statistically significant (Student's t-test, $P = 0.211$).

Representative Case (Patient 7). The patient was a 16-year-old female with osteosarcoma of the left distal femur (Figure 2(a)). She underwent neoadjuvant chemotherapy with adriamycin, cisplatin, and ifosfamide, and reduction in the size of the tumor was noted (Figures 2(b) and 2(c)). Intercalary wide resection was performed and the length of the bone defect was 20 cm. This was reconstructed using a composite graft comprising a frozen autograft and a vascularized fibula placed into the medullary canal of the frozen autograft. Microvascular anastomoses were performed and the composite graft was finally fixed to the host bone with a locking plate and screws (Figures 3(a) and 3(b)). Postoperatively, adjuvant chemotherapy with the same agents was performed. There were no postoperative complications or local recurrence. At 9 months after surgery, bone union at the host-devitalized autograft junction and host-fibula graft junction was achieved (Figure 3(c)). Hypertrophy of the inlaid fibula and subsequent integration with the frozen autograft became evident on CT at 39 months after surgery (Figure 4). The patient was able to walk without a walking aid and enjoy mild sports activity at 75 months after surgery. The MSTS score at the time of last follow-up was 100%.

4. Discussion

Reconstruction options following intercalary resection of lower extremity malignancy have included the use of massive allografts [22–24], autoclaved autografts [25], pasteurized

TABLE 3: Treatment, oncologic, and functional outcomes.

Number	Time to callus formation (months)	Time to bone union (months)	Postoperative complications	Additional surgery for complications	Graft removal or amputation	Local recurrence	Metastasis	Oncologic outcome	Follow-up period (months)
1	3	7	Graft displacement resulting from screw breakage (11 months)	Reduction and refixation	Amputation due to recurrence	Yes	Lung, bone	DOD	44
2	4	12	None		No	No	No	CDF	131
3	3	13	None		Amputation due to recurrence	Yes	No	NED	129
4	11	14	None		No	No	Lung	DOD	39
5	6	12	Fracture (21 months) Infection (32 months)	Reduction and refixation Graft removal	Removal due to deep infection	No	No	CDF	104
6	4	10	None		No	No	No	CDF	81
7	3	9	None		No	No	No	CDF	75
8	NA	NA	Infection (2 months)	Graft removal and external fixation	Removal due to deep infection	No	Lung	AWD	56
9	4	10	None		No	No	Lung	AWD	37
10	3	8	None		No	No	Lung	AWD	31
11	3	4	None		No	No	No	CDF	25

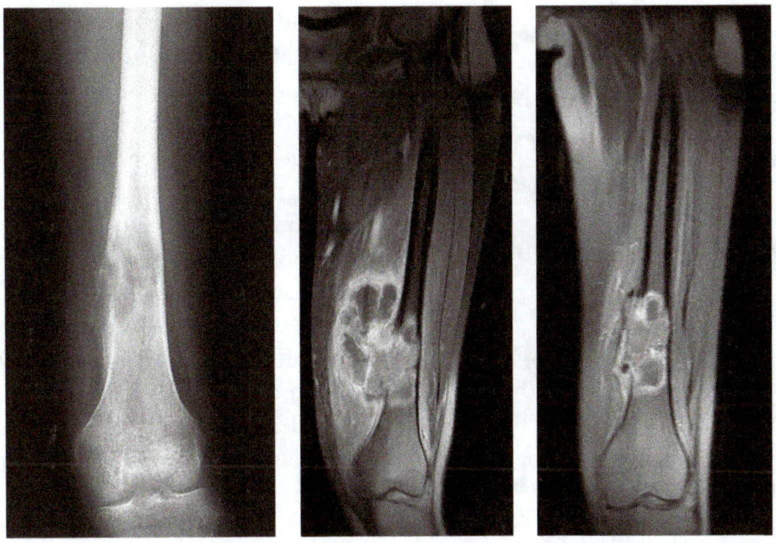

FIGURE 2: A plain radiograph of the left distal femur demonstrates an osteolytic lesion with destruction of the cortex and intratumoral ossification (a). Coronal MR images demonstrate a large extraosseous mass with destruction of the cortex (b). Reduction in size of the tumor was noted after preoperative chemotherapy (c).

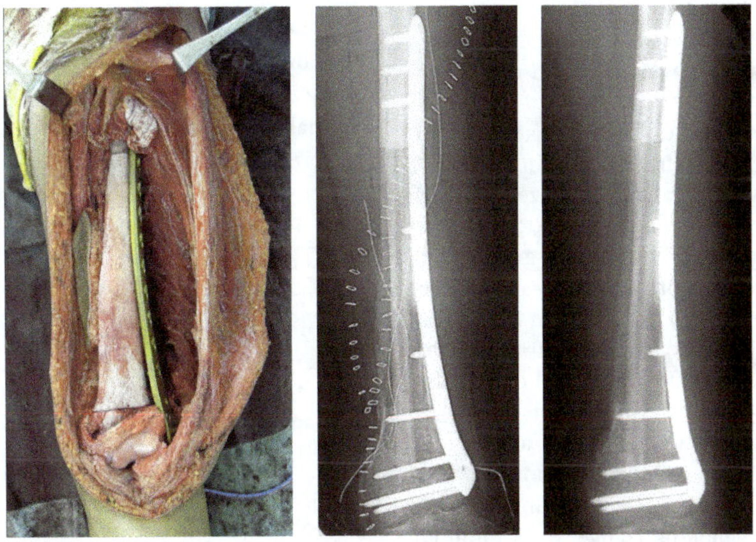

FIGURE 3: The composite graft was rigidly fixed to the host bone with a locking plate and screws ((a) operative photograph, (b) postoperative plain radiograph). A plain radiograph 9 months after surgery. Bone union was achieved (c).

autografts [8], irradiated autografts [26], and segmental prostheses [9, 27]. Each procedure has its own shortcomings and no standardized method has been established. The complication rate associated with intercalary allograft reconstruction has been considerably high. The complications of intercalary allografts have included nonunion (12–57%), fracture (17–30%), and infection (10–15%) [1–6, 22–24, 28]. One of the main disadvantages of devitalized autografts such as autoclaved, pasteurized, or irradiated autografts is that it takes a long time for them to be revascularized and incorporated into the surrounding bone. In addition, several investigators have reported high rates of infections, fractures, nonunions, and bone resorption associated with the procedure [8, 25, 26, 28]. For example, reconstruction using a pasteurized autograft was associated with high rate (52%) of complications including primary nonunion (20%), infection (20%), fracture (12%), and massive bone resorption (8%) [8]. Reconstruction using an autograft frozen with liquid nitrogen was reported to be a simple and effective method of biological reconstruction [7]. However, it still has some problems similar to those of allografts or other types of devitalized autografts, including infection (11%),

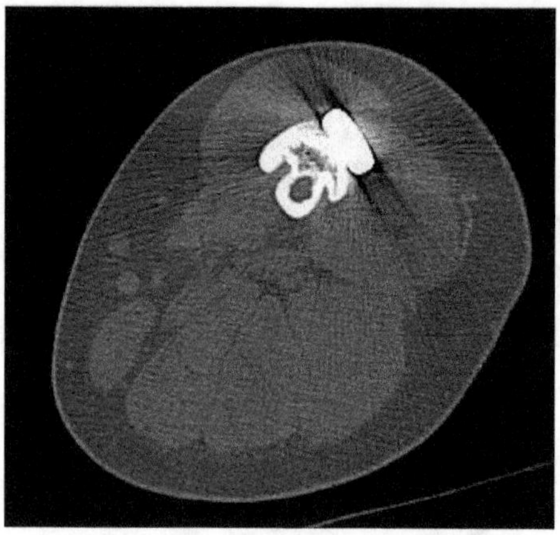

Figure 4: A CT scan at 39 months after surgery. Bridging bone formation from the hypertrophic inlaid fibula to the frozen autograft is evident.

fracture (7%), or nonunion (7%) [7], and there is an urgent need to develop an optimal reconstruction to decrease these problems.

Recently, a composite graft technique that combines an allograft or a devitalized autograft with a vascularized fibula graft for reconstruction of large bony defects has been developed [10, 16–18, 29, 30]. The rationale for use of a composite graft is that it combines the advantages of immediate mechanical endurance of a massive allograft or a devitalized autograft with the long-standing biological properties of a vascularized fibula graft. The allograft or devitalized autograft provides a massive bone stock and early stabilization, whereas the vascularized fibular graft facilitates host-graft union. Chang and Weber [18] reported 6 primary intercalary reconstructions with composite use of a vascularized fibula graft and an allograft. All of the 6 studied patients (100%) achieved successful bone union, and the mean time until bone union was 6 months (range, 3–8 months). Sugiura et al. [10] reported 15 intercalary reconstructions with composite use of a vascularized fibula graft and a pasteurized autograft. Bone union was achieved in 13 cases (87%) and the mean period until bone union was 13.5 months (range, 7–25 months). Postoperative complications included fractures in 2 patients and infection in another 2. There were no local recurrences. Krieg et al. [17] reported 13 intercalary reconstructions with composite use of a vascularized fibula graft and an extracorporeal irradiated autograft. Nonunion was found in 16% of host-donor junctions and they required additional surgical procedures. The median time until primary bone union was 7.5 months at metaphyseal junctions and 11.1 months at diaphyseal junctions. Postoperative complications included 1 fracture. There were no cases of infection. Although direct comparison is difficult due to the lack of statistical power and the heterogeneity of the population, the bone union rate in the present study (91%) was comparable to these reports (84–100%) and postoperative complication rate (27%) seemed relatively high compared with these reports (0–27%) [10, 17, 18].

In addition to reconstruction with a previously reported combination of a vascularized fibula graft and a pasteurized autograft, we performed a novel reconstruction method combining a vascularized fibula graft with a frozen autograft for large segmental bone defects. Although there were no significant differences, perhaps as a result of limited statistical power, the frozen autograft group tended to have a shorter operation time, less blood loss, a lower postoperative complication rate, and better functional outcome. Out of 3 postoperative complications in 2 patients in the pasteurized autograft group, 1 fracture and 1 implant failure were related to insufficient internal fixation, and hence they may have been avoided by rigid fixation using a locking plate, as used in recent cases involving frozen autografts. The better functional outcome in the frozen autograft group may have been associated with earlier bone union, resulting in early mobilization of the reconstructed limb postoperatively. Another major point with regard to the use of a frozen autograft in composite graft reconstruction is its ability to be used anywhere and the simplicity of the procedure.

However, reconstruction using a composite graft has several disadvantages. First, it is impossible to perform histological analysis of the whole specimen for determining the effects of chemotherapy and the adequacy of the surgical margins. Second, it takes a longer operation time and requires specialist plastic surgeons. Third, the majority of the cases in the present study consisted of the reconstruction of the femur, which is considered to be less challenging than that of the tibia. Further investigation is required to show the applicability to expand this technique to patients with reconstruction of the tibia. Finally, some donor site complications which require surgical intervention such as claw toe deformity or peroneal nerve palsy may occur after the harvesting of vascularized fibula graft although there were no cases of such complications requiring surgical intervention in our series.

5. Conclusions

In conclusion, although some complications were noted especially in early cases involving a pasteurized autograft, our results suggest that a devitalized autograft combined with a vascularized fibula graft is a promising biological alternative for intercalary reconstruction after wide resection of malignant bone tumors of the lower extremity, especially in younger patients for whom longer life expectancy and increased physical activity make fractures and infections more likely. In addition, our novel method involving a combination of a frozen autograft with a vascularized fibula graft and rigid fixation with a locking plate may offer better outcomes than previously reported allografts or devitalized autografts, although longer follow-up of a greater number of patients will be required to confirm this.

Acknowledgments

This study was funded by a Grant-in-Aid for Scientific Research from the Ministry of Education and Science (B, no. 22390296) and by the National Cancer Center Research and Development Fund (23-A-10).

References

[1] D. Donati, M. di Liddo, M. Zavatta et al., "Massive bone allograft reconstruction in high-grade osteosarcoma," *Clinical Orthopaedics and Related Research*, no. 377, pp. 186–194, 2000.

[2] M. C. Gebhardt, D. I. Flugstad, D. S. Springfield, and H. J. Mankin, "The use of bone allografts for limb salvage in high-grade extremity osteosarcoma," *Clinical Orthopaedics and Related Research*, no. 270, pp. 181–196, 1991.

[3] W. Mnaymneh, T. I. Malinin, R. D. Lackman, F. J. Hornicek, and L. Ghandur-Mnaymneh, "Massive distal femoral osteoarticular allografts after resection of bone tumors," *Clinical Orthopaedics and Related Research*, no. 303, pp. 103–115, 1994.

[4] D. L. Muscolo, M. A. Ayerza, L. Aponte-Tinao, M. Ranalletta, and E. Abalo, "Intercalary femur and tibia segmental allografts provide an acceptable alternative in reconstructing tumor resections," *Clinical Orthopaedics and Related Research*, no. 426, pp. 97–102, 2004.

[5] E. Ortiz-Cruz, M. C. Gebhardt, L. C. Jennings, D. S. Springfield, and H. J. Mankin, "The results of transplantation of intercalary allografts after resection of tumors. A long-term follow-up study," *The Journal of Bone and Joint Surgery—Americasn Volume*, vol. 79, no. 1, pp. 97–106, 1997.

[6] R. A. V. Griend, "The effect of internal fixation on the healing of large allografts," *The Journal of Bone and Joint Surgery Series A*, vol. 76, no. 5, pp. 657–663, 1994.

[7] H. Tsuchiya, S. L. Wan, K. Sakayama, N. Yamamoto, H. Nishida, and K. Tomita, "Reconstruction using an autograft containing tumour treated by liquid nitrogen," *Journal of Bone and Joint Surgery—Series B*, vol. 87, no. 2, pp. 218–225, 2005.

[8] J. Manabe, A. R. Ahmed, N. Kawaguchi, S. Matsumoto, and H. Kuroda, "Pasteurized autologous bone graft in surgery for bone and soft tissue sarcoma," *Clinical Orthopaedics and Related Research*, no. 419, pp. 258–266, 2004.

[9] M. D. Sewell, S. A. Hanna, A. McGrath et al., "Intercalary diaphyseal endoprosthetic reconstruction for malignant tibial bone tumours," *The Journal of Bone and Joint Surgery—British Volume*, vol. 93, no. 8, pp. 1111–1117, 2011.

[10] H. Sugiura, M. Takahashi, K. Nakanishi, Y. Nishida, and Y. Kamei, "Pasteurized intercalary autogenous bone graft combined with vascularized fibula," *Clinical Orthopaedics and Related Research*, no. 456, pp. 196–202, 2007.

[11] J. G. del Pino, E. B. del Valle, G. L. Graña, and J. F. Villanova, "Free vascularized fibular grafts have a high union rate in atrophic nonunions," *Clinical Orthopaedics and Related Research*, no. 419, pp. 38–45, 2004.

[12] A. Maghari, K. S. Forootan, S. A. Emami, and C. Melow, "Microvascular reconstruction of soft tissue and bone loss in war wounds," *Scandinavian Journal of Plastic and Reconstructive Surgery and Hand Surgery*, vol. 26, no. 1, pp. 91–96, 1992.

[13] A. Minami, T. Kasashima, N. Iwasaki, H. Kato, and K. Kaneda, "Vascularised fibular grafts. An experience of 102 patients," *Journal of Bone and Joint Surgery—Series B*, vol. 82, no. 7, pp. 1022–1025, 2000.

[14] R. Pollock, P. Stalley, K. Lee, and D. Pennington, "Free vascularized fibula grafts in limb-salvage surgery," *Journal of Reconstructive Microsurgery*, vol. 21, no. 2, pp. 79–84, 2005.

[15] H. Yajima, S. Tamai, S. Mizumoto, and H. Ono, "Vascularised fibular grafts for reconstruction of the femur," *The Journal of Bone and Joint Surgery—British Volume*, vol. 75, no. 1, pp. 123–128, 1993.

[16] O. Brunet, P. Anract, S. Bouabid et al., "Intercalary defects reconstruction of the femur and tibia after primary malignant bone tumour resection. A series of 13 cases," *Orthopaedics & Traumatology: Surgery & Research*, vol. 97, no. 5, pp. 512–519, 2011.

[17] A. H. Krieg, A. W. Davidson, and P. D. Stalley, "Intercalary femoral reconstruction with extracorporeal irradiated autogenous bone graft in limb-salvage surgery," *The Journal of Bone and Joint Surgery—British Volume*, vol. 89, no. 3, pp. 366–371, 2007.

[18] D. W. Chang and K. L. Weber, "Use of a vascularized fibula bone flap and intercalary allograft for diaphyseal reconstruction after resection of primary extremity bone sarcomas.," *Plastic and Reconstructive Surgery*, vol. 116, no. 7, pp. 1918–1925, 2005.

[19] H. Sugiura, S. Yamamura, K. Sato et al., "Remodelling and healing process of moderately heat-treated bone grafts after wide resection of bone and soft-tissue tumors," *Archives of Orthopaedic and Trauma Surgery*, vol. 123, no. 10, pp. 514–520, 2003.

[20] Y. Rong, K. Sato, H. Sugiura et al., "Effect of elevated temperature on experimental swarm rat chondrosarcoma," *Clinical Orthopaedics and Related Research*, no. 311, pp. 227–231, 1995.

[21] W. F. Enneking, W. Dunham, M. C. Gebhardt, M. Malawar, and D. J. Pritchard, "A system for the functional evaluation of reconstructive procedures after surgical treatment of tumors of the musculoskeletal system," *Clinical Orthopaedics and Related Research*, no. 286, pp. 241–246, 1993.

[22] R. L. M. Deijkers, R. M. Bloem, H. M. Kroon, J. B. van Lent, R. Brand, and A. H. M. Taminiau, "Epidiaphyseal versus other intercalary allografts for tumors of the lower limb," *Clinical Orthopaedics and Related Research*, no. 439, pp. 151–160, 2005.

[23] C. F. Lord, M. C. Gebhardt, W. W. Tomford, and H. J. Mankin, "Infection in bone allografts. Incidence, nature, and treatment," *The Journal of Bone and Joint Surgery—American Volume*, vol. 70, no. 3, pp. 369–376, 1988.

[24] H. J. Mankin, M. C. Gebhardt, L. C. Jennings, D. S. Springfield, and W. W. Tomford, "Long-term results of allograft replacement in the management of bone tumors," *Clinical Orthopaedics and Related Research*, no. 324, pp. 86–97, 1996.

[25] M. J. Khattak, M. Umer, and M. Umar, "Autoclaved tumor bone for reconstruction: an alternative in developing countries," *Clinical Orthopaedics and Related Research*, no. 447, pp. 138–144, 2006.

[26] D. Sabo, D. R. C. Brocai, M. Eble, M. Wannenmacher, and V. Ewerbeck, "Influence of extracorporeal irradiation on the reintegration of autologous grafts of bone and joint," *The Journal of Bone and Joint Surgery—British Volume*, vol. 82, no. 2, pp. 276–282, 2000.

[27] E. Y. S. Chao, B. Fuchs, C. M. Rowland, D. M. Ilstrup, D. J. Pritchard, and F. H. Sim, "Long-term results of segmental prosthesis fixation by extracortical bone-bridging and ingrowth," *The Journal of Bone and Joint Surgery—American Volume*, vol. 86, no. 5, pp. 948–955, 2004.

[28] B. Fuchs, C. Ossendorf, T. Leerapun, and F. H. Sim, "Intercalary segmental reconstruction after bone tumor resection," *European Journal of Surgical Oncology*, vol. 34, no. 12, pp. 1271–1276, 2008.

[29] D. W. Chang and K. L. Weber, "Segmental femur reconstruction using an intercalary allograft with an intramedullary vascularized fibula bone flap," *Journal of Reconstructive Microsurgery*, vol. 20, no. 3, pp. 195–199, 2004.

[30] K. Muramatsu, K. Ihara, T. Hashimoto, S. Seto, and T. Taguchi, "Combined use of free vascularised bone graft and extracorporeally-irradiated autograft for the reconstruction of massive bone defects after resection of malignant tumour," *Journal of Plastic, Reconstructive and Aesthetic Surgery*, vol. 60, no. 9, pp. 1013–1018, 2007.

8

Consumptive Coagulopathy in Angiosarcoma: A Recurrent Phenomenon?

Mohamad Farid, Linda Ahn, Andrew Brohl, Angela Cioffi, and Robert G. Maki

Mount Sinai Medical Center, One Gustave L. Levy Place, P.O. Box 1128, New York, NY 10029-6574, USA

Correspondence should be addressed to Robert G. Maki; robert.maki@mssm.edu

Academic Editor: Andrea Deyrup

Objectives. To report the prevalence of consumptive coagulopathy in angiosarcoma patients seen at a single center. *Methods.* We retrospectively reviewed case records of 42 patients diagnosed with angiosarcoma at Mount Sinai Hospital between 2000 and 2013. *Results.* Seven patients (17%) met clinical criteria for disseminated intravascular coagulation (DIC) in absence of concomitant clinical states known to cause coagulopathy or myelosuppression. In all patients who received systemic antineoplastic therapy with resultant disease response or stability, DIC resolved in tandem with clinical improvement. DIC recurred at time of disease progression in all cases. Two patients had bulky disease, defined as diameter of largest single or contiguous tumor mass measuring 5 cm or more. All patients demonstrated an aggressive clinical course with short duration of disease control and demise within 1 year. In contrast, evaluation over the same period of 17 epithelioid hemangioendothelioma patients serving as a clinical control group revealed no evidence of DIC. *Conclusion.* Angiosarcomas can be associated with a consumptive coagulopathy arising in tandem with disease activity. Vigilance for this complication will be needed in the course of often aggressive multimodality therapy. The potential utility of coagulopathy as a prognostic biomarker will need to be explored in future studies.

1. Introduction

Hypercoagulability is a well-characterized association of malignancy which can manifest in one of several clinical syndromes, including disseminated intravascular coagulation (DIC). DIC is characterized by aberrant activation of the coagulation cascade leading to initial hypercoagulability, then progressing to a secondary hypocoagulable state resulting from consumptive coagulopathy and secondary fibrinolysis. In patients with cancer, DIC can be proximately related to altered levels of various mediators of hemostasis (procoagulants, cytokines, and fibrinolytic mediators), in addition to tumor-related endothelial cell alterations and systemic depressions in hemostatic defenses [1]. DIC is known to complicate up to 15% of leukemias [2] and up to 7% of solid tumors, with data suggesting an association with adverse cancer prognosis [3].

Sarcomas comprise 1% of adult malignancies, and can take the form of more than 70 different histologic subtypes, each describing unique natural histories and clinical behavior [4]. The prevalence of coagulation abnormalities across the different sarcoma histotypes has not been well characterized. In a large series of more than 1000 patients with solid tumors, only 41 patients had sarcoma, of whom 2 were assessed to have DIC [3].

Angiosarcomas are aggressive malignancies of vascular origin that comprise 2–5% of sarcomas. They arise in virtually any anatomic site, including skin, breast, bone, extremities, deep soft tissues, and viscera [5]. Angiosarcomas are associated with a variety of environmental carcinogenic factors, including dyes, chronic lymphedema, and radiation, but most commonly arise sporadically. In advanced disease, effective therapies are limited and prognosis is dismal, with median survival of less than 1 year [5].

Epithelioid hemangioendotheliomas represent another group of vascular sarcomas derived from endothelial cells. Affecting less that 1 person per million of the population, these tumors most often involve the liver, usually multifocally. Distinct from angiosarcoma, they can be associated with an indolent clinical course and prolonged disease control, even in the absence of any therapy in some cases [6].

There are sporadic case reports describing the coexistence of a consumptive coagulopathy with angiosarcoma [7–11]. These have been characterized as variants of Kasabach-Merritt Phenomenon (KMP), the eponymous syndrome first described in 1941 in an infant with a giant capillary hemangioma, and henceforth sometimes loosely defined as a thrombocytopenic consumptive coagulopathy associated with an enlarging vascular neoplasm or malformation. The diagnosis of KMP, however, should be restricted only to severe thrombocytopenia concomitant with fibrinolysis and microangiopathic anemia as arising in 2 very specific tumors in young children—kaposiform hemangioendothelioma (KHE) and tufted angioma (TE)—pathophysiologically underpinned by DIC precipitated by platelet and clotting factor sequestration [12]. There has yet been no systematic characterization of coagulation abnormalities in angiosarcomas, a phenomenon with undoubted therapeutic and potentially prognostic significance for this tumor. We were thus keen to better define the incidence and clinical course of DIC amongst patients with this rare but often fatal disease, with concomitant evaluation for consumptive coagulopathy in epithelioid hemangioendotheliomas as a clinical comparator group.

Table 1: International Society of Thrombosis and Hemostasis criteria for overt DIC.

Laboratory test	Result	Score*
Platelet count ($\times10^3$/L)	>100	0
	>50 but <100	1
	<50	2
Increase in fibrinogen degradation products (FDP)	None	0
	Moderate[@]	2
	Strong[@]	3
Prolongation of prothrombin time (PT) over upper limit normal (s)	<3	0
	>3 but <5.9	1
	>6	2
Fibrinogen level (g/dL)	≥1	0
	<1	1

*Scores ≥5 compatible with overt DIC.

[@]A level of <0.5 μg/mL (the upper limit of normal of the D-dimer assay in this study) was considered normal, a level between 0.5 and 5.0 μg/mL was considered moderately increased, and a level of >5.0 μg/mL was considered strongly increased.

2. Methods

Consent was obtained from the Institutional Review Board of the Mount Sinai School of Medicine and Hospital (MSSM) for retrospective analysis. All cases with the diagnosis of "angiosarcoma" seen at MSSM between 1 January 2000 and 31 June 2013 were identified through the institutional diagnostic records system. Clinical data were retrieved from patients' clinical notes and the MSSM electronic patient medical records. The cutoff date for reporting data was 31 June 2013. Survival data was determined from medical charts and cross referenced against the death registry.

Overt DIC was defined according to the International Society of Thrombosis and Hemostasis (ISTH) guidelines, evaluating 4 parameters (platelet counts, fibrinogen degradation products, prothrombin time, and fibrinogen levels) and assigning points to particular values (Table 1) [13]. This metric was chosen amongst the several clinical criteria available to define DIC in view of its simplicity and widespread use. Patients with pertinent laboratory derangements were then evaluated for the presence of other causes of coagulopathy or DIC including trauma, sepsis, pharmacotherapeutic myelosuppression, and bone marrow involvement with disease. Patients in whom these causes had been excluded, or in whom these causes existed but were unable to fully account for the hematological abnormalities seen, then had further elements of their clinical course characterized. Patients were designated as having bulky disease if the largest single or contiguous tumor mass measured 5 cm or more in diameter. We evaluated this clinical characteristic as we postulated that the size of singular or contiguous masses (as distinct from the sum total size of multiple disseminated tumor masses) in vascular tumors may influence the likelihood of consumptive coagulopathy putatively because smaller such masses are less likely to trap platelets in sufficient quantity to cause significant platelet trapping and destruction. The 5 cm cutoff was chosen based upon a previous evaluation of KHE in which all patients developing KMP had primary tumors larger than 5 cm [14]. The same process of case identification and evaluation for DIC was then repeated for patients with the diagnosis "epithelioid hemangioendothelioma" (EHE).

3. Results

Forty-two patients with angiosarcoma were identified from our institutional database. The median age was 62 years (range 16–86 years); 22 patients (52%) were male. Twenty patients (48%) had advanced disease, defined as either metastatic or unresectable AS. Eighteen patients (43%) had bulky disease, of whom 12 had advanced disease. The five commonest anatomical primary sites include breast (12 patients), liver (5), mediastinum (4), upper limb (3), and scalp or face (3). Twelve patients (29%) had radiation-associated AS, the majority of which developed following radiation for early breast cancer (6 developing breast AS and 2 developing chest wall AS).

Out of this cohort of AS patients, 11 patients were identified to have evidence of DIC during the course of their illness. Four of these patients were deemed to have had their coagulopathy probably attributable to pharmacotherapy (including chemotherapy) or sepsis, leaving 7 patients (17%) with unexplained DIC. The clinical features of these patients are described in Table 2. The trend of selected hematological and coagulation parameters for 2 representative patients is detailed in Figure 1.

Six patients fulfilled the ISTH criteria for overt DIC; patient 7, whose clinical data was incomplete, scored the maximum 4 points based on the hematologic and coagulation data available. Three patients manifested either clinical thrombosis or hemorrhage during the course of their illness; patients 2 and 4 manifested clinically apparent hemorrhage

Table 2: Hematologic and coagulation parameters associated with clinical features of the 7 angiosarcoma patients with DIC.

No.	Age (yrs), sex (M/F), anatomic sites	Systemic therapy in metastatic disease	ISTH score	DIC in 1st 30 days^	DIC resolved with disease response/ stability	DIC recurred at progression	Bone marrow involvement	Tumor burden@	Clinical thrombosis/ hemorrhage	Survival in metastatic disease	Remarks
1	37 M liver with metastasis to spleen	Pegylated liposomal doxorubicin	7	Yes	Yes	Yes	No	Nonbulky	No	9 months	Metastatic at first presentation. No evidence of clinically significant portal hypertension
2	42 F breast (de novo) with metastasis to chest wall, ribs, lung	Pegylated liposomal doxorubicin plus carboplatin, sirolimus, pazopanib, abraxane, bevacizumab plus vinorelbine	5	No	NA	Yes	Not done	Nonbulky	Yes	11 months	Localized to right breast at first presentation, had mastectomy, then 6 cycles adjuvant gemcitabine plus docetaxel followed by radiation. Developed metastatic relapse within 11 months
3	39 M mediastinal with metastasis to bone, lung, brain	Doxorubicin plus paclitaxel, ifosfamide plus cisplatin, gemcitabine plus vinorelbine	5	Yes	Yes	Yes	Not done	Bulky	Yes	5 months	Metastatic at first presentation
4	54 F cardiac with metastasis to lung, pleura, bones, bone marrow	Doxorubicin plus ifosfamide	7	Yes	Yes	Yes	Yes	Bulky	Yes	6 months	Metastatic at first presentation
5	70 F breast (radiation related) with metastasis to lymph nodes, lung	Doxorubicin plus ifosfamide	6	Yes	Yes	Yes	No	Nonbulky	No	11 months	Metastatic at first presentation; developed angiosarcoma 9 years following lumpectomy and radiation for early stage breast adenocarcinoma
6	66 F skull and meninges with metastasis to spinal cord, lungs, bone	Nil	6	Yes	NA	NA	Not done	Nonbulky	No	1 month	Metastatic at first presentation; poor performance status precluded any therapy
7	78 M foot (bony) with metastasis to lungs	Nil	4*	Yes	NA	NA	Not done	Nonbulky	No	2 months	Metastatic at first presentation; poor performance status precluded any therapy

*Data available only for prothrombin time and platelets, giving a maximum possible ISTH score of 4.
@Bulky tumor is defined as the largest single or contiguous tumor mass 5 cm or more in diameter.
^Development of DIC within 30 days of presentation with metastatic disease.

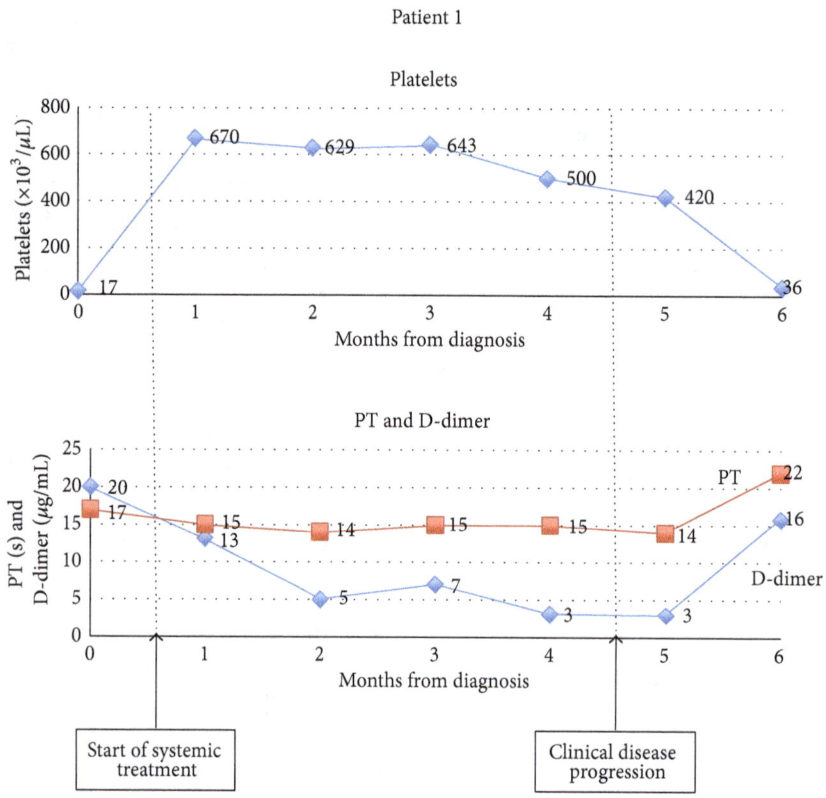

FIGURE 1: Variation in hematological and coagulation parameters showing coagulopathy at diagnosis that improved with therapy but recurred at disease relapse.

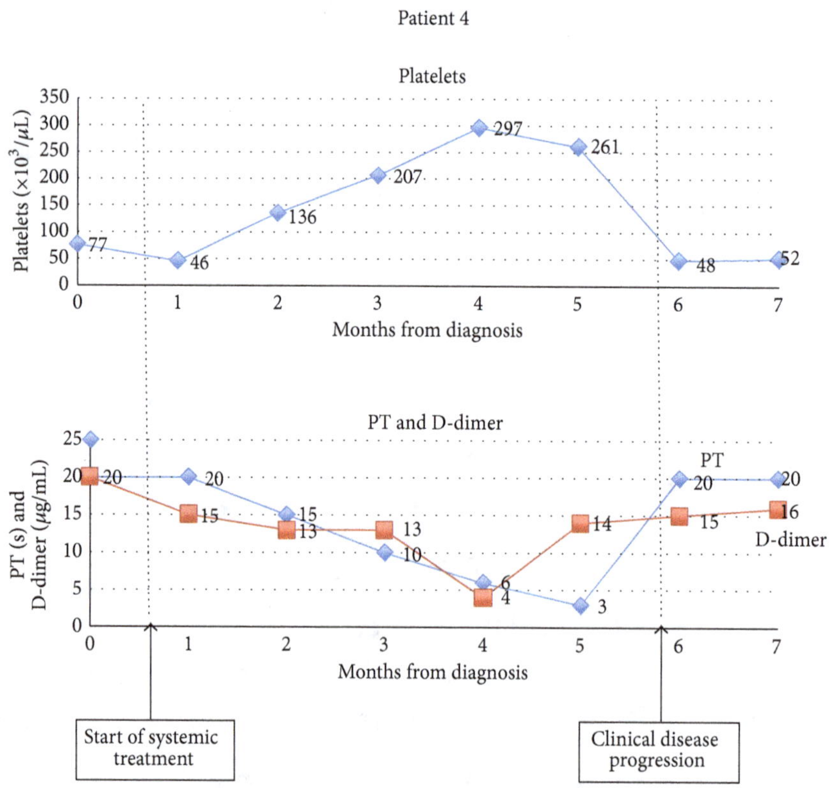

FIGURE 2: Variation in hematological and coagulation parameters showing coagulopathy at diagnosis that improved with therapy but recurred at disease relapse.

necessitating local therapy (surgical ablation or radiotherapy); and patient 3 had superior vena caval thrombosis. All but one patient manifested coagulopathy within the first month of diagnosis; all patients who demonstrated clinico-radiologic response or stability to systemic therapy (patients 1, 3, 4 and 5) also demonstrated improvement in their coagulation and hematological parameters in tandem with their clinical response. All patients demonstrated worsening coagulopathy coincident with disease progression. The depth and trend of this coagulopathy for two representative patients is depicted in Figure 2. Only two patients (patients 3 and 4) had bulky disease. All patients had very short survival, with limited duration of disease control, if any.

We conducted an identical review of patients with EHE. There were 17 patients in total. The median age was 51 years (range 23–80 years), and 9 patients (53%) were female. Fourteen patients (82%) had disease arising in the liver, of whom 8 had metastatic disease (primarily to lungs and bone) and 6 had multifocal liver disease. Of the remaining 3 patients (18%) with extrahepatic primary disease, 2 had advanced EHE. Only 3 patients (18%) had bulky disease according to our definition. Patients were variably treated with a range of sequential therapies including orthotopic liver transplantation, hepatic ablative therapies, systemic therapies, or expectant management. Half of the patients were free of disease progression for more than 2 years, and 4 patients were stable for more than 5 years. No patient demonstrated evidence of DIC.

4. Discussion

Amongst the malignant mesenchymal tumors, angiosarcomas have a particularly aggressive clinical course. Even in the context of early disease receiving aggressive multimodality therapy, relapses are frequent and often early; in the setting of advanced disease, treatment, responses are uncommon and usually short-lived [5, 15, 16]. Systemic therapy in advanced disease often involves the use of anthracyclines and taxanes, putatively the most active agents in this disease [17]. The value of therapy directed against the vascular endothelial growth factor (VEGF), often overexpressed in this endothelium-derived tumor, remains unsettled. A recent study reported 2 out of 23 angiosarcoma patients achieving a partial response to single agent bevacizumab [18]; these therapies continue to be evaluated actively in this disease. What is not in doubt is the well-documented propensity of anti-VEGF therapies to cause vascular toxicities. Bevacizumab has been associated with bleeding in up to 40% of patients, with the rate for such events with the tyrosine kinase inhibitor sunitinib reported to be 16%; the risk of both arterial and venous thromboembolism can also be increased with use of these agents [19]. The potential for significant myelotoxicity with cytotoxic therapy, as well as the risk of hemorrhage and hemostatic derangements with anti-VEGF therapies, in this aggressive malignancy with few effective therapies, brings into sharp relief the significant therapeutic implications of any disease-associated coagulopathy.

Few systematic data exist on the prevalence of DIC in sarcomas; as mentioned earlier, one series found DIC in 2 out of 41 (4%) sarcoma patients evaluated [3]. More generally, with the possible exception of nonislet cell tumor hypoglycemia seen in a proportion of sarcoma subtypes such as solitary fibrous tumor [20], sarcomas are not known to be consistently associated with particular paraneoplastic phenomena. Whether this is due to a dearth of systematic evaluation in an uncommon and biologically diverse group of diseases, or rather the consequence of a genuine lack of association between sarcomas and the triggering factors of paraneoplastic syndromes, is unknown at this time. Specific to angiosarcoma, the occurrence of consumptive coagulopathy has been documented in several case reports. Two reports described bulky de novo breast angiosarcomas [8, 11], two others reported nonbulky scalp angiosarcomas in elderly Asian males [9, 10], and one case described a bulky hepatic angiosarcoma [7]. The two patients with breast disease and one with scalp disease had concomitant hemorrhage or thrombosis. In the only report that described delivery of antineoplastic therapy, chemoradiotherapy resulted in resolution of DIC for the other patient with scalp disease [9]. In all other cases, patients experienced rapid clinical deterioration and eventual demise.

Seventeen percent of patients in our series developed DIC, with all patients with complete data meeting the ISTH criteria for overt DIC. DIC affected patients across a range of anatomic primary sites, manifested early in the disease, improved with effective therapy, and recurred at the time of disease progression. Importantly, these derangements were assessed to be independent of concomitant clinical conditions known to cause similar laboratory abnormalities, such as sepsis or bone marrow failure. Half the patients developed clinically apparent thrombosis or hemorrhage; given the clear presence of a consumptive coagulopathic process in all patients, it is possible that an occult clot or bleeding diathesis was present in the remaining patients that was merely not assessed for or detected clinically. The clinical course of these patients was not inconsistent with the known dismal prognosis of patients with visceral angiosarcoma, with no patients living beyond 1 year [21].

We did not find any evidence of this coagulopathy in the EHE patients. Notwithstanding clear distinctions in clinical behavior described earlier, EHE is arguably the closest clinical analogue of angiosarcoma. Both are malignant vascular neoplasms of endothelial origin that commonly overexpress similar mitogens like VEGF and have been studied together in therapeutic trials [18]. While the sample sizes in both groups were too small to allow for statistically meaningful comparisons, the disparity in the occurrence of coagulopathy between angiosarcomas and EHEs may point towards underlying biological features unique to the former, as distinct from a feature common to vascular neoplasms.

It is interesting to speculate on the particular features of specific subtypes of mesenchymal tumors that lend them more prone to DIC than others. In the case of KMP, it is speculated that the unique vessel architecture of Kaposiform hemangioendothelioma (KHE) and tufted angiomas (TA) promotes platelet trapping and the resultant consumptive coagulopathy; in contrast to the ordered tree-like vasculature of infantile hemangioma, convoluted capillaries arise directly off large vessels in KHE and TA resulting in turbulent flow-promoting platelet activation and aggregation [12]. The observation of KMP in young infants may suggest the additional role of developmental differences in infantile endothelial structure and composition that increase the likelihood of coagulopathy [12]. Not dissimilarly in angiosarcomas, it is possible that as yet undefined derangements in the physiology and function of the endothelium, the histologic cell of origin in this disease contributes to the platelet adhesion and activation that leads to consequent DIC.

In our series, 71% of patients (5 out of 7) developing DIC had angiosarcoma where no single or contiguous mass was larger than 5 cm. Notably, all patients who developed DIC had metastatic disease. The necessarily tentative nature of any conclusions drawn from this small sample of patients notwithstanding, these data may be interpreted to suggest the limited importance of local physical factors (specifically size of single largest tumor mass) as compared with systemic factors, such as hormonal and cytokine elements associated with disseminated disease, in the development of DIC in angiosarcoma. Furthermore, the apparent correlation with disease activity, in as much as the manner the DIC waxed and waned in tandem with clinical disease, suggests concordance between the processes driving the angiosarcoma with those causing the coagulopathy and hints at the potential utility of the latter as a biomarker for the former. Indeed, though not evaluated in the context of DIC, D-dimer, the final degradation product of cross-linked fibrin that is one of the markers of activated clotting and fibrinolysis, has been shown to have independent prognostic value in sarcomas [22], as in several other solid tumors.

We suggest that these cases represent an addition to the literature linking angiosarcoma to derangements in hemostatic control. Undoubtedly, the severity and clinical manifestations of the coagulopathy vary widely even within this small group, and their prognostic implications remain to be rigorously defined. The precise mechanisms underlying the occurrence of this phenomenon also remain to be elucidated. Nevertheless, we think that this data importantly highlights the presence of a clinical syndrome with clear potential implications for therapy. Angiosarcoma patients are often subjected to aggressive oncologic therapy, often including extensive surgery and intensive chemotherapy; vigilance for the development of DIC and hemorrhage appears critical to minimize the morbidities of these therapies. As consistent with the treatment of DIC in cancer in general, therapy involves addressing the underlying malignant disease with appropriate antineoplastic therapy. In addition, the intriguing hints at potential alterations in tandem with disease burden speak to the possibility of utilizing these parameters as convenient biomarkers of disease status.

5. Conclusions

Our data systematically complements previous reports linking angiosarcoma to consumptive coagulopathy. This association appears unique to this histologic subtype amongst the vascular tumors and has clear implications for the safe and effective delivery of therapy. We suggest that a baseline coagulation screen be performed for newly diagnosed patients with angiosarcoma; if abnormal, these tests should be repeated regularly to assess the trend with disease and therapy. Further studies should assess this association in larger data sets with a view to evaluating its true prognostic value, if any.

References

[1] H. I. Saba, G. A. Morelli, and R. I. Saba, "Disseminated Intravascular Coagulation (DIC) in cancer," *Cancer Treatment and Research*, vol. 148, pp. 137–156, 2009.

[2] M. Franchini, M. N. Di Minno, and A. Coppola, "Disseminated intravascular coagulation in hematologic malignancies," *Seminars in Thrombosis and Hemostasis*, vol. 36, no. 4, pp. 388–403, 2010.

[3] S. Sallah, J. Y. Wan, N. P. Nguyen, L. R. Hanrahan, and G. Sigounas, "Disseminated intravascular coagulation in solid tumors: clinical and pathologic study," *Thrombosis and Haemostasis*, vol. 86, no. 3, pp. 828–833, 2001.

[4] M. A. Clark, C. Fisher, I. Judson, and J. Meirion Thomas, "Soft-tissue sarcomas in adults," *The New England Journal of Medicine*, vol. 353, no. 7, pp. 701–711, 2005.

[5] R. J. Young, N. J. Brown, M. W. Reed, D. Hughes, and P. J. Woll, "Angiosarcoma," *The Lancet Oncology*, vol. 11, no. 10, pp. 983–991, 2010.

[6] A. M. Mistry, D. L. Gorden, J. F. Busler, A. C. Coogan, and B. S. Kelly, "Diagnostic and therapeutic challenges in hepatic epithelioid hemangioendothelioma," *Journal of Gastrointestinal Cancer*, vol. 43, no. 4, pp. 521–525, 2012.

[7] C. Alliot, B. Tribout, M. Barrios, and M.-F. Gontier, "Angiosarcoma variant of Kasabach-Merritt syndrome," *European Journal of Gastroenterology and Hepatology*, vol. 13, no. 6, pp. 731–734, 2001.

[8] S. H. Y. Moussa, A. L. K. Oliveira, A. P. de Amorim, D. Scandiuzzi, E. F. C. Murta, and S. Soares, "Angiosarcoma of the breast associated with Kasabach-Merritt syndrome," *Archives of Gynecology and Obstetrics*, vol. 267, no. 1, pp. 43–45, 2002.

[9] S. Imafuku, C. Hosokawa, Y. Moroi, and M. Furue, "Kasabach-Merritt syndrome associated with angiosarcoma of the scalp successfully treated with chemoradiotherapy," *Acta Dermato-Venereologica*, vol. 88, no. 2, pp. 193–194, 2008.

[10] S. M. Tans, Y. K. Tay, T. T. Liu, and K. Mancer, "Cutaneous angiosarcoma associated with the Kasabach-Merritt syndrome," *Annals of the Academy of Medicine Singapore*, vol. 39, no. 12, pp. 941–942, 2010.

[11] M. Bernathova, W. Jaschke, C. Pechlahner, B. Zelger, and G. Bodner, "Primary angiosarcoma of the breast associated Kasabach-Merritt syndrome during pregnancy," *Breast*, vol. 15, no. 2, pp. 255–258, 2006.

[12] M. Kelly, "Kasabach-merritt phenomenon," *Pediatric Clinics of North America*, vol. 57, no. 5, pp. 1085–1089, 2010.

[13] K. Bakhtiari, J. C. M. Meijers, E. de Jonge, and M. Levi, "Prospective validation of the International Society of Thrombosis and Haemostasis scoring system for disseminated intravascular coagulation," *Critical Care Medicine*, vol. 32, no. 12, pp. 2416–2421, 2004.

[14] M. Sarkar, J. B. Mulliken, H. P. W. Kozakewich, R. L. Robertson, and P. E. Burrows, "Thrombocytopenic coagulopathy (Kasabach-Merritt Phenomenon) is associated with Kaposiform

hemangioendothelioma and not with common infantile hemangioma," *Plastic and Reconstructive Surgery*, vol. 100, no. 6, pp. 1377–1386, 1997.

[15] M. G. Fury, C. R. Antonescu, K. J. Van Zee, M. F. Brennan, and R. G. Maki, "A 14-year retrospective review of angiosarcoma: clinical characteristics, prognostic factors, and treatment outcomes with surgery and chemotherapy," *The Cancer Journal*, vol. 11, no. 3, pp. 241–247, 2005.

[16] M. Schlemmer, P. Reichardt, J. Verweij et al., "Paclitaxel in patients with advanced angiosarcomas of soft tissue: a retrospective study of the EORTC soft tissue and bone sarcoma group," *European Journal of Cancer*, vol. 44, no. 16, pp. 2433–2436, 2008.

[17] A. Italiano, A. Cioffi, N. Penel et al., "Comparison of doxorubicin and weekly paclitaxel efficacy in metastatic angiosarcomas," *Cancer*, vol. 118, no. 13, pp. 3330–3336, 2012.

[18] M. Agulnik, J. L. Yarber, S. H. Okuno et al., "An open-label, multicenter, phase II study of bevacizumab for the treatment of angiosarcoma and epithelioid hemangioendotheliomas," *Annals of Oncology*, vol. 24, no. 1, pp. 257–263, 2013.

[19] D. Keefe, J. Bowen, R. Gibson, T. Tan, M. Okera, and A. Stringer, "Noncardiac vascular toxicities of vascular endothelial growth factor inhibitors in advanced cancer: a review," *Oncologist*, vol. 16, no. 4, pp. 432–444, 2011.

[20] J. W. B. de Groot, B. Rikhof, J. van Doorn et al., "Non-islet cell tumour-induced hypoglycaemia: a review of the literature including two new cases," *Endocrine-Related Cancer*, vol. 14, no. 4, pp. 979–993, 2007.

[21] J. Fayette, E. Martin, S. Piperno-Neumann et al., "Angiosarcomas, a heterogeneous group of sarcomas with specific behavior depending on primary site: a retrospective study of 161 cases," *Annals of Oncology*, vol. 18, no. 12, pp. 2030–2036, 2007.

[22] S. D. Raj, X. Zhou, C. E. Bueso-Ramos et al., "Prognostic significance of elevated D-dimer for survival in patients with sarcoma," *American Journal of Clinical Oncology*, vol. 35, no. 5, pp. 462–467, 2012.

9

Clinical Activity and Tolerability of a 14-Day Infusional Ifosfamide Schedule in Soft-Tissue Sarcoma

Juan Martin-Liberal,[1] Salma Alam,[1] Anastasia Constantinidou,[1] Cyril Fisher,[2] Komel Khabra,[3] Christina Messiou,[4] David Olmos,[5] Scott Mitchell,[6] Omar Al-Muderis,[1] Aisha Miah,[1] Mark Linch,[1] Robin L. Jones,[1] Michelle Scurr,[1] Ian Judson,[1] and Charlotte Benson[1]

[1] *Sarcoma Unit, The Royal Marsden Hospital, Fulham Road, London SW3 6JJ, UK*
[2] *Department of Histopathology, The Royal Marsden Hospital, Fulham Road , London SW3 6JJ, UK*
[3] *Department of Statistics, The Royal Marsden Hospital, Downs Road, Sutton SM2 5PT, UK*
[4] *Department of Radiodiagnostics, The Royal Marsden Hospital, Fulham Road, London SW3 6JJ, UK*
[5] *Spanish National Cancer Research Centre (CNIO), Clinical Research Programme, 3 Melchor Fernandez Almagro, 28029 Madrid, Spain*
[6] *Department of Pharmacy, The Royal Marsden Hospital, Fulham Road, London SW3 6JJ, UK*

Correspondence should be addressed to Juan Martin-Liberal; juan.martin@rmh.nhs.uk

Academic Editor: Shreyaskumar Patel

Background. Soft-tissue sarcomas (STS) are a heterogeneous group of diseases with lack of effective treatments in most cases. Previous data suggest that continuous infusional ifosfamide regimens might improve cytotoxicity and tolerability compared to standard schedules. *Methods.* We retrospectively report the outcome of 35 patients affected by STS treated with a 14-day infusional ifosfamide regimen (1000 mg/m^2/day) in our institution. Predictive factors for toxicity were also explored. *Results.* Median age was 53 years. There were 16 males and 19 females. Classification by histology was dedifferentiated liposarcoma (DDLPS): 22 (62.8%), synovial sarcoma: 7 (20%), myxoid/round-cell liposarcoma: 3 (8.5%), and others: 3 (8.5%). Overall, 7 patients (20%) achieved partial response (PR) and 10 patients (29%) achieved stable disease (SD). DDLPS showed special sensitivity: 5 patients (22.7%) had PR, 7 patients (31.8%) had SD, and disease control rate was 54.5%. Median progression-free survival and overall survival were 4.2 and 11.2 months, respectively. The most common toxicities were fatigue, nausea, and vomiting (all grades: 85.7%, 83%, and 54.3%, resp.). Neither hypoalbuminaemia nor gender was found to predict toxicity, although encephalopathy predominantly affected females. *Conclusion.* Ifosfamide administered as a 14-day continuous infusion is a safe regimen in STS with notable activity in DDLPS.

1. Introduction

Soft-tissue sarcomas (STS) are a group of rare tumours of mesenchymal origin. They encompass more than 50 different malignancies with different molecular features, clinical behavior, and prognosis. With respect to systemic therapy the most active agents achieve response rates of approximately 20–30% or less depending on the series [1, 2] and the median overall survival (OS) of patients with metastatic disease is only around 1 year [3]. With such disappointing data, the implementation of new active therapeutic strategies is an imperative.

One specific subtype of STS, dedifferentiated liposarcoma (DDLPS), responds especially poorly to chemotherapy with no reliably effective treatment being identified to date [4]. These tumours most commonly occur in the retroperitoneum. Primary surgical resection, where technically possible, is the mainstay of treatment, often involving extensive surgical procedures in specialist units, with en bloc multivisceral resections [5]. On development of disease recurrence further surgical excision may be performed after taking into account the disease extent and time since primary surgery but until recently treatment options in multiply recurrent, inoperable, or metastatic disease have been limited [6].

Experience with standard sarcoma chemotherapy regimens such as doxorubicin has been disappointing, although activity has been reported with trabectedin [7]. This intrinsic drug resistance makes the prognosis of a patient with advanced DDLPS very poor.

Ifosfamide may be used in the treatment of STS given either as a single agent [8] or in combination with doxorubicin [9]. The most commonly used regimen is three daily divided doses with doses ranging from 2 to 4 g/m^2/day given as an inpatient over 4 hours. There is some evidence that a more prolonged infusion may have an improved cytotoxicity and tolerability profile although it is associated with worse urothelial toxicity compared with the three day infusion [10]. There is good stability data for the use of ifosfamide in disposable infusion pumps, used in the outpatient setting, and the longest stability data available is over a 9-day period [11–13]. Furthermore, continuous infusional ifosfamide is given in the outpatient setting and so is an attractive option to patients, lessening the impact on healthcare resources.

Since 2008, we have been using continuous infusional ifosfamide for patients with inoperable STS, especially DDLPS [13–15], at The Royal Marsden Hospital (United Kingdom).

This study assesses the toxicity and efficacy of infusional ifosfamide in all STS patients treated in our institution between September 2008 and December 2012.

2. Methods

2.1. Population. Clinical data from all STS patients who were treated with infusional ifosfamide in either the first or second line setting at The Royal Marsden Hospital from September 2008 to December 2012 were retrospectively collected. Cases were identified using the prospectively maintained Sarcoma Unit database and institutional ethical approval was obtained.

The patients all had histologically proven, inoperable, or metastatic progressing STS. Tumours were diagnosed according to the WHO Classification of Tumours of Soft Tissue and Bone [16]. The diagnosis of DDLPS was made where a pleomorphic component was found adjacent to well-differentiated liposarcoma or in intra-abdominal undifferentiated pleomorphic sarcomas that expressed Cyclin-Dependent Kinase 4 (CDK4) and p16 on immunohistochemistry and Mouse Double Minute 2 (MDM2) gene amplification using FISH. All patients were required to have adequate renal function as determined by either 24-hour creatinine clearance or EDTA, PS < 2, albumin > 30 g/L. The patients were treated with this infusional schedule because of histology, as there is some preliminary evidence to suggest activity in liposarcomas and synovial sarcoma.

2.2. Treatment. Continuous infusional ifosfamide was administered over 14 consecutive days in cycles of 28 days. The planned maximum number of cycles per patient was 6. Treatment was administered in an outpatient setting at a dose of 1000 mg/m^2/day utilising a Baxter LV1.5 ambulatory pump, filled to a volume of 255 mL. Each pump was designed to infuse over 7 days and contained 7000 mg/m^2 of ifosfamide. Mesna was also given to ameliorate urothelial toxicity. The total dose of mesna was equal to that of ifosfamide, either completely added to the pump or, depending on volume constraints, supplemented by oral tablets (rounded to the nearest measurable tablet). The oral dose of mesna was based on the assumption of a 2 : 1 oral to intravenous ratio. Patients attended hospital on day 8 for toxicity assessment and pump change. Every patient was given urine dipsticks and advised to test pH and blood with each void. Oral sodium bicarbonate 500 mg was used to alkalinise urine when urine dipstick showed pH < 6.5 and additional doses of mesna 1000 mg/m^2 were to be taken if blood was present in the urine. Patients were advised to drink at least 1.5 litres of fluids daily to ensure an adequate diuresis. Also, thiamine 100 mg three times daily (tds) was prescribed to try and prevent encephalopathy and metoclopramide 10 mg tds was advised to be taken as required for nausea. Dose reduction of 20% in both ifosfamide and mesna was applied if the patient experienced grade 3-4 toxicity or persistent grade 2 toxicity.

2.3. Toxicity and Efficacy Evaluation. Toxicities were recorded and graded according to Common Terminology Criteria for Adverse Events (CTCAE) version 4.0 [17].

Computerized tomography (CT) scanning of the thorax, abdomen, and pelvis was performed at baseline and subsequently after every 2 cycles of treatment. Response assessment was evaluated according to RECIST criteria v 1.1 [18] by a named Sarcoma Unit radiologist. In the cohort of patients affected by DDLPS, the target lesions were selected by focussing on the dense dedifferentiated component in the knowledge that these areas behave most aggressively and are what the chemotherapy targets. Disease control was defined as partial response (PR) rate and stable disease (SD) rate.

Progression-free survival (PFS) was defined from date of starting treatment to date of objective progressive disease (PD) or death from disease. Any surviving progression-free patients were censored at last followup. OS was defined from date of starting treatment to date of death from any cause and any surviving patients were censored at last followup. Kaplan-Meier methods were used to calculate OS and PFS and the inverse Kaplan-Meier method was used to calculate median followup. SPSS version 21.0 was used to summarise any descriptive statistics and to determine OS and PFS.

3. Results

3.1. Patient Characteristics. A total of 35 consecutive patients received at least one cycle of continuous infusional ifosfamide between September 2008 and December 2012. The median age of the patients was 53 years (range 27–76 years) and there was a slight preponderance of females (54.3%). The predominant histology subtype was DDLPS (62.8%), followed by synovial sarcoma (20%). Two-thirds of patients were chemonaive and one-quarter had received a priorifosfamide-containing regimen. More detailed demographics and baseline characteristics are summarised in Table 1.

3.2. Toxicity. The total number of cycles of treatment administered was 35, with a median of 2 cycles given per patient

TABLE 1: Patient characteristics.

Total	35
Age (median, range)	53 (27–76)
	n (%)
Sex	
Male	16 (45.7%)
Female	19 (54.3%)
ECOG performance status at baseline	
0	1 (2.8%)
1	30 (85.7%)
2	4 (11.4%)
Histology	
De-differentiated liposarcoma	22 (62.8%)
Synovial sarcoma	7 (20%)
Myxoid/round-cell liposarcoma	3 (8.5%)
Other	3 (8.5%)
Previous chemotherapy	
Chemotherapy naive	23 (65.7%)
Ifosfamide-containing regimen	9 (25.7%)
Nonifosfamide-containing regimen	3 (8.5%)
Previous surgery	
Yes	23 (65.7%)
No	12 (34.3%)
Baseline creatinine clearance (Cockroft-Gault formula)	
Median	97 mL/min (51.9–215.8)
Baseline albumin	
Median	35 g/L (21–43)

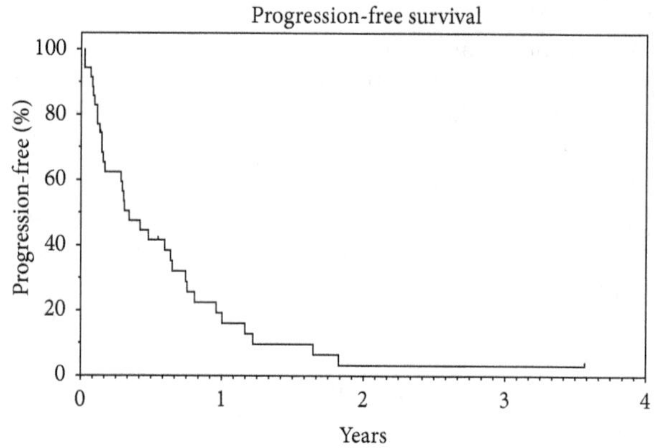

FIGURE 1: Median PFS: 4.2 months (95% CI: 2.0–6.3). PFS rate at 1 year: 19.2%. Median followup: 6.7 months.

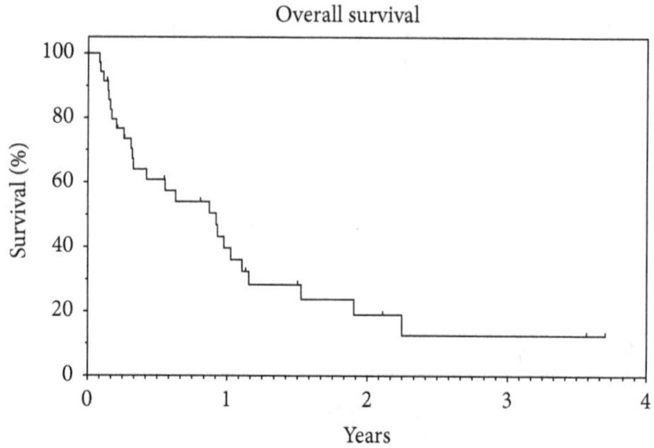

FIGURE 2: Median OS: 11.2 months (95% CI: 5.7–16.7). OS rate at 1 year: 39.6%. Median followup: 11.8 months.

TABLE 2: Toxicity—number of patients.

Toxicity	Grade 1-2	Grade 3-4	Total
Fatigue	28 (80%)	2 (5.7%)	30 (85.7%)
Nausea	24 (68.6%)	5 (14.3%)	29 (83%)
Vomiting	16 (45.7%)	3 (8.6%)	19 (54.3%)
Myelosuppression	14 (40%)	2 (5.7%)	16 (45.7%)
Encephalopathy	6 (17.1%)	6 (17.1%)	12 (34.2%)
Constipation	10 (28.6%)	0	10 (28.6%)
Diarrhoea	4 (11.4%)	2 (5.7%)	6 (17.1%)
Renal function impairment	5 (14.3%)	0	5 (14.3%)
Liver function tests alteration	1 (2.8%)	0	1 (2.8%)

(range 1–9). Twenty-six patients (74%) had to stop treatment early, while 9 patients (26%) reached 6 cycles. Among the patients who stopped treatment early, toxicity was the cause in 11 cases (42%), while 15 patients (58%) discontinued treatment due to disease progression. Dose reductions were necessary in 8 patients (22.8%) and 5 patients (14.3%) received only 1 cycle due to toxicity: grade 3-4 encephalopathy in 4 patients and 1 patient with gastrointestinal toxicity resulting in acute renal impairment secondary to dehydration.

All patients had toxicities attributable to the regimen. However, most side effects were mild (grade 1 or 2) and the majority of toxicities reported occurred from day 3 to day 12. The most common toxicities were fatigue (all grades, 85.7%), nausea (all grades, 83%), and vomiting (all grades, 54.3%).

For this regimen the most significant toxicity was encephalopathy with 12 patients (34.2%) having clinically significant symptoms, grade 3-4 in 6 patients. This led to discontinuation of treatment for 4 of these patients. Interestingly, all but one episode of encephalopathy occurred during the first treatment period. There is no data regarding the compliance of patients with the use of thiamine during treatment. There was one death in this cohort of patients, due to neutropenic sepsis; however overall myelotoxicity was acceptable with only 2 episodes of grade 3-4 myelosuppression for all cycles reported. Urothelial toxicity is an established toxicity for ifosfamide, with some reports suggesting prolonged infusions may increase this risk, but there was no significant urothelial toxicity seen, with no episodes of frank haematuria recorded. Renal toxicity was also mild with only 5 patients (14.3%) developing reversible grade 1-2 renal impairment. The toxicity data are summarized in Table 2.

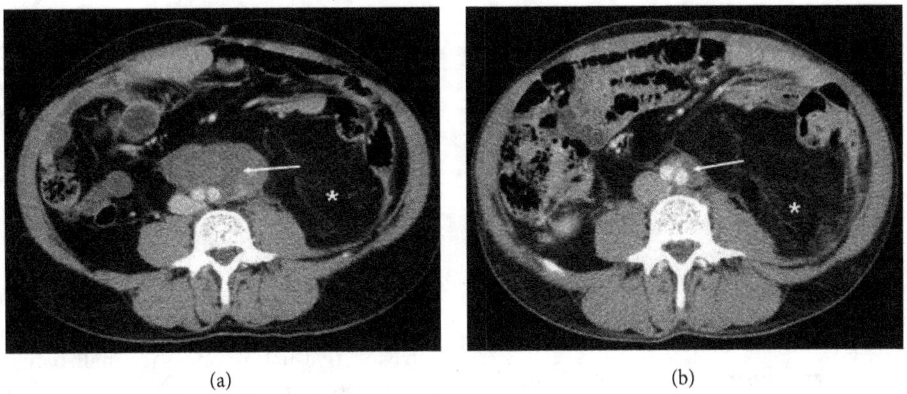

FIGURE 3: Axial contrast enhanced CT images of the abdomen in a 63-year-old male with retroperitoneal liposarcoma at baseline (a) and following 5 months therapy (b). Although the well-differentiated component filling the left side of the retroperitoneum (∗) showed little change, the dedifferentiated component (arrows) surrounding the aortic bifurcation reduced in size from 7.9 cm to 2.5 cm (PR).

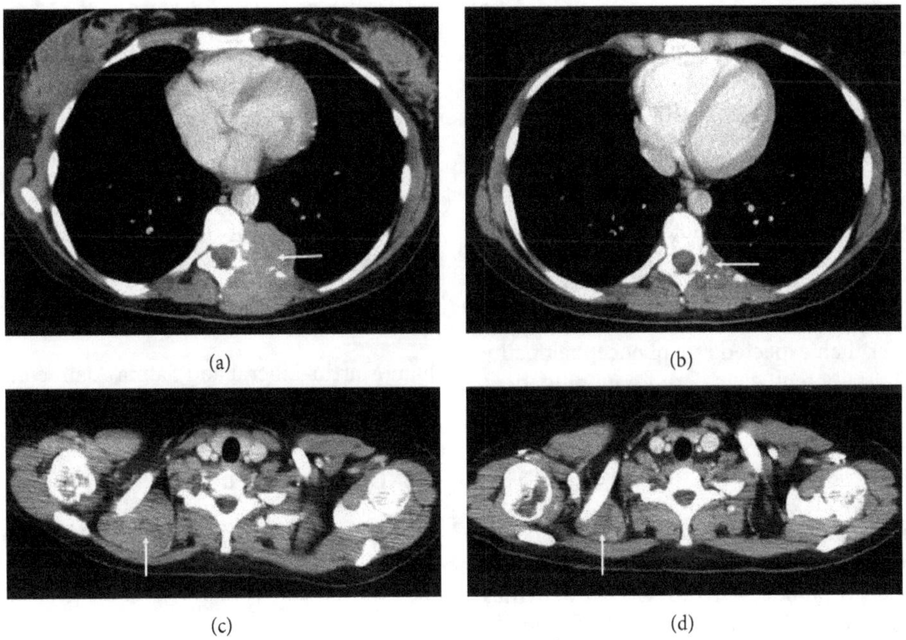

FIGURE 4: Axial contrast enhanced CT images of the lower and upper thorax in a 37-year-old female with metastatic synovial sarcoma at baseline ((a) and (c)) and following 2-month therapy ((b) and (d)). The 5.6 cm left sided paravertebral mass which was causing destruction of the posterior rib ((a), arrow) showed a dramatic reduction in size with only a thin plaque of indeterminate low attenuation tissue remaining at this site ((b), arrow). A further site of disease behind the right clavicle ((b), arrow) reduced in size from 6.5 cm to 3.6 cm ((d), arrow).

Patient baseline demographics, renal function, and albumen level were analysed as potential predictors for toxicity, in particular encephalopathy, as this may allow for the identification of patients for whom a dose reduction may be useful in lessening the risk of developing significant encephalopathy. In this cohort baseline renal function, albumen, and gender were not statistically significant predictors for toxicity. Grade 3-4 encephalopathy did occur more frequently in females (5 versus 1 male) but due to sample size was not statistically significant.

3.3. *Efficacy.* Overall, 7 patients (20%) achieved PR and 10 patients (29%) achieved SD, in 7 cases lasting for more than 24 weeks. The median duration of response was 7 months (range 4–14) and the median duration of disease control (PR + SD) was 8.5 months (range 4–22). PD as best response was reported in 14 patients (40%), with 9 of these patients progressing during the first cycle of treatment. Among the patients that had previously received an ifosfamide-containing regimen, 1 SD and 2 PR were observed. Four patients had incomplete radiology for response assessment.

DDLPS proved to have particular sensitivity to the treatment: PR was seen in 5 out of 22 patients (22.7%) and 7 patients (31.8%) achieved SD, 5 of them (71.4%) for more than 24 weeks. In total, the disease control rate in this cohort was 54.5%. Activity was also seen in the synovial sarcoma cohort with 2 out of 7 patients achieving PR (28.6%) and a further patient had SD for 20 weeks. Amongst the other subtypes, 1 patient with myxoid liposarcoma out of 3 demonstrated SD and further disease stabilization was seen in 1 patient with pleomorphic sarcoma.

In terms of survival, median PFS was 4.2 months (95% CI: 2.0–6.3) and PFS rate at 1 year was 19.2% with a median followup of 6.7 months (Figure 1). The median OS was 11.2 months (95% CI: 5.7–16.7) and 1 year OS rate was 39.6% with a median followup of 11.8 months (Figure 2). In the DDLPS cohort, median PFS was 3.7 months (95% CI: 0.0–7.8) and median OS was 10.5 months (95% CI: 3.3–17.6) with a median followup of 25.3 months.

Radiological responses are illustrated in Figures 3 and 4.

4. Discussion

Our report demonstrates that ifosfamide administered as a 14-day continuous infusion is a safe outpatient regimen for STS. The majority of toxicities observed were mild and easily manageable and usually appeared within the first few days of treatment, allowing early intervention with effective symptomatic treatment. Haematuria did not appear to be a significant toxicity with this regimen and the rate of clinically significant neutropenia was acceptable. Moreover, this regimen has also the advantage of not requiring planned inpatient hospital admission. This has a direct impact on the quality of life of patients, especially important as this treatment regimen is usually given in the palliative setting.

There was a higher than expected rate of encephalopathy in our cohort, which is a potential concern for an outpatient regimen. Although not statistically significant, we found that female gender was a predictor for developing encephalopathy. One possible explanation might be the intrinsic pharmacokinetic difference between genders. An increased CYP3A4 expression in females may explain the differences in sex-dependent drug clearance [19]. These differences had no consequences on the ifosfamide 4-hydroxylation activities of liver microsomes *in vitro*. In contrast, in the ifosfamide N-dechloroethylation reaction, a statistically significant difference between the liver microsomes of male and female patients was found [20]. The relative greater production of chloroacetaldehyde in the female liver might explain the relative increase in neurotoxicity observed. Whatever the reason, delivery of cycle one at a lower dose (for instance, 750 mg/m^2/day) and dose escalation should be taken into consideration if treatment is tolerated in female patients, given the increased risk of encephalopathy observed. Interestingly, this toxicity profile differs from the one previously reported by Meazza et al. [12]. In their paediatric population, only 4 out of 14 patients experienced mild nausea, and antiemetic prophylaxis was required in only a minority of patients. Moreover, no neurological or renal toxicity was observed, which illustrates the different tolerance to this treatment in adults.

Our regimen also showed evidence of antitumour activity, particularly in DDLPS, synovial sarcoma, and myxoid/round-cell liposarcoma. Synovial sarcoma is known to be particularly sensitive to ifosfamide, even upon rechallenge [21]. In contrast, DDLPS is not sensitive to conventional chemotherapy, although trabectedin has shown some activity [7]. Investigational novel drugs such as inhibitors of MDM2 or CDK4 have recently been assessed in this histological subtype with encouraging results [22, 23]. Our efficacy data show that infusional ifosfamide might be a treatment option especially in DDLPS, with a disease control rate of 54.5% in patients with confirmed PD prior to starting treatment.

In conclusion, our data suggest that infusional ifosfamide is a feasible schedule in STS. However, due to the retrospective nature and the small patient numbers of our report, prospective validation is clearly required. The European Organization for Research and Treatment of Cancer (EORTC) is planning to conduct a prospective randomized phase II trial that will compare infusional ifosfamide with cabazitaxel in patients affected by DDLPS. This study will hopefully provide us with more reliable information in a near future.

5. Conclusions

Infusional ifosfamide is a safe treatment in STS, with notable activity in dedifferentiated liposarcoma. This regimen deserves further investigation.

Authors' Contribution

Juan Martin-Liberal and Salma Alam contributed equally in this paper.

Acknowledgment

The authors acknowledge support from the NIHR RM/ICR Biomedical Research Centre.

References

[1] M. van Glabbeke, A. T. Van Oosterom, J. W. Oosterhuis et al., "Prognostic factors for the outcome of chemotherapy in advanced soft tissue sarcoma: an analysis of 2,185 patients treated with anthracycline- containing first-line regimens—a European organization for research and treatment of cancer soft tissue and bone sarcoma group study," *Journal of Clinical Oncology*, vol. 17, no. 1, pp. 150–157, 1999.

[2] A. T. van Oosterom, H. T. Mouridsen, O. S. Nielsen et al., "Results of randomised studies of the EORTC Soft Tissue and Bone Sarcoma Group (STBSG) with two different ifosfamide regimens in first- and second-line chemotherapy in advanced soft tissue sarcoma patients," *European Journal of Cancer*, vol. 38, no. 18, pp. 2397–2406, 2002.

[3] M. Leahy, X. Garcia Del Muro, P. Reichardt, I. Judson, A. Staddon, and J. Verweij, "Chemotherapy treatment patterns and clinical outcomes in patients with metastatic soft tissue sarcoma. The SArcoma treatment and Burden of Illness in North America and Europe (SABINE) study," *Annals of Oncology*, vol. 23, no. 10, pp. 2763–2770, 2012.

[4] R. L. Jones, C. Fisher, O. Al-Muderis, and I. R. Judson, "Differential sensitivity of liposarcoma subtypes to chemotherapy," *European Journal of Cancer*, vol. 41, no. 18, pp. 2853–2860, 2005.

[5] S. J. Neuhaus, P. Barry, M. A. Clark, A. J. Hayes, C. Fisher, and J. M. Thomas, "Surgical management of primary recurrent liposarcoma," *British Journal of Surgery*, vol. 92, no. 2, pp. 246–252, 2005.

[6] A. M. Crago and S. Singer, "Clinical and molecular approaches to well differentiated and dedifferentiated liposarcoma," *Current Opinion in Oncology*, vol. 23, no. 4, pp. 373–378, 2011.

[7] B. L. Samuels, S. Chawla, S. Patel, M. von Mehren, J. Hamm, and P. E. Kaiser, "Clinical outcomes and safety with trabectedin therapy in patients with advanced soft tissue sarcomas following failure of prior chemotherapy: results of a worldwide expanded access program study," *Annals of Oncology*, vol. 24, no. 6, pp. 1703–1709, 2013.

[8] S. Sleijfer, M. Ouali, M. van Glabbeke et al., "Prognostic and predictive factors for outcome to first-line ifosfamide-containing chemotherapy for adult patients with advanced soft tissue sarcomas. An exploratory, retrospective analysis on large series from the European Organization for Research and Treatment of Cancer-Soft Tissue and Bone Sarcoma Group (EORTC-STBSG)," *European Journal of Cancer*, vol. 46, no. 1, pp. 72–83, 2010.

[9] I. Judson, W. van der Graaf, J. Verweij et al., "Results of a randomised phase III trial (EORTC 2012) of single agent doxorubicin versus doxorubicin plus ifosfamide as first line chemotherapy for patients with advanced or metastatic soft tissue sarcoma: a survival study by the EORTC Soft Tissue and Bone Sarcoma Group [Abstract LBA7]," in *Proceedings of the ESMO Annual Meeting*.

[10] P. Lorigan, J. Verweij, Z. Papai et al., "Phase III trial of two investigational schedules of ifosfamide compared with standard-dose doxorubicin in advanced or metastatic soft tissue sarcoma: a European Organisation for Research and Treatment of Cancer Soft Tissue and Bone Sarcoma Group study," *Journal of Clinical Oncology*, vol. 25, no. 21, pp. 3144–3150, 2007.

[11] A. V. Boddy, S. M. Yule, R. Wyllie, L. Price, A. D. J. Pearson, and J. R. Idle, "Pharmacokinetics and metabolism of ifosfamide administered as a continuous infusion in children," *Cancer Research*, vol. 53, no. 16, pp. 3758–3764, 1993.

[12] C. Meazza, M. Casanova, R. Luksch et al., "Prolonged 14-day continuous infusion of high-dose ifosfamide with an external portable pump: feasibility and efficacy in refractory pediatric sarcoma," *Pediatric Blood and Cancer*, vol. 55, no. 4, pp. 617–620, 2010.

[13] J. A. Radford, J. M. Margison, R. Swindell, M. J. Lind, P. M. Wilkinson, and N. Thatcher, "The stability of ifosfamide in aqueous solution and its suitability for continuous 7-day infusion by ambulatory pump," *Journal of Cancer Research and Clinical Oncology*, vol. 117, no. 4, pp. 154–156, 1991.

[14] R. S. Benjamin, S. S. Legha, S. R. Patel, and C. Nicaise, "Single-agent ifosfamide studies in sarcomas of soft tissue and bone. The M.D. Anderson Experience," *Cancer Chemotherapy and Pharmacology*, vol. 31, supplement, no. 2, pp. S174–S179, 1993.

[15] L. Leone, A. Comandone, C. Oliva et al., "Stability of ifosfamide in solutions for multiday infusion by external pump," *Anti-Cancer Drugs*, vol. 6, no. 4, pp. 604–607, 1995.

[16] C. D. Fletcher and F. Mertens, Eds., *WHO Classification of Tumour: Pathology and Genetics of Tumours of Soft Tissue and Bone*, IARC Press, Lyon, France, 2002.

[17] http://evs.nci.nih.gov/ftp1/CTCAE/CTCAE_4.03_2010-06-14_QuickReference_5x7.pdf.

[18] E. A. Eisenhauer, P. Therasse, J. Bogaerts et al., "New response evaluation criteria in solid tumours: revised RECIST guideline (version 1.1)," *European Journal of Cancer*, vol. 45, no. 2, pp. 228–247, 2009.

[19] R. Wolbold, K. Klein, O. Burk et al., "Sex is a major determinant of CYP3A4 expression in human liver," *Hepatology*, vol. 38, no. 4, pp. 978–988, 2003.

[20] R. Schmidt, F. Baumann, H. Hanschmann, F. Geissler, and R. Preiss, "Gender difference in ifosfamide metabolism by human liver microsomes," *European Journal of Drug Metabolism and Pharmacokinetics*, vol. 26, no. 3, pp. 193–200, 2001.

[21] A. Constantinidou and R. L. Jones, "Ifosfamide re-challenge in soft-tissue sarcoma," in *Proceedings of the 16th Annual Meeting Connective Tissue Oncology Society (CTOS '10)*, 2010.

[22] I. Ray-Coquard, J. Y. Blay, A. Italiano, A. Le Cesne, N. Penel, and J. Zhi, "Effect of the MDM2 antagonist RG7112 on the P53 pathway in patients with MDM2-amplified, well-differentiated or dedifferentiated liposarcoma: an exploratory proof-of-mechanism study," *The Lancet Oncology*, vol. 13, no. 11, pp. 1133–1140, 2012.

[23] M. A. Dickson, W. D. Tap, M. L. Keohan et al., "Phase II trial of the CDK4 inhibitor PD0332991 in patients with advanced CDK4-amplified well-differentiated or dedifferentiated liposarcoma," *Journal of Clinical Oncology*, vol. 31, no. 16, pp. 2024–2028, 2013.

10

Cost-Effectiveness of Pazopanib in Advanced Soft Tissue Sarcoma in the United Kingdom

Jordan Amdahl,[1] Stephanie C. Manson,[2] Robert Isbell,[2] Ayman Chit,[3,4] Jose Diaz,[2] Lily Lewis,[5] and Thomas E. Delea[1]

[1] *Policy Analysis Inc. (PAI), Four Davis Court, Brookline, MA 02445, USA*
[2] *GlaxoSmithKline, Stockley Park West, Uxbridge, Middlesex UB11 1BT, UK*
[3] *GlaxoSmithKline, 7333 Mississauga Road, Mississauga, ON, Canada L5N 6L4*
[4] *University of Toronto, 144 College Street, Toronto, ON, Canada M5S 3M2*
[5] *York Health Economics Consortium, Level 2, Market Square, University of York, Heslington, York YO10 5NH, UK*

Correspondence should be addressed to Thomas E. Delea; tdelea@pai2.com

Academic Editor: Antoine Italiano

In the phase III PALETTE trial, pazopanib improved progression-free survival (PFS) compared with placebo in patients with advanced/metastatic soft tissue sarcomas (mSTS) who had received prior chemotherapy. We used a multistate model to estimate expected PFS, overall survival (OS), lifetime STS treatment costs, and quality-adjusted life-years (QALYs) for patients receiving pazopanib, placebo, trabectedin, ifosfamide, or gemcitabine plus docetaxel as second-line mSTS therapies. The cost-effectiveness of pazopanib was expressed as the incremental costs per QALY gained. Estimates of PFS/OS, adverse events, and utilities for pazopanib and placebo were from the PALETTE trial. Estimates of relative effectiveness of the other comparators were from an unadjusted indirect comparison versus pazopanib. Costs were from published sources. Pazopanib is estimated to increase QALYs by 0.128 and costs by £7,976 versus placebo; cost per QALY gained with pazopanib versus placebo is estimated to be £62,000. Compared with the other chemotherapies, pazopanib provides similar QALYs at a lower cost. Pazopanib may not be cost-effective versus placebo but may be cost-effective versus the most commonly used active treatments, although this conclusion is uncertain. Given the unmet need for effective treatments for mSTS, pazopanib may be an appropriate alternative to some currently used medications in the United Kingdom.

1. Introduction

Soft tissue sarcomas (STS) are a rare group of solid tumors originating from mesenchymal cells and their precursors. STS includes more than 50 histological subtypes but accounts for less than 1% of all new malignancies in adults and approximately 2% of total cancer-related mortality [1, 2]. In 2010, 3,272 persons in the United Kingdom (UK) were diagnosed with cancer of connective and soft tissue [3].

Surgery, often combined with radiation therapy, offers the only potential cure for localized STS; however, approximately one-half of all patients with STS eventually develop local recurrence or metastases following surgery, radiotherapy, or both [4, 5]. Advanced STS is typically treated with palliative chemotherapy, and the median overall survival (OS) from the time metastases are found is 14 months [6].

Doxorubicin, alone or combined with ifosfamide, is the standard of care for first-line treatment of STS [5, 7, 8]. Although there is no standard of care following first-line chemotherapy, treatments recommended as second-line therapy by the British Sarcoma Group and the European Society for Medical Oncology are trabectedin, ifosfamide, gemcitabine plus docetaxel, taxanes (including docetaxel), gemcitabine, and dacarbazine [5, 7, 8]. Results from the Sarcoma Treatment and Burden of Illness in North America and Europe (SABINE) trial, a retrospective chart review of patients with metastatic STS, reported that gemcitabine plus docetaxel was the most frequently used second-line therapy, followed by ifosfamide monotherapy. Trabectedin was the most frequently used third-line therapy, followed by investigational drugs [9]. Current UK treatment guidelines recommend treatment with trabectedin, gemcitabine, gemcitabine plus docetaxel, or ifosfamide for patients who fail initial chemotherapy with doxorubicin-based therapy [5, 7].

Pazopanib (GW786034, Votrient, GlaxoSmithKline, Research Triangle Park, NC, USA), a multiple tyrosine kinase inhibitor, is approved for use in the United States, Canada, and the European Union for the treatment of advanced (unresectable and/or metastatic) STS (aSTS) in patients who have received prior chemotherapy [10–12]. Pazopanib was investigated in the PALETTE trial (ClinicalTrials.gov identifier: NCT00753688), a randomized, phase III investigation of pazopanib versus placebo in 369 patients with aSTS who had received prior chemotherapy [12]. Results of the PALETTE trial showed pazopanib improved progression-free survival (PFS) versus placebo (median 4.6 versus 1.6 months, resp.; hazard ratio [HR], 0.35; 95% confidence interval [CI], 0.26–0.48; $P < 0.001$) [10]. Median OS, a secondary objective of the trial, was 12.6 versus 10.7 months, respectively (HR, 0.87; 95% CI, 0.67–1.12; $P = 0.26$) [10]. However, posttreatment anticancer therapy (PTACT) was received by 62% in the placebo group compared with 45% in the pazopanib group at the data cutoff date [12], which may have diluted the survival benefit of pazopanib. Patients in the pazopanib arm were more likely to experience at least one on-therapy adverse event (AE) (99% versus 89%) and at least one serious AE (SAE) (41% versus 24%) compared with patients in the placebo arm [13]. The most frequently reported on-treatment AEs in the pazopanib group included fatigue, diarrhea, nausea, decreased weight, hypertension, and decreased appetite.

The primary objective of this study was to evaluate the cost-effectiveness of pazopanib versus best supportive care (BSC) from a UK healthcare system perspective when used in patients with aSTS who have received prior anthracycline-based chemotherapy.

2. Methods

2.1. Model Description. A multistate model was used to estimate expected PFS, OS, lifetime costs of treatment of aSTS, and quality-adjusted life-years (QALYs) in patients who had received prior treatment with chemotherapy and who were assumed to receive pazopanib, placebo, or chemotherapy. The model was developed in Microsoft Excel (Microsoft Corporation, Redmond, WA, USA).

Consistent with the modeling approach used in a multitude of other evaluations of treatments for advanced oncology indications [14–16], patients in the model were assumed to be in one of three mutually exclusive heath states at any given time: alive with no progression (PFS), alive with disease progression (postprogression survival [PPS]), or dead. The model was designed to permit two alternative approaches to estimate the proportion of patients in each health state over time. With the "partitioned-survival analysis" approach, survival distributions for PFS and OS were entered into the model, and the proportion of patients in the PPS state was calculated as the difference between OS and PFS. Alternatively, with the "Markov cohort analysis" approach, survival distributions for PFS and PPS were entered into the model, along with the estimated proportion of PFS events that are deaths. Transition probabilities were then derived from these inputs and combined to calculate the survival distribution for OS. With both approaches, expected costs and QALYs for each strategy were calculated as the product of the expected PFS and PPS and corresponding cost and utility value estimates for pre- and postprogression survival time, adjusted for "one-off" decrements in costs and quality of life associated with treatment initiation, AEs, progression, and death.

Expected lifetime outcomes and costs were evaluated over a 10-year timeframe, approximating a lifetime projection for patients with aSTS (i.e., virtually all patients were projected to be dead after 10 years). The model periodicity (i.e., the minimum duration of time a patient might remain in any disease state) was one week. Effectiveness measures were calculated on a discounted and undiscounted basis; costs were calculated on a discounted basis only. A 3.5% annual discount rate was employed beginning at the end of the first year of the model [17]. A UK healthcare system perspective was employed.

The primary analysis focused on direct comparisons of pazopanib versus BSC. In this analysis, data on PFS and OS for placebo patients from PALETTE were used without any adjustment of OS for the differential receipt of PTACT in the two groups. Utilization (and therefore costs) of PTACT was assumed to differ between groups as observed in PALETTE. For this analysis, the partitioned-survival analysis modeling approach was employed (i.e., the model took as inputs the distribution of OS rather than the distribution of PPS).

In a secondary analysis, pazopanib was compared with trabectedin (1.5 mg/m^2), ifosfamide (3 g/m^2), and gemcitabine plus docetaxel (900 mg/m^2, 100 mg/m^2). These therapies were the most relevant chemotherapy comparators in the UK based on treatment patterns reported in the SABINE study and consultation with clinical experts. In this analysis, a Markov cohort approach was employed, and it was assumed that PPS and PTACT utilization and costs would be the same for chemotherapy and pazopanib. Because PPS was assumed to be the same for pazopanib and chemotherapy, the difference between treatment strategies in mean OS was assumed to be equal to the difference in PFS (i.e., the benefits in PFS for pazopanib were assumed to translate directly to benefits of equal magnitude in OS). This approach was used because there was insufficient data from controlled trials to conduct robust adjusted indirect treatment comparisons of PFS and OS [18]. Accordingly, these comparisons were based on naive or unadjusted indirect comparisons. Because data on OS is more likely to be impacted by differences in patient populations and trial design than data on PFS, it was believed that the comparisons would be more reliable if based on PFS alone rather than PFS and OS. Also, there is no reason to believe that PPS would be different for patients receiving pazopanib versus chemotherapy.

TABLE 1: Survival distribution inputs.

	Pazopanib	Placebo	Reference
Weibull survival function parameters			
PFS (months)			
Lambda	0.1279	0.3714	PALETTE
Gamma	1.1252	1.0809	PALETTE
OS (months)			
Lambda	0.0282	0.0469	PALETTE
Gamma	1.2341	1.1027	PALETTE
PPS (months)			
Lambda	0.104	0.118	PALETTE
Gamma	0.902	0.898	PALETTE
Probability of death without disease progression (required for Markov cohort model)[a]	0.053	0	PALETTE
HR for PFS for pazopanib versus comparator			
Ifosfamide	0.91 (95% CI, 0.73–1.14)		Sharma et al. 2013 [18] van Oosterom et al. 2002 [43]
Trabectedin	0.90 (95% CI, 0.76–1.07)		Sharma et al. 2013 [18] Demetri et al. 2009 [44] Garcia-Carbonero et al. 2005 [45] le Cesne et al. 2005 [46] Yovine et al. 2004 [47]
Gemcitabine + docetaxel	0.99 (95% CI, 0.70–1.40)		Sharma et al. 2013 [18] Hensley et al. 2008 [48] Pautier et al. 2012 [33]

CI: confidence interval; HR: hazard ratio; OS: overall survival; PFS: progression-free survival; PPS: postprogression survival.
[a]Same value was assumed for chemotherapies in indirect comparison.

2.2. Model Estimation. A summary of model inputs can be found in Table 1. PFS, OS, and PPS were estimated for pazopanib and placebo by fitting parametric survival functions to patient-level data from PALETTE using accelerated failure time regression (Figure 1) [19]. Investigator-assessed PFS (including clinical progression) was used as it was considered most likely to reflect PFS in clinical practice. OS was based on intent-to-treat analyses. Survival distributions for pazopanib and placebo were estimated independently. Exponential, Weibull, and log-logistic models were considered. Based on visual inspection and comparison of the restricted mean (i.e., area under the curve) for the empirical versus fitted distributions, the Weibull distribution provided the best fit for all distributions and was used in base-case analyses. Because the OS distribution for pazopanib derived from the PFS and PPS distributions in the Markov cohort analysis approach did not match the tail end of the empirical OS distribution well, the parameters of the PPS Weibull distribution were adjusted by calibrating the parameters of the distribution to minimize the differences between the model projections of expected OS and those obtained from the Weibull distribution fit to OS directly.

PFS for the other comparators was estimated by applying to the estimated PFS distribution for pazopanib estimates of the HRs for these treatments versus pazopanib using the formula

$$PFS_{Comparator}[t] = PFS_{Pazopanib}[t]^{HR_{Comparator\ versus\ Pazopanib}}. \quad (1)$$

HRs for PFS for each comparator versus pazopanib were estimated using data from published studies of the comparators of interest that were identified based on a systematic review of the literature (Table 2). HRs were calculated by comparing the published Kaplan-Meier curves for PFS (or time to progression if PFS was unavailable) for the comparator(s) of interest in each study with the Kaplan-Meier PFS curve for pazopanib from PALETTE [20].

In PALETTE, the EuroQol 5-dimension (EQ-5D) health questionnaire was assessed only at baseline and at 4 weeks, whereas the European Organization for Research and Treatment of Cancer Quality of Life Questionnaire (EORTC QLQ-C30) was also assessed at 8 and 12 weeks [12, 13]. Therefore, a mapping algorithm was developed using data for the EQ-5D and QLQ-C30 at baseline and four weeks to predict EQ-5D utility values at 8 and 12 weeks given the responses to the EORTC QLQ-C30 at those later assessments [21]. The observed and mapped utility values were then combined to calculate mean utility values for each group for all pre- and postprogression assessments. Because the mean time from progression to postprogression utility assessment in PALETTE was only approximately one week in both groups, the mean differences in utility post- versus preprogression from PALETTE reflect declines in utility values immediately following progression only and do not reflect the declines in utility that would be expected over the entire postprogression period [22–25]. Accordingly, postprogression utility values for pazopanib and placebo were obtained by combining

TABLE 2: Studies used in indirect treatment comparison of progression-free survival.

Study	Design	Treatment	Control	Number of patients		Population	Outcomes assessed		
				Treatment	Control		TTP	PFS	OS
van der Graaf et al. 2012 [12]	Phase III RCT	Pazopanib 800 mg 1q1d	Placebo	246	123	Intermediate-/high-grade malignant STS excluding GIST and adipocytic subtypes, WHO PS 0/1, ≤4 prior systemic therapies for advanced disease and ≤2 combination regimens, age 18–83 y	No	Yes IRC and INV	Yes
Demetri et al. 2009 [44]	Phase II RCT	Trabectedin 1.5 mg/m^2 1q3w 24 h	Trabectedin 0.58 mg/m^2 1q1w 3 h	136	134	Unresectable and/or metastatic liposarcoma or LMS, ECOG PS 0/1, ≤2 prior cytotoxic regimens, age 20–80 y	IRC and INV	IRC, but KM curve not reported	Yes
Garcia-Carbonero et al. 2005 [45]	Phase II nonrandomized trial	Trabectedin 1.5 mg/m^2 1q3w 24 h		36		Histologically confirmed recurrent or metastatic STS with disease progression despite prior CT with ≤2 prior regimens for advanced disease, ECOG PS ≤ 1, age ≥ 18 y	Yes	No	Yes
le Cesne et al. 2005 [46]	Phase II nonrandomized trial	Trabectedin 1.5 mg/m^2 1q3w 24 h		104		Bidimensionally measurable metastatic or unresectable locoregional recurrent histologically proven advanced STS, ≥1 prior AC-based CT (±ifosfamide), PS ≤ 2, age < 75 y	Yes	No	Yes
Yovine et al. 2004 [47]	Phase II nonrandomized trial	Trabectedin 1.5 mg/m^2 1q3w 24 h		54		Advanced or metastatic, histologically proven STS, previous treatment with at least one line of either single-agent or combination CT, WHO PS ≤ 1, age ≥ 18 y	Yes	No	Yes
van Oosterom et al. 2002 [43]	Phase II RCT	Ifosfamide 5 g/m^2 × 1q3w	Ifosfamide 3 g/m^2 × 3q3w	36	40	Locally recurrent STS not amenable to treatment or metastatic STS, WHO PS 0–2, age 22–75 y	Yes	No	Yes
Hensley et al. 2008 [48]	Phase II nonrandomized trial	Gemcitabine 900 mg/m^2 2q3w + DOC 100 mg/m^2 1q3w		48		Women with advanced or recurrent uterine LMS progressed after 1 cytotoxic regimen, no prior therapy with gemcitabine or DOC, GOG PS 0–2	Yes	No	Yes
Pautier et al. 2012 [33]	Phase II RCT	Gemcitabine 900 mg/m^2 2q3w + DOC 100 mg/m^2 1q3w	Gemcitabine 1,000 mg/m^2 3q4w	69	52	Metastatic or unresectable LMS, PS ≤ 2, ≥1 prior AC-based regimen, age 41–80 y	No	Yes	Yes

AC: anthracycline; CT: chemotherapy; DOC: docetaxel; ECOG: Eastern Cooperative Oncology Group; GIST: gastrointestinal stroma tumor; GOG: Gynecologic Oncology Group; INV: investigator; IRC: institutional review committee; KM: Kaplan-Meier; LMS: leiomyosarcoma; OS: overall survival; PFS: progression-free survival; PS: performance status; RCT: randomized clinical trial; STS: soft tissue sarcoma; TTP: time to progression; WHO: World Health Organization.

TABLE 3: Utility values used in the model.

	Mean (SE)	Source
Utility values for PFS and PPS, mean (SE)		
Preprogression		
Pazopanib	0.674 (0.015)	PALETTE
Placebo	0.678 (0.024)	PALETTE
Postprogression		
Pazopanib	0.568 (0.044)	PALETTE
Placebo	0.636 (0.040)	PALETTE
Estimated disutility values for AEs (SE)		
Alopecia	0.045 (0.015)	Nafees et al. 2008 [27]
Anemia/hemoglobin	0.119 (0.023)	Swinburn et al. 2010 [28]
Asthenia/fatigue	0.262 (0.027)	Shingler et al. 2013 [26]
Cardiovascular (cardiac toxicity/left ventricular dysfunction)	0.2 (0)	Assumption
Decreased appetite/anorexia/weight decreased	0.2 (0)	Assumption
Diarrhea	0.327 (0.028)	Shingler et al. 2013 [26]
Edema	0.2 (0)	Assumption
Febrile neutropenia	0.09 (0.016)	Nafees et al. 2008 [27]
Leucopoenia/neutropenia/neutrophils/thrombocytopenia/low platelets	0.09 (0.015)	Nafees et al. 2008 [27]
Liver toxicity (ALT/AST elevation)	0	Assumption
Hypertension	0.153 (0.024)	Swinburn et al. 2010 [28]
Myalgia/muscle pain/neurotoxicity/peripheral sensory neuropathy	0.236 (0.025)	Shingler et al. 2013 [26]
Nausea/vomiting	0.357 (0.026)	Shingler et al. 2013 [26]
Pulmonary (dyspnea/pleural effusion/pneumothorax/pulmonary toxicity)	0.242 (0.026)	Shingler et al. 2013 [26]

AEs: adverse events; ALT: alanine aminotransferase; AST: aspartate aminotransferase; HR: hazard ratio; OS: overall survival; PFS: progression-free survival; PPS: postprogression survival; SE: standard error.

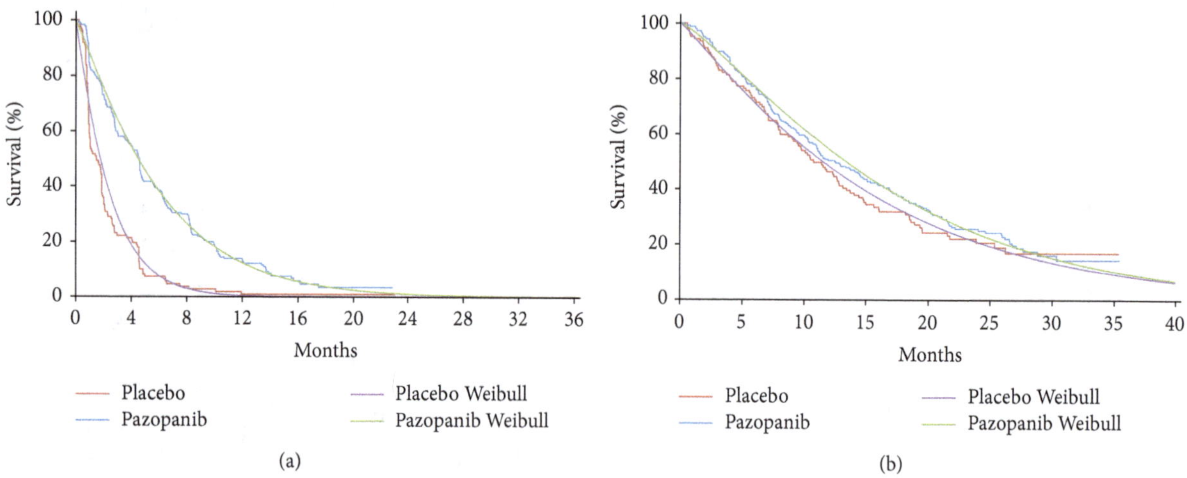

FIGURE 1: Weibull versus Kaplan-Meier survival distributions for (a) progression-free survival and (b) overall survival of pazopanib and placebo for patients in the PALETTE trial.

treatment group-specific estimates of the mean decrement in utility postprogression in PALETTE (reflecting the period immediately following progression) with an estimate of utility in the terminal phase of the disease. The latter was based on the estimated utility value for progressive disease from a vignettes study by Shingler and colleagues (mean [standard error], 0.263 [0.0231]) [26]. For the comparisons of pazopanib with chemotherapies, QALYs were adjusted for differences between treatments in the incidence of AEs using data on the incidence of AEs from PALETTE and the studies of chemotherapies noted above as well as disutility values for AEs that were obtained from published vignettes studies [26–28]. Utility values used in the model are reported in Table 3.

TABLE 4: Cost estimates used in the model.

Estimate	Costs, £	Reference
Medications unit costs		
Pazopanib, 200 mg tablet (no discount)	18.68	British National Formulary [32]
Pazopanib, 200 mg tablet (with discount)	16.35	
Trabectedin (per mg)[a]	1,366	
Ifosfamide (per mg)	0.04	
Gemcitabine (per mg)	0.14	
Docetaxel (per mg)	5.14	
Lenograstim (per mg)	238	
Mesna (per mg)	0.010	
Total costs of poststudy chemotherapy		
Placebo	11,493	PALETTE, British National Formulary [32]
Pazopanib[b]	8,531	NHS 2010-2011 Reference Costs [35]
Administration/dispensing		
Pazopanib	12.00	NHS 2010-2011 Reference Costs [35]
Ifosfamide	331.49	
Trabectedin	331.49	
Gemcitabine plus docetaxel	204.68	
Management costs[c]		
Preprogression monthly cost	92	Judson et al. 2007 [36]
Postprogression monthly cost	185	

[a]Costs are capped after five cycles; [b]poststudy costs are assumed to be the same for pazopanib, ifosfamide, trabectedin, and gemcitabine + docetaxel in the indirect comparison; [c]costs are updated to 2010/11 prices; preprogression costs are assumed to be half of postprogression costs.

In the model, patients receiving pazopanib were assumed to incur the cost of a 28-day supply of pazopanib each 28-day cycle if they remained alive and progression-free. Any medication supplied but not taken was assumed to be discarded. Drug utilization was adjusted for dosage adjustment, early discontinuation, and interruptions. It was assumed that pazopanib would be provided to the UK National Health Service (NHS) at a 12.5% discount to the list price consistent with a published patient access scheme (PAS) agreement between the NHS and GlaxoSmithKline [29]. The cost of trabectedin medication was calculated assuming that the acquisition cost of trabectedin to the NHS would be capped at five cycles of treatment, consistent with a PAS agreement between the manufacturer of trabectedin (PharmaMar, Colmenar Viejo, Spain) and the NHS [30]. However, administration costs after five cycles were included in the cost estimate.

Expected costs of PTACT for each treatment group were calculated by combining Kaplan-Meier sample average estimates of the mean number of lines of PTACT received and treatment group-specific estimates of the distribution of PTACTs in PALETTE with corresponding estimates of the cost per course of each PTACT (for details, see Table 7) [31]. The mean duration of PTACT was assumed to be 4 months, which was an average of the mean PFS in the placebo and pazopanib arms in PALETTE (2.5 and 6 months, resp.). This value is similar to the mean time between lines of PTACT for patients who received more than one PTACT in PALETTE (4.5 months). Dosages for PTACTs were based on published studies and prescribing information.

Medication unit costs were obtained from the 63rd edition of the British National Formulary (details on drug and administration costs are listed in Table 4) [32]. Patients treated with ifosfamide were assumed to receive concomitant treatment with mesna to prevent urotoxicity. Patients receiving gemcitabine plus docetaxel were assumed to receive treatment with lenograstim to prevent neutropenic complications; those with prior pelvic irradiation were assumed to receive a 25% dose reduction of gemcitabine plus docetaxel [33]. Administration costs included the cost of dispensing pazopanib based on the hourly cost of a hospital pharmacist (as reported by Personal Social Services Research Unit) [34] and assumed each dispensation requires 15 minutes. Facility costs for administering trabectedin and ifosfamide were based on a weighted average of the outpatient and day case 2010/2011 NHS reference costs for HRG SB14Z, "delivery of complex chemotherapy (including prolonged infusional treatment at first attendance)" [35].

The costs of treatment of AEs were calculated by multiplying estimates of the incidence of AEs with estimates of the cost of treatment for each event (Table 8). Only grade 3–5 AEs for which the difference in incidence between pazopanib and placebo was ≥2% or that were considered by clinical experts to be of special interest were considered. Estimates of the incidence of AEs for pazopanib and placebo were from the PALETTE trial. Estimates of the incidence of AEs for chemotherapies were based on reported values in the literature. In the absence of a reported value, AE incidence was assumed to be equal to the AE incidence in the placebo arm of the PALETTE trial. All AEs were assumed to require one additional consultant visit, the cost of which was based on the NHS reference costs for HRG 800 "Clinical Oncology, Consultant Led: Follow up Attendance Non-Admitted Face to Face" [35]. The proportions of patients requiring hospitalization for each AE were estimated separately for pazopanib and placebo and were based on the proportions of events that were serious in each arm of PALETTE. Lacking similar data for trabectedin, ifosfamide, and gemcitabine plus docetaxel, the proportions of events resulting in hospitalization for these therapies were assumed to be the same as those for pazopanib. The costs of hospitalizations for AEs were based on 2010/11 NHS reference costs for nonelective inpatient stays for these events (long stay and short stay) [35] (Table 9).

Other STS-related direct medical costs were estimated based on a retrospective study of the cost of the management of metastatic STS in the UK by Judson and colleagues [36].

2.3. Sensitivity Analyses. Deterministic and probabilistic sensitivity analyses were undertaken to explore the effect of

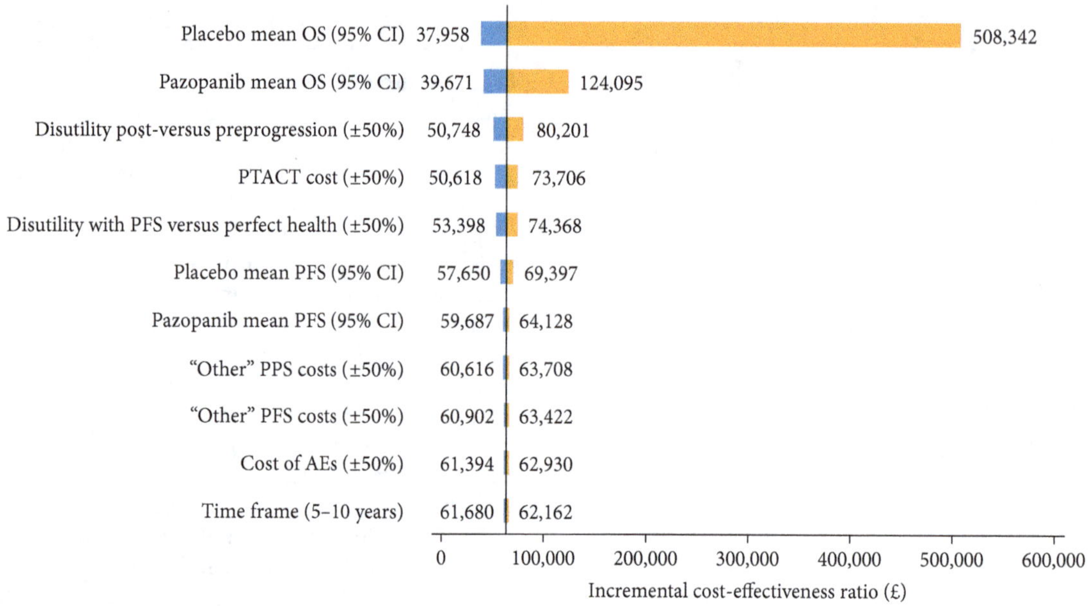

FIGURE 2: Tornado diagram showing result of deterministic sensitivity analysis for the direct comparison of cost-effectiveness of pazopanib versus placebo. Parameters were varied by 0.5 or 1.5 and shown on either side of the graph. AE: adverse events; CI: confidence interval; OS: overall survival; PFS: progression-free survival; PPS: postprogression survival; PTACT: posttreatment anticancer therapy.

TABLE 5: Base-case results for direct comparison of cost-effectiveness of pazopanib versus placebo.

	Pazopanib	Placebo	Pazopanib versus placebo
Effectiveness (discounted)			
LYs	1.375	1.262	0.113
PFLYs	0.503	0.211	0.292
PPLYs	0.872	1.051	−0.179
QALYs	0.719	0.591	0.128
Costs (discounted), £			
Study medication	10,733	0	10,733
Administration	81	0	81
Adverse events	251	54	197
Other costs PFS	557	234	323
Other costs PPS	10,463	13,822	−3,359
Total	**22,086**	**14,110**	**7,976**
Cost per QALY gained			62,162

LYs: life-years; PFLYs: progression-free life-years; PFS: progression-free survival; PPLYs: postprogression life-years; PPS: postprogression survival; QALYs: quality-adjusted life-years.

changing assumptions concerning key model parameter values on model results and cost-effectiveness acceptability curves generated [37, 38].

3. Results

3.1. Direct Comparison. In the base-case analyses (Table 5), pazopanib was estimated to increase QALYs by 0.128 and costs by £7,976 compared with placebo. The incremental cost-effectiveness ratio (ICER) of pazopanib versus placebo was estimated to be £62,162 per QALY gained.

Results for the deterministic sensitivity analysis are presented in Figure 2. In this analysis, the most influential variables were mean OS in the placebo group (range: £37,958–£508,342) and mean OS in the pazopanib group (range: £39,671–£124,095). For most parameters, the ICER changed <30% with ±50% changes in the parameter value.

Probabilistic sensitivity analysis and acceptability curves for the comparison of pazopanib and placebo are presented in Figures 3(a) and 3(b), respectively. A high concentration of simulations was present in the north-eastern quadrant of the cost-effectiveness plane. Given a threshold value of £30,000 per QALY gained, there is an estimated 2.2% probability that pazopanib is preferred (i.e., considered to be cost-effective) versus placebo.

3.2. Indirect Comparisons. Results for comparisons of pazopanib versus ifosfamide, trabectedin, and gemcitabine plus docetaxel are summarized in Table 6. Pazopanib was estimated to gain 0.040, 0.029, and 0.001 QALYs versus ifosfamide, trabectedin, and gemcitabine plus docetaxel, respectively. Pazopanib was less costly than ifosfamide (£3,957 savings), trabectedin (£6,729 savings), and gemcitabine plus docetaxel (£2,692 savings). These results suggest pazopanib is dominant (i.e., lower costs and greater QALYs) compared with each comparator. In probabilistic sensitivity analyses, there was an estimated 100% probability that pazopanib is cost-effective versus ifosfamide or trabectedin and 98% probability versus gemcitabine plus docetaxel.

TABLE 6: Base-case results for pairwise indirect comparisons versus pazopanib (PPS-based analysis).

	Pazopanib[a]	Trabectedin	Ifosfamide	Gemcitabine + docetaxel	Pazopanib versus trabectedin	Pazopanib versus ifosfamide	Pazopanib versus gemcitabine + docetaxel
Effectiveness (discounted)							
LYs	1.375	1.334	1.336	1.373	0.041	0.039	0.003
PFLYs	0.503	0.461	0.463	0.500	0.042	0.040	0.003
PPLYs	0.872	0.874	0.873	0.872	−0.001	−0.001	0.000
QALYs	0.692	0.663	0.652	0.691	0.029	0.040	0.001
Costs (discounted), £							
Study medication	10,733	11,699	5,675	9,769	−965	5,059	964
Administration	81	2,491	6,516	2,707	−2,411	−6,435	−2,627
Adverse events	653	3,481	2,706	1,685	−2,828	−2,053	−1,033
Other costs PFS	557	1,080	1,082	554	−522	−525	3
Other costs PPS	10,464	10,466	10,466	10,464	−3	−3	0
Total	**22,488**	**29,217**	**26,445**	**25,180**	**−6,729**	**−3,957**	**−2,692**
Cost per QALY gained					Dominant	Dominant	Dominant

LYs: life-years; PFLYs: progression-free life-years; PFS: progression-free survival; PPLYs: postprogression life-years; PPS: postprogression survival; QALYs: quality-adjusted life-years.
[a]Because a Markov methodology was used for the indirect comparison, the effectiveness and cost results are similar but not identical to the direct comparison with placebo.

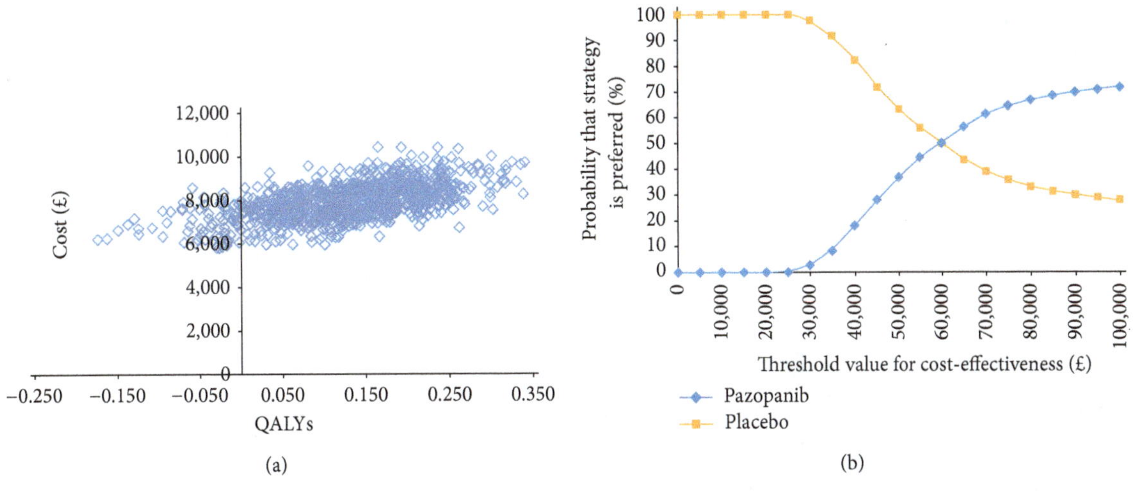

FIGURE 3: (a) Probabilistic sensitivity analyses for comparison of cost-effectiveness of pazopanib versus placebo. (b) Acceptability curve for comparison of cost-effectiveness of pazopanib versus placebo. QALYs: quality-adjusted life-years.

4. Discussion

This study was a cost-effectiveness evaluation of pazopanib in the treatment of patients with aSTS who have received prior chemotherapy from the perspective of the UK healthcare system. The primary analysis focused on a comparison of pazopanib and placebo. Based on cost-effectiveness criteria used by the National Institute for Health and Care Excellence (NICE), the results of our analysis suggest pazopanib is not cost-effective compared with placebo or BSC in these patients from a UK healthcare system perspective [39]. However, pazopanib might be cost-effective compared with trabectedin, ifosfamide, or gemcitabine when used in combination with docetaxel.

There is a dearth of information regarding the cost-effectiveness of other systemic agents to treat aSTS in the UK. Soini and colleagues [40] evaluated the cost-effectiveness of trabectedin versus end-stage treatment in Finland and reported ICERs ranging from €42,633 to €47,735/QALY depending on the utility values used in the model. A NICE

TABLE 7: Calculation of costs of posttreatment anticancer therapy.

Treatment	Medication cost[a]						Administration costs[b]			Total cost per course of therapy, £
	Mg per tab or vial	Cost per tab or vial, £	Cost per mg, £	Cost per administration, £	Expected days of use per course	Cost per course of therapy, £	Cost per administration, £	Expected days of use per course	Cost per course of therapy, £	
Cyclophosphamide	500	6	0	30	6.14	187	330	6.14	2,027	2,214
Dacarbazine	1,000	32	0	68	3.35	229	205	3.35	686	915
Doxorubicin	200	275	1	181	2.85	515	205	2.85	583	1,098
Etoposide	100	12	0	13	30.68	400	205	30.68	6,280	6,681
Etoposide + ifosfamide (+mesna)										
Etoposide	100	12	0	13	26.30	343	205	26.30	5,383	—
Ifosfamide	1,000	44	0	217	15.78	3,430	302	15.78	1,539	—
Mesna	400	4	0	46	15.78	725	—	15.78	—	—
Total	—	—	—	—	—	**4,499**	—	—	**6,922**	**11,421**
Gemcitabine	1,500	214	0.14	197	13.57	2,674	205	13.57	2,778	5,451
Gemcitabine + docetaxel (+lenograstim)										
Gemcitabine	1,500	214	0.14	185	8.90	1,643	205	8.90	1,821	—
Docetaxel	140	720	5.14	676	4.45	3,007	—	4.45	—	—
Lenograstim	0.263	62.54	238	64	31.14	1,988	0.57	31.14	18	—
Total	—	—	—	—	—	**6,639**	—	—	**1,839**	**8,478**
Ifosfamide (+mesna)										
Ifosfamide	1,000	44	0	217	15.78	3,430	302	15.78	4,769	—
Mesna	400	4	0	46	15.78	725	—	15.78	—	—
Total	—	—	—	—	—	**4,156**	—	—	**4,769**	**8,924**
Sorafenib	200	27	0	71	114.37	8,096	12	4.08	49	8,145
Sunitinib	12.5	28	2	99	65.33	6,489	12	1.56	19	6,508
Temozolomide	250	136	0.54304	109	23.67	2,570	12	0.85	10	2,580
Trabectedin	1	1,366	1,366	3,167	3.40	10,768	330	3.40	1,123	11,891

Tab: tablet; [a]unit costs of medications based on British National Formulary [32, 35]; [b]facility costs for administration of intravenous therapies are based on a weighted average of the outpatient, day case, and other 2010/2011 NHS Reference Costs for delivery of a chemotherapy cycle (SB12Z deliver simple parenteral chemotherapy at first attendance, and SB14Z deliver complex chemotherapy, including prolonged infusional treatment at first attendance for infusion of more than 24 hours) [35]. Assume dispensing costs of oral medications are based on the cost of a community pharmacist (15 minutes) [34].

TABLE 8: Random effects estimates of the probabilities of grade 3–5 AEs for each comparator based on Freeman-Tukey transformation (%)[a].

Description of adverse event (% [SE])	Pazopanib	BSC	Trabectedin	Ifosfamide 3 g/m^2	GEM/DOC
General					
Alopecia	0.1 (6.4)	0.2 (9.0)	0.5 (13.5)	64.6 (15.6)	0.5 (14.3)
Asthenia/fatigue	13.9 (6.4)	5.2 (9.0)	6.9 (15.5)	5.2 (9.0)	3.0 (14.3)
Hypertension	6.8 (6.4)	0.2 (9.0)	0.2 (9.0)	0.2 (9.0)	0.2 (9.0)
Myalgia/muscle pain	2.3 (6.4)	0.2 (9.0)	0.2 (9.0)	0.2 (9.0)	0.2 (9.0)
Neurotoxicity/peripheral sensory neuropathy	0.6 (6.4)	1.2 (9.0)	1.2 (9.0)	6.0 (15.6)	0.5 (14.3)
Edema	2.3 (6.4)	2.0 (9.0)	4.1 (16.7)	2.0 (9.0)	19.4 (14.3)
Liver toxicity					
ALT elevation	9.9 (6.5)	3.6 (9.0)	43.2 (12.5)	1.2 (9.0)	1.2 (9.0)
AST elevation	8.2 (6.5)	2.0 (9.0)	35.3 (8.2)	1.2 (9.0)	0.5 (14.3)
Cardiovascular					
Cardiac toxicity	0.1 (6.4)	0.2 (9.0)	0.2 (9.0)	0.2 (9.0)	0.2 (9.0)
Left ventricular dysfunction	1.9 (6.4)	0.2 (9.0)	0.2 (9.0)	0.2 (9.0)	0.2 (9.0)
Pulmonary					
Dyspnea	6.4 (6.4)	6.0 (9.0)	4.2 (8.7)	6.0 (9.0)	0.5 (14.3)
Pleural effusion	2.3 (6.4)	0.2 (9.0)	0.2 (8.7)	0.2 (9.0)	0.5 (14.3)
Pneumothorax	2.3 (6.4)	0.2 (9.0)	0.2 (9.0)	0.2 (9.0)	0.2 (9.0)
Pulmonary toxicity	0.1 (6.4)	0.2 (9.0)	0.2 (9.0)	0.2 (9.0)	9.2 (14.3)
Gastrointestinal					
Decreased appetite/anorexia	6.0 (6.4)	0.2 (9.0)	1.5 (7.3)	0.2 (9.0)	0.2 (9.0)
Diarrhea	4.8 (6.4)	1.2 (9.0)	0.9 (7.3)	1.2 (9.0)	1.2 (9.0)
Nausea/vomiting	6.8 (6.4)	2.8 (9.0)	13.5 (5.6)	18.3 (15.6)	3.0 (14.3)
Weight decreased	3.9 (6.4)	0.2 (9.0)	0.2 (9.0)	0.2 (9.0)	0.2 (9.0)
Hematologic abnormalities					
Febrile neutropenia	0.1 (6.4)	0.2 (9.0)	5.3 (14.5)	0.2 (9.0)	0.2 (9.0)
Anemia/hemoglobin	6.4 (6.4)	2.0 (9.0)	13.6 (9.9)	20.7 (15.6)	25.5 (14.3)
Leucopenia	1.4 (6.4)	0.2 (9.0)	43.2 (7.2)	64.6 (15.6)	23.5 (14.3)
Neutropenia/neutrophils	4.4 (6.4)	0.2 (9.0)	49.2 (8.7)	50.0 (15.6)	21.4 (14.3)
Thrombocytopenia/low platelets	3.9 (6.4)	0.2 (9.0)	15.7 (5.6)	15.8 (15.6)	39.8 (14.3)

AE: adverse event; ALT: alanine aminotransferase; AST: aspartate aminotransferase; BSC: best supportive care; GEM/DOC: gemcitabine + docetaxel; SE: standard error.
[a]SE on Freeman-Tukey transformation scale.
Note: if there is no information on AE then probability [SE] is assumed to be the same as placebo in PALETTE.

Table 9: Costs of adverse events.

AE	Probability that AE is serious		Cost per AE, £		Weighted average cost per AE, £	
	Pazopanib	Placebo	Nonserious	Serious	Pazopanib	Placebo
General						
Alopecia	100	0	0	0	0	0
Asthenia/fatigue	15	17	122	122	122	122
Hypertension	0	0	122	2,234	122	122
Myalgia/muscle pain	40	0	122	122	122	122
Neurotoxicity/peripheral sensory neuropathy	100	100	122	1,320	1,320	1,320
Edema	0	0	122	1,602	122	122
Liver toxicity						
ALT elevation	100	0	122	2,664	2,664	122
AST elevation	100	100	122	2,664	2,664	2,664
Cardiovascular						
Cardiac toxicity	100	0	122	3,843	3,843	122
Left ventricular dysfunction	100	0	122	3,843	3,843	122
Pulmonary						
Dyspnea	75	0	122	878	689	122
Pleural effusion	0	0	122	1,974	122	122
Pneumothorax	100	25	122	1,974	1,974	585
Pulmonary toxicity	100	0	122	1,713	1,713	122
Gastrointestinal						
Decreased appetite/anorexia	60	0	122	122	122	122
Diarrhea	0	0	122	1,171	122	122
Nausea/vomiting	7	0	122	1,171	195	122
Weight decreased	9	0	122	122	122	122
Hematologic abnormalities						
Febrile neutropenia	100	67	122	4,417	4,417	2,999
Anemia/hemoglobin	0	0	122	1,482	122	122
Leucopenia	0	0	122	4,417	122	122
Neutropenia/neutrophils	100	100	122	4,417	4,417	4,417
Thrombocytopenia/low platelets	50	50	122	2,051	1,086	1,086

AE: adverse event; ALT: alanine aminotransferase; AST: aspartate aminotransferase.

evaluation of trabectedin versus end-stage treatment based on the same model reported an ICER of £56,985/QALY [41]. However, criticism of this model [42] has suggested that the incremental mean survival benefit of 21.1 months for trabectedin versus 7.2 months for end-stage treatment is clinically implausible and might be overestimated.

In the PALETTE study, there was a 3-month gain in PFS for pazopanib compared with BSC [12]. However, an imbalance in the use of PTACT between the two treatment arms may have affected the translation of the PFS benefit to OS. Of the 94% of patients who were off-protocol at the data cutoff date, 62% of patients in the placebo group and 45% of patients in the pazopanib group received additional chemotherapy, and 14% of patients in the placebo group versus 10% in the pazopanib group received targeted therapies. Given limitations in the data available from the PALETTE trial, it was infeasible to reliably adjust for differences in PTACT use. Therefore, we used OS data as observed and included the estimated costs of PTACT in each group. While this approach is internally consistent with respect to estimates of effectiveness and costs, it may not be generalizable to other settings, where treatment with placebo followed by PTACT is not a widely used treatment strategy.

While the PALETTE trial provided relatively robust information on utility values during PFS for patients treated with pazopanib and BSC, there was relatively little information on utility values after disease progression. Data from the PALETTE trial were combined with data from a vignettes study to estimate utility values for the PPS state [13, 23]. The model was relatively sensitive to the assumed decrement in utility following progression. Although utilities from vignettes studies have been used in numerous prior cost-effectiveness analyses of oncology therapies, the validity of the values obtained from such studies has never been formally assessed.

It is debatable whether placebo represents an appropriate treatment strategy given that the majority of patients in PALETTE went on to receive other active therapies. We therefore conducted a secondary analysis in which we compared pazopanib with other widely used chemotherapies. In this analysis, pazopanib was estimated to be dominant (i.e., provides greater QALYs at a lower cost) compared with trabectedin, ifosfamide, and gemcitabine plus docetaxel. However, the estimated differences in PFS and OS between pazopanib and these treatments were small and based on an unadjusted or naive indirect treatment comparison. Given the small differences and inherent uncertainty associated with these comparisons, no firm conclusion can be drawn with respect to the relative cost-effectiveness of pazopanib versus these treatments.

There may be other important factors besides cost-effectiveness that should be considered in reimbursement decisions regarding pazopanib in this indication. In particular, STS is an ultra-rare, incurable disease with short life expectancy and for which existing therapies are inadequate. Pazopanib represents a novel therapeutic class for the treatment of this condition. As an oral therapy, pazopanib may be an option for patients who wish to receive treatment at home.

5. Conclusion

From a UK healthcare system perspective, taking into account the threshold of £30,000/QALY, pazopanib is not cost-effective compared with BSC (base-case); however, pazopanib might be cost-effective compared with trabectedin, ifosfamide, or gemcitabine when used in combination with docetaxel.

Appendix

Model Inputs and Parameters

See Tables 7, 8, and 9.

Acknowledgments

Funding for this study was provided to Policy Analysis Inc. by GlaxoSmithKline (GSK). All listed authors meet the criteria for authorship set forth by the International Committee for Medical Journal Editors. The authors wish to acknowledge Nate Connors, Ph.D., and Nancy Price, Ph.D., of AOI Communications, L.P., for medical writing and editorial support (assembling tables and figures, collating author comments, copyediting, fact checking, and referencing) and graphic services, which were funded by GSK.

References

[1] N. B. Jones, H. Iwenofu, T. Scharschmidt, and W. Kraybill, "Prognostic factors and staging for soft tissue sarcomas: an update," *Surgical Oncology Clinics of North America*, vol. 21, no. 2, pp. 187–200, 2012.

[2] R. Benjamin, P. W. T. Pisters, L. J. Helman, V. H. C. Bramwell, B. P. Rubin, and B. O'Sullivan, "Sarcomas of soft tissue," in *Clinical Oncology*, M. D. Abeloff, J. O. Armitage, J. E. Niederhuber et al., Eds., pp. 2009–2056, Churchill Livingstone, Philadelphia, Pa, USA, 2008.

[3] Cancer Research UK, "Soft tissue sarcoma incidence statistics," http://www.cancerresearchuk.org/cancer-info/cancerstats/types/soft-tissue-sarcoma/incidence/.

[3] Cancer Research UK, "Soft tissue sarcoma incidence statistics," http://www.cancerresearchuk.org/cancer-info/cancerstats/types/soft-tissue-sarcoma/incidence/.

[4] J. M. Coindre, P. Terrier, L. Guillou et al., "Predictive value of grade for metastasis development in the main histologic types of adult soft tissue sarcomas: a study of 1240 patients from the French Federation of Cancer Centers Sarcoma Group," *Cancer*, vol. 91, no. 10, pp. 1914–1926, 2001.

[5] R. Grimer, I. Judson, D. Peake, and B. Seddon, "Guidelines for the management of soft tissue sarcomas," *Sarcoma*, vol. 2010, Article ID 506182, 15 pages, 2010.

[6] A. Italiano, S. Mathoulin-Pelissier, A. le Cesne et al., "Trends in survival for patients with metastatic soft-tissue sarcoma," *Cancer*, vol. 117, no. 5, pp. 1049–1054, 2011.

[7] P. G. Casali, L. Jost, S. Sleijfer, J. Verweij, and J.-Y. Blay, "Soft tissue sarcomas: ESMO clinical recommendations for diagnosis, treatment and follow-up," *Annals of Oncology*, vol. 20, no. 4, pp. iv132–iv136, 2009.

[8] The ESMO/European Sarcoma Network Working Group, "Soft tissue and visceral sarcomas: ESMO Clinical Practice Guidelines for diagnosis, treatment and follow-up," *Annals of Oncology*, vol. 23, supplement 7, pp. vii92–vii99, 2012.

[9] M. Leahy, X. G. del Muro, P. Reichardt et al., "Chemotherapy treatment patterns and clinical outcomes in patients with metastatic soft tissue sarcoma. The SArcoma treatment and Burden of Illness in North America and Europe (SABINE) study," *Annals of Oncology*, vol. 23, no. 10, pp. 2763–2770, 2012.

[10] US Food and Drug Administration, "Votrient (pazopanib) tablets: for treatment of patients with soft tissue sarcoma," FDA Oncologic Drugs Advisory Committee Briefing Document (NDA 22-465), 2012.

[11] Votrient Summary of Product Characteristics, 2012, http://www.ema.europa.eu/docs/en_GB/document_library/EPAR_-_Product_Information/human/001141/WC500094272.pdf.

[12] W. T. van der Graaf, J. Y. Blay, S. P. Chawla et al., "Pazopanib for metastatic soft-tissue sarcoma (PALETTE): a randomized, double-blind, placebo-controlled phase 3 trial," *The Lancet*, vol. 379, no. 9829, pp. 1879–1886, 2012.

[13] GlaxoSmithKline, "A randomised double blind phase III trial of pazopanib versus placebo in patients with soft tissue sarcoma whose disease has progressed during or following prior therapy," http://www.gsk-clinicalstudyregister.com/study/VEG110727#rs.

[14] T. E. Delea, P. Tappenden, O. Sofrygin et al., "Cost-effectiveness of lapatinib plus capecitabine in women with HER2+ metastatic breast cancer who have received prior therapy with trastuzumab," *The European Journal of Health Economics*, vol. 13, no. 5, pp. 589–603, 2012.

[15] T. E. Delea, K. el Ouagari, J. Rotter, A. Wang, S. Kaura, and G. J. Morgan, "Cost-effectiveness of zoledronic acid compared with clodronate in multiple myeloma," *Current Oncology*, vol. 19, no. 6, pp. e392–e403, 2012.

[16] T. E. Delea, J. Amdahl, A. Chit, and M. M. Amonkar, "Cost-effectiveness of lapatinib plus letrozole in HER2-positive, hormone receptor-positive metastatic breast cancer in Canada," *Current Oncology*, vol. 20, no. 5, pp. e371–e387, 2013.

[16] T. E. Delea, J. Amdahl, A. Chit, and M. M. Amonkar, "Cost-effectiveness of lapatinib plus letrozole in HER2-positive, hormone receptor-positive metastatic breast cancer in Canada," *Current Oncology*, vol. 20, no. 5, pp. e371–e387, 2013.

[17] National Institute for Health and Care Excellence (NICE), "Guide to the methods of technology appraisal," 2013, http://publications.nice.org.uk/guide-to-the-methods-of-technology-appraisal-2013-pmg9/the-reference-case.

[18] S. Sharma, S. Takyar, S. C. Manson, S. Powell, and N. Penel, "Efficacy and safety of pharmacological interventions in second- or later-line treatment of patients with advanced soft tissue sarcoma: a systematic review," *BMC Cancer*, vol. 13, article 385, 2013.

[19] J. D. Kalbfleisch and R. L. Prentice, *The Statistical Analysis of Failure Time Data*, Wiley, New York, NY, USA, 1980.

[20] J. F. Tierney, L. A. Stewart, D. Ghersi, S. Burdett, and M. R. Sydes, "Practical methods for incorporating summary time-to-event data into meta-analysis," *Trials*, vol. 8, article 16, 2007.

[21] J. Amdahl, S. C. Manson, R. Isbell, A. Chit, and T. E. Delea, "Utility mapping of the EORTC QLQ-C30 onto EQ-5D in patients with soft tissue sarcoma," *Value in Health*, vol. 16, no. 7, p. A419, 2013.

[22] J. M. Giesinger, L. M. Wintner, A. S. Oberguggenberger et al., "Quality of life trajectory in patients with advanced cancer during the last year of life," *Journal of Palliative Medicine*, vol. 14, no. 8, pp. 904–912, 2011.

[23] B. Mayrbäurl, L. M. Wintner, J. M. Giesinger et al., "Chemotherapy line-associated differences in quality of life in patients with advanced cancer," *Supportive Care in Cancer*, vol. 20, no. 10, pp. 2399–2405, 2012.

[24] M. A. Elmqvist, M. S. Jordhøy, K. Bjordal, S. Kaasa, and M. Jannert, "Health-related quality of life during the last three months of life in patients with advanced cancer," *Supportive Care in Cancer*, vol. 17, no. 2, pp. 191–198, 2009.

[25] S. S. Hwang, V. T. Chang, D. L. Fairclough, J. Cogswell, and B. Kasimis, "Longitudinal quality of life in advanced cancer patients: pilot study results from a VA Medical Cancer Center," *Journal of Pain and Symptom Management*, vol. 25, no. 3, pp. 225–235, 2003.

[26] S. L. Shingler, P. Swinburn, A. Lloyd et al., "Elicitation of health state utilities in soft tissue sarcoma," *Quality of Life Research*, vol. 22, no. 7, pp. 1697–1706, 2013.

[27] B. Nafees, M. Stafford, S. Gavriel, S. Bhalla, and J. Watkins, "Health state utilities for non small cell lung cancer," *Health and Quality of Life Outcomes*, vol. 6, article 84, 2008.

[28] P. Swinburn, A. Lloyd, P. Nathan, T. K. Choueiri, D. Cella, and M. P. Neary, "Elicitation of health state utilities in metastatic renal cell carcinoma," *Current Medical Research and Opinion*, vol. 26, no. 5, pp. 1091–1096, 2010.

[29] NHS National Institute for Health and Care Excellence (NICE), "Pazopanib for the first-line treatment of advanced renal cell carcinoma," National Institute for Health and Care Excellence (NICE) Technology appraisal guidance 215, http://www.nice.org.uk/nicemedia/live/13346/53304/53304.pdf.

[30] National Institute for Health and Care Excellence (NICE), "Tabectedin patient access scheme submission," Technology Appraisals, National Institute for Health and Care Excellence (NICE), PharmaMar, 2009.

[31] T. A. Young, "Estimating mean total costs in the presence of censoring: a comparative assessment of methods," *PharmacoEconomics*, vol. 23, no. 12, pp. 1229–1242, 2005.

[32] *British National Formulary (BNF) 63*, British Medical Journal Publishing Group and Pharmaceutical Press, 2012.

[33] P. Pautier, A. Floquet, N. Penel et al., "Randomized multicenter and stratified phase II study of gemcitabine alone versus gemcitabine and docetaxel in patients with metastatic or relapsed leiomyosarcomas: a Fédération Nationale des Centres de Lutte Contre le Cancer (FNCLCC) French Sarcoma Group Study (TAXOGEM study)," *The Oncologist*, vol. 17, no. 9, pp. 1213–1220, 2012.

[34] L. Curtis, *Unit Costs of Health and Social Care 2010*, University of Kent, 2010.

[35] NHS Reference Costs 2010-2011, "NHS trust and PCT combined reference cost schedules," 2012, http://www.dh.gov.uk/en/Publicationsandstatistics/Publications/PublicationsPolicyAndGuidance/DH_131140.

[36] I. Judson, O. al-Muderis, D. Scott, A. Lloyd, F. Alonso, and B. Garcia, "Cost of management of metastatic soft tissue sarcoma," in *Proceedings of the National Cancer Research Institute (NCRI) Cancer Conference*, NCRI, Birmingham, UK, October 2007.

[37] A. H. Briggs, "Handling uncertainty in cost-effectiveness models," *PharmacoEconomics*, vol. 17, no. 5, pp. 479–500, 2000.

[38] M. Lothgren and N. Zethraeus, "Definition, interpretation and calculation of cost-effectiveness acceptability curves," *Health Economics*, vol. 9, no. 7, pp. 623–630, 2000.

[39] M. D. Rawlins and A. J. Culyer, "National institute for clinical excellence and its value judgments," *British Medical Journal*, vol. 329, no. 7459, pp. 224–227, 2004.

[40] E. J. O. Soini, B. G. san Andrés, and T. Joensuu, "Trabectedin in the treatment of metastatic soft tissue sarcoma: cost-effectiveness, cost-utility and value of information," *Annals of Oncology*, vol. 22, no. 1, pp. 215–223, 2011.

[41] C. Blomqvist, R. Johansson, and M. Tarkkanen, "Trabectedin in the treatment of metastatic soft-tissue sarcoma: cost-effectiveness and cost-utility are yet to be proved," *Annals of Oncology*, vol. 22, no. 4, p. 988, 2011.

[42] NHS National Institute for Health and Clinical Excellence (NICE), "Trabectedin for the treatment of advanced soft tissue sarcoma," http://www.nice.org.uk/nicemedia/live/12813/47472/47472.pdf.

[43] A. T. van Oosterom, H. T. Mouridsen, O. S. Nielsen et al., "Results of randomised studies of the EORTC Soft Tissue and Bone Sarcoma Group (STBSG) with two different ifosfamide regimens in first- and second-line chemotherapy in advanced soft tissue sarcoma patients," *European Journal of Cancer*, vol. 38, no. 18, pp. 2397–2406, 2002.

[44] G. D. Demetri, S. P. Chawla, M. von Mehren et al., "Efficacy and safety of trabectedin in patients with advanced or metastatic liposarcoma or leiomyosarcoma after failure of prior anthracyclines and ifosfamide: results of a randomized phase II study of two different schedules," *Journal of Clinical Oncology*, vol. 27, no. 25, pp. 4188–4196, 2009.

[45] R. Garcia-Carbonero, J. G. Supko, R. G. Maki et al., "Ecteinascidin-743 (ET-743) for chemotherapy-naive patients with advanced soft tissue sarcomas: multicenter phase II and pharmacokinetic study," *Journal of Clinical Oncology*, vol. 23, no. 24, pp. 5484–5492, 2005.

[46] A. le Cesne, J. Y. Blay, I. Judson et al., "Phase II study of ET-743 in advanced soft tissue sarcomas: a European Organisation for the Research and Treatment of Cancer (EORTC) Soft Tissue and Bone Sarcoma Group trial," *Journal of Clinical Oncology*, vol. 23, no. 3, pp. 576–584, 2005.

[47] A. Yovine, M. Riofrio, J. Y. Blay et al., "Phase II study of ecteinascidin-743 in advanced pretreated soft tissue sarcoma patients," *Journal of Clinical Oncology*, vol. 22, no. 5, pp. 890–899, 2004.

[48] M. L. Hensley, J. A. Blessing, K. DeGeest, O. Abulafia, P. G. Rose, and H. D. Homesley, "Fixed-dose rate gemcitabine plus docetaxel as second-line therapy for metastatic uterine leiomyosarcoma: a Gynecologic Oncology Group phase II study," *Gynecologic Oncology*, vol. 109, no. 3, pp. 323–328, 2008.

11

Potential Therapeutic Targets in Uterine Sarcomas

Tine Cuppens,[1] Sandra Tuyaerts,[1] and Frédéric Amant[1,2,3]

[1] *Department of Oncology, Gynaecologic Oncology, KU Leuven (University of Leuven), 3000 Leuven, Belgium*
[2] *Department of Obstetrics and Gynaecology, University Hospitals Leuven, 3000 Leuven, Belgium*
[3] *Center for Gynaecologic Oncology Amsterdam (CGOA), Antoni van Leeuwenhoek-Netherlands Cancer Institute, 1066 CX Amsterdam, Netherlands*

Correspondence should be addressed to Frédéric Amant; frederic.amant@uzleuven.be

Academic Editor: Silvia Stacchiotti

Uterine sarcomas are rare tumors accounting for 3,4% of all uterine cancers. Even after radical hysterectomy, most patients relapse or present with distant metastases. The very limited clinical benefit of adjuvant cytotoxic treatments is reflected by high mortality rates, emphasizing the need for new treatment strategies. This review summarizes rising potential targets in four distinct subtypes of uterine sarcomas: leiomyosarcoma, low-grade and high-grade endometrial stromal sarcoma, and undifferentiated uterine sarcoma. Based on clinical reports, promising approaches for uterine leiomyosarcoma patients include inhibition of VEGF and mTOR signaling, preferably in combination with other targeted or cytotoxic compounds. Currently, the only targeted therapy approved in leiomyosarcoma patients is pazopanib, a multitargeted inhibitor blocking VEGFR, PDGFR, FGFR, and c-KIT. Additionally, preclinical evidence suggests effect of the inhibition of histone deacetylases, tyrosine kinase receptors, and the mitotic checkpoint protein aurora kinase A. In low-grade endometrial stromal sarcomas, antihormonal therapies including aromatase inhibitors and progestins have proven activity. Other potential targets are PDGFR, VEGFR, and histone deacetylases. In high-grade ESS that carry the YWHAE/FAM22A/B fusion gene, the generated 14-3-3 oncoprotein is a putative target, next to c-KIT and the Wnt pathway. The observation of heterogeneity within uterine sarcoma subtypes warrants a personalized treatment approach.

1. Introduction

Although uterine sarcomas only account for 3,4% of all uterine corpus malignancies, they entail a high mortality rate [1, 2]. Reported risk factors are unopposed estrogen stimulation, tamoxifen treatment, obesity, and diabetes [3–5]. However, little is known about their precise etiology, mainly due to their highly divergent genetic aberrations. Together with the rarity of the disease, this contributes to the current lack of optimal treatment modalities. Next to standard hysterectomy (often with bilateral salpingo-oophorectomy), adjuvant treatment options are scarce and depend on the histologic subtype [2]. In this review, we discuss new potential therapeutic approaches in uterine leiomyosarcoma (uLMS), low-grade endometrial stromal sarcomas (LGESS), high-grade endometrial stromal sarcomas (HGESS), and undifferentiated uterine sarcomas (UUS).

2. Uterine Leiomyosarcoma

Uterine leiomyosarcomas, arising from the myometrium, are generally high-grade tumors accounting for 60% of all uterine sarcomas [1]. Due to lack of evidence of clinical benefit, adjuvant chemotherapy is not standardly administered in patients with local disease [6]. At least 50% of patients diagnosed with stage I/II uLMS relapse and/or present with distant metastases [7]. For patients with localized metastases, complete metastasectomy enhances disease-specific survival [7]. Adjuvant cytotoxic treatment options are scarce and generally result in limited clinical benefit. The management of advanced uterine LMS has recently been summarized in an extensive review by Amant et al. [8]. The standard first-line treatment consists of doxorubicin ± ifosfamide [8]. The use of gemcitabine ± docetaxel has yielded inconsistent response rates in different studies and is used mostly as a second-line treatment option [9–11]. Interestingly, a randomized phase III study is currently ongoing, assessing the efficacy of gemcitabine + docetaxel, followed by doxorubicin in stage I uterine LMS patients after hysterectomy (ClinicalTrials.gov Identifier: NCT01533207). Another approach in advanced disease is trabectedin, a marine-derived drug that has shown minor first-line and second-line activity in LMS patients, but is currently not approved by the Food and Drug Administration (FDA) [8, 12, 13].

Uterine LMS show multiple and varied genetic aberrations and very complex, often aneuploid or polyploid, karyotypes [14, 15]. This heterogeneity complicates the identification of driver mutations and therapeutic targets. While point mutations are rather scarce in uLMS, its genome is characterized by dispersed large amplifications and deletions, with gains of up to 15% of the genome and losses of up to 45% of the genome [14–16].

2.1. Receptor Tyrosine Kinase Signaling. Mutations in receptor tyrosine kinases (RTK), leading to aberrant pathway activation, have often been reported in cancer. Amplifications, mutations, and rearrangements of platelet-derived growth factor (*PDGF*) and its receptor *PDGFR* have been implicated in the pathophysiology of multiple tumor types including gastrointestinal stromal tumor (GIST), glioblastoma, and dermatofibrosarcoma protuberans [17–19]. Although PDGF(R) aberrations have not been studied thoroughly in uLMS, one study reported on PDGFR-β amplifications in uLMS [20]. Furthermore, taking together results from three expression studies, 49/215 (23%) uLMS samples (from 128 patients) showed positivity for PDGFR-β [7, 21, 22]. Similarly, of 239 uLMS samples retrieved from 128 patients, 108 samples (45%) were moderately to strongly positive for PDGFR-α, while no activating mutations have been found in the gene [7, 21, 23]. Despite the finding of strong PDGFR expression in a subgroup of uLMS patients, there are very few reports on targeting this receptor in uLMS. PDGF signaling can be blocked by multitargeted kinase inhibitors, such as imatinib, sunitinib, sorafenib, and pazopanib. Only one report was found on treatment of a uLMS patient with imatinib, which inhibits PDGFR and KIT. The patient was progressive on imatinib treatment and ultimately died due to complications of hypereosinophilia. Sunitinib and sorafenib are multitargeted tyrosine kinase inhibitors that also inhibit vascular endothelial growth factor receptor 2 (VEGFR2) and vascular endothelial growth factor receptor 3 next to PDGFR. Sorafenib is currently used to treat carcinomas but has been tested in a phase II study including LMS patients. However, of 12 uLMS patients, only 4 had stable disease [24]. Sunitinib was suggested by Mahmood et al. to have some activity in LMS but also proved insufficient for treatment of uLMS in a phase II trial by the Gynecologic Oncology Group [25, 26]. Pazopanib inhibits VEGFR, PDGFR, fibroblast growth factor receptor (FGFR), and c-KIT. After a recent successful placebo-controlled phase III trial, the PALETTE study, it was approved by the FDA (April 2012) for use in soft-tissue sarcomas, including leiomyosarcomas [27]. An earlier phase II study reported a progression-free survival rate of 44% at 12 weeks in LMS patients [28].

Although *VEGF* expression in uLMS has been previously explored in IHC studies, results are highly inconsistent. In summary, more than half of the samples (total $n = 73$) were scored positive for VEGF [29–32]. In addition, *VEGFR1* and *VEGFR2* are frequently expressed in uLMS [29, 31]. In case reports, the anti-VEGF monoclonal antibody bevacizumab has resulted in stable disease in one of two uLMS patients [33]. Remarkably, in a case report of epithelioid uLMS, a combination of bevacizumab and the alkylating agent temozolomide resulted in complete remission [34]. Furthermore, a decrease in tumor cell proliferation and angiogenesis and increased apoptosis have been described in *in vitro* and *in vivo* uLMS models after treatment with vandetanib, a VEGFR2/epidermal growth factor receptor (EGFR) inhibitor [35]. Moreover, a recently published phase I study, combining the VEGFR inhibitor cediranib with an inhibitor of γ-secretase (an important player in the Notch signaling pathway), reported prolonged stable disease in one of three LMS patients (the responding patient had the uterine subtype; others were not further specified) [36]. In contrast, aflibercept, a VEGF binding and blocking recombinant protein, showed only modest response in a phase II study: 11/41 (27%) uLMS patients had stable disease [37].

Overexpression of *ERBB2/HER-2*, belonging to the ERBB family of tyrosine kinase receptors, is of great clinical importance in breast cancer, where it is tackled by the monoclonal antibody trastuzumab [38]. It has been shown to be amplified in uLMS, but only in one study [20]. Three studies have assessed ERBB2 protein expression in uLMS, with variable results [39–41]. In total, 35 uLMS and 11 uterine sarcomas, not otherwise specified (NOS), were included, of which 12 cases (26%) showed at least moderate staining [39–41]. Hence, a selected group of uLMS patients may benefit from ERBB2 inhibition. However, at present, trastuzumab or other inhibitors have not been tested in uterine sarcomas in preclinical settings, nor in case reports.

Another important cell growth regulator of the ERBB family is *EGFR*. EGFR has been shown to be upregulated in uLMS when compared to normal controls [7]. One study, including 199 tissue microarray samples of 109 uLMS patients, found 72/199 samples to be EGFR-positive [7]. Two other groups compared EGFR expression between uLMS and uterine leiomyomas (LM). Although one group reported significantly increased immunoreactivity in uLMS versus LM, the other group only detected EGFR expression in 1/25 uLMS and in 1/19 LM [23, 31]. A recent report described the activation of the EGFR pathway in uLMS cell cultures, as shown by high receptor phosphorylation levels. Also downstream AKT and mitogen-activated protein kinase (MAPK) pathways were activated, as AKT, EPH receptor B2 (also termed ERK), and ribosomal protein S6 were highly phosphorylated [42]. Interestingly, targeting EGFR with gefitinib rendered uLMS cells sensitive to cytotoxic treatment, *in vitro* as well as in an *in vivo* xenograft model [42].

Insulin-like growth factor 2 (*IGF2*), which activates IGF 1/2 receptors (IGF1/2R), has been reported to be upregulated in uLMS [43, 44]. Some clinical studies using agents that block IGF1R have included LMS patients. A phase II study tested the efficacy of cixutumumab, a selective IGF1R blocker, in sarcoma patients. Only 3/22 (13,6%) LMS patients (NOS) had stable disease at 12 weeks, while other patients were progressive [45]. A phase I study by Macaulay et al. described a partial response in 2/4 LMS patients upon treatment with the anti-IGF1R antibody AVE1642, although patients simultaneously received gemcitabine and erlotinib, an EGFR inhibitor [46]. Another phase I study combined the IGF1R inhibitor figitumumab with the mTOR inhibitor everolimus. A small decrease in tumor size was detected in 1 out of 4 LMS patients (NOS), while another patient had stable disease [47]. Hence, it may be of use to further test combination therapies of IGF receptor blockers with other compounds in uLMS.

Lastly, brain-derived neurotrophic factor (*BDNF*) and its tyrosine kinase receptor, neurotrophic tyrosine kinase receptor type 2 (*NTRK2*, also termed TRKB), have recently been reported to be upregulated in uLMS compared to LM and myometrium. Treatment of MES-SA cells, which are derived from uterine sarcoma, with the multikinase inhibitor K252a or the NTRK2 ectodomain suppressed proliferation and induced apoptosis. Moreover, in MES-SA-injected mouse models, administration of K252a resulted in smaller tumors, lower proliferation rates, and more apoptosis [48].

2.2. Upregulated Pathways. Hyperactivation of the phosphatidylinositol 3-kinase/AKT/mammalian target of rapamycin (*PIK3/AKT/mTOR*) pathway has been implicated in uLMS and may play a role in its etiology (Figure 1 displays the discussed pathways and targeted treatments) [49, 50]. The PIK3/AKT/mTOR pathway controls cell growth, proliferation, and survival through regulation of gene transcription and protein synthesis [51]. Phosphorylation of AKT and mTOR has been detected in most uLMS, with phosphorylation of downstream molecules such as eukaryotic translation initiation factor 4E-binding (eIF-4E) and 4E-binding protein 1 (4E-BP1) [49, 52]. Inhibiting the pathway with the natural herb curcumin resulted in apoptosis and reduced cell growth in the uLMS cell lines SKN and SK-UT-1 [53, 54]. These *in vitro* findings were later confirmed *in vivo* [55]. Recently, the clinical response of the rapamycin-analog ridaforolimus was tested in a phase III trial in 711 sarcoma patients, including 231 LMS patients (NOS). While the progression-free survival was modestly increased in patients receiving ridaforolimus, no significant improvement in the overall survival was reached [56]. The FDA did not approve this mTOR inhibitor for the treatment of sarcoma patients, also taking into account its notable toxicity. Another rapamycin-analog, temsirolimus, has led to a partial response (for 17 months) in a uLMS patient, in a phase II trial including 9 LMS patients (NOS) [57]. However, the administration of mTOR inhibitors in combination with a second targeted or cytotoxic agent will likely achieve higher response. For example, combining the mTOR inhibitor rapamycin with the cytotoxic gemcitabine led to cell cycle arrest *in vitro* and this combination was recently confirmed to strongly inhibit tumor growth *in vivo* by an independent group [58, 59]. Furthermore, clinical response was achieved on gemcitabine + rapamycin treatment in an extrauterine LMS patient [60]. After a dose-finding phase I trial for advanced solid tumors, a phase II trial has been completed recently and the results are eagerly awaited [58]. Also, combined targeting of the mTOR pathway and the mitotic checkpoint protein aurora kinase A, using rapamycin + MLN8237, synergistically reduced uLMS cell growth *in vitro*, as well as tumor growth in an *in vivo* model [61].

Next to the mTOR pathway, *Wnt/β-catenin* signaling may be upregulated in uLMS (Figure 1). The Wnt pathway is highly conserved throughout evolution and plays a key role in development [62]. An extensive study by Lusby et al. showed increased expression of β-catenin in uLMS compared to normal smooth muscle controls [7]. The authors used 203 samples from 109 uLMS patients and studied β-catenin expression in the cytoplasm (low expression in 36% and high expression in 64% of samples) and on the membrane (low expression in 80% and high expression in 20% of samples) [7]. Other groups reported on nuclear expression in 22% and cytoplasmic expression in 87% of 238 uLMS cases [63, 64]. The Wnt/β-catenin pathway is targetable through many different pathway players with commercially available inhibitors, but this approach has not yet been tested in uLMS [65].

Moreover, a portion of uLMS tumors are characterized by expression of receptor tyrosine kinase-like orphan receptor 2 (*ROR2*), which is involved in noncanonical Wnt signaling (Figure 1) [62, 66]. ROR2 suppression reduced invasiveness of an LMS cell line *in vitro* and ROR2 knockdown resulted in smaller tumor volumes in xenograft models [66].

In addition to Wnt and mTOR pathways, also transforming growth factor beta/bone morphogenetic protein (*TGF-β/BMP*) signaling may play a role in uLMS (Figure 1). Recently, *endoglin*, a coreceptor in TGF-β/BMP signaling, was found to be expressed in 9/22 uLMS. Interestingly, *in vitro* knockdown of endoglin resulted in reduced migration, invasion, and VEGF secretion [67].

2.3. Other Targets. In a recent genome-wide study of 12 uLMS, aurora kinase A (*AURKA*) was found to be highly overexpressed. Of note, almost all genes with >9-fold increase in expression were involved in regulating chromosomal homeostasis and spindle assembly, suggesting that proteins involved in these functions could be useful therapeutic targets. Indeed, the single targeting of AURKA with siRNA or MK-5108 inhibited uLMS cell proliferation *in vitro* and decreased the number and size of tumor implants *in vivo* [68]. Similarly, the aurora kinase inhibitor VE465 induced cytotoxicity in the MES-SA uterine sarcoma cell line [69]. Of note, a phase II trial evaluating the AURKA inhibitor alisertib (MLN8237) in pretreated LMS patients has been activated [70].

MDM2 is an oncogene that negatively regulates p53 function by three mechanisms: (1) targeting p53 for ubiquitin-based degradation, (2) blocking the p53 transcriptional activation domain, and (3) shuttling p53 from the nucleus to the cytoplasm [71]. Blocking MDM2 enhances p53 function and hence provides a therapeutic strategy for many cancer types. Amplifications have been reported in uLMS and in extrauterine LMS [20, 72, 73]. Moreover, MDM2 is overexpressed in 10% of uLMS [74, 75]. MDM2 inhibitors have proven efficient in preclinical settings and, at present, agents

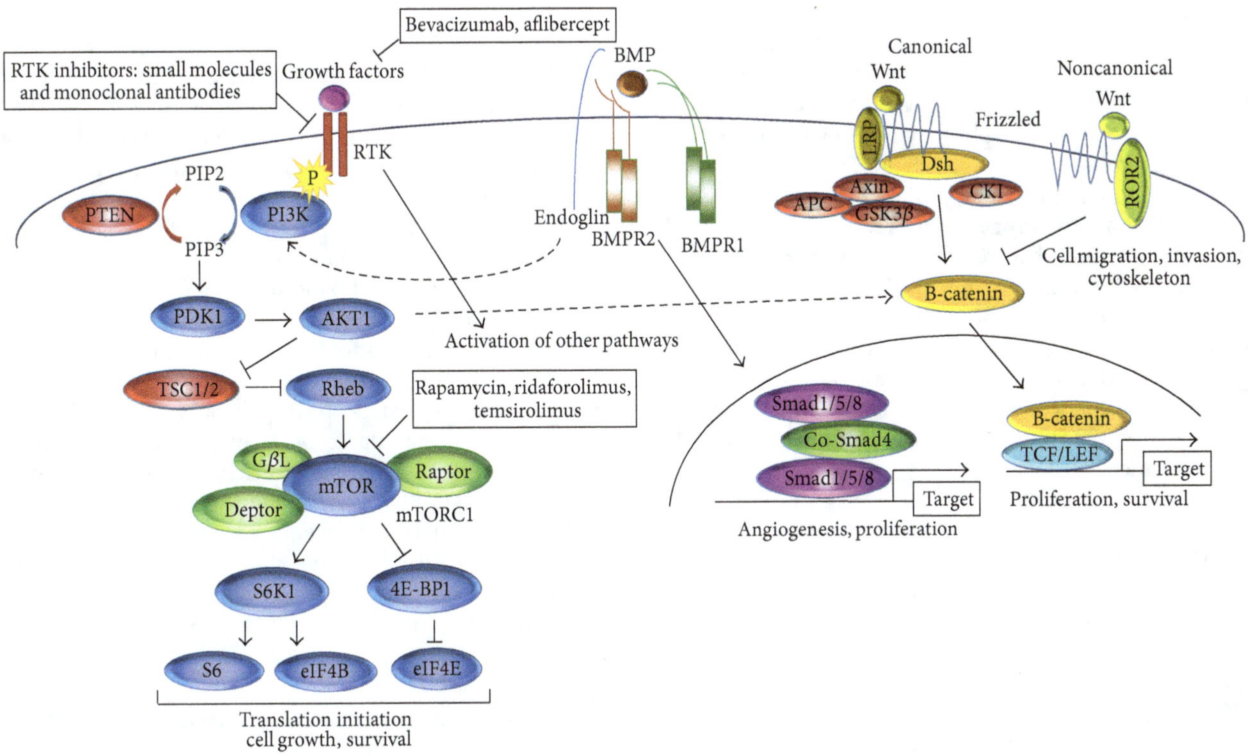

FIGURE 1: Left: the PI3K/AKT/mTOR pathway is mainly activated by nutrients (not shown) and growth factors, binding to receptor tyrosine kinases and activating PI3K. As PIP2 (phosphatidylinositol 4,5-bisphosphate) is converted to PIP3 (phosphatidylinositol 3,4,5-trisphosphate), PDK1 (pyruvate dehydrogenase kinase, isozyme 1) phosphorylates AKT1 (v-akt murine thymoma viral oncogene homolog 1) upon PIP3-mediated recruitment to the plasma membrane. AKT1 inhibits TSC1/2 (tuberous sclerosis 1/2), relieving the inhibition of Rheb (Ras homolog enriched in brain), which activates mTOR. The recruitment of Raptor (regulatory associated protein of MTOR, complex 1), Deptor (DEP domain containing MTOR-interacting protein), and GβL (mLST8; G protein beta subunit-like MTOR associated protein, LST8 homolog) gives rise to the mTOR complex 1 (mTORC1). Upon activation of S6K1 (ribosomal protein S6 kinase 1) and inhibition of 4EBP-1 (EIF4EBP1; eukaryotic translation initiation factor 4E binding protein 1), protein translation is stimulated by activation of ribosomal protein S6 and eIF4B and E (eukaryotic translation initiation factor 4B and E). Additionally, AKT1 activates β-catenin signaling. Middle: BMP (bone morphogenetic protein) signaling is modulated through binding of BMPs to BMPR1 and BMPR2 (bone morphogenetic protein receptor type I/II) and the coreceptor endoglin, activating Smad1/5/8 and leading to transcription of target genes involved in angiogenesis and proliferation. Endoglin may also activate PI3K/AKT signaling. Right: canonical Wnt signaling is activated by binding of Wnt to the Frizzled receptor and the LRP (low-density lipoprotein receptor-related protein) coreceptor. Upon recruitment of Dsh (dishevelled) and Axin to the plasma membrane, the β-catenin destruction complex, which contains Axin, APC (adenomatosis polyposis coli), GSK3 (glycogen synthase kinase 3), and CKI (casein kinase 1), is inactivated, leading to β-catenin accumulation and transcription of target genes after association with TCF/LEF (transcription factor/lymphoid enhancer-binding factor). Noncanonical signaling plays a role in cell migration, invasion, and cytoskeleton arrangement and is mediated through binding of Wnt to Frizzled and other coreceptors such as ROR2 (receptor tyrosine kinase-like orphan receptor 2) or without coreceptors.

such as AMG232 and RG7112 are clinically being explored in various cancer types, although not yet in uterine sarcomas [76–78]. To tackle the problem of resistance to single-agent therapy, Saiki et al. tested potential synergistic combinations of MDM2 antagonists with other compounds *in vitro* in 40 cell lines. Synergy was observed upon simultaneous inhibition of MDM2 and MEK and/or PI3K. Interestingly, this effect was not dependent on the mutation status of genes in the PI3K pathway, and the highest inhibitory effect was noted when all three molecules were blocked [79].

Furthermore, MDM2 inhibitors were found to greatly synergize with histone deacetylase (*HDAC*) inhibitors, as detected by a tremendous increase in apoptosis and decrease in cell proliferation [79]. Histone deacetylases control gene transcription through deacetylation of nucleosomal histones [80]. Of note, HDAC9 was reported to be amplified in 73% of 15 uLMS samples and HDAC8 has been designated as a marker of smooth muscle differentiation and hence may be involved in uLMS, which arises from smooth muscle cells [15, 81]. HDAC inhibition using vorinostat or valproate resulted in growth suppression of the uterine sarcoma cell line MES-SA *in vitro* [69, 82]. Moreover, vorinostat treatment has led to tumor growth reduction of MES-SA-induced tumors *in vivo* [82]. Also, combining vorinostat with the PI3K/AKT/mTOR pathway inhibitors rapamycin or LY294002 showed a synergistic effect on growth inhibition in MES-SA cells [83]. While HDAC inhibitors are clinically being tested in various cancers, mainly in combination regimens with other targeted or cytotoxic treatments, no uLMS patients have been included in these studies to our knowledge [84, 85].

Recently, Edris et al. reported on the use of an antibody against *CD47* for LMS treatment. The antibodies abolish the suppression of phagocytosis that is controlled by macrophage interaction. Interestingly, treatment of uLMS cells with anti-CD47 antibodies increased phagocytosis *in vitro* and reduced uLMS tumor volumes *in vivo* [86].

Further, approximately 50% of uLMS express estrogen receptor (ER) and/or progesterone receptors (PR), [7, 87–90]. A recently published retrospective study on the use of the aromatase inhibitor letrozole in 16 ER/PR positive uLMS patients revealed clinical benefit in 10/16 patients (partial response in 2/16 and stable disease in 8/16 patients). Also the use of the aromatase inhibitor exemestane in second line resulted in clinical benefit in 50% of patients [91]. However, no prospective trials testing hormonal therapy in uLMS have been performed.

2.4. Loss of Tumor Suppressor Genes and Synthetic Lethality. In uLMS, recurrent regions of loss often include tumor suppressor genes (TSG) such as phosphatase and tensin homolog (PTEN), tumor protein p53 (TP53), retinoblastoma 1 (RB1), and cyclin-dependent kinase inhibitor 2A (CDKN2A) [15, 92–94].

CDKN2A encodes the p16 protein, which controls cell proliferation by inhibiting cell cycle progression. When p16 is absent, cyclin-dependent kinases bind to cyclins, enabling them to phosphorylate RB1. Upon phosphorylation, RB1 releases the transcription factor E2F, stimulating cell cycle progression [94]. In uLMS, several aberrations can alter the cell cycle process. Kawaguchi et al. reported on the inactivation of CDKN2A in soft-tissue LMS by promoter hypermethylation (11/49 cases) and homozygous deletion (3/49 cases). Moreover, 15/49 samples showed decreased p16 expression [94].

Further, the *RB1* gene is frequently deleted in uLMS [15, 93]. The *RB1* gene is named after the corresponding cancer type hereditary retinoblastoma, where the gene is homozygously deleted. It was shown recently that retinoblastoma patients with the hereditary type (RB1 deletion) have an increased risk of uLMS; 3,2% of patients developed uLMS, which corresponds to an excess risk of 3,9/10000 women [95].

PTEN is a negative regulator of the PI3K-AKT-mTOR pathway, and loss of PTEN is associated with increased pathway activity, as found in many cancers (Figure 1) [96, 97]. Also in uLMS cells, low levels of PTEN have been associated with high levels of phosphorylated EGFR, AKT, ERK, and S6 ribosomal protein, indicating mTOR pathway activity [42]. Of note, mice that carry homozygous deletions at the *PTEN* locus spontaneously develop LMS, suggesting a strong tumor suppressor role for PTEN in LMS [49]. In preclinical models, loss of PTEN has often been shown to be predictive for response to mTOR pathway inhibition [98–100]. Hence, selection of patients for treatment with PI3K/mTOR inhibitors based on PTEN loss could be a useful strategy in uLMS.

Another tumor suppressor gene, which is mutated in approximately 50% of cancers and frequently deleted in uLMS, is *TP53* [15, 75, 93, 101]. P53 functions in various ways, with major roles in regulating the cell cycle and thus preventing uncontrolled proliferation, and in apoptosis when cells carry highly damaged DNA [101]. Conditional knockout of *TP53* in the reproductive tract of female mice has led to the development of uterine tumors with the uLMS morphology [102]. Additionally, simultaneous loss of the TSG breast cancer 1, early onset (*BRCA1*), and *TP53* accelerated tumor progression in this mouse model. Further, the authors described downregulation of *BRCA1* in 29% of uLMS, most likely due to promoter methylation [102].

Tumor cells that display loss of tumor suppressor function can be tackled by the inhibition of another protein that has become indispensable after loss of the first tumor suppressor, that is, the synthetic lethality principle [103]. For example, inhibition of poly ADP-ribose polymerase (PARP), which is involved in the repair of DNA single-strand breaks, selectively kills cells that are deficient in tumor suppressor protein BRCA1 or BRCA2, which repair double-strand breaks [104]. Similarly, PTEN deficiency has been shown to predict response to PARP inhibitors [105]. However, until present, this approach has not been explored in any uterine sarcoma type. The most important discussed targets in uLMS are displayed in Table 1.

3. Low-Grade Endometrial Stromal Sarcoma

Low-grade endometrial stromal sarcomas comprise about 20% of uterine sarcomas [1]. They are myometrium-infiltrating tumors with a notable resemblance to proliferative endometrial stroma [106, 107]. They are often characterized by a less aggressive disease course compared to uLMS, with delayed recurrences [2]. Since LGESS often express ER/PR receptors, patients can benefit from hormonal treatment, for example, by removal of adnexa and progestin therapy, but recurrence rates remain higher than 30% [108, 109]. Unlike uLMS, most LGESS are translocation-related sarcomas [107].

3.1. Receptor Tyrosine Kinase Signaling. From IHC studies, the *PDGF* signaling pathway has proven interesting to explore in LGESS. Taking together seven studies, 71/141 (50%) of LGESS cases showed expression of PDGFR-α and 53/127 (42%) of LGESS were positive for PDGFR-β [21, 110–115]. Interestingly, two case reports of LGESS patients treated with imatinib have shown objective responses [116, 117]. One case was immunohistochemically assessed for the expression of imatinib targets. Whereas the tumor was negative for c-KIT, it was strongly positive for PDGFR-α and PDGFR-β, designating this receptor as a potential therapeutic target in LGESS and warranting further research [117]. Sardinha et al. investigated *c-KIT* expression in 52 cases and summarized previous studies, revealing only 16 c-KIT positive cases in 203 included LGESS (8% positive), suggesting c-KIT is not a valuable target in LGESS [114]. The only exception is the study by Park et al., where 32/39 LGESS were scored positive for c-KIT [113, 117].

Further, in a total of 156 LGESS samples, *EGFR* expression has been detected in 35 cases (22%), with substantial differences between studies, varying from 0/39 to 14/20 positive cases [110, 111, 113–115, 118, 119]. Hence, the expression and activity of this receptor should be further investigated in

TABLE 1: Overview of potential therapeutic targets and corresponding treatments in uterine sarcomas.

	Therapeutic target	Targeted agents
uLMS	HER-2	HER-2 inhibitors (e.g., trastuzumab, CP-724714, CUDC-101)
	EGFR	EGFR inhibitors (e.g., gefitinib, erlotinib, cetuximab, vandetanib)
	PDGFR	PDGFR inhibitors (e.g., pazopanib, imatinib, sunitinib, sorafenib)
	VEGF-VEGFR	VEGF-VEGFR inhibitors (e.g., bevacizumab, aflibercept, vandetanib, cediranib)
	IGFIR	Figitumumab, cixutumumab, AVE1642
	BDNF-NTRK2	BDNF-NTRK2 inhibitors (e.g., K252a)
	PIK3/AKT/mTOR Loss of PTEN	PIK3/AKT/mTOR pathway inhibitors (e.g., curcumin, rapamycin, ridaforolimus)
	AURKA	AURKA inhibitors (e.g., MLN8237, MK-5108, VE465)
	Wnt/β-catenin	β-catenin inhibitors (e.g., LGK-974, PKF118-310, PNU-74654)
	ROR2	ROR2 inhibitors (not yet developed)
	Endoglin/CD105	Anti-CD105 antibodies (in development)
	MDM2	MDM2 inhibitors (e.g., AMG232, RG7112)
	HDAC	HDAC inhibitors (e.g., vorinostat, valproate)
	CD47	Anti-CD47 antibodies (in development)
	ER, PR	Aromatase inhibitors (e.g., letrozole, exemestane) Progestins (e.g., medroxyprogesterone acetate, megestrol acetate)
	Loss of TSG	Synthetic lethality principle (e.g., PARP inhibitors)
LGESS	PDGFR	PDGFR inhibitors (e.g., pazopanib, imatinib, sunitinib, sorafenib)
	EGFR	EGFR inhibitors (e.g., gefitinib, erlotinib, cetuximab, vandetanib)
	VEGF-VEGFR	VEGF-VEGFR inhibitors (e.g., bevacizumab, aflibercept, vandetanib, cediranib)
	HDAC	HDAC inhibitors (e.g., vorinostat, valproate)
	Wnt/β-catenin	β-catenin inhibitors (e.g. LGK-974, PKF118-310, PNU-74654)
	ER, PR	Aromatase inhibitors (e.g., letrozole) Progestins (e.g., medroxyprogesterone acetate, megestrol acetate)
HGESS	14-3-3 oncoprotein	14-3-3 oncoprotein inhibitors (not yet developed)
	PDGFR	PDGFR inhibitors (e.g., pazopanib, imatinib, sunitinib, sorafenib)
	HER-2	HER-2 inhibitors (e.g., trastuzumab, CP-724714, CUDC-101)
	EGFR	EGFR inhibitors (e.g., gefitinib, erlotinib, cetuximab, vandetanib)
	c-KIT	c-KIT inhibitors (e.g., imatinib, pazopanib)
HGESS/UUS	Tyrosine kinases	Cabozantinib

LGESS. Overexpression is not the result of gene amplification in LGESS [120]. No studies including LGESS targeting EGFR have been reported to our knowledge.

Combining three studies, with a total of 22 LGESS patients, 60% of tumors expressed *VEGF* [29, 110, 118]. VEGF receptors have not been explored in ESS, except in one study that included 4 samples. All 4 LGESS cases were positive for VEGFR1 and 2/4 tumors showed VEGFR2 staining [29]. A recently published phase I study, combining the VEGFR inhibitor cediranib with a γ-secretase inhibitor, reported partial response in a LGESS patient [36]. This promising result warrants further clinical studies with VEGF/VEGFR-targeting agents.

3.2. Other Targets. Histone deacetylases and the inhibition thereof are under investigation in many cancer types. In LGESS, overexpression of *HDAC2* has been reported. Although treatment of the ESS-1 cell line with a HDAC inhibitor resulted in cell cycle arrest and cell differentiation *in vitro*, the results failed to translate into clinical response: in a phase II trial exploring the effect of the HDAC inhibitor panobinostat, no responses were observed in 3 LGESS patients [121, 122]. On the other hand, the HDAC inhibitor vorinostat induced cell death via autophagy and it affected mTOR signaling as it reduced mTOR, phospho-S6, p-p70S6K, and p-4E-BP1 levels [83, 123]. Interestingly, further blocking the PI3K/AKT/mTOR pathway using rapamycin or LY294002 in combination with vorinostat showed a synergistic effect on growth inhibition in the ESS-1 cell line [83]. One report by Wu et al. described mTOR expression in 7 of 54 (13%) LGESS samples, but the PI3K/AKT/mTOR pathway is further underexplored in LGESS [124].

Also little is known on the *Wnt/β-catenin* pathway in endometrial stromal tumors. Taking together results from 4 independent studies, 75/121 LGESS show positive β-catenin-staining [64, 125–127]. However, expression of cyclin D1, a direct transcriptional target of β-catenin that allows cell cycle progression and contributes to cell proliferation, is only rarely detected in LGESS [115, 126, 128].

Hormone receptors are expressed in 70–80% of LGESS, with proven therapeutic importance for over a decade [124, 129–132]. Partial responses have been noted in LGESS patients upon treatment with the aromatase inhibitor letrozole and even complete responses have been achieved on treatment with the progestins medroxyprogesterone acetate and megestrol acetate [133–137]. The antiprogesterone mifepristone resulted in stable disease in 1/2 LGESS patients in a phase II trial [138]. Of note, withdrawing estrogen replacement therapy (ERT) and tamoxifen has also resulted in stable disease [137]. Retrospective studies have shown superior survival rates in patients on progestin therapy compared to patients who received other hormonal treatments, pelvic radiation, or no adjuvant treatment [109, 133]. However, due to the rareness of ESS, no prospective randomized placebo-controlled trials have been published on the use of hormone-directed treatment. All targets in LGESS are summarized in Table 1.

4. High-Grade Endometrial Stromal Sarcoma and Undifferentiated Uterine Sarcoma

High-grade ESS (HGESS) arise from the endometrial stroma, but unlike LGESS, they show a high-grade round-cell morphology and are clinically more aggressive [107, 139]. They should be distinguished from undifferentiated uterine sarcomas (UUS), which can arise from the myometrium as well as from the endometrium and show no specific differentiation. While being not considered in the WHO 2003 edition, UUS originating in the myometrium most likely represent the previously described "dedifferentiated uLMS," supporting their inclusion in the latest WHO 2014 classification [107]. Before, HGESS were frequently categorized as "undifferentiated endometrial sarcoma with nuclear uniformity" (UES-U), while most currently termed UUS cases were designated "undifferentiated endometrial sarcoma with nuclear pleomorphism" (UES-P) [107, 130]. Due to the rarity of the disease, no randomized prospective trials have been completed. Although responses have been observed on treatment with gemcitabine/docetaxel or single-agent doxorubicin, the median overall survival is only 11,8 months [140].

4.1. The 14-3-3 Oncoprotein. Recently, the translocation t(10; 17)(q22;p13) has been described in HGESS [128, 141–145]. The translocation results in the fusion gene YWHAE/FAM22A/B, which gives rise to a *14-3-3 oncoprotein* [145]. Interestingly, knockdown of the oncoprotein by shRNA or siRNA reduced cell growth and migration in an ESS cell line, defining it as a potential therapeutic target [145]. At present, no small molecule inhibitor has been developed. Interestingly, a strong correlation has been reported between the YWHAE rearrangement and the HGESS (UES-U) morphology, confirming that HGESS and UUS are different entities [146].

4.2. Receptor Tyrosine Kinase Signaling. Similar to LGESS, *PDGFR* signaling may be involved in HGESS and UUS. Both PDGFR-α and PDGFR-β have been detected in 37% of 30 reported samples, warranting studies on its clinical relevance [111, 114, 115].

Only one group has studied *ERBB2* in HGESS/UUS. In a single study by Amant et al., one of four (25%) cases showed amplification and overexpression in the primary and the recurrent tumor [39]. Hence, trastuzumab treatment may be an option for selected patients. *EGFR* overexpression has been reported more frequently in HGESS/UUS. Taken together, 16/33 (48%) cases were EGFR-positive by IHC [111, 114, 115, 119]. A low-level EGFR amplification has only been described in one report. This patient responded temporarily to imatinib, although no c-KIT expression and no genetic aberrations in c-KIT and PDGFR were detected (expression of PDGFR was not assessed) [147]. Another response to imatinib was reported in a patient with *c-KIT* overexpression [148]. C-KIT was recently reported to be overexpressed in 12/12 HGESS carrying the YWHAE/FAM22A/B fusion [149]. Lastly, a phase II clinical trial was recently started by EORTC, testing cabozantinib as a maintenance therapy in high-grade uterine sarcoma patients (ClinicalTrials.gov Identifier: NCT01979393). Cabozantinib is a multikinase inhibitor targeting VEGFR2, c-Met, Ret, Kit, Flt-1/3/4, Tie2, and AXL, which has been approved for treatment of progressive metastatic medullary thyroid cancer [150]. In the current trial, only patients showing response or having stable disease after chemotherapy (doxorubicin ± ifosfamide) are eligible for maintenance treatment with cabozantinib, which will be compared to a placebo arm.

4.3. Other Targets. *Cyclin D1* expression has been detected exclusively in UES-U, whereas all reported UES-P cases were negative [126, 146]. Cyclin D1 expression was confirmed specifically in UES that carried the YWHAE/FAM22A/B rearrangement [128]. Hence, cyclin D1 is correlated with the HGESS-subtype carrying the t(10;17) translocation. The presence of cyclin D1 indicates activation of the *Wnt/β-catenin* pathway (Figure 1). Indeed, expression of β-catenin has been demonstrated in 6/7 (85%) UES-U cases and only in 2/6 (33%) UES-P cases [130]. Expression of β-catenin has been reported in 9/12 additional HGESS/UUS cases, but these were not further classified [125, 151]. As inhibitors for the Wnt/β-catenin pathway are available, it may be valuable to test this approach in translocation-related HGESS cases.

UES-U and UES-P also differ in the expression of *sex hormone receptors*. Kurihara et al. found that ER and PR are present in at least half of UES-U cases, while they were not detected in any UES-P cases [130]. The presence of hormone receptors could confer sensitivity to hormonal treatment. The only group reporting on the administration of progestins in a HGESS/UUS patient with weak ER expression, noted a partial response [140]. A summary of all targets is displayed in Table 1.

5. Conclusions

In this review, we summarize the latest reported aberrations with potential therapeutic applicability in uterine leiomyosarcomas, low-grade and high-grade endometrial stromal sarcomas, and undifferentiated uterine sarcomas.

Among the scarce clinical reports on targeted treatments in uterine leiomyosarcoma patients, a promising approach involves tackling the PI3K/AKT/mTOR pathway. However, mTOR inhibition leads to activation of AKT through upstream receptor tyrosine kinase signaling, due to interruption of feedback inhibition [152]. Therefore, we propose mTOR inhibition should be considered mainly in combination with other agents. Preclinical responses have been noted upon combination of mTOR pathway inhibition with aurora kinase A inhibitors, MDM2 inhibitors, or histone deacetylase inhibitors [61, 79, 83]. Interestingly, the recently developed small molecule inhibitor CUDC-907, targeting both HDAC and PI3K, shows activity in many human cancer cell lines and xenografts and, additionally, the molecule seems to block treatment escape of cancer cells by also blocking the RAF-MEK-MAPK pathway [153]. Since synergistic effects of blocking HDAC and mTOR have already been described in uterine sarcoma cells, CUDC-907 may be effective in uterine sarcomas [83]. Similarly, another new small molecule inhibitor, CUDC-101, acts on EGFR, ERBB2, and HDAC, which are all potential targets in uterine sarcomas [154]. CUDC-101 has shown strong activity in human cancer cell lines and it also overcomes resistance by simultaneously tackling escape routes [154]. These findings support preclinical research on CUDC-101 in uterine sarcomas.

Another promising approach in uLMS is the interruption of VEGF signaling. Although most responses are published in case reports, sorafenib and aflibercept made it to a phase II trial, resulting in a minor response: stable disease was reached in 4/12 (33%) and 11/41 (27%) uLMS patients, respectively [24, 37]. So far, pazopanib, a multikinase inhibitor targeting VEGFR, PDGFR, FGFR, and c-KIT, is the only FDA-approved targeted treatment in LMS [27]. Combination treatments should be further tested, for example, combination of VEGF(R) inhibition with an EGFR- or γ-secretase inhibitor or chemotherapeutics such as temozolomide [34–36].

In low-grade endometrial stromal sarcomas, particularly aromatase inhibitors and progestins have proven their effectiveness. Further, PDGF and VEGF signaling seem to be potential targets in LGESS, but at the moment only case reports have been published. HDAC inhibitors have been shown to be effective *in vitro*, but combination regimens may be necessary to reach efficacy *in vivo*.

High-grade endometrial stromal sarcomas often carry the translocation t(10;17)(q22;p13), giving rise to the fusion gene YWHAE/FAM22A/B [145]. The resulting gene product, a 14-3-3 oncoprotein, was put forward as a therapeutic target when Lee et al. found that its knockdown leads to reduced cell growth and migration in an ESS cell line [145]. 14-3-3 proteins are expressed in all normal cells and they affect signaling pathways, transcription, and survival [145]. Although at present no inhibitors for the oncoprotein are available, this may be a target to look out for in the coming years.

Moreover, Wnt pathway players have been detected specifically in this HGESS subgroup [126, 128, 130, 146]. Hence, the effect of Wnt pathway blocking should be investigated. Also detected in translocation-related HGESS is c-KIT overexpression [149]. Significant tumor regression upon imatinib treatment in a c-KIT-overexpressing HGESS case supports further use in the clinic [148].

Undifferentiated uterine sarcomas appear to be underexplored, as no targets could be identified from literature. Although partly due to their rarity, the recent reclassification of the tumor subtypes by the World Health Organization also impedes the identification of the UUS subtype in older publications [107].

In conclusion, combinations of treatments and multitargeted compounds such as pazopanib overall generate higher clinical benefit than single agents, partly by tackling escape routes that lead to resistance. While multiple promising targets were identified for uterine leiomyosarcoma and low/high-grade endometrial stromal sarcoma, the lack of studies on undifferentiated sarcomas warrants more multicentric studies on these rare tumors. Since randomized trials are scarce for uterine sarcoma patients, we support a personalized therapy approach. Preclinical studies testing the rational combination of existing inhibitors on cell lines and xenografts might pave the way to use these inhibitors in off-label use or repurposed drugs in uterine sarcoma patients, corresponding to their genetic profile.

Acknowledgments

Tine Cuppens is aspirant of the Research Fund Flanders (FWO) and Frédéric Amant is senior researcher for the Research Fund Flanders (FWO). Sandra Tuyaerts is financially supported by the Anticancer Fund and the Verelst Uterine Cancer Fund Leuven.

References

[1] V. M. Abeler, O. Røyne, S. Thoresen, H. E. Danielsen, J. M. Nesland, and G. B. Kristensen, "Uterine sarcomas in Norway. A histopathological and prognostic survey of a total population from 1970 to 2000 including 419 patients," *Histopathology*, vol. 54, no. 3, pp. 355–364, 2009.

[2] F. Amant, A. Coosemans, M. Debiec-Rychter, D. Timmerman, and I. Vergote, "Clinical management of uterine sarcomas," *The Lancet Oncology*, vol. 10, no. 12, pp. 1188–1198, 2009.

[3] M. Arenas, A. Rovirosa, V. Hernández et al., "Uterine sarcomas in breast cancer patients treated with tamoxifen," *International Journal of Gynecological Cancer*, vol. 16, no. 2, pp. 861–865, 2006.

[4] A. S. Felix, L. S. Cook, M. M. Gaudet et al., "The etiology of uterine sarcomas: a pooled analysis of the epidemiology of endometrial cancer consortium," *British Journal of Cancer*, vol. 108, no. 3, pp. 727–734, 2013.

[5] S. M. Schwartz, N. S. Weiss, J. R. Daling et al., "Exogenous sex hormone use, correlates of endogenous hormone levels, and the incidence of histologic types of sarcoma of the uterus," *Cancer*, vol. 77, no. 4, pp. 717–724, 1996.

[6] R. Mancari, M. Signorelli, A. Gadducci et al., "Adjuvant chemotherapy in stage I-II uterine leiomyosarcoma: a multicentric retrospective study of 140 patients," *Gynecologic Oncology*, vol. 133, no. 3, pp. 531–536, 2014.

[7] K. Lusby, K. B. Savannah, E. G. Demicco et al., "Uterine leiomyosarcoma management, outcome, and associated molecular biomarkers: a single institution's experience," *Annals of Surgical Oncology*, vol. 20, no. 7, pp. 2364–2372, 2013.

[8] F. Amant, D. Lorusso, A. Mustea, F. Duffaud, and P. Pautier, "Management strategies in advanced uterine leiomyosarcoma: focus on trabectedin," *Sarcoma*, vol. 2015, Article ID 704124, 14 pages, 2015.

[9] M. L. Hensley, R. Maki, E. Venkatraman et al., "Gemcitabine and docetaxel in patients with unresectable leiomyosarcoma: results of a phase II trial," *Journal of Clinical Oncology*, vol. 20, no. 12, pp. 2824–2831, 2002.

[10] M. L. Hensley, J. A. Blessing, K. Degeest, O. Abulafia, P. G. Rose, and H. D. Homesley, "Fixed-dose rate gemcitabine plus docetaxel as second-line therapy for metastatic uterine leiomyosarcoma: a Gynecologic Oncology Group phase II study," *Gynecologic Oncology*, vol. 109, no. 3, pp. 323–328, 2008.

[11] D. M. Hyman, R. N. Grisham, and M. L. Hensley, "Management of advanced uterine leiomyosarcoma," *Current Opinion in Oncology*, vol. 26, no. 4, pp. 422–427, 2014.

[12] G. D. Demetri, S. P. Chawla, M. von Mehren et al., "Efficacy and safety of trabectedin in patients with advanced or metastatic liposarcoma or leiomyosarcoma after failure of prior anthracyclines and ifosfamide: results of a randomized phase II study of two different schedules," *Journal of Clinical Oncology*, vol. 27, no. 25, pp. 4188–4196, 2009.

[13] B. J. Monk, J. A. Blessing, D. G. Street, C. Y. Muller, J. J. Burke, and M. L. Hensley, "A phase II evaluation of trabectedin in the treatment of advanced, persistent, or recurrent uterine leiomyosarcoma: a gynecologic oncology group study," *Gynecologic Oncology*, vol. 124, no. 1, pp. 48–52, 2012.

[14] W. Kildal, V. M. Abeler, G. B. Kristensen, M. Jenstad, S. Ø. Thoresen, and H. E. Danielsen, "The prognostic value of DNA ploidy in a total population of uterine sarcomas," *Annals of Oncology*, vol. 20, no. 6, pp. 1037–1041, 2009.

[15] M. Raish, M. Khurshid, M. A. Ansari et al., "Analysis of molecular cytogenetic alterations in uterine leiomyosarcoma by array-based comparative genomic hybridization," *Journal of Cancer Research and Clinical Oncology*, vol. 138, no. 7, pp. 1173–1186, 2012.

[16] S. Murray, H. Linardou, G. Mountzios et al., "Low frequency of somatic mutations in uterine sarcomas: a molecular analysis and review of the literature," *Mutation Research*, vol. 686, no. 1-2, pp. 68–73, 2010.

[17] T. P. Fleming, A. Saxena, W. C. Clark et al., "Amplification and/or overexpression of platelet-derived growth factor receptors and epidermal growth factor receptor in human glial tumors," *Cancer Research*, vol. 52, no. 16, pp. 4550–4553, 1992.

[18] M. C. Heinrich, C. L. Corless, G. D. Demetri et al., "Kinase mutations and imatinib response in patients with metastatic gastrointestinal stromal tumor," *Journal of Clinical Oncology*, vol. 21, no. 23, pp. 4342–4349, 2003.

[19] C. L. Sawyers, "Imatinib GIST keeps finding new indications: successful treatment of dermatofibrosarcoma protuberans by targeted inhibition of the platelet-derived growth factor receptor," *Journal of Clinical Oncology*, vol. 20, no. 17, pp. 3568–3569, 2002.

[20] Y. L. Cho, S. Bae, M. S. Koo et al., "Array comparative genomic hybridization analysis of uterine leiomyosarcoma," *Gynecologic Oncology*, vol. 99, no. 3, pp. 545–551, 2005.

[21] S. F. Adams, J. A. Hickson, J. Y. Hutto, A. G. Montag, E. Lengyel, and S. D. Yamada, "PDGFR-α as a potential therapeutic target in uterine sarcomas," *Gynecologic Oncology*, vol. 104, no. 3, pp. 524–528, 2007.

[22] J. J. Caudell, M. T. Deavers, B. M. Slomovitz et al., "Imatinib mesylate (gleevec)-targeted kinases are expressed in uterine sarcomas," *Applied Immunohistochemistry and Molecular Morphology*, vol. 13, no. 2, pp. 167–170, 2005.

[23] S. E. Anderson, D. Nonaka, S. Chuai et al., "p53, epidermal growth factor, and platelet-derived growth factor in uterine leiomyosarcoma and leiomyomas," *International Journal of Gynecological Cancer*, vol. 16, no. 2, pp. 849–853, 2006.

[24] R. G. Maki, D. R. D'Adamo, M. L. Keohan et al., "Phase II study of sorafenib in patients with metastatic or recurrent sarcomas," *Journal of Clinical Oncology*, vol. 27, no. 19, pp. 3133–3140, 2009.

[25] M. L. Hensley, M. W. Sill, D. R. Scribner Jr. et al., "Sunitinib malate in the treatment of recurrent or persistent uterine leiomyosarcoma: a Gynecologic Oncology Group phase II study," *Gynecologic Oncology*, vol. 115, no. 3, pp. 460–465, 2009.

[26] S. T. Mahmood, S. Agresta, C. E. Vigil et al., "Phase II study of sunitinib malate, a multitargeted tyrosine kinase inhibitor in patients with relapsed or refractory soft tissue sarcomas. Focus on three prevalent histologies: leiomyosarcoma, liposarcoma and malignant fibrous histiocytoma," *International Journal of Cancer*, vol. 129, no. 8, pp. 1963–1969, 2011.

[27] W. T. A. Van Der Graaf, J.-Y. Blay, S. P. Chawla et al., "Pazopanib for metastatic soft-tissue sarcoma (PALETTE): a randomised, double-blind, placebo-controlled phase 3 trial," *The Lancet*, vol. 379, no. 9829, pp. 1879–1886, 2012.

[28] S. Sleijfer, I. Ray-Coquard, Z. Papai et al., "Pazopanib, a multikinase angiogenesis inhibitor, in patients with relapsed or refractory advanced soft tissue sarcoma: a phase II study from the European organisation for research and treatment of cancer-soft tissue and bone sarcoma group (EORTC Study 62043)," *Journal of Clinical Oncology*, vol. 27, no. 19, pp. 3126–3132, 2009.

[29] S. Arita, F. Kikkawa, H. Kajiyama et al., "Prognostic importance of vascular endothelial growth factor and its receptors in the uterine sarcoma," *International Journal of Gynecological Cancer*, vol. 15, no. 2, pp. 329–336, 2005.

[30] K. Mayerhofer, P. Lozanov, K. Bodner et al., "Ki-67 and vascular endothelial growth factor expression in uterine leiomyosarcoma," *Gynecologic Oncology*, vol. 92, no. 1, pp. 175–179, 2004.

[31] M. Sanci, C. Dikis, S. Inan, E. Turkoz, N. Dicle, and C. Ispahi, "Immunolocalization of VEGF, VEGF receptors, EGF-R and Ki-67 in leiomyoma, cellular leiomyoma and leiomyosarcoma," *Acta Histochemica*, vol. 113, no. 3, pp. 317–325, 2011.

[32] C. Poncelet, R. Fauvet, G. Feldmann, F. Walker, P. Madelenat, and E. Darai, "Prognostic value of von Willebrand factor, CD34, CD31, and vascular endothelial growth factor expression in women with uterine leiomyosarcomas," *Journal of Surgical Oncology*, vol. 86, no. 2, pp. 84–90, 2004.

[33] J. D. Wright, M. A. Powell, J. S. Rader, D. G. Mutch, and R. K. Gibb, "Bevacizumab therapy in patients with recurrent uterine neoplasms," *Anticancer Research*, vol. 27, no. 5, pp. 3525–3528, 2007.

[34] M. Takano, Y. Kikuchi, N. Susumu et al., "Complete remission of recurrent and refractory uterine epithelioid leimyosarcoma

using weekly administration of bevacizumab and temozolomide," *European Journal of Obstetrics Gynecology & Reproductive Biology*, vol. 157, no. 2, pp. 236–238, 2011.

[35] W. Ren, B. Korchin, G. Lahat et al., "Combined vascular endothelial growth factor receptor/epidermal growth factor receptor blockade with chemotherapy for treatment of local, uterine, and metastatic soft tissue sarcoma," *Clinical Cancer Research*, vol. 14, no. 17, pp. 5466–5475, 2008.

[36] S. Sahebjam, P. L. Bedard, V. Castonguay et al., "A phase i study of the combination of ro4929097 and cediranib in patients with advanced solid tumours (PJC-004/NCI 8503)," *British Journal of Cancer*, vol. 109, no. 4, pp. 943–949, 2013.

[37] H. J. MacKay, R. J. Buckanovich, H. Hirte et al., "A phase II study single agent of aflibercept (VEGF Trap) in patients with recurrent or metastatic gynecologic carcinosarcomas and uterine leiomyosarcoma. A trial of the Princess Margaret Hospital, Chicago and California Cancer Phase II Consortia," *Gynecologic Oncology*, vol. 125, no. 1, pp. 136–140, 2012.

[38] J. S. Ross and J. A. Fletcher, "The HER-2/neu oncogene in breast cancer: prognostic factor, predictive factor, and target for therapy," *Oncologist*, vol. 3, no. 4, pp. 237–252, 1998.

[39] F. Amant, V. Vloeberghs, H. Woestenborghs et al., "ERBB-2 gene overexpression and amplification in uterine sarcomas," *Gynecologic Oncology*, vol. 95, no. 3, pp. 583–587, 2004.

[40] L. J. Layfield, K. Liu, R. Dodge, and S. H. Barsky, "Uterine smooth muscle tumors: utility of classification by proliferation, ploidy, and prognostic markers versus traditional histopathology," *Archives of Pathology and Laboratory Medicine*, vol. 124, no. 2, pp. 221–227, 2000.

[41] M. Zafrakas, L. Zepiridis, T. D. Theodoridis et al., "ERBB2 (HER2) protein expression in uterine sarcomas," *European Journal of Gynaecological Oncology*, vol. 30, no. 3, pp. 292–294, 2009.

[42] G. Sette, V. Salvati, L. Memeo et al., "EGFR inhibition abrogates leiomyosarcoma cell chemoresistance through inactivation of survival pathways and impairment of CSC potential," *PLoS ONE*, vol. 7, no. 10, Article ID e46891, 2012.

[43] T. Gloudemans, I. Prinsen, J. A. M. Van Unnik, C. J. M. Lips, W. Den Otter, and J. S. Sussenbach, "Insulin-like growth factor gene expression in human smooth muscle tumors," *Cancer Research*, vol. 50, no. 20, pp. 6689–6695, 1990.

[44] T. H. Vu, C. Yballe, S. Boonyanit, and A. R. Hoffman, "Insulin-like growth factor II in uterine smooth-muscle tumors: maintenance of genomic imprinting in leiomyomata and loss of imprinting in leiomyosarcomata," *Journal of Clinical Endocrinology and Metabolism*, vol. 80, no. 5, pp. 1670–1676, 1995.

[45] P. Schöffski, D. Adkins, J.-Y. Blay et al., "An open-label, phase 2 study evaluating the efficacy and safety of the anti-IGF-1R antibody cixutumumab in patients with previously treated advanced or metastatic soft-tissue sarcoma or Ewing family of tumours," *European Journal of Cancer*, vol. 49, no. 15, pp. 3219–3228, 2013.

[46] V. M. Macaulay, M. R. Middleton, A. S. Protheroe et al., "Phase I study of humanized monoclonal antibody AVE1642 directed against the type 1 insulin-like growth factor receptor (IGF-1R), administered in combination with anticancer therapies to patients with advanced solid tumors," *Annals of Oncology*, vol. 24, no. 3, pp. 784–791, 2013.

[47] R. Quek, Q. Wang, J. A. Morgan et al., "Combination mTOR and IGF-1R inhibition: phase I trial of everolimus and figitumumab in patients with advanced sarcomas and other solid tumors," *Clinical Cancer Research*, vol. 17, no. 4, pp. 871–879, 2011.

[48] K. Makino, K. Kawamura, W. Sato, N. Kawamura, T. Fujimoto, and Y. Terada, "Inhibition of uterine sarcoma cell growth through suppression of endogenous tyrosine kinase B signaling," *PLoS ONE*, vol. 7, no. 7, Article ID e41049, 2012.

[49] E. Hernando, E. Charytonowicz, M. E. Dudas et al., "The AKT-mTOR pathway plays a critical role in the development of leiomyosarcomas," *Nature Medicine*, vol. 13, no. 6, pp. 748–753, 2007.

[50] S. Dhingra, M. E. Rodriguez, Q. Shen et al., "Constitutive activation with overexpression of the mTORC2-phospholipase D1 pathway in uterine leiomyosarcoma and STUMP: morphoproteomic analysis with therapeutic implications," *International Journal of Clinical and Experimental Pathology*, vol. 4, no. 2, pp. 134–146, 2011.

[51] N. Hay and N. Sonenberg, "Upstream and downstream of mTOR," *Genes and Development*, vol. 18, no. 16, pp. 1926–1945, 2004.

[52] N. Setsu, H. Yamamoto, K. Kohashi et al., "The Akt/mammalian target of rapamycin pathway is activated and associated with adverse prognosis in soft tissue leiomyosarcomas," *Cancer*, vol. 118, no. 6, pp. 1637–1648, 2012.

[53] B. Li, T. Takeda, K. Tsuiji et al., "Curcumin induces cross-regulation between autophagy and apoptosis in uterine leiomyosarcoma cells," *International Journal of Gynecological Cancer*, vol. 23, no. 5, pp. 803–808, 2013.

[54] T. F. Wong, T. Takeda, B. Li et al., "Curcumin disrupts uterine leiomyosarcoma cells through AKT-mTOR pathway inhibition," *Gynecologic Oncology*, vol. 122, no. 1, pp. 141–148, 2011.

[55] T. F. Wong, T. Takeda, B. Li et al., "Curcumin targets the AKT-mTOR pathway for uterine leiomyosarcoma tumor growth suppression," *International Journal of Clinical Oncology*, vol. 19, no. 2, pp. 354–363, 2014.

[56] G. D. Demetri, S. P. Chawla, I. Ray-Coquard et al., "Results of an international randomized phase III trial of the mammalian target of rapamycin inhibitor ridaforolimus versus placebo to control metastatic sarcomas in patients after benefit from prior chemotherapy," *Journal of Clinical Oncology*, vol. 31, no. 19, pp. 2485–2492, 2013.

[57] S. Okuno, H. Bailey, M. R. Mahoney et al., "A phase 2 study of temsirolimus (CCI-779) in patients with soft tissue sarcomas: a study of the Mayo phase 2 consortium (P2C)," *Cancer*, vol. 117, no. 15, pp. 3468–3475, 2011.

[58] J. Martin-Liberal, M. Gil-Martín, M. Sáinz-Jaspeado et al., "Phase I study and preclinical efficacy evaluation of the mTOR inhibitor sirolimus plus gemcitabine in patients with advanced solid tumours," *British Journal of Cancer*, vol. 111, no. 5, pp. 858–865, 2014.

[59] O. Merimsky, Y. Gorzalczany, and R. Sagi-Eisenberg, "Molecular impacts of rapamycin-based drug combinations: combining rapamycin with gemcitabine or imatinib mesylate (Gleevec) in a human leiomyosarcoma model," *International Journal of Oncology*, vol. 31, no. 1, pp. 225–232, 2007.

[60] O. Merimsky, "Targeting metastatic leiomyosarcoma by rapamycin plus gemcitabine: an intriguing clinical observation," *International Journal of Molecular Medicine*, vol. 14, no. 5, pp. 931–935, 2004.

[61] K. J. Brewer Savannah, E. G. Demicco, K. Lusby et al., "Dual targeting of mTOR and Aurora-A kinase for the treatment of uterine leiomyosarcoma," *Clinical Cancer Research*, vol. 18, no. 17, pp. 4633–4645, 2012.

[62] K. Saito-Diaz, T. W. Chen, X. Wang et al., "The way Wnt works: components and mechanism," *Growth Factors*, vol. 31, no. 1, pp. 1–31, 2013.

[63] M. A. de Graaff, A.-M. Cleton-Jansen, K. Szuhai, and J. V. M. G. Bovée, "Mediator complex subunit 12 exon 2 mutation analysis in different subtypes of smooth muscle tumors confirms genetic heterogeneity," *Human Pathology*, vol. 44, no. 8, pp. 1597–1604, 2013.

[64] W. Kildal, M. Pradhan, V. M. Abeler, G. B. Kristensen, and H. E. Danielsen, "Beta-catenin expression in uterine sarcomas and its relation to clinicopathological parameters," *European Journal of Cancer*, vol. 45, no. 13, pp. 2412–2417, 2009.

[65] A. Voronkov and S. Krauss, "Wnt/beta-catenin signaling and small molecule inhibitors," *Current Pharmaceutical Design*, vol. 19, no. 4, pp. 634–664, 2013.

[66] B. Edris, I. Espinosa, T. Mühlenberg et al., "ROR2 is a novel prognostic biomarker and a potential therapeutic target in leiomyosarcoma and gastrointestinal stromal tumour," *The Journal of Pathology*, vol. 227, no. 2, pp. 223–233, 2012.

[67] H. Mitsui, K. Shibata, Y. Mano et al., "The expression and characterization of endoglin in uterine leiomyosarcoma," *Clinical and Experimental Metastasis*, vol. 30, no. 6, pp. 731–740, 2013.

[68] W. Shan, P. Y. Akinfenwa, K. B. Savannah et al., "A small-molecule inhibitor targeting the mitotic spindle checkpoint impairs the growth of uterine leiomyosarcoma," *Clinical Cancer Research*, vol. 18, no. 12, pp. 3352–3365, 2012.

[69] Y. Li, T. Liu, C. Ivan et al., "Enhanced cytotoxic effects of combined valproic acid and the aurora kinase inhibitor VE465 on gynecologic cancer cells," *Frontiers in Oncology*, vol. 3, article 58, 2013.

[70] Hyman and National Cancer Institute (NCI), "Alisertib in treating patients with recurrent or persistent leiomyosarcoma of the uterus," Tech. Rep. NCT01637961, 2014.

[71] A. J. Levine and M. Oren, "The first 30 years of p53: growing ever more complex," *Nature Reviews Cancer*, vol. 9, no. 10, pp. 749–758, 2009.

[72] P. Ragazzini, G. Gamberi, L. Pazzaglia et al., "Amplification of CDK4, MDM2, SAS and GLI genes in leiomyosarcoma, alveolar and embryonal rhabdomyosarcoma," *Histology and Histopathology*, vol. 19, no. 3, p. 1013, 2004.

[73] U. N. M. Rao, S. D. Finkelstein, and M. W. Jones, "Comparative immunohistochemical and molecular analysis of uterine and extrauterine leiomyosarcomas," *Modern Pathology*, vol. 12, no. 11, pp. 1001–1009, 1999.

[74] R. Blom, C. Guerrieri, O. Stål, H. Malmström, and E. Simonsen, "Leiomyosarcoma of the uterus: a clinicopathologic, DNA flow cytometric, p53, and mdm-2 analysis of 49 cases," *Gynecologic Oncology*, vol. 68, no. 1, pp. 54–61, 1998.

[75] K. L. Hall, M. G. Teneriello, R. R. Taylor et al., "Analysis of Ki-ras, p53, and MDM2 genes in uterine leiomyomas and leiomyosarcomas," *Gynecologic Oncology*, vol. 65, no. 2, pp. 330–335, 1997.

[76] J.-C. Carry and C. Garcia-Echeverria, "Inhibitors of the p53/hdm2 protein-protein interaction-path to the clinic," *Bioorganic and Medicinal Chemistry Letters*, vol. 23, no. 9, pp. 2480–2485, 2013.

[77] Q. Ding, Z. Zhang, J.-J. Liu et al., "Discovery of RG7388, a potent and selective p53-MDM2 inhibitor in clinical development," *Journal of Medicinal Chemistry*, vol. 56, no. 14, pp. 5979–5983, 2013.

[78] D. Sun, Z. Li, Y. Rew et al., "Discovery of AMG 232, a potent, selective, and orally bioavailable MDM2-p53 inhibitor in clinical development," *Journal of Medicinal Chemistry*, vol. 57, no. 4, pp. 1454–1472, 2014.

[79] A. Y. Saiki, S. Caenepeel, D. Yu et al., "MDM2 antagonists synergize broadly and robustly with compounds targeting fundamental oncogenic signaling pathways," *Oncotarget*, vol. 5, no. 8, pp. 2030–2043, 2014.

[80] M. Grunstein, "Histone acetylation in chromatin structure and transcription," *Nature*, vol. 389, no. 6649, pp. 349–352, 1997.

[81] L. de Leval, D. Waltregny, J. Boniver, R. H. Young, V. Castronovo, and E. Oliva, "Use of histone deacetylase 8 (HDAC8), a new marker of smooth muscle differentiation, in the classification of mesenchymal tumors of the uterus," *American Journal of Surgical Pathology*, vol. 30, no. 3, pp. 319–327, 2006.

[82] A. Hrzenjak, F. Moinfar, M.-L. Kremser et al., "Histone deacetylase inhibitor vorinostat suppresses the growth of uterine sarcomas in vitro and in vivo," *Molecular Cancer*, vol. 9, article 49, 2010.

[83] P. Quan, F. Moinfar, I. Kufferath et al., "Effects of targeting endometrial stromal sarcoma cells via histone deacetylase and PI3K/AKT/mTOR signaling," *Anticancer Research*, vol. 34, no. 6, pp. 2883–2897, 2014.

[84] A. Atmaca, S.-E. Al-Batran, A. Maurer et al., "Valproic acid (VPA) in patients with refractory advanced cancer: a dose escalating phase I clinical trial," *British Journal of Cancer*, vol. 97, no. 2, pp. 177–182, 2007.

[85] P. Münster, D. Marchion, E. Bicaku et al., "Phase I trial of histone deacetylase inhibition by valproic acid followed by the topoisomerase II inhibitor epirubicin in advanced solid tumors: a clinical and translational study," *Journal of Clinical Oncology*, vol. 25, no. 15, pp. 1979–1985, 2007.

[86] B. Edris, K. Weiskopf, A. K. Volkmer et al., "Antibody therapy targeting the CD47 protein is effective in a model of aggressive metastatic leiomyosarcoma," *Proceedings of the National Academy of Sciences of the United States of America*, vol. 109, no. 17, pp. 6656–6661, 2012.

[87] N. Ü. Çomunoğlu, H. Durak, C. Çomunoğlu et al., "Expression of cyclooxygenase-2, c-kit, progesterone and estrogen receptors in uterine smooth muscle tumors: differential diagnosis," *APMIS*, vol. 115, no. 6, pp. 726–735, 2007.

[88] C.-H. Lee, D. A. Turbin, Y.-C. V. Sung et al., "A panel of antibodies to determine site of origin and malignancy in smooth muscle tumors," *Modern Pathology*, vol. 22, no. 12, pp. 1519–1531, 2009.

[89] M. M. Leitao, R. A. Soslow, D. Nonaka et al., "Tissue microarray immunohistochemical expression of estrogen, progesterone, and androgen receptors in uterine leiomyomata and leiomyosarcoma," *Cancer*, vol. 101, no. 6, pp. 1455–1462, 2004.

[90] Y. Rodríguez, D. Báez, F. M. de Oca et al., "Comparative analysis of the ERalpha/ERbeta ratio and neurotensin and its high-affinity receptor in myometrium, uterine leiomyoma, atypical leiomyoma, and leiomyosarcoma," *International Journal of Gynecological Pathology*, vol. 30, no. 4, pp. 354–363, 2011.

[91] E. Thanopoulou, K. Thway, K. Khabra, and I. Judson, "Treatment of hormone positive uterine leiomyosarcoma with aromatase inhibitors," *Clinical Sarcoma Research*, vol. 4, article 5, 2014.

[92] J. Hu, V. Khanna, M. Jones, and U. Surti, "Genomic alterations in uterine leiomyosarcomas: potential markers for clinical

diagnosis and prognosis," *Genes Chromosomes and Cancer*, vol. 31, no. 2, pp. 117–124, 2001.

[93] Y.-L. Zhai, T. Nikaido, A. Orii, A. Horiuchi, T. Toki, and S. Fujii, "Frequent occurrence of loss of heterozygosity among tumor suppressor genes in uterine leiomyosarcoma," *Gynecologic Oncology*, vol. 75, no. 3, pp. 453–459, 1999.

[94] K. Kawaguchi, Y. Oda, T. Saito et al., "Mechanisms of inactivation of the p16INK4a gene in leiomyosarcoma of soft tissue: decreased p16 expression correlates with promoter methylation and poor prognosis," *The Journal of Pathology*, vol. 201, no. 3, pp. 487–495, 2003.

[95] J. H. Francis, R. A. Kleinerman, J. M. Seddon, and D. H. Abramson, "Increased risk of secondary uterine leiomyosarcoma in hereditary retinoblastoma," *Gynecologic Oncology*, vol. 124, no. 2, pp. 254–259, 2012.

[96] M. C. Hollander, G. M. Blumenthal, and P. A. Dennis, "PTEN loss in the continuum of common cancers, rare syndromes and mouse models," *Nature Reviews Cancer*, vol. 11, no. 4, pp. 289–301, 2011.

[97] V. Stambolic, A. Suzuki, J. L. de la Pompa et al., "Negative regulation of PKB/Akt-dependent cell survival by the tumor suppressor PTEN," *Cell*, vol. 95, no. 1, pp. 29–39, 1998.

[98] M. S. Neshat, I. K. Mellinghoff, C. Tran et al., "Enhanced sensitivity of PTEN-deficient tumors to inhibition of FRAP/mTOR," *Proceedings of the National Academy of Sciences of the United States of America*, vol. 98, no. 18, pp. 10314–10319, 2001.

[99] M. Patel, N. C. Gomez, A. W. McFadden et al., "PTEN deficiency mediates a reciprocal response to IGFI and mTOR inhibition," *Molecular Cancer Research*, vol. 12, no. 11, pp. 1610–1620, 2014.

[100] L. S. Steelman, P. M. Navolanic, M. L. Sokolosky et al., "Suppression of PTEN function increases breast cancer chemotherapeutic drug resistance while conferring sensitivity to mTOR inhibitors," *Oncogene*, vol. 27, no. 29, pp. 4086–4095, 2008.

[101] S. Nag, J. Qin, K. S. Srivenugopal, M. Wang, and R. Zhang, "The MDM2-p53 pathway revisited," *Journal of Biomedical Research*, vol. 27, no. 4, pp. 254–271, 2013.

[102] D. Xing, G. Scangas, M. Nitta et al., "A role for BRCA1 in uterine leiomyosarcoma," *Cancer Research*, vol. 69, no. 21, pp. 8231–8235, 2009.

[103] S. M. B. Nijman and S. H. Friend, "Cancer: potential of the synthetic lethality principle," *Science*, vol. 342, no. 6160, pp. 809–811, 2013.

[104] P. C. Fong, D. S. Boss, T. A. Yap et al., "Inhibition of poly(ADP-ribose) polymerase in tumors from BRCA mutation carriers," *The New England Journal of Medicine*, vol. 361, no. 2, pp. 123–134, 2009.

[105] K. J. Dedes, D. Wetterskog, A. M. Mendes-Pereira et al., "PTEN deficiency in endometrioid endometrial adenocarcinomas predicts sensitivity to PARP inhibitors," *Science Translational Medicine*, vol. 2, no. 53, Article ID 53ra75, 2010.

[106] I. Chew and E. Oliva, "Endometrial stromal sarcomas: a review of potential prognostic factors," *Advances in Anatomic Pathology*, vol. 17, no. 2, pp. 113–121, 2010.

[107] E. Oliva, M. L. Carcangiu, S. G. Carinelli et al., "Tumours of the uterine corpus—mesenchymal tumours," in *WHO Classification of Tumours of Female Reproductive Organs*, R. J. Kurman, Ed., pp. 135–147, 4th edition, 2014.

[108] F. Amant, A. De Knijf, B. Van Calster et al., "Clinical study investigating the role of lymphadenectomy, surgical castration and adjuvant hormonal treatment in endometrial stromal sarcoma," *British Journal of Cancer*, vol. 97, no. 9, pp. 1194–1199, 2007.

[109] T. L. Beck, P. K. Singhal, H. M. Ehrenberg et al., "Endometrial stromal sarcoma: analysis of recurrence following adjuvant treatment," *Gynecologic Oncology*, vol. 125, no. 1, pp. 141–144, 2012.

[110] X. Cheng, G. Yang, K. M. Schmeler et al., "Recurrence patterns and prognosis of endometrial stromal sarcoma and the potential of tyrosine kinase-inhibiting therapy," *Gynecologic Oncology*, vol. 121, no. 2, pp. 323–327, 2011.

[111] P. Cossu-Rocca, M. Contini, M. G. Uras et al., "Tyrosine kinase receptor status in endometrial stromal sarcoma: an immunohistochemical and genetic-molecular analysis," *International Journal of Gynecological Pathology*, vol. 31, no. 6, pp. 570–579, 2012.

[112] B. Liegl, O. Reich, F. F. Nogales, and S. Regauer, "PDGF-α and PDGF-β are expressed in endometrial stromal sarcoma: a potential therapeutic target for tyrosine kinase inhibitors?" *Histopathology*, vol. 49, no. 5, pp. 545–546, 2006.

[113] J.-Y. Park, K.-R. Kim, and J.-H. Nam, "Immunohistochemical analysis for therapeutic targets and prognostic markers in low-grade endometrial stromal sarcoma," *International Journal of Gynecological Cancer*, vol. 23, no. 1, pp. 81–89, 2013.

[114] R. Sardinha, T. Hernández, S. Fraile et al., "Endometrial stromal tumors: immunohistochemical and molecular analysis of potential targets of tyrosine kinase inhibitors," *Clinical Sarcoma Research*, vol. 3, article 3, 2013.

[115] S.-I. Iwasaki, T. Sudo, M. Miwa et al., "Endometrial stromal sarcoma: clinicopathological and immunophenotypic study of 16 cases," *Archives of Gynecology and Obstetrics*, vol. 288, no. 2, pp. 385–391, 2013.

[116] M. E. Kalender, A. Sevinc, M. Yilmaz, C. Ozsarac, and C. Camci, "Detection of complete response to imatinib mesylate (Glivec/Gleevec) with ^{18}F-FDG PET/CT for low-grade endometrial stromal sarcoma," *Cancer Chemotherapy and Pharmacology*, vol. 63, no. 3, pp. 555–559, 2009.

[117] A. Trojan, M. Montemurro, M. Kamel, and G. Kristiansen, "Successful PDGFR-α/β targeting with imatinib in uterine sarcoma," *Annals of Oncology*, vol. 20, no. 11, pp. 1898–1899, 2009.

[118] C. Lan, X. Huang, S. Lin, M. Cai, and J. Liu, "Endometrial stromal sarcoma arising from endometriosis: a clinicopathological study and literature review," *Gynecologic and Obstetric Investigation*, vol. 74, no. 4, pp. 288–297, 2012.

[119] F. Moinfar, M. Gogg-Kamerer, A. Sommersacher et al., "Endometrial stromal sarcomas frequently express epidermal growth factor receptor (EGFR, HER-1): potential basis for a new therapeutic approach," *The American Journal of Surgical Pathology*, vol. 29, no. 4, pp. 485–489, 2005.

[120] G. Capobianco, F. Pili, M. Contini et al., "Analysis of epidermal growth factor receptor (EGFR) status in endometrial stromal sarcoma," *European Journal of Gynaecological Oncology*, vol. 33, no. 6, pp. 629–632, 2012.

[121] P. A. Cassier, A. Lefranc, E. Y Amela et al., "A phase II trial of panobinostat in patients with advanced pretreated soft tissue sarcoma. A study from the French Sarcoma Group," *British Journal of Cancer*, vol. 109, no. 4, pp. 909–914, 2013.

[122] A. Hrzenjak, F. Moinfar, M.-L. Kremser et al., "Valproate inhibition of histone deacetylase 2 affects differentiation and

decreases proliferation of endometrial stromal sarcoma cells," *Molecular Cancer Therapeutics*, vol. 5, no. 9, pp. 2203–2210, 2006.

[123] A. Hrzenjak, M.-L. Kremser, B. Strohmeier, F. Moinfar, K. Zatloukal, and H. Denk, "SAHA induces caspase-independent, autophagic cell death of endometrial stromal sarcoma cells by influencing the mTOR pathway," *Journal of Pathology*, vol. 216, no. 4, pp. 495–504, 2008.

[124] T.-I. Wu, H.-H. Chou, C.-J. Yeh et al., "Clinicopathologic parameters and immunohistochemical study of endometrial stromal sarcomas," *International Journal of Gynecological Pathology*, vol. 32, no. 5, pp. 482–492, 2013.

[125] C.-K. Jung, J.-H. Jung, A. Lee et al., "Diagnostic use of nuclear β-catenin expression for the assessment of endometrial stromal tumors," *Modern Pathology*, vol. 21, no. 6, pp. 756–763, 2008.

[126] S. Kurihara, Y. Oda, Y. Ohishi et al., "Coincident expression of β-catenin and cyclin D1 in endometrial stromal tumors and related high-grade sarcomas," *Modern Pathology*, vol. 23, no. 2, pp. 225–234, 2010.

[127] T. L. Ng, A. M. Gown, T. S. Barry et al., "Nuclear beta-catenin in mesenchymal tumors," *Modern Pathology*, vol. 18, no. 1, pp. 68–74, 2005.

[128] C.-H. Lee, R. H. Ali, M. Rouzbahman et al., "Cyclin D1 as a diagnostic immunomarker for endometrial stromal sarcoma with YWHAE-FAM22 rearrangement," *American Journal of Surgical Pathology*, vol. 36, no. 10, pp. 1562–1570, 2012.

[129] Y. J. Ioffe, A. J. Li, C. S. Walsh et al., "Hormone receptor expression in uterine sarcomas: prognostic and therapeutic roles," *Gynecologic Oncology*, vol. 115, no. 3, pp. 466–471, 2009.

[130] S. Kurihara, Y. Oda, Y. Ohishi et al., "Endometrial stromal sarcomas and related high-grade sarcomas: immunohistochemical and molecular genetic study of 31 cases," *American Journal of Surgical Pathology*, vol. 32, no. 8, pp. 1228–1238, 2008.

[131] O. Reich, S. Regauer, W. Urdl, M. Lahousen, and R. Winter, "Expression of oestrogen and progesterone receptors in low-grade endometrial stromal sarcomas," *British Journal of Cancer*, vol. 82, no. 5, pp. 1030–1034, 2000.

[132] A. Yoon, J.-Y. Park, J.-Y. Park et al., "Prognostic factors and outcomes in endometrial stromal sarcoma with the 2009 FIGO staging system: a multicenter review of 114 cases," *Gynecologic Oncology*, vol. 132, no. 1, pp. 70–75, 2014.

[133] M. C. Chu, G. Mor, C. Lim, W. Zheng, V. Parkash, and P. E. Schwartz, "Low-grade endometrial stromal sarcoma: hormonal aspects," *Gynecologic Oncology*, vol. 90, no. 1, pp. 170–176, 2003.

[134] M. C. Lim, S. Lee, and S.-S. Seo, "Megestrol acetate therapy for advanced low-grade endometrial stromal sarcoma," *Onkologie*, vol. 33, no. 5, pp. 260–262, 2010.

[135] M. Mizuno, Y. Yatabe, A. Nawa, and T. Nakanishi, "Long-term medroxyprogesterone acetate therapy for low-grade endometrial stromal sarcoma," *International Journal of Clinical Oncology*, vol. 17, no. 4, pp. 348–354, 2012.

[136] K. Nakayama, M. Ishikawa, Y. Nagai, N. Yaegashi, Y. Aoki, and K. Miyazaki, "Prolonged long-term survival of low-grade endometrial stromal sarcoma patients with lung metastasis following treatment with medroxyprogesterone acetate," *International Journal of Clinical Oncology*, vol. 15, no. 2, pp. 179–183, 2010.

[137] D. Pink, T. Lindner, A. Mrozek et al., "Harm or benefit of hormonal treatment in metastatic low-grade endometrial stromal sarcoma: single center experience with 10 cases and review of the literature," *Gynecologic Oncology*, vol. 101, no. 3, pp. 464–469, 2006.

[138] L. M. Ramondetta, A. J. Johnson, C. C. Sun et al., "Phase 2 trial of mifepristone (RU-486) in advanced or recurrent endometrioid adenocarcinoma or low-grade endometrial stromal sarcoma," *Cancer*, vol. 115, no. 9, pp. 1867–1874, 2009.

[139] G. Garg, J. P. Shah, E. P. Toy, C. S. Bryant, S. Kumar, and R. T. Morris, "Stage IA vs. IB endometrial stromal sarcoma: does the new staging system predict survival?" *Gynecologic Oncology*, vol. 118, no. 1, pp. 8–13, 2010.

[140] E. J. Tanner, K. Garg, M. M. Leitao Jr., R. A. Soslow, and M. L. Hensley, "High grade undifferentiated uterine sarcoma: surgery, treatment, and survival outcomes," *Gynecologic Oncology*, vol. 127, no. 1, pp. 27–31, 2012.

[141] F. Amant, T. Tousseyn, L. Coenegrachts, J. Decloedt, P. Moerman, and M. Debiec-Rychter, "Case report of a poorly differentiated uterine tumour with t(10;17) translocation and neuroectodermal phenotype," *Anticancer Research*, vol. 31, no. 6, pp. 2367–2371, 2011.

[142] K. Leunen, F. Amant, M. Debiec-Rychter et al., "Endometrial stromal sarcoma presenting as postpartum haemorrhage: report of a case with a sole t(10;17)(q22;p13) translocation," *Gynecologic Oncology*, vol. 91, no. 1, pp. 265–271, 2003.

[143] F. Micci, C. U. Walter, M. R. Teixeira et al., "Cytogenetic and molecular genetic analyses of endometrial stromal sarcoma: nonrandom involvement of chromosome arms 6p and 7p and confirmation of JAZF1/JJAZ1 gene fusion in t(7;17)," *Cancer Genetics and Cytogenetics*, vol. 144, no. 2, pp. 119–124, 2003.

[144] S. Regauer, W. Emberger, O. Reich, and R. Pfragner, "Cytogenetic analyses of two new cases of endometrial stromal sarcoma—non-random reciprocal translocation t(10;17)(q22; p13) correlates with fibrous ESS," *Histopathology*, vol. 52, no. 6, pp. 780–783, 2008.

[145] C. H. Lee, W. B. Ou, A. Mariño-Enriquez et al., "14-3-3 fusion oncogenes in high-grade endometrial stromal sarcoma," *Proceedings of the National Academy of Sciences of the United States of America*, vol. 109, no. 3, pp. 929–934, 2012.

[146] S. Croce, I. Hostein, A. Ribeiro et al., "YWHAE rearrangement identified by FISH and RT-PCR in endometrial stromal sarcomas: genetic and pathological correlations," *Modern Pathology*, vol. 26, no. 10, pp. 1390–1400, 2013.

[147] T. Mitsuhashi, M. Nakayama, S. Sakurai et al., "KIT-negative undifferentiated endometrial sarcoma with the amplified epidermal growth factor receptor gene showing a temporary response to imatinib mesylate," *Annals of Diagnostic Pathology*, vol. 11, no. 1, pp. 49–54, 2007.

[148] A. Salvatierra, A. Tarrats, C. Gomez, J. M. Sastre, and C. Balaña, "A case of c-kit positive high-grade stromal endometrial sarcoma responding to Imatinib Mesylate," *Gynecologic Oncology*, vol. 101, no. 3, pp. 545–547, 2006.

[149] C.-H. Lee, L. N. Hoang, S. Yip et al., "Frequent expression of KIT in endometrial stromal sarcoma with YWHAE genetic rearrangement," *Modern Pathology*, vol. 27, no. 5, pp. 751–757, 2014.

[150] 2012, http://www.fda.gov/drugs/informationondrugs/approveddrugs/ucm330213.htm.

[151] A. Hrzenjak, M. Tippl, M.-L. Kremser et al., "Inverse correlation of secreted frizzled-related protein 4 and β-catenin expression in endometrial stromal sarcomas," *Journal of Pathology*, vol. 204, no. 1, pp. 19–27, 2004.

[152] K. E. O'Reilly, F. Rojo, Q.-B. She et al., "mTOR inhibition induces upstream receptor tyrosine kinase signaling and activates Akt," *Cancer Research*, vol. 66, no. 3, pp. 1500–1508, 2006.

[153] C. Qian, C.-J. Lai, R. Bao et al., "Cancer network disruption by a single molecule inhibitor targeting both histone deacetylase activity and phosphatidylinositol 3-kinase signaling," *Clinical Cancer Research*, vol. 18, no. 15, pp. 4104–4113, 2012.

[154] C.-J. Lai, R. Bao, X. Tao et al., "CUDC-101, a multitargeted inhibitor of histone deacetylase, epidermal growth factor receptor, and human epidermal growth factor receptor 2, exerts potent anticancer activity," *Cancer Research*, vol. 70, no. 9, pp. 3647–3656, 2010.

12

Medication Exposures and Subsequent Development of Ewing Sarcoma

Judith U. Cope,[1] Gregory H. Reaman,[2] and Joseph M. Tonning[3]

[1]*Office of Pediatric Therapeutics, Office of Special Medical Programs, Office of the Commissioner/Food and Drug Administration, Building 32, Room 5156, 10903 New Hampshire Avenue, Silver Spring, MD 20993, USA*
[2]*Office of Hematology and Oncology Products, OND, Center for Drug Evaluation and Research, U.S. Food and Drug Administration, White Oak Bldg. 22, Room 2202, 10903 New Hampshire Avenue, Silver Spring, MD 20993, USA*
[3]*U.S. Public Health Service Commissioned Corps, Office of Translational Sciences, Center for Drug Evaluation and Research, U.S. Food and Drug Administration, White Oak Bldg. 22, Room 3410, 10903 New Hampshire Avenue, Silver Spring, MD 20993, USA*

Correspondence should be addressed to Judith U. Cope; judith.cope@fda.hhs.gov

Academic Editor: Cyril Fisher

Background. Ewing sarcoma family of tumors (ESFT) are rare but deadly cancers of unknown etiology. Few risk factors have been identified. This study was undertaken to ascertain any possible association between exposure to therapeutic drugs and ESFT. *Methods.* This is a retrospective, descriptive study. A query of the FDA Adverse Event Reporting System (FAERS) was conducted for all reports of ESFT, January 1, 1998, through December 31, 2013. Report narratives were individually reviewed for patient characteristics, underlying conditions and drug exposures. *Results.* Over 16 years, 134 ESFT reports were identified, including 25 cases of ESFT following therapeutic drugs and biologics including immunosuppressive agents and hormones. Many cases were confounded by concomitant medications and other therapies. *Conclusions.* This study provides a closer look at medication use and underlying disorders in patients who later developed ESFT. While this study was not designed to demonstrate any clear causative association between ESFT and prior use of a single product or drug class, many drugs were used to treat immune-related disease and growth or hormonal disturbances. Further studies may be warranted to better understand possible immune or neuroendocrine abnormalities or exposure to specific classes of drugs that may predispose to the later development of ESFT.

1. Introduction and Study Objective

Ewing sarcoma family of tumors (ESFT) is a group of small, round blue cell tumors that arise in the bone or soft tissue. ESFT include classic Ewing sarcoma (ES) of bone, extraskeletal ES, skin tumors of the chest wall, and primitive neuroectodermal tumors (PNET) of the bone or soft tissue. About 90% of ESFT cases are characterized by the chromosome translocation t(11;22)(q24;q12) which involves the EWS/FLI-1 fusion gene and may share a common neural histogenesis [1–4]. While ESFT is rare, it is the second most common primary malignant bone tumor occurring in children and young adults and accounts for 10–15% of all primary bone tumors and 3% of all pediatric malignancies. ESFT occurs with a male predominance and highest incidence rates among whites with considerably lower rates in Blacks and East Asian populations. Age of onset is normally in the second decade of life, with 80% occurring in the first 2 decades of life and 80% occur in the skeleton [2–5]. Each year up to 400 patients in the US will be diagnosed with ESFT. The incidence has been steady over the past few decades [6].

While few risk factors for ESFT have been identified, the racial difference and specific chromosomal translocation might suggest a genetic predisposition [1, 7]. However, unlike other bone cancers (e.g., osteosarcoma) and soft tissue sarcomas (e.g., rhabdomyosarcoma) ESFT has not been found to be associated with any genetic disease or hereditary cancer syndrome [2, 7, 8]. Epidemiological studies have examined a wide array of possible risk factors, including childhood conditions and various parental exposures [9–16]. There is limited data about drug exposures as possible risk factors for ESFT. One study reported a possible association with poison or overdose of medications [11]. Another study by Valery et al. 2003 [16] found medication use to be more prevalent in controls than cases. While few if any studies have found an association with medications and ESFT (with exposure to medications), two studies [10, 16] found an inverse association with asthma, but this has not been confirmed by the other studies [9, 11, 12, 16]. Despite continuing efforts to identify risk factors for ESFT, its etiology is still unknown.

The aim of this study was to review all cases of ESFT that have been reported to FDA from January 1, 1998, through December 31, 2013, and to assess any possible association with therapeutic products. (FAERS includes therapeutic agents which include drugs and also biologics.) We also conducted an extensive literature search of articles that pertained to the epidemiology of ESFT.

2. Methods

All case reports for drug products that included ESFT from the FDA Adverse Event Reporting System (FAERS) database were analyzed. The FAERS database, including foreign and domestic reports and all age groups, was searched for the time period, January 1, 1998, through December 31, 2013. The following Medical Dictionary for Regulatory Activities (MedDRA) search terms (MedDRA website, http://www.meddra.org/ see [17]) were used to identify any reports of cases with ESFT: Ewing's sarcoma, Ewing's sarcoma metastatic, Ewing's sarcoma recurrent, extraosseous Ewing's sarcoma, extraosseous Ewing's sarcoma metastatic, extraosseous Ewing's sarcoma nonmetastatic, extraosseous Ewing's sarcoma recurrent, neuroectodermal neoplasm, primitive neuroectodermal tumour, primitive neuroectodermal tumour metastatic, and peripheral primitive neuroectodermal tumour of soft tissue. Cases were stratified by year of occurrence and defined by the reporter as definite, probable, possible, and unlikely in terms of the diagnosis of ES and potential association with drug exposure. Reports of ESFT as a secondary malignancy, as a primary tumor preceding a secondary malignancy, adverse events related to chemotherapy, and other treatments for ESFT and report duplications were excluded. Case reports of medication use pre-ESFT were analyzed by two independent reviewers.

Data Source. This study utilized the FAERS database of adverse event (AE) reports. Since 1969, FDA has maintained this passive surveillance system to detect problems with drugs and biological products used by humans. Manufacturers are required by US law to report AEs associated with their products, and AEs may also be spontaneously reported by health care professionals and consumers. The database contains reports from the US and non-US countries. Reports that the reporter thought to be related to the use of a product are reviewed, coded, and accumulated into an electronic database. The adverse events are codified by MedDRA terminology. This passive surveillance program functions as an early warning system for the detection of serious AEs not identified during the premarket testing or clinical trials. A special feature of this program includes follow-up reports of cases following FDA's request for further information. Some of the reports in this database may also be found in the published literature.

3. Results

3.1. Overall FAERS Reports Summary. Over the 16-year time period, 134 reports were retrieved with mention of ESFT. After clinical review of the narrative reports 25 cases were identified with a history of medication use prior to ESFT diagnosis, most with a history of ≥18 months. Age range was 5–68 years of age (median 24 years) (Table 1). Many of our cases were outside the adolescent age group.

Primary ESFT after Drug Use (n = 25) (Table 2). A total of 25 out of 134 reports revealed the use of various suspect drug products with subsequent development of ESFT. Reports were excluded if ESFT occurred as a secondary malignancy, drug adverse events occurred with ESFT therapy, or ESFT occurred as a primary cancer before a secondary cancer occurred that followed drug therapies. The 25 cases of ESFT ranged in age from 4 to 68 years (median 24 years). There was no age information for 4 cases. Thirteen were US cases. Latency to ESFT diagnosis was ≥1 year for 14 cases, <1 year for 5, and unknown for 4. The reported medications included immunosuppressive drugs or drugs used for immune-related disorders (e.g., interferon beta-1, peginterferon alpha-2A and ribavirin, tumor necrosis factor (TNF) blockers, methotrexate, cyclosporine, and azathioprine), isotretinoin, recombinant growth hormone (rGH), and psychotropic medications including antiepileptics (AEDs), atypical antipsychotics, and psychostimulants. Many of the incident cases were confounded by concomitant medications that are labeled for possible carcinogenicity risk.

Twelve cases were treated with immunosuppressive products for a variety of conditions including 3 Crohn's, 3 multiple sclerosis (MS), 1 renal transplant, 1 rheumatoid arthritis (RA) and 1 each of ankylosing spondylitis, psoriasis vulgaris, chronic hepatitis C genotype 1b, and nephrotic syndrome. Use of more than one immunosuppressant drug was mentioned in 6 of the 12 reports.

Three cases received growth hormone (GH) and were diagnosed with ESFT 18 months to 4 years after beginning therapy. One child was treated with somatropin for microsomia due to neurosecretory GH disorder and a second child was treated for GH deficiency. The third case was a patient with Crohn's disease who received immunosuppressants and GH (this case is included in the 12 immunosuppressant cases above).

Three cases received other hormonal products, including parathyroid hormone, combined estrogen/progesterone, and etonogestrel implant. The one case treated with recombinant human parathyroid hormone had failed several earlier therapies for osteoporosis. The one case taking combined estrogen/medroxyprogesterone was a menopausal woman who was diagnosed with ESFT 10 months later, and the third case with the etonogestrel implant was a morbidly obese young woman (268 pounds, body mass index (BMI) = 42).

Six cases were treated with psychotropic medications, including 2 with atypical antipsychotics (1 olanzapine for

TABLE 1: Summary of FAERS reports of medication use prior to Ewing Sarcoma Family of Tumor (ESFT) diagnosis, 1997–2013. Total = 25; 13 US, 12 foreign; 16 females, 9 males. Ages 4–68 years (median age 24 years; mean 30 years). Known latency for 20 patients: 3 months–12 years (median 27 months; mean 3.2 years); 5 unknown.

(a)

Report year	Number of cases
1997–1999	1
2000–2004	6
2005–2009	9
2010–2013	9

(b)

Drug use	Number of cases	Patient age (yrs)	Latency
Immunosuppressive*	12	5–68	Mean 4.2 years, median 4 years
Growth hormone (GH)	2*	11, 16	4 months after 5 years therapy, 18 months
Estrogen/progestin	2	24, 47	10 months, 2.5 years
CNS depressant	2	34, 42	22 months, unknown
Atypical antipsychotic	1	17	No information
Antiepileptic	1	8	8 years
Antipsychotic and AED	1	19	3 months
ADHD	1	8	No information
Isotretinoin	1	20	10 months
Statin for hyperlipidemia	1	9	>2 years
rPTH**	1	49	1 year

*1 Crohn's patient also received GH.
**rPTH, recombinant parathyroid hormone.

(c)

Underlying conditions		
12	Immune-related	3 Crohn's disease, 3 multiple sclerosis, 1 renal transplant, 1 rheumatoid arthritis, 1 nephrotic syndrome, 1 ankylosing spondylitis, 1 psoriasis vulgaris, and 1 chronic hepatitis B
5	Endocrine	2 growth disorders, 1 menopause, 1 osteoporosis, and 1 birth control (patient morbidly obese but no underlying condition reported)
3	Neurologic	1 each of narcolepsy, seizure disorder, and fibromyalgia with sciatica/neuropathic pain
3	Psychiatric	1 each of unspecified depression, psychoses, and ADHD
2	Other	1 each of familial hypercholesterolemia, acne

unspecified condition, 1 olanzapine and antiepileptic drugs (AED), clonazepam, for depression), 1 attention deficit hyperactivity disorder (ADHD) drug, methylphenidate, 1 case taking 3 AEDs (ethosuximide, valproic acid, and clobazam), 1 case treated with sodium oxylate for narcolepsy, and 1 case treated with another AED, pregabalin, for neuropathic pain.

There were 2 additional cases that received other medications and then developed ESFT, including 1 young adult treated with isotretinoin for acne and developed ESFT 9 months later and 1 young child treated with atorvastatin for familial hypercholesterolemia.

4. Discussion

The FAERS is a passive surveillance system that collects data on adverse events possibly related to drugs and biologics that are reported to FDA by manufacturers, user facilities, and voluntary reporters, such as health care professionals and consumers. Importantly this system may capture rare and serious events that may not be detected in clinical trials and other studies and may lead to further understanding of possible associations of drugs and other risk factors for various diseases.

While few studies have found any association of exposure to medications with ESFT, our retrospective review of FAERS reports identified 25 cases of ES that followed drug therapy for various conditions. The majority were immunosuppressive agents used to treat autoimmune disorders. Most of the other reported drugs included hormones and psychotropic medications. We also reviewed the published literature to see if our findings might be consistent with other studies and case reports.

While various other malignancies have been reported in association with each of the drugs reported in the FAERS cases, there have been few literature reports of ESFT with the use of these medications. Many of the immunosuppressant drugs and some of the psychotropic and hormonal products are labeled with warnings of increased risk for malignancy or have product labeling for carcinogenicity based on animal studies (Table 3).

While the possible carcinogenic effects would differ for all these products, it may be important that most of the drugs in our case series may affect the hypothalamus and pituitary axis causing growth and neuroendocrine disturbance.

4.1. ESFT Cases following Immunosuppressive Agents. Nine of the 25 (36%) ESFT cases had been previously treated with immunosuppressive agents for autoimmune disorders including Crohn's disease, MS, RA, psoriasis, and ankylosing spondylitis. Three other cases receiving immunosuppressive therapy included 1 each for renal transplant, chronic hepatitis C, and nephrotic syndrome. Most were older individuals who had received immunosuppressive products two years or more prior to developing ESFT. While many of the case reports did not provide detailed information about duration of therapy and dosage, several reports indicated the use of combination or multimodal therapy with a variety of agents including cytotoxic drugs (e.g., cyclophosphamide, azathioprine, and

TABLE 2: Characteristics of 25 FDA case reports of pre-ESFT drug exposures.

	Age/sex	Disease	latency	Site	Drug	Type	Concomitant meds	Other
1	13 f	Crohn's	>2 yrs	Pelvis	Infliximab	Immune	None reported	
2	26 f	Crohn's	4 yrs	Calf	Infliximab	Immune	Mesalamine, GH	Severe Crohn's, registry azathioprine lansoprazole
3	39 m	Crohn's	2.5 yrs	Unknown	Infliximab	Immune	Mesalamine, Azathioprine	
4	f	MS	9-10 mos	Clavicle	Interferon	Immune	Potassium	pmh: clavicle fibrodysplasia, beta-1A, FMH positive for cancer
5	68 f	MS	>5 yrs	Shoulder	Interferon	Immune	No information	beta-1A
6	54 f	MS	3 mos	Brain	Natalizumab	immune	No information	
7	m	Ankylosing spondylitis	unknown	Unknown	Infliximab	Immune	No information	
8	50 f	RA	4 yrs	Unknown	Etanercept	Immune	No information	Canada
9	20 m	Psoriasis	6 yrs	Unknown	Infliximab	Immune	Methotrexate, cyclosporine, etanercept	Acitretin, efalizumab >6 yrs
10	52 m	transplant	8 yrs	Abdomen	Cyclosporine	Immune	steroids, azathioprine	Lliterature case [18] patient had OKT3 ab 2 transplants, nephrosclerosis
11	65 m	Chronic hepatitis C	12 yrs	Unknown	Peginterferon	Immune		Cholecystectomy, cirrhosis, esophageal varices alfa-2b and ribavirin
12	5 f	Nephrotic sx	18 mos	Spine	Cyclosporine	Immune	Dipyramidole, warfarin, prednisolone, cyclosporin	
13	11 f	GH def	18 mos	Thigh	r-somatropin	Hormone		Dose 0.7 mg sq should have been 0.47
14	16 f	GH def	Unknown	Clavicle	r-somatropin	Hormone		Patient grew 2.5 cm after GH
15	47 f	Menopause	10 mos	Spine	Estrogen/progestin	hormone	No information	Medical history—negative
16	24 f	Contraception	2.5 yrs	Unknown	Etonogestrel	Hormone	No information	Patient wt 268 lbs, ht 66.9″, BMI = 42
17	49 f	Osteoporosis	4 mos	Shoulder	Teriparatide	Hormone		Other osteoporosis drugs, family history—breast cancer
18	17 m	Unspecified psychiatric condition	unknown	Unknown	Olanzapine	Psychotropic	Acetaminophen	
19	19 m	Depression	3 mos	Unknown	Olanzapine	Psychotropic	Clonazepam	Unspecified depression
20	8 m	Epilepsy	8 yrs	metastatic	Ethosuximide	Psychotropic	Clobazam, valproic acid	CNS depressant
21	8 f	ADHD	Unknown	Mnknown	Methylphenidate	Psychotropic		
22	34 f	Narcolepsy	22 mos	Unknown	Sodium oxybate	Psychotropic	None	
23	42 f	Sciatica	Unknown	Unknown	Pregabalin	Psychotropic	Lisinopril for high blood pressure	Fibromyalgia, CNS depressant peripheral neuropathy
24	24 f	Acne	10 mos	Unknown	Isotretinoin	Others	No information	
25	9 m	High cholesterol	23 mos	Mandible	Atorvastatin	Cholesterol Lowering	Ezetimibe	3-year trial

TABLE 3: Product labeling information on carcinogenicity for medications reported in FAERS that were used pre-ESFT diagnosis (Drugs@fda)*.

Black box warning:	Adalimumab, azathioprine, cyclosporine, etanercept, everolimus, infliximab, teriparatide
Warning and precautions:	Recombinant human growth hormone or somatropin, methotrexate, estrogen/medroxyprogesterone
Cancer occurrence in mice or rat studies	Isotretinoin, olanzapine, atorvastatin, methylphenidate, pregabalin, valproic acid
No increase in tumor growth rates or metastasis in mouse xenograft transplant studies	Natalizumab
No carcinogenic risk detected in long-term studies:	Clozapine
No carcinogenic risk in animal studies conducted:	Mesalamine, etonogestrel implant, xyrem
No information on carcinogenicity in labeling:	Ethosuximide
Carcinogenicity testing not adequately addressed:	Clobazam
Carcinogenicity testing not done:	Interferon beta-1a, clonazepam, peginterferon alfa-2b

* http://www.accessdata.fda.gov/scripts/cder/drugsatfda/.

methotrexate), antibodies and other drug and biologic products for example, interferons, TNF blockers (infliximab, etanercept, and adalimumab), also mesalamine (aminosalicylate, an anti-inflammatory), and 1 case with glucocorticoids.

While ESFT per se has not been reported in association with immunosuppressant drugs, increased exposure to immunosuppressive agents has been found to be related to other cancers [21, 22]. In particular patients receiving higher potency and dosing of therapies for organ transplants have increased cancer risk of non-Hodgkin's lymphoma (NHL), Kaposi's sarcoma, nonmelanoma skin cancer, and other malignancies [23, 24]. While the literature highlights the accumulating evidence for elevated cancer risks with some of the immunosuppressant drugs, further studies are needed especially for the newer biologic treatments for immune-mediated inflammatory diseases. It is unclear whether there may be an elevated risk of extraintestinal solid cancers with the newer biologic agents including TNF blockers [25]. There are several limitations in the studies evaluating cancer risk among patients with exposure to immunosuppressive drugs. While no increase in risk of malignancies overall or in cancer subgroups may be found in clinical trials, study patients may not be a representative sample population and the length of follow-up might not be sufficiently long for malignancies to occur [26]. It is not always clear if it is the underlying autoimmune condition, the immunosuppressive therapy (a specific agent, dosage, or number of therapies) [27], or even potentially oncogenic viruses that play a major role in causing these cancers [28]. Several studies have found consistent increased cancer risk for patients with various underlying inflammatory immune diseases, including Crohn's and RA [29–32]. While the overall cancer incidence and mortality risk are similar to the general population in inflammatory bowel disease, there is an increased cancer risk for Crohn's and slightly increased risk for RA and psoriasis [21]. Studies have been less consistent in showing increased cancer risk associated with MS [33–35] and ankylosing spondylitis. For ankylosing spondylitis increased cancer risk seems to be associated with radiotherapy [36, 37]. Particularly with newer biologic agents including TNF blockers, further studies are needed to better determine if there is an increased cancer risk with the therapies themselves, with the higher doses, and longer treatments, or whether any increased cancer risk is due to underlying severe disease.

In our case series, most reports had incomplete information with regard to dosage and what additional past therapies had been given for the underlying diseases. While most cases had latency periods over a year, 2 of the MS cases had very short latencies of 3 and 10 months. It seems likely that these may have been misdiagnoses for what was later identified to be ESFT. With ESFT, compared to other malignancies, there is frequently a long period of time after initial symptoms until a diagnosis is made. Studies have shown the mean time to be 19–37 weeks [38–40]. One of the FAERS cases had a history of fibrous dysplasia of the clavicle and then later developed ES at the clavicular site. ES has been reported to mimic fibrous dysplasia [41–43].

From a regulatory perspective, FDA classifies carcinogenic risk of drugs and biologics based on their mechanism of action and hazard identification from in vivo and in vitro nonclinical assays [43]. In our series of 25 FAERS cases, 8 had received immunosuppressive products which are labeled with Box Warnings for carcinogenicity and the other 4 reports included immunosuppressants interferon beta-1a (2 FAERS reports), peginterferon alfa-2b (1 FAERS report), and natalizumab (1 FAERS report) which are not labeled for carcinogenicity. Three of these have not undergone carcinogenicity testing. Despite the clear association between immunosuppressant drugs and increased risk of cancer, many products may fail to predict an increased risk in the preclinical studies [44]. Identification of cancer risk with postmarketing pharmacovigilance is crucial. With regard to ESFT, not only is it a rare malignancy, but unlike other bone cancers such as osteosarcoma, there is no animal model.

We also conducted an extensive literature search for additional cases of ESFT reported with underlying autoimmune disorders or immunosuppressive therapy. In addition to the one renal transplant case in our series which was a case report by Balakrishnan et al. [18], we found three additional ESFT cases following renal transplant in the literature, 1 in a 34-year-old female with vaginal PNET [45], a 15-year-old female with PNET of uterus 9 years after renal transplant for end stage renal disease [46], and a case of unknown age with ESFT of the sacrum following renal transplant [47]. A higher risk of developing malignancy in transplant recipients has been reported [48]. No additional published cases of ESFT associated with other autoimmune disorders or immunosuppressant agents were found.

4.2. ESFT Cases following Hormonal Drugs. There were three reports of ESFT following GH therapy, including two with GH deficiency and an additional case with Crohn's disease who received both GH and immunosuppressants (included in the 12 immunosuppressant drug reports above). It remains unclear if GH is a carcinogen. Studies have conflicting results regarding any association with GH and cancer. A French population-based cohort study, The French Safety and Appropriateness of Growth Hormone treatments in Europe (SAGhE), of patients treated with recombinant GH reported an increased risk of bone cancers ($n = 3$ cases observed versus 0.6 expected; SMR 5.00; 95% CI, 1.01–14.63), both osteosarcoma (2 cases, statistically nonsignificant) and Ewing sarcoma (1 case, statistically significant) [49]. The selected population for the study included low risk patients who were treated for conditions of idiopathic isolated GH deficiency, idiopathic short stature, short stature in children born short for gestational age, or isolated GH deficiency associated with a minor craniofacial malformation, such as cleft lip. Patients in the middle risk category with pediatric syndromes such as Turner and Noonan syndrome were excluded. The authors of the study thought the elevated bone cancer risk was biologically plausible as bone cancers occur during rapid bone growth of puberty that relate to the insulin-like growth factor 1 (IGF-1) system. It is known that GH and IGF-I do have mitogenic and antiapoptotic activity and that there is a theoretical risk that GH treatment may be associated with cancer [50]. However, interpretation of the study results is limited by the select patient population, the relatively short-term follow-up, and lack of information on the administered GH doses. Other subsequent studies did not demonstrate any increased cancer risks [51–56]. Currently, while GH does not appear to increase the risk for new malignancy in children without known risk factors, an increased risk of a second neoplasm, mostly intracranial tumors in those with prior radiation, has been reported in childhood cancer survivors treated with GH compared with those not treated [51, 55, 57] and this is in the labeling for GH products. Overall, there remain concerns about the possibility of delayed posttreatment effects of heightened GH and IGF-1 on cancer risk. It is unknown if GH treatment may increase the risk of cancer in patients with short stature. Further ongoing surveillance and longer-term studies are needed.

ESFT is thought to be of neural origin and while neurogenic cancers such as neuroblastoma have been reported after GH, we could find no additional literature reports of ESFT following GH. In our ESFT cases one might wonder about the possible risk factor for cancer: is it the GH or is it related to the underlying growth disorder itself?

The other therapeutic hormonal drugs prior to ESFT diagnosis in our series included progestin, combined estrogen/progestin, and parathyroid hormone in nonadolescent females. Our literature review revealed one case report of ES in a young woman four months following abortion [58]. Her only reported drug exposure was four years of oral contraceptive (levonorgestrel 0.05 mg and ethinylestradiol 0.03 mg). (Pregnancy itself leads to decreased circulating GH and slightly increased IGF.)

4.3. Growth and Neuroendocrine Effects of the Drugs Used Pre-ESFT. It is of interest that 16 of the 25 FAERS reports involved various drugs that all have an influence or effect on the hypothalamic-pituitary axis. In particular interferons may be associated growth suppression. Some studies showed that immunosuppressive agents, such as TNF blockers (e.g., infliximab), can also affect the hypothalamic-pituitary-adrenal axis [59]. One of the cases treated with a TNF blocker had also received growth hormone. Many of the psychotropic drugs cause hyperprolactinemia. Antipsychotic drugs may be prone to causing hyperprolactinemia [60] and patients treated with psychostimulants may experience slowing of growth or growth retardation. Small transient decreases in serum IGF-1 may occur early in the treatment of patients with methylphenidate. This is less common in females [61]. Seizure medications, especially valproic acid and ethosuximide, have been known to be associated with hyperandrogenism, menstrual disorders, and polycystic ovary syndrome [62]. Isotretinoin has an effect on the pituitary adrenal axis with mild suppression of pituitary hormones. While long-term studies are needed, Karadag et al. [63] found that isotretinoin appeared to have a negative influence on the GH/IGF-1 axis, with a significant decrease in IGF-1 and IGFBP3 levels after 3 months of isotretinoin treatment. Also, steroids used to treat Crohn's may cause suppression of the HPA axis.

Epilepsy itself [62] has sex-specific effects on hormone levels and reproductive function. Women with seizures have hypothalamic disorders, amenorrhea and reproductive/endocrine disorders, and ovarian cysts [64, 65].

4.4. ESFT Cases following Psychotropic Drugs. The other category of pre-ESFT therapies included psychotropic drugs. There was only 1 case of each therapy in this category. Currently, most antipsychotic drugs are not considered to increase the risk of cancer [66]. One product, clozapine, has a separate status given that this molecule shows antiproliferative effects implied in agranulocytosis as well as a potential increased risk for leukemia [67].

4.5. Literature Review of Studies and Case Reports of ESFT. Few studies have closely examined drug exposures in children who later develop ESFT. Past registry, case-control studies and case series that collected data on medication use [9, 10, 12, 16] have not consistently identified any specific drug therapy as a risk factor for ESFT (see Table 4). Due to the rarity of ESFT, many studies examining possible risk factors lack the statistical power to definitely prove or disprove any association with medication exposures, underlying diseases or genetic disorders. Several studies and literature reports have found a wide array of different medical conditions, anomalies, and even genetic syndromes in patients who developed ESFT (Table 4). More than one study reported congenital genitourinary and renal anomalies (e.g., cryptorchidism, duplication

TABLE 4: ESFT-related studies.

Author/publication year/age group	Number of cases	Number of controls/cohort	Findings
		Case-control studies	
Buckley et al., 1998 [10], (<21 yrs)	153	153	Inverse association with asthma. Looked at diseases and treatments, but not specifically medications. Earlier growth spurt and lower gain in weight and height among males but ES females no differences between cases and controls during growth spurt associations between GU anomalies and ES could not be confirmed.
Hartley et al., 1988 [9], (<15 yrs)	43 soft tissue & bone cancers (16 ES)	146	Developmental anomalies in 5 ES children: 1 meningomyelocele; 1 with an absent kidney and ureter. Medications were evaluated first month of life, 1–5 months, ≥6 months and grouped as antibiotics, anticonvulsants, corticosteroids, anti-allergic, bronchodilators, decongestants, cough suppressants and expectorants, and drugs for GI disorders.
Holly et al., 1992 [11], (<31 yrs)	43	193	Agricultural exposures, overdose of medications or accidental ingestion of poisonings
Winn et al., 1992 [12], (5 mos–22 yrs)	208	395	Hernias ~6 times more than expected, (OR 5.7; 95% Cl, 1.7–19.3) and also excess of cardiac conditions which however were mostly functional heart murmurs
Valery et al., 2003 [16], (most <20 yrs, ~75%)	106	344	Disorders of the digestive tract, behavioral hyperactivity and disorder of male organs (hydrocele and cryptorchidism) were also more frequent in cases but were not statistically significant. Only hernia excess achieved statistical significance (OR 3.1, 95% CI 1.2–7.6). Inverse association with asthma; deficit of bone disorders in cases (mostly fractures); also less frequent family history of stomach and neuroectodermal cancers. Authors state inverse association with medications: Use of medication and medical procedures steroids 9 cases, 30 controls 1.2 (0.5–2.9) anti-epileptic 1 case, 4 controls 0.9 (0.1–9.3) antibiotic 95 cases, 324 controls 0.6 (0.3–1.5) vermicide 62 cases, 246 controls 0.5 (0.3–0.8) hormone 6 cases, 51 controls 0.5 (0.2–1.5)
		Cohort studies: case series or registries	
Pendergrass et al. 1984 [19], (≤18 yrs)	291	n/a	No strong association with stature
Cope et al. 2000 [13], (<46 yrs)	306	n/a	13 inguinal hernias, also 14 bony anomalies, 5 undescended testes, 1 abnormal kidney, 6 duplication of ureters, Zollinger-Ellison syndrome (which is associated with pituitary tumors)
Narod et al., 1997 [14], (<15),	396 ES (out of 20,304 cancers)	23 (5.8% anomalies)	National Registry Britain for Childhood Tumors (NRCT) and the BC British Registry for anomalies for presence of anomalies note in this study CNS PNETs were classified with medulloblastomas not part of ES. 2 cases osteogenic imperfecta. (confirmed previous associations that McKeen et al. [15] found)
McKeen et al., 1983 [15], (<46 yrs)	154 (23 cases ES)		Genitourinary, musculoskeletal. 56 development anomalies, 19 GU, of 99 males, 2 with unilateral cryptorchidism, 2 hypospadias, 5 of 55 females with unilateral ureter duplications, 8 rib anomalies, 7 vertebral defects, 4 with benign bone neoplasms (2 at primary ESFT site were bone cyst and enchondroma)
Glass and Fraumeni 1970 [20] (<15 yrs)	146 (out of 396 childhood cancers)		Hospital series, 2 spina bifida (1 with café au lait spots), osteoid osteoma, bone cysts, cryptorchidism, varicocele, Meckel's diverticulum, colonic polyps w/accessory spleen, congenital pulmonic stenosis, pulmonic valve 4 cusps, 1 mongolism (Down syndrome), 2 mothers of ES pts had multiple sclerosis; thyroidectomy for goiters in 2 mothers of ES pts.
Beyaert et al., 2013 [21]			Rib anomalies ES with high incidence of cervical ribs. 17.1% (not confirmed by other studies)

Table 4: Continued.

Author/publication year/age group	Number of cases	Number of controls/cohort	Findings
Pooled analysis and meta-analysis of studies regarding hernias in association with ESFT			
Valery et al. 2003 [16]	199 cases	1,451 controls	Association with hernias, umbilical, inguinal, and congenital. The primary endpoint was development of a tumor from the Ewing's sarcoma family. 138 patients with such a tumor and 574 controls were included in the pooled analysis, and 357 patients with these tumors and 745 controls were included in the meta-analysis.

of ureters and collecting system, and inguinal hernias) and musculoskeletal and spinal anomalies (e.g., cervical ribs, spina bifida, and myelomeningocele) [9, 12–15, 20, 68, 69]. It is of interest that many of these conditions are known to be associated with growth and neuroendocrine dysfunction. Our literature review found reports of ESFT in patients with other genetic syndromes including 4 articles with 5 cases with Down syndrome [20, 70–72], 1 case with chromosome 18q-deletion syndrome [73], and 2 cases with osteogenesis imperfecta [14]. While these syndromes are not uncommon and it might be expected that ESFT would occur, it is of interest that all these syndromes are known to be associated with short stature with abnormal pubertal growth and GH deficiency or pituitary dysfunction. Unlike osteosarcoma there has been no consistent association with tall stature or pubertal bone growth in patients with ESFT [10, 16, 19, 74]. Perhaps it is the hormonal changes and interference with growth aspects of puberty that are awry in the development of ESFT.

While our FAERS reports were submitted to FDA in association with drug use, the reported therapies were used to treat autoimmune disorders and childhood conditions that, especially if severe, might lead to growth and/or endocrine disturbance. Crohn's disease, renal failure (especially posttransplant), psychoses, and epilepsy [62, 64] may all cause or be associated with hyperprolactinemia, growth disturbance, and/or pituitary dysfunction during childhood and adolescence. Thus, these cases might also support that there is an underlying endocrine disturbance in patients with ESFT. Also, the various inflammatory conditions that were treated with immunosuppressants in our FAERS case series may also affect bone health (e.g., RA, Crohn's, and MS) and alter pubertal development. Mood disorders such as anxiety, bipolar disorder, insomnia, and fibromyalgia also involve the HPA axis and GH deficiency is associated with high cholesterolemia, osteoporosis, and short stature.

4.6. Limitations. The observation of a small number of cases of an uncommon cancer occurring in association with certain exposures does not provide evidence of any causal link. This study using the FDA database has several limitations including reporting biases for cases from manufacturers as well as health care professionals and consumers. FAERS cases may be reported to FDA from postmarket surveillance studies with incomplete enrollment and reporting is dependent upon physician investigator compliance with submitting forms consistently and accurately, and whether the reported disease is related or unrelated to the therapy is subjective. Submitted reports may lack important information on the underlying disease, comorbid conditions, and prior therapies. These reports do not provide histopathologic confirmation of the cancer diagnosis. Another limitation of this study is that it is a retrospective analysis. However, epidemiological studies on patient populations also have limited value because of the long latency period for most cancers and because most studies lack sensitivity. Most studies approach bone cancers as a group without breakdown into subtypes of osteosarcoma and ESFT which are thought to have very different etiologies. Nonetheless, FAERS is the largest postmarketing drug safety database in the world maintained by a single country, containing more than 9 million reports of "drug-related" (but not necessarily causal) adverse event reports since 1969. Because of its potential comprehensiveness in capturing rare drug-associated adverse events from all over the world, the FAERS data may be useful in generating hypotheses relating to possible causes of a specific rare cancer, which later if warranted may be tested in formal and more rigorous epidemiological studies.

5. Conclusions

ESFT is known for its striking unimodal incident peak during puberty and few risk factors have been identified as to its etiology. In this present study we found ESFT cases following the use of immunosuppressant agents as well as hormonal medications. These medications as well as the reported underlying immune disorders and neuroendocrine conditions are associated with abnormal growth and hormonal disturbance. These findings may provide insight as to why this cancer has a peak incidence during adolescence. Perhaps the neuroendocrine abnormalities might even be linked to a common gene. Formal epidemiological or clinical studies should be conducted to further evaluate any possible role of neuroendocrine disturbances with these underlying conditions and drugs in the development of ESFT.

Disclosure

All authors are government employees of the Food and Drug Administration, HHS.

References

[1] M. U. Jawad, M. C. Cheung, E. S. Min, M. M. Schneiderbauer, L. G. Koniaris, and S. P. Scully, "Ewing sarcoma demonstrates racial disparities in incidence-related and sex-related differences in outcome: an analysis of 1631 cases from the SEER database, 1973–2005," *Cancer*, vol. 115, no. 15, pp. 3526–3536, 2009.

[2] Z. Burningham, M. Hashibe, L. Spector, and J. D. Schiffman, "The epidemiology of sarcoma," *Clinical Sarcoma Research*, vol. 2, no. 1, article 14, 2012.

[3] M. Ladanyi, "EWS-FLI1 and Ewing's sarcoma: recent molecular data and new insights," *Cancer Biology & Therapy*, vol. 1, no. 4, pp. 330–336, 2002.

[4] I. M. Ambros, P. F. Ambros, S. Strehl, H. Kovar, H. Gadner, and M. Salzer-Kuntschik, "MIC2 is a specific marker for ewing's sarcoma and peripheral primitive neuroectodermal tumors. Evidence for a common histogenesis of ewing's sarcoma and peripheral primitive neuroectodermal tumors from MIC2 expression and specific chromosome aberration," *Cancer*, vol. 67, no. 7, pp. 1886–1893, 1991.

[5] O. Javery, K. Krajewski, K. O'Regan et al., "A to Z of extraskeletal Ewing sarcoma family of tumors in adults: imaging features of primary disease, metastatic patterns, and treatment responses," *The American Journal of Roentgenology*, vol. 197, no. 6, pp. W1015–W1022, 2011.

[6] N. Esiashvili, M. Goodman, and R. B. Marcus, "Changes in incidence and survival of ewing sarcoma patients over the past 3 decades: surveillance epidemiology and end results data," *Journal of Pediatric Hematology/Oncology*, vol. 30, no. 6, pp. 425–430, 2008.

[7] J. Worch, K. K. Matthay, J. Neuhaus, R. Goldsby, and S. G. Dubois, "Ethnic and racial differences in patients with ewing sarcoma," *Cancer*, vol. 116, no. 4, pp. 983–988, 2010.

[8] R. L. Randall, S. L. Lessnick, K. B. Jones et al., "Is there a predisposition gene for ewing's sarcoma?" *Journal of Oncology*, vol. 2010, Article ID 397632, 6 pages, 2010.

[9] A. L. Hartley, J. M. Birch, P. A. McKinney et al., "The Inter-Regional Epidemiological Study of Childhood Cancer (IRESCC): case control study of children with bone and soft tissue sarcomas," *British Journal of Cancer*, vol. 58, no. 6, pp. 838–842, 1988.

[10] J. D. Buckley, T. W. Pendergrass, C. M. Buckley et al., "Epidemiology of osteosarcoma and Ewing's sarcoma in childhood: a study of 305 cases by the children's cancer group," *Cancer*, vol. 83, no. 7, pp. 1440–1448, 1998.

[11] E. A. Holly, D. A. Aston, D. K. Ahn, and J. J. Kristiansen, "Ewing's bone sarcoma, paternal occupational exposure, and other factors," *American Journal of Epidemiology*, vol. 135, no. 2, pp. 122–129, 1992.

[12] D. M. Winn, F. P. Li, L. L. Robison, J. J. Mulvihill, A. E. Daigle, and J. F. Fraumeni Jr., "A case-control study of the etiology of Ewing's sarcoma," *Cancer Epidemiology Biomarkers and Prevention*, vol. 1, no. 7, pp. 525–532, 1992.

[13] J. U. Cope, M. Tsokos, L. J. Helman, G. Gridley, and M. A. Tucker, "Inguinal hernia in patients with Ewing sarcoma: a clue to etiology," *Medical and Pediatric Oncology*, vol. 34, no. 3, pp. 195–199, 2000.

[14] S. A. Narod, M. M. Hawkins, C. M. Robertson, and C. A. Stiller, "Congenital anomalies and childhood cancer in Great Britain," *American Journal of Human Genetics*, vol. 60, no. 3, pp. 474–485, 1997.

[15] E. A. McKeen, M. R. Hanson, J. J. Mulvihill, and D. L. Glaubiger, "Birth defects with Ewing's sarcoma," *The New England Journal of Medicine*, vol. 309, no. 24, pp. 1522–1523, 1983.

[16] P. C. Valery, W. McWhirter, A. Sleigh, G. Williams, and C. Bain, "A national case-control study of Ewing's sarcoma family of tumours in Australia," *International Journal of Cancer*, vol. 105, no. 6, pp. 825–830, 2003.

[17] MedDRA, November 2014, http://www.meddra.org/.

[18] R. Balakrishnan, Q. T. Khairullah, A. Giraldo, and R. Provenzano, "Extraskeletal Ewing's sarcoma in a kidney transplant patient," *American Journal of Kidney Diseases*, vol. 33, no. 6, pp. 1164–1167, 1999.

[19] T. W. Pendergrass, M. A. Foulkes, L. L. Robison, and M. E. Nesbit, "Stature and Ewing's sarcoma in childhood," *American Journal of Pediatric Hematology/Oncology*, vol. 6, no. 1, pp. 33–39, 1984.

[20] A. G. Glass and J. F. Fraumeni Jr., "Epidemiology of bone cancer in children," *Journal of the National Cancer Institute*, vol. 44, no. 1, pp. 187–199, 1970.

[21] R. Beyaert, L. Beaugerie, G. van Assche et al., "Cancer risk in immune-mediated inflammatory diseases (IMID)," *Molecular Cancer*, vol. 12, no. 1, article 98, 2013.

[22] L. A. Habel and G. D. Friedman, "Chapter 25. Phaamaceuticals other than hormones," in *Textbook of Cancer Epidemiology and Prevention*, D. Schottenfeld and J. F. Fraumeni, Eds., pp. 248–268, University Press, New York, NY, USA, 3rd edition, 2006.

[23] E. A. Engels, R. M. Pfeiffer, J. F. Fraumeni Jr. et al., "Spectrum of cancer risk among US solid organ transplant recipients," *Journal of the American Medical Association*, vol. 306, no. 17, pp. 1891–1901, 2011.

[24] G. Opelz and R. Henderson, "Incidence of non-Hodgkin lymphoma in kidney and heart transplant recipients," *The Lancet*, vol. 342, no. 8886-8887, pp. 1514–1516, 1993.

[25] D. Hudesman, S. Lichtiger, and B. Sands, "Risk of extraintestinal solid cancer with anti-TNF therapy in adults with inflammatory bowel disease: review of the literature," *Inflammatory Bowel Diseases*, vol. 19, no. 3, pp. 644–649, 2013.

[26] L. Peyrin-Biroulet, P. Deltenre, N. de Suray, J. Branche, W. J. Sandborn, and J.-F. Colombel, "Efficacy and safety of tumor necrosis factor antagonists in Crohn's disease: meta-analysis of placebo-controlled trials," *Clinical Gastroenterology and Hepatology*, vol. 6, no. 6, pp. 644–653, 2008.

[27] T. Vial and J. Descotes, "Immunosuppressive drugs and cancer," *Toxicology*, vol. 185, no. 3, pp. 229–240, 2003.

[28] I. Penn, "Sarcomas in organ allograft recipients," *Transplantation*, vol. 60, no. 12, pp. 1485–1491, 1995.

[29] G. Gridley, J. K. McLaughlin, A. Ekbom et al., "Incidence of cancer among patients with rheumatoid arthritis," *Journal of the National Cancer Institute*, vol. 85, no. 4, pp. 307–311, 1993.

[30] L. Mellemkjær, M. S. Linet, G. Gridley, M. Frisch, H. Møller, and J. H. Olsen, "Rheumatoid arthritis and cancer risk," *European Journal of Cancer Part A*, vol. 32, no. 10, pp. 1753–1757, 1996.

[31] L. J. Kinlen, "Incidence of cancer in rheumatoid arthritis and other disorders after immunosuppressive treatment," *The American Journal of Medicine*, vol. 78, no. 1, pp. 44–49, 1985.

[32] E. Zintzaras, M. Voulgarelis, and H. M. Moutsopoulos, "The risk of lymphoma development in autoimmune diseases: a meta-analysis," *Archives of Internal Medicine*, vol. 165, no. 20, pp. 2337–2344, 2005.

[33] C. Lebrun, M. Debouverie, P. Vermersch et al., "Cancer risk and impact of disease-modifying treatments in patients with

multiple sclerosis," *Multiple Sclerosis*, vol. 14, no. 3, pp. 399–405, 2008.

[34] N. M. Nielsen, K. Rostgaard, S. Rasmussen et al., "Cancer risk among patients with multiple sclerosis: a population-based register study," *International Journal of Cancer*, vol. 118, no. 4, pp. 979–984, 2006.

[35] E. Kingwell and H. Tremlett, "Interferons and multiple sclerosis: is it plausible that β-IFN treatment could influence the risk of cancer among MS patients?" *Expert Review of Neurotherapeutics*, vol. 9, no. 9, pp. 1263–1265, 2009.

[36] S. C. Darby, E. Nakashima, and H. Kato, "A parallel analysis of cancer mortality among atomic bomb survivors and patients with ankylosing spondylitis given X-ray therapy," *Journal of the National Cancer Institute*, vol. 75, no. 1, pp. 1–21, 1985.

[37] H. A. Weiss, S. C. Darby, and R. Doll, "Cancer mortality following x-ray treatment for ankylosing spondylitis," *International Journal of Cancer*, vol. 59, no. 3, pp. 327–338, 1994.

[38] B. Widhe and T. Widhe, "Initial symptoms and clinical features in osteosarcoma and Ewing sarcoma," *The Journal of Bone & Joint Surgery—American Volume*, vol. 82, no. 5, pp. 667–674, 2000.

[39] F. J. Frassica, D. A. Frassica, D. J. Pritchard, P. J. Schomberg, L. E. Wold, and F. H. Sim, "Ewing sarcoma of the pelvis. Clinicopathological features and treatment," *The Journal of Bone and Joint Surgery—American Volume*, vol. 75, no. 10, pp. 1457–1465, 1993.

[40] T. A. Damron, F. H. Sim, M. I. O'Connor, D. J. Pritchard, and W. A. Smithson, "Ewing's sarcoma of the proximal femur," *Clinical Orthopaedics & Related Research*, vol. 322, pp. 232–244, 1996.

[41] M. Sundaram, C. Y. Inwards, T. E. Shives, and P. M. Anderson, "Ewing's sarcoma of the humerus mimicking fibrous dysplasia on imaging and biological behavior," *Skeletal Radiology*, vol. 34, no. 5, pp. 285–289, 2005.

[42] K. Kato, T. Hayashi, K. Tabuchi et al., "Concurrent Ewing sarcoma family of tumors and fibrous dysplasia: possible diagnostic pitfall," *Journal of Pediatric Hematology/Oncology*, vol. 29, no. 1, pp. 15–18, 2007.

[43] A. Jacobs and D. Jacobson-Kram, "Human carcinogenic risk evaluation, part III: assessing cancer hazard and risk in human drug development," *Toxicological Sciences*, vol. 81, no. 2, pp. 260–262, 2004.

[44] P. J. Bugelski, A. Volk, M. R. Walker, J. H. Krayer, P. Martin, and J. Descotes, "Critical review of preclinical approaches to evaluate the potential of immunosuppressive drugs to influence human neoplasia," *International Journal of Toxicology*, vol. 29, no. 5, pp. 435–466, 2010.

[45] P. Gaona-Luviano, E. Unda-Franco, L. González-Jara, P. Romero, and H. Medina-Franco, "Primitive neuroectodermal tumor of the vagina," *Gynecologic Oncology*, vol. 91, no. 2, pp. 456–458, 2003.

[46] E. Peres, T. K. Mattoo, J. Poulik, and I. Warrier, "Primitive neuroectodermal tumor (PNET) of the uterus in a renal allograft patient: a case report," *Pediatric Blood and Cancer*, vol. 44, no. 3, pp. 283–285, 2005.

[47] I. Penn, "Post-transplant malignancy: the role of immunosuppression," *Drug Safety*, vol. 23, no. 2, pp. 101–113, 2000.

[48] P. Ruangkanchanasetr, B. Lauhawatana, S. Leawseng, S. Kitpanich, A. Lumpaopong, and P. Thirakhupt, "Malignancy in renal transplant recipients: a single-center experience in Thailand," *Journal of the Medical Association of Thailand*, vol. 95, supplement 5, pp. S12–S16, 2012.

[49] J.-C. Carel, E. Ecosse, F. Landier et al., "Long-term mortality after recombinant growth hormone treatment for isolated growth hormone deficiency or childhood short stature: preliminary report of the French SAGhE study," *The Journal of Clinical Endocrinology & Metabolism*, vol. 97, no. 2, pp. 416–425, 2012.

[50] I. Banerjee and P. E. Clayton, "Growth hormone treatment and cancer risk," *Endocrinology and Metabolism Clinics of North America*, vol. 36, no. 1, pp. 247–263, 2007.

[51] J. Bell, K. L. Parker, R. D. Swinford, A. R. Hoffman, T. Maneatis, and B. Lippe, "Long-term safety of recombinant human growth hormone in children," *Journal of Clinical Endocrinology and Metabolism*, vol. 95, no. 1, pp. 167–177, 2010.

[52] L. Sävendahl, M. Maes, K. Albertsson-Wikland et al., "Long-term mortality and causes of death in isolated GHD, ISS, and SGA patients treated with recombinant growth hormone during childhood in Belgium, The Netherlands, and Sweden: preliminary report of 3 countries participating in the EU SAGhE study," *The Journal of Clinical Endocrinology & Metabolism*, vol. 97, no. 2, pp. E213–E217, 2012.

[53] A. L. Ogilvy-Stuart and H. Gleeson, "Cancer risk following growth hormone use in childhood: implications for current practice," *Drug Safety*, vol. 27, no. 6, pp. 369–382, 2004.

[54] Y. Nishi, T. Tanaka, K. Takano et al., "Recent status in the occurrence of leukemia in growth hormone-treated patients in Japan," *The Journal of Clinical Endocrinology & Metabolism*, vol. 84, no. 6, pp. 1961–1965, 1999.

[55] C. A. Sklar, A. C. Mertens, P. Mitby et al., "Risk of disease recurrence and second neoplasms in survivors of childhood cancer treated with growth hormone: a report from the childhood cancer survivor study," *Journal of Clinical Endocrinology and Metabolism*, vol. 87, no. 7, pp. 3136–3141, 2002.

[56] D. Mo, D. S. Hardin, E. M. Erfurth, and S. Melmed, "Adult mortality or morbidity is not increased in childhood-onset growth hormone deficient patients who received pediatric GH treatment: an analysis of the Hypopituitary Control and Complications Study (HypoCCS)," *Pituitary*, vol. 17, no. 5, pp. 477–485, 2014.

[57] W. Chemaitilly and L. L. Robison, "Safety of growth hormone treatment in patients previously treated for cance," *Endocrinology and Metabolism Clinics of North America*, vol. 41, no. 4, pp. 785–792, 2012.

[58] Z. J. Hagay, R. J. Leiberman, M. Katz, and A. Witznitzer, "Oral contraceptives and focal nodular hyperplasia of the liver," *Archives of Gynecology and Obstetrics*, vol. 243, no. 4, pp. 231–234, 1988.

[59] G. Valesini and M. Cutolo, "Effects of TNF antagonists on immune and neuroendocrine system," *Reumatismo*, vol. 57, no. 4, supplement, pp. 3–7, 2005.

[60] S. Madhusoodanan, S. Parida, and C. Jimenez, "Hyperprolactinemia associated with psychotropics—a review," *Human Psychopharmacology*, vol. 25, no. 4, pp. 281–297, 2010.

[61] C. U. Corell and H. E. Carlson, "Endocrine and metabolic adverse effects of psychotropic medications in children and adolescents," *Journal of the American Academy of Child and Adolescent Psychiatry*, vol. 45, no. 7, pp. 771–791, 2006.

[62] A. G. Herzog and K. M. Fowler, "Sexual hormones and epilepsy: threat and opportunities," *Current Opinion in Neurology*, vol. 18, no. 2, pp. 167–172, 2005.

[63] A. S. Karadag, D. T. Ertugrul, E. Tutal, and K. O. Akin, "Isotretinoin influences pituitary hormone levels in acne patients," *Acta Dermato-Venereologica*, vol. 91, no. 1, pp. 31–34, 2011.

[64] L. Bilo, R. Meo, R. Valentino, C. Di Carlo, S. Striano, and C. Nappi, "Characterization of reproductive endocrine disorders in women with epilepsy," *The Journal of Clinical Endocrinology & Metabolism*, vol. 86, no. 7, pp. 2950–2956, 2001.

[65] N. W. Jacobsen, B. Halling-Sørensen, and F. K. Birkved, "Inhibition of human aromatase complex (CYP19) by antiepileptic drugs," *Toxicology in Vitro*, vol. 22, no. 1, pp. 146–153, 2008.

[66] G. Fond, A. Macgregor, J. Attal et al., "Antipsychotic drugs: pro-cancer or anti-cancer? A systematic review," *Medical Hypotheses*, vol. 79, no. 1, pp. 38–42, 2012.

[67] J. Nielsen and A. Boysen, "Clozapine treatment associated with increased risk of acute myeloid leukemia (AML)," *Schizophrenia Research*, vol. 123, no. 2-3, pp. 270–272, 2010.

[68] P. C. Valery, E. A. Holly, A. C. Sleigh, G. Williams, N. Kreiger, and C. Bain, "Hernias and Ewing's sarcoma family of tumours: a pooled analysis and meta-analysis," *The Lancet Oncology*, vol. 6, no. 7, pp. 485–490, 2005.

[69] R. Schumacher, A. Mai, and P. Gutjahr, "Association of rib anomalies and malignancy in childhood," *European Journal of Pediatrics*, vol. 151, no. 6, pp. 432–434, 1992.

[70] R. W. Miller, "Childhood cancer and congenital defects. A study of U.S. death certificates during the period 1960–1966," *Pediatric Research*, vol. 3, no. 5, pp. 389–397, 1969.

[71] L. Casorzo, L. Fessia, A. Sapino, G. Ponzio, and G. Bussolati, "Extraskeletal Ewing's tumor with translocation t(11;22) in a patient with Down syndrome," *Cancer Genetics and Cytogenetics*, vol. 37, no. 1, pp. 79–84, 1989.

[72] J. A. Bridge, J. R. Neff, D. A. Borek, and D. A. Hackbarth, "Primary skeletal Ewing's sarcoma in Down syndrome," *Cancer Genetics and Cytogenetics*, vol. 47, no. 1, pp. 61–68, 1990.

[73] M. Machin Valtueña, J. M. Garcia-Sagredo, A. Muñoz Villa, C. Lozano Giménez, and J. M. Aparicio Meix, "18q-syndrome and extraskeletal Ewing's sarcoma," *Journal of Medical Genetics*, vol. 24, no. 7, pp. 426–428, 1987.

[74] S. J. Cotterill, C. M. Wright, M. S. Pearce, and A. W. Craft, "Stature of young people with malignant bone tumors," *Pediatric Blood and Cancer*, vol. 42, no. 1, pp. 59–63, 2004.

13

Phase II Trial of Gemcitabine and Docetaxel with Bevacizumab in Soft Tissue Sarcoma

Mark A. Dickson,[1] David R. D'Adamo,[2] Mary L. Keohan,[1] Sandra P. D'Angelo,[1] Richard D. Carvajal,[3] Mrinal M. Gounder,[1] Robert G. Maki,[4] Li-Xuan Qin,[5] Robert A. Lefkowitz,[6] Olivia R. McKennon,[1] Catherine M. Hirst,[1] Gary K. Schwartz,[3] and William D. Tap[1]

[1]*Department of Medicine, Memorial Sloan-Kettering Cancer Center and Weill Cornell Medical College, New York, NY, USA*
[2]*Eisai, Inc., Woodcliff Lake, NJ, USA*
[3]*Department of Medicine, Columbia University, New York, NY, USA*
[4]*Departments of Medicine and Pediatrics, Mount Sinai School of Medicine, New York, NY, USA*
[5]*Department of Biostatistics, Memorial Sloan-Kettering Cancer Center and Weill Cornell Medical College, New York, NY, USA*
[6]*Department of Radiology, Memorial Sloan-Kettering Cancer Center and Weill Cornell Medical College, New York, NY, USA*

Correspondence should be addressed to Mark A. Dickson; dicksonm@mskcc.org

Academic Editor: Peter C. Ferguson

Gemcitabine (G) and docetaxel (D) are commonly used to treat recurrent/metastatic soft tissue sarcoma. This study tested the hypothesis that outcomes would be improved by addition of bevacizumab (B). The initial design was randomized double-blind trial of G + D + B versus G + D + placebo. Due to slow accrual this was modified to single-arm open-label G + D + B. Eligible patients had diagnosis of leiomyosarcoma, pleomorphic undifferentiated sarcoma, pleomorphic liposarcoma, or angiosarcoma. Treatment was B 15 mg/kg on d1, G 900 mg/m^2 on d1 and d8, and D 75 mg/m^2 on d8, q21d. Primary endpoint was progression-free survival (PFS) at 6 months and would be met if ≥17 patients were progression-free at 6 m. Secondary endpoints are response rate, PFS at 3 m, overall survival, and toxicity. Of 44 patients enrolled, 35 were treated with GDB and evaluable for safety and efficacy. Median age was 55, 50% male, most ECOG 0. Toxicity is mostly myelosuppression with one deep vein thrombosis and one small bowel perforation possibly related to B. There were 17 partial responses (49%) by RECIST 1.1. Among 35 patients, the number who remained on study and progression-free was 24 at 3 m and 15 at 6 m. 9 withdrew prior to 6 m for reasons other than toxicity or progression. PFS at 6 m was 65% (95% CI: 51–85%). The primary endpoint of 6 m PFS was not met due to censoring of patients who withdrew. However PFS at 3 m (76%) was promising and response rate was higher than expected from G + D.

1. Introduction

The combination of gemcitabine and docetaxel for soft tissue sarcoma has been widely adopted over the last decade. This regimen was first examined in a phase 2 study in leiomyosarcoma which showed a high RECIST response rate of 53% [1]. A subsequent large retrospective analysis supported the activity of this regimen in multiple sarcoma subtypes but the reported response rate was lower at 18% [2]. A randomized prospective phase 2 study confirmed that gemcitabine and docetaxel combination was superior to gemcitabine alone in unselected histologies, with a response rate of 16% in the 73 patients treated with the combination [3]. Based on these data, gemcitabine and docetaxel combination has been widely adopted to treat recurrent sarcoma. In the published studies, most of the responses were in two histologies—leiomyosarcoma and undifferentiated pleomorphic sarcoma (UPS; previously known as malignant fibrous histiocytoma)—although responses were also seen in pleomorphic liposarcoma, rhabdomyosarcoma, and angiosarcoma [3].

This study attempted to improve on the standard gemcitabine and docetaxel regimen by adding the antiangiogenic drug bevacizumab. Bevacizumab is a humanized monoclonal antibody that binds vascular endothelial growth factor-A (VEGF-A). Bevacizumab enhances the effect of chemotherapy in multiple solid tumors and is FDA-approved for the treatment of lung, kidney, and colon cancer and glioblastoma.

Previous efforts at treating sarcoma with bevacizumab have met with limited success. Bevacizumab has some activity as a single agent in vascular sarcomas, for which it is a form of targeted therapy. The response rate is ~9% in angiosarcoma [4]. Bevacizumab has also been tested in combination with doxorubicin, which for many years has been the standard first-line regimen for recurrent sarcoma. In a phase II study, the response rate was modest at 12% but the study was closed due to excessive cardiac toxicity [5].

The current study tested the hypothesis that the addition of bevacizumab would enhance the activity of gemcitabine and docetaxel. The initial trial design was a double-blind, placebo-controlled, randomized trial of gemcitabine and docetaxel given with or without bevacizumab. Due to slow accrual, the trial was changed to a single-arm, open-label, nonrandomized study of gemcitabine, docetaxel, and bevacizumab, which we term here GDB.

2. Patient Eligibility

Eligible patients met the following criteria: histologically confirmed metastatic or locally recurrent leiomyosarcoma, undifferentiated pleomorphic sarcoma (UPS, formerly known as malignant fibrous histiocytoma, MFH), pleomorphic liposarcoma, pleomorphic rhabdomyosarcoma, or angiosarcoma, no more than 1 prior chemotherapy regimen for metastatic disease, measurable disease as defined by RECIST 1.1, ECOG performance status 0 or 1, age 18 to 75, and adequate hematologic, hepatic, and renal function. Patients with recent myocardial infarction, transient ischemic attack or stroke, congestive heart failure, brain metastases, uncontrolled hypertension, significant vascular disease, proteinuria, and recent abdominal fistula, perforation, or abscess were excluded. The protocol was approved by the Institutional Review Board of Memorial Sloan-Kettering Cancer Center and all patients provided written informed consent (Clinicaltrials.gov identifier NCT00887809).

3. Treatment Plan

Patients were treated with bevacizumab 15 mg/kg on day 1 of each 21-day cycle intravenously over 30 minutes. For cycles 1 through 6, patients were treated with gemcitabine 900 mg/m^2 over 90 minutes on days 1 and 8 and docetaxel 75 mg/m^2 over 60 minutes on day 8. Chemotherapy was started up to 60 minutes after the bevacizumab infusion. Treatment was followed by either 5 days of filgrastim or a single injection of pegfilgrastim. To improve tolerability for cycles 7 and beyond, gemcitabine was reduced to 800 mg/m^2 over 30 minutes on days 1 and 8 and docetaxel was given at 35 mg/m^2 over 30 minutes, also on days 1 and 8. Growth factors were not routinely used for patients receiving these doses beyond cycle 7.

4. Evaluation

A physical exam was done on day 1 and day 8 of the first two cycles and on day 1 of each subsequent cycle. Blood tests (complete blood count, serum chemistries, and liver enzymes) were performed prior to the start of every cycle and a complete blood count was repeated on day 8. Urinalysis was performed at every two cycles. Radiology assessments (CT or MRI) were performed every two cycles for the first 6 cycles, every 3 cycles for cycles 7–18, and every 4 cycles thereafter. Response was assessed by RECIST 1.1 [6].

5. Statistical Analysis

The initial study design involved a sample size of 72 patients, with 36 patients in the bevacizumab arm and 36 in the placebo arm. This study design would have allowed detection of a 75% improvement in median PFS in the bevacizumab arm, with type 1 and 2 error both set at 0.2. Due to slow accrual, the study was changed to a single-arm, nonrandomized trial of gemcitabine, docetaxel, and bevacizumab (GDB). For the revised study, a one-stage design was used with a sample size of 34. Patients previously enrolled in the randomized study were unblinded and only those who had received bevacizumab were included in the analysis. Accrual then continued until at least 34 evaluable patients had been treated with gemcitabine, docetaxel, and bevacizumab.

The primary endpoint for this study was progression-free survival (PFS) at 6 months. PFS includes both disease progression (as defined by RECIST 1.1) and death from any cause. Based on historical controls, a PFS of >60% at 6 months is considered promising, and a PFS of <40% is considered not promising [3, 7–9]. The study would be claimed to be positive if there were 17 or more who were progression-free at 6 months. This design has a type I error rate of 0.15 and a type II error rate of 0.09 based on an exact binomial test. Secondary endpoints included response rate by RECIST 1.1, PFS at 3 months, overall survival, and toxicity.

6. Results

Between June 2009 and April 2010, 17 patients were enrolled in the randomized trial. At the time the study was changed to single-arm study of GDB, those 17 patients were unblinded. 9 had received placebo and were excluded from the safety and efficacy analysis. 8 had received bevacizumab. Between February 2011 and April 2012, an additional 27 patients were enrolled and treated with gemcitabine, docetaxel, and bevacizumab. Thus a total of 35 patients were treated with the combination and this population was used for the safety and efficacy analysis. The flow of these patients is shown in the CONSORT diagram in Figure 1.

The characteristics of all 44 patients enrolled are shown in Table 1. The median age was 55 (range 24–75) and 50% were male. Most patients had ECOG score of 0. The most common tumor types were leiomyosarcoma and UPS of the extremity or abdomen. Most patients (77%) had received no prior chemotherapy. The remainder had received one prior regimen of either doxorubicin or liposomal doxorubicin alone

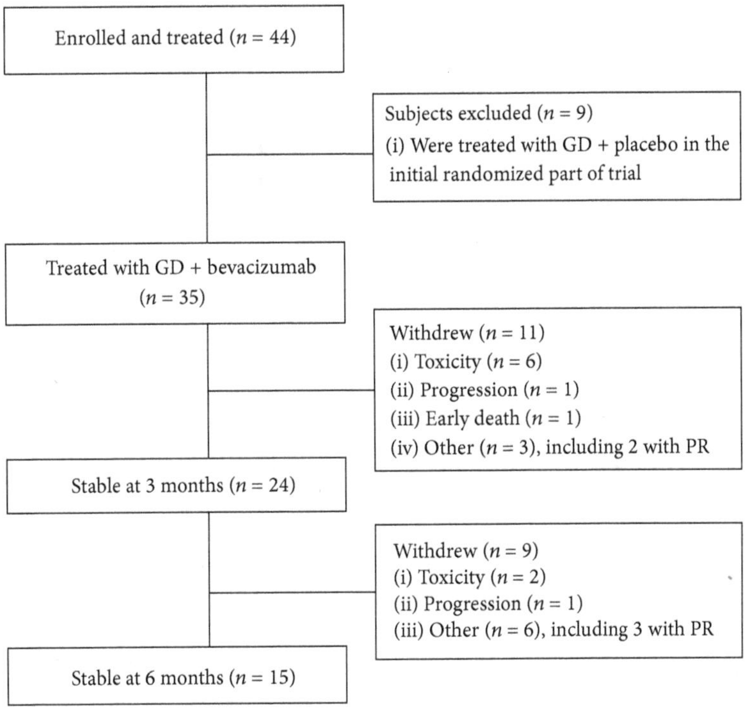

FIGURE 1: CONSORT diagram. Patients who received gemcitabine + docetaxel (GD) and placebo were excluded from the toxicity and efficacy analysis of GD + bevacizumab.

(5), doxorubicin with ifosfamide (4), doxorubicin + ifosfamide + dacarbazine (1), or sorafenib + dacarbazine (2—on a prior clinical trial).

6.1. Toxicity. The rates of adverse events are shown in Table 2. The most common adverse events were myelosuppression, consistent with prior reports of gemcitabine and docetaxel. One patient had a deep vein thrombosis that was likely related to metastatic sarcoma. One patient had a grade 2 small bowel perforation from diverticular disease that required a partial colectomy. This was considered possibly related to bevacizumab.

6.2. Efficacy. Of 35 patients, there were 17 partial responses, for an overall response rate of 49% (95% CI 31–66%). Responses were seen in all histologies: leiomyosarcoma (8/17 = 47%), undifferentiated pleomorphic sarcoma (5/11 = 45%), angiosarcoma (3/5 = 60%), and pleomorphic liposarcoma (1/1). Within the leiomyosarcoma group, 2/5 patients with uterine leiomyosarcoma had partial responses. In addition to the 17 partial responses, 9 patients had decrease in target lesions of at least 10% but not sufficient to meet criteria for PR. The best response by RECIST for each evaluable patient is shown in a waterfall plot in Figure 2.

Twenty four patients remained on treatment and progression-free at 3 months. The 11 patients who went off study before 3 months include 6 who stopped for toxicity, 3 who withdrew consent (see Figure 1 and Table 3), 1 who progressed, and 1 who died. Thus, when the patients who withdrew consent are censored, the PFS at 3 months is 76% (95% CI: 63–92%), based on the Kaplan-Meier method.

TABLE 1: Patient characteristics.

Characteristic	All patients	GDB patients
Total	44	35
Male	22 (50%)	15 (43%)
Female	22 (50%)	20 (57%)
Age		
Median	54.5	54
Range	24–75	39–72
ECOG		
Median	0	0
Range	0-1	0-1
Tumor type		
Leiomyosarcoma	20 (45%)	18 (51%)
Uterine	5	5
Nonuterine	15	13
Undifferentiated pleomorphic sarcoma	17 (39%)	11 (31%)
Angiosarcoma (liver, bone, soft tissue)	6 (14%)	5 (14%)
Pleomorphic liposarcoma	1 (2%)	1 (3%)
Prior treatment		
Doxorubicin (or liposomal doxorubicin)	8	5
Ifosfamide	5	3
Dacarbazine	3	2
Sorafenib	2	1
None	34 (77%)	29 (83%)

(The outcomes of the 3 patients who withdrew consent before 3 months are described in Table 3. Two of the patients had PR by RECIST, and one was stable. Two underwent surgery

TABLE 2: Adverse events occurring in more than 1 patient and all grade 3-4 adverse events.

Adverse event	Grade 2	Grade 3	Grade 4
Anemia	17	7	1
Neutropenia	7	7	6
Leukopenia	6	8	3
Hyperglycemia	12	3	1
Hypoalbuminemia	13	1	
Lymphopenia		11	2
Thrombocytopenia	1	4	5
Elevated ALT	9		1
Elevated AST	7	1	
Fatigue	1	5	
Hypophosphatemia	2	3	
Elevated alkaline phosphatase	2	2	
Hypokalemia		2	
Edema		2	
Diverticulitis		1	
Kidney stone		1	
Cellulitis		1	
Neck pain		1	
Pneumonia		1	
Mucositis	3		
Hemorrhage, nose	1		
Perforation, GI-small bowel NOS	1		
Thrombosis/thrombus/embolism			1

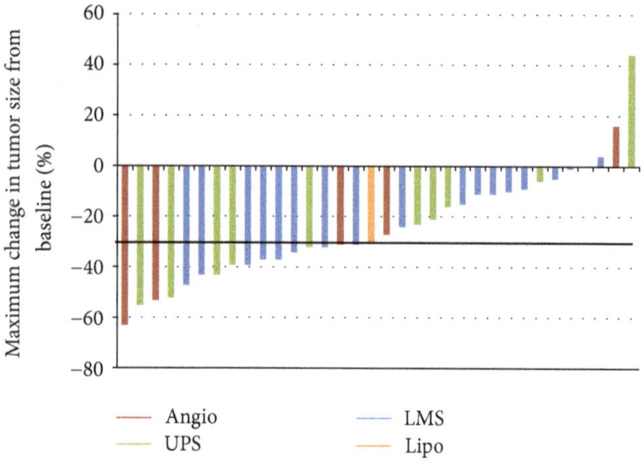

FIGURE 2: Waterfall plot showing tumor response in patients treated with gemcitabine + docetaxel + bevacizumab.

and all 3 are without evidence of disease.) Between 3 and 6 months, an additional 2 patients stopped for toxicity, 6 withdrew consent (see Figure 1 and Table 3), and 1 progressed, resulting in 15 patients remaining on treatment and progression-free at 6 months. However the study required 17 patients to be progression-free at 6 months, so the primary endpoint was not reached.

A Kaplan-Meier curve of progression-free survival for all 35 patients is shown in Figure 3. The PFS at 6 months is

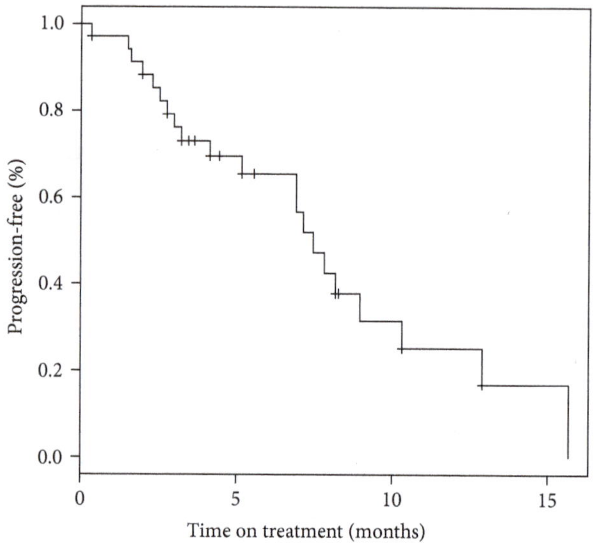

FIGURE 3: Progression-free survival.

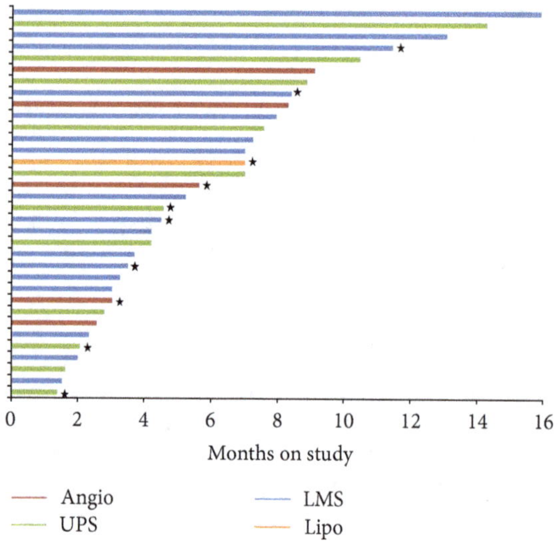

FIGURE 4: Duration on study for each patient treated with gemcitabine + docetaxel + bevacizumab. Patients marked by stars discontinued treatment on study because of good response and elected to have surgery.

65% (95% CI: 51–85%); however this includes censoring for patients who withdrew. Note that 13 patients who had stable disease or partial response chose to stop protocol treatment for reasons other than progression or toxicity. Their outcomes are shown in Table 3. This group includes 9 patients who stopped treatment before reaching 6 months progression-free. The time on study for each evaluable patient is shown in Figure 4. Patients who were responding and elected to stop treatment so they could have surgery are indicated by stars. Patients who withdrew consent were censored for PFS analysis at the time of withdrawal. With this in mind, the median PFS for the 35 patients was 7.5 months (95% CI: 6.9-NR). The median overall survival was 2.4 years (95% CI: 1.9-NR).

Table 3: Outcomes of patients who withdrew from treatment with GDB for reasons other than toxicity or progression (AWD = alive with disease; NED = no evidence of disease; DOD = died of disease).

	Time on treatment (months)	Best response (RECIST)	Maximal change of tumor (%)	Treatment after GDB	Pathology from surgery	Outcome
63 y male with recurrent UPS of thigh	1.4	PR	−39	Resection of local recurrence	Treatment effect but viable tumor	NED at 3.1 y
55 y female with recurrent UPS of thigh	2.1	SD	0	Limb perfusion and then surgery	30–40% necrosis and fibrosis	NED at 3.5 y
44 y female with angiosarcoma of vagina	3.0	PR	−63	Observation since biopsy showed no tumor	No tumor detected	NED at 1.3 y
55 y male with metastatic LMS	3.5	PR	−31	Resection of lung metastases	Necrosis and histiocytic infiltration (70%)	DOD at 1.4 y
50 y female with large pelvic (nonuterine) LMS	3.7	SD	−11	Evaluated for surgery but unresectable	N/A	AWD at 2.5 y
39 y male with metastatic LMS	4.2	SD	−15	Radio-frequency ablation of liver metastases	N/A	DOD at 2.4 y
69 y female with metastatic uterine LMS	4.5	SD	−24	Resection of pelvic metastases	Predominantly viable	AWD at 2.2 y
40 y male with metastatic UPS	4.6	PR	−32	Resection of lung metastases	Viable tumor	DOD at 1 y
52 y male with metastatic angiosarcoma	5.6	PR	−31	Resection of lung metastases	Viable but microscopic tumor	AWD at 11 m
56 y male with metastatic pleomorphic liposarcoma	7.0	SD	−30	Resection of solitary bone metastasis	>99% necrosis, rare viable cells	NED at 3.1 y
52 y male with metastatic LMS	8.4	PR	−32	Resection of lung metastases	95% treatment effect	AWD at 2.2 y
72 y female with metastatic UPS	8.9	PR	−55	Observation and then further chemotherapy	N/A	AWD at 2.6 y
57 y female with metastatic uterine LMS	11.4	PR	−43	Resection of lung metastases	30% treatment effect	DOD at 1.9 y

7. Discussion

This study demonstrated the safety and potential efficacy of the combination of GDB for selected soft tissue sarcomas. The combination was generally tolerable and the most common toxicities were hematologic. This is consistent with the expected toxicity profile of gemcitabine and docetaxel. There did not appear to be a significant increase in toxicity due to the addition of bevacizumab, although conclusions drawn from a single-arm trial are limited. Several patients did withdraw from treatment due to toxicity. Although there was one episode of thrombosis and one episode of gastrointestinal perforation, overall the frequency of these events was not markedly higher than what has been reported in other solid tumors.

The objective RECIST response rate was 49% which compares favorably to what would be expected from gemcitabine and docetaxel alone, again taking into account the limitations of a single-arm phase 2 study. Only the initial phase 2 study in leiomyosarcoma reported a higher response rate (of 53% in 34 patients) [1]; however this was never replicated in subsequent studies. The pivotal randomized phase 2 study of gemcitabine and docetaxel versus gemcitabine alone showed a response rate of just 16% in 73 patients treated with the combination [3]. A second randomized phase 2 study in leiomyosarcoma showed a response rate of 24% for uterine and 5% for nonuterine LMS in a total of 90 patients [10].

A prior phase IB study of gemcitabine, docetaxel, and bevacizumab has been performed with a response rate of 31% in 36 patients [11]. In that study, however, the dose of bevacizumab was lower (5 mg/kg every 2 weeks, compared to 15 mg/kg every 3 weeks in this study) and the chemotherapy was given on an unusual schedule (gemcitabine 1500 mg/m^2 and docetaxel 50 mg/m^2 every two weeks). In contrast, the results of our study demonstrate that a higher dose of bevacizumab can be given with the standard doses of gemcitabine (days 1 and 8) and docetaxel (day 8) on an every-3-week schedule usually used in clinical practice.

After 6 cycles of treatment, we reduced the dose of docetaxel in all patients. It is our clinical practice to do this often in patients treated with conventional gemcitabine and docetaxel; however it has not been formally studied. The potential toxicity and efficacy of "split-dose" docetaxel warrant further study.

Radiographic responses occurred in all histological subtypes of sarcoma that were treated on this study. The results were particularly notable in visceral angiosarcoma where 4 of 5 patients had demonstrable tumor shrinkage and 3 met criteria for PR. This is a potentially encouraging result since the response rate of bevacizumab alone is low, and a recent randomized phase II study in angiosarcoma showed no benefit from the addition of bevacizumab to chemotherapy with paclitaxel [12]. Thus GDB may be a good option for angiosarcoma; however this hypothesis would have to be tested in a randomized trial.

This study also highlights the importance of choosing endpoints in phase II trials in sarcoma. Although this study did not meet its primary endpoint (17 evaluable patients progression-free at 6 months), this may have been due to the high withdrawal rate of patients for reasons other than progression. In particular, several patients who responded well elected to have surgery to resect residual metastatic disease, while others withdrew due to toxicity. Thus many patients became inevaluable for the primary endpoint of PFS at 6 months, confounding the results. A more standard benchmark for evaluating chemotherapy regimens in sarcoma is PFS at 3 months. By this standard, a 3-month PFS of at least 40% is considered promising in the second-line setting [9]. Although this was not the benchmark used in this study, the 3-month PFS of 76% would have compared favorably, except that most patients in this study were treated in the first-line setting and would therefore be expected to do better. In sum, this study suggests some favorable activity of GDB in certain sarcoma subtypes and also highlights the challenges of performing randomized trials in rare diseases and the importance of choosing consistent endpoints.

Authors' Contribution

Mark A. Dickson and David R. D'Adamo, Gary K. Schwartz, and William D. Tap contributed equally to the work.

Acknowledgment

The study was sponsored by Genentech.

References

[1] M. L. Hensley, R. Maki, E. Venkatraman et al., "Gemcitabine and docetaxel in patients with unresectable leiomyosarcoma: results of a phase II trial," *Journal of Clinical Oncology*, vol. 20, no. 12, pp. 2824–2831, 2002.

[2] J.-O. Bay, I. Ray-Coquard, J. Fayette et al., "Docetaxel and gemcitabine combination in 133 advanced soft-tissue sarcomas: a retrospective analysis," *International Journal of Cancer*, vol. 119, no. 3, pp. 706–711, 2006.

[3] R. G. Maki, J. K. Wathen, S. R. Patel et al., "Randomized phase II study of gemcitabine and docetaxel compared with gemcitabine alone in patients with metastatic soft tissue sarcomas: results of sarcoma alliance for research through collaboration study 002 [corrected]," *Journal of Clinical Oncology*, vol. 25, pp. 2755–2763, 2007.

[4] M. Agulnik, J. L. Yarber, S. H. Okuno et al., "An open-label, multicenter, phase II study of bevacizumab for the treatment of angiosarcoma and epithelioid hemangioendotheliomas," *Annals of Oncology*, vol. 24, no. 1, pp. 257–263, 2013.

[5] D. R. D'Adamo, S. E. Anderson, K. Albritton et al., "Phase II study of doxorubicin and bevacizumab for patients with metastatic soft-tissue sarcomas," *Journal of Clinical Oncology*, vol. 23, no. 28, pp. 7135–7142, 2005.

[6] E. A. Eisenhauer, P. Therasse, J. Bogaerts et al., "New response evaluation criteria in solid tumours: revised RECIST guideline (version 1.1)," *European Journal of Cancer*, vol. 45, no. 2, pp. 228–247, 2009.

[7] M. L. Hensley, J. A. Blessing, K. DeGeest, O. Abulafia, P. G. Rose, and H. D. Homesley, "Fixed-dose rate gemcitabine plus docetaxel as second-line therapy for metastatic uterine

leiomyosarcoma: a Gynecologic Oncology Group phase II study," *Gynecologic Oncology*, vol. 109, no. 3, pp. 323–328, 2008.

[8] M. L. Hensley, J. A. Blessing, R. Mannel, and P. G. Rose, "Fixed-dose rate gemcitabine plus docetaxel as first-line therapy for metastatic uterine leiomyosarcoma: a Gynecologic Oncology Group phase II trial," *Gynecologic Oncology*, vol. 109, no. 3, pp. 329–334, 2008.

[9] M. Van Glabbeke, J. Verweij, I. Judson, and O. S. Nielsen, "Progression-free rate as the principal end-point for phase II trials in soft-tissue sarcomas," *European Journal of Cancer*, vol. 38, no. 4, pp. 543–549, 2002.

[10] P. Pautier, A. Floquet, N. Penel et al., "Randomized multicenter and stratified phase II study of gemcitabine alone versus gemcitabine and docetaxel in patients with metastatic or relapsed leiomyosarcomas: a fédération nationale des centres de lutte contre le cancer (FNCLCC) French Sarcoma Group Study (TAXOGEM study)," *Oncologist*, vol. 17, no. 9, pp. 1213–1220, 2012.

[11] C. F. Verschraegen, H. Arias-pulido, S.-J. Lee et al., "Phase IB study of the combination of docetaxel, gemcitabine, and bevacizumab in patients with advanced or recurrent soft tissue sarcoma: the Axtell regimen," *Annals of Oncology*, vol. 23, no. 3, pp. 785–790, 2012.

[12] N. Penel, J. Y. Blay, O. Mir et al., "ANGIOTAX-PLUS trial: a randomized phase II trial assessing the activity of weekly paclitaxel plus or minus bevacizumab in advanced angiosarcoma," *Journal of Clinical Oncology*, vol. 32, abstract 10501, 2014.

14

Myeloablative Chemotherapy with Autologous Stem Cell Transplant for Desmoplastic Small Round Cell Tumor

Christopher J. Forlenza,[1] Brian H. Kushner,[1] Nancy Kernan,[1] Farid Boulad,[1] Heather Magnan,[1] Leonard Wexler,[1] Suzanne L. Wolden,[2] Michael P. LaQuaglia,[1,3] and Shakeel Modak[1]

[1] *Department of Pediatrics, Memorial Sloan-Kettering Cancer Center, 1275 York Avenue, New York, NY 10065, USA*
[2] *Department of Radiation Oncology, Memorial Sloan-Kettering Cancer Center, 1275 York Avenue, New York, NY 10065, USA*
[3] *Department of Surgery, Memorial Sloan-Kettering Cancer Center, 1275 York Avenue, New York, NY 10065, USA*

Correspondence should be addressed to Shakeel Modak; modaks@mskcc.org

Academic Editor: Cyril Fisher

Desmoplastic small round cell tumor (DSRCT), a rare, aggressive neoplasm, has a poor prognosis. In this prospective study, we evaluated the role of myeloablative chemotherapy, followed by autologous stem cell transplant in improving survival in DSRCT. After high-dose induction chemotherapy and surgery, 19 patients with chemoresponsive DSRCT underwent autologous stem cell transplant. Myeloablative chemotherapy consisted of carboplatin (400–700 mg/m^2/day for 3 days) + thiotepa (300 mg/m^2/day for 3 days) ± topotecan (2 mg/m^2/day for 5 days). All patients were engrafted and there was no treatment-related mortality. Seventeen patients received radiotherapy to sites of prior or residual disease at a median of 12 weeks after transplant. Five-year event-free and overall survival were 11 ± 7% and 16 ± 8%, respectively. Two patients survive disease-free 16 and 19 years after transplant (both in complete remission before transplant). 14 patients had progression and died of disease at a median of 18 months following autologous transplant. These data do not justify the use of myeloablative chemotherapy with carboplatin plus thiotepa in patients with DSRCT. Alternative therapies should be considered for this aggressive neoplasm.

1. Introduction

First described as a distinct entity in 1989 [1], desmoplastic small round cell tumor (DSRCT) remains a relatively poorly understood neoplasm. It is mainly a disease of adolescent and young adult males, usually presenting with widespread intra-abdominal tumors not restricted to particular organs, but related to serosal surfaces [2]. Pleural [3] or paratesticular [4] involvement can also occur but is less common. Rare sites include orbit [5], bone [6], kidney [7], lung [8], ovary [9], and soft tissues of hand [10] and neck [11]. There is often disseminated disease at the time of diagnosis. Metastatic sites include lymph nodes, liver, and lung [12]. DSRCT has a characteristic histological appearance: nests of undifferentiated, moderately pleomorphic small round cells are surrounded by abundant desmoplastic stroma [2]. Epithelial, neural, and muscle markers are typically coexpressed on immunohistochemistry [13]. Besides the typical histological features, DSRCT is distinguished from other small round blue tumors by the presence of the t(11;22)(p13:q12) chromosomal translocation [14]. This translocation leads to the fusion of the EWS gene to the tumor suppressor gene WT1 [15]. The resultant chimeric protein acts as an aberrant transcription factor and is probably tumorigenic [16].

Despite the demonstrated chemosensitivity, optimal therapy for this rare disease remains to be determined, and prognosis is currently extremely poor. We previously reported on an aggressive multimodality therapeutic approach including high-dose, multiagent chemotherapy (the P6 protocol), surgery, and radiation therapy for DSRCT [17]. Tumors consistently responded to alkylator-based chemotherapy, although complete remissions were usually not obtained with chemotherapy alone. In order to exploit this demonstrated chemosensitivity and possibly improve survival in patients with DSRCT, we dose-intensified chemotherapy using autologous hematopoietic stem cells to reverse the associated myeloablation. Patients were treated with high-dose carboplatin and thiotepa taking advantage of the known responsiveness of DSRCT to alkylator-based therapy, dose-response behavior of these agents, and manageable extra medullary toxicities. Topotecan was later included for three patients, in an attempt to take advantage of possible potentiation of activity of alkylating agents, as well as favorable toxicity profile. We report on the results achieved with this strategy.

2. Patients and Methods

Patients with DSRCT treated at Memorial Sloan-Kettering Cancer Center (MSKCC) were given the option to consent to this study. All patients, except for two, were enrolled on an IRB-approved therapeutic protocol (ClinicalTrials.gov identifier NCT00002515) designed to evaluate myeloablative chemotherapy (MA) followed by autologous stem cell infusion (ASCT) in patients with rare high-risk solid tumors between 1993 and 2004. Patients that are not enrolled in study were treated as per protocol (patients 6, 17, Table 1) after obtaining written informed consent for protocol chemotherapy and ASCT. Records from the latter were accessed after obtaining permission from MSKCC Institutional Review Board. The diagnosis of DSRCT was established by histological evaluation of tumor specimens at MSKCC.

All patients had received induction chemotherapy followed by surgical resection with the objective of achieving remission prior to ASCT. Eligibility criteria for ASCT included: (A) demonstration of "chemosensitive" disease: patients needed to be in complete remission (CR) defined as no radiological evidence of disease or have ≥50% decrease in one measurable parameter attributable to prior chemotherapy without evidence of progressive disease by any other parameter, (B) availability of $\geq 2 \times 10^6$ CD34+ autologous hematopoietic stem cells harvested peripherally via leukapheresis or $\geq 10^8$ nucleated cells/kg via bone marrow (BM) harvest and (C) adequate renal, hepatic, pulmonary, and cardiac function.

Planned MA for 16 patients was thiotepa 300 mg/m^2 by 3-hour intravenous (IV) infusion on days −8, −7, and −6 (total, 900 mg/m^2) and carboplatin by 4-hour IV infusion on days −5, −4, and −3. Carboplatin was dosed for an area under the curve (AUC) of 7 mg/mL/min using the Calvert formula with a maximum daily carboplatin dose of 700 mg/m^2 [18]. Following protocol amendments, for a further three patients (patients 3, 14, and 19, Table 2), topotecan 2 mg/m^2/day via 30 min IV infusion was added on days −8, −7, −6, −5, and −4.

ASCT was carried out on day 0 with autologous bone marrow (BM) or peripheral blood stem cells (PBSCs). Granulocyte colony-stimulating factor (G-CSF) 5-to-10 μg/kg/day was started on day +1. Standard post-ASCT care was provided including the prophylactic use of antibiotics, parenteral nutrition, and blood product support. Toxicities were recorded according to the Children's Cancer Group Toxicity and Complications Criteria based on NCI common toxicity criteria.

Patients underwent the extent of disease evaluation approximately four to six weeks after ASCT with computed tomography (CT) or magnetic resonance imaging (MRI) of the primary site and potential sites of metastases. For patients with evaluable disease before ASCT, response was classified as follows: CR; good partial response: >90% decrease in all disease parameters; partial response (PR): >50% decrease in all disease parameters, mixed response: >50% decrease in ≥1 disease parameters but not in all; stable disease (SD) <50% decrease in all disease parameters; and progressive disease (PD): new lesions or >25% increase in any disease parameter. These criteria are in continuity with our previous report and were chosen due to the disseminated nature of DSRCT [17].

Planned therapy after hematopoietic recovery after ASCT included maximally tolerated radiotherapy to sites at high risk for progressive disease. Other therapies could be administered after radiotherapy at the discretion of the treating physician.

Survival curves were generated according to the Kaplan-Meier method and comparisons between groups performed using log-rank test using SPSS (IBM, Armonk, NY).

3. Results

3.1. Patient Demographics. Nineteen patients with DSRCT, (16 male, 3 female) with a median age at diagnosis of 18.5 years (range 10–42 years) were treated with ASCT. Patient characteristics before ASCT are presented in Table 1. Sixteen patients did not have relapse or PD prior to MA: eight were in first CR and eight had chemosensitive but persistent disease. Three patients were treated after first relapse: one was in second CR and two had persistent disease that was chemosensitive to salvage therapy prior to ASCT.

3.2. Prior Therapy. 16 patients had received induction therapy with P6 protocol as previously described [17]. Briefly, this consisted of 4 cycles of high-dose cyclophosphamide, doxorubicin, and vincristine, followed by 3 cycles of ifosfamide and etoposide. One patient (#9) was initially thought to have neuroblastoma and received therapy with ifosfamide, carboplatin, and etoposide prior to correction of diagnosis to DSCRT whereupon he received P6 protocol. Another patient (#17) was initially diagnosed with testicular germ cell tumor and was observed without further therapy after initial surgical excision; he received P6 protocol at relapse. A third patient (#14) was treated with 6 cycles of high-dose chemotherapy as induction: three with high-dose cyclophosphamide plus doxorubicin and vincristine followed by three with high-dose cyclophosphamide plus topotecan and vincristine.

3.3. MA and ASCT. All patients received planned MA at a median of 9.1 (range 5.7–25.3) months from diagnosis (Table 1). Median carboplatin dose was 500 mg/m^2/day. The source of autologous hematopoietic stem cells was PBSCs for 9, BM for 7, and combination of PB+BM for 3 patients in whom insufficient number of PBSCs were available. Median

Table 1: Patient characteristics before ASCT.

Pt#	Sex	Age at diagnosis (years)	Initial disease sites	Initial/induction therapy	Response to induction	Second line therapy	Diagnosis to ASCT (months)
First complete remission before ASCT							
1	F	11.9	Abdomen, pelvis	P6	CR	None	7.6
2	M	14.8	Abdomen, pelvis	P6	CR	None	7.6
3	M	15.0	Abdomen, pelvis	P6	CR	None	5.8
4	M	16.1	Abdomen, mediastinum	P6	CR	None	9.5
5	M	22.4	Abdomen, pelvis	P6	CR	None	5.7
6	M	24.1	Abdomen, pelvis	P6	CR	None	10.2
7	M	24.3	Abdomen, pelvis	P6	CR	None	6.8
8	F	47.7	Abdomen, mediastinum	P6	CR	None	10.1
Persistent but chemosensitive disease before ASCT							
9	M	10.0	Abdomen, pelvis	NB therapy followed by P6	PR	None	16.1
10	M	13.0	Abdomen, pelvis	P6	PR	None	7.8
11	F	13.6	Abdomen, pelvis, mediastinum, neck	P6	PR	None	9.8
12	M	16.3	Abdomen, pelvis	P6	PR	None	6.1
13	M	17.1	Abdomen, pelvis	P6	PR	None	9.1
14	M	20.7	Abdomen, pelvis, mediastinum	CAV/CTV	PR	None	7.9
15	M	31.7	Abdomen, pelvis, mediastinum	P6	PR	None	6.8
16	M	32.5	Abdomen, pelvis, neck	P6	PR	High-dose cyclophosphamide	10.7
Relapse before ASCT							
17	M	18.5	Testes	Surgery; observation	Not applicable	P6	25.3
18	M	22.4	Abdomen, mediastinum	P6	CR	High-dose cyclophosphamide; surgery	22.4
19	M	26.9	Abdomen, pelvis, neck	P6	PD	High-dose cyclophosphamide + topotecan	12.5

ASCT: autologous stem cell transplant; CAV: high-dose cyclophosphamide plus doxorubicin and vincristine; CR: complete remission; CTV: high-dose cyclophosphamide plus topotecan and vincristine; F: female; M: male; NB: neuroblastoma; P6: P6 protocol; PD: progressive disease; PR: partial remission.

TABLE 2: Myeloablative chemotherapy and autologous stem cell transplant: toxicities and response.

Pt#	Residual disease before ASCT	MA	Carboplatin dose (per m^2)	Source of SC	Dose of SC ($\times 10^6$ CD34+ cells/kg)	Time (days) to ANC >500	Time (days) to platelet count >20 K	Major acute nonhematological toxicities	Response to ASCT
First complete remission before ASCT									
1	None	CT	700	PB + BM	3.0	13	51	Grade 3 hyperbilirubinemia, grade 3 hematuria	N/A
2	None	CT	500	BM	4.1	14	48	Grade 3 sepsis	N/A
3	None	CTT	700	PB	17.5	13	11	Grade 4 mucositis, grade 3 SGOT elevation	N/A
4	None	CT	700	PB + BM	3.4	13	34	None	N/A
5	None	CT	600	BM	5.6	9	28	Grade 3 diarrhea	N/A
6	None	CT	500	BM	3.2	13	26	Grade 3 hyperbilirubinemia, grade 3 mucositis	N/A
7	None	CT	450	PB	4.4	9	9	Grade 3 mucositis	N/A
8	None	CT	400	PB	UA	12	15	Grade 3 diarrhea, grade 3 vomiting	N/A
Persistent but chemosensitive disease before ASCT									
9	Abdomen	CT	500	BM	2.4	23	57	None	SD
10	Abdomen	CT	400	BM	2.6	11	16	Grade 3 mucositis	SD
11	Abdomen, pelvis, mediastinum	CT	425	PB	2.1	12	13	Grade 4 hyperbilirubinemia, grade 3 mucositis	Minor
12	Abdomen, mediastinum	CT	600	PB	7.2	9	14	Grade 4 sepsis	SD
13	Abdomen	CT	700	BM	3.1	14	41	Grade 4 hyperbilirubinemia	Lost to followup
14	Abdomen, mediastinum	CTT	500	PB	6.2	10	10	Grade 3 mucositis	SD
15	Abdomen, pelvis, mediastinum	CT	500	PB	4.1	6	13	Grade 3 hyperbilirubinemia, grade 3 vomiting	SD
16	Abdomen	CT	500	BM	2.4	10	11	Grade 3 hypertension, grade 3 mucositis	PD
Relapse before ASCT									
17	Mediastinum	CT	600	PB	5.1	9	15	Grade 3 vomiting	SD
18	None	CT	500	PB	5.0	10	13	Grade 3 mucositis, grade 3 diarrhea, grade 3 hematuria	N/A
19	Abdomen, axilla	CTT	600	PB + BM	UA	11	16	Grade 3 hyperbilirubinemia, grade 4 sepsis, grade 4 hearing loss, grade 4 hematuria, grade 3 mucositis	SD

ANC: absolute neutrophil count; ASCT: autologous stem cell transplant; BM: bone marrow; CT: carboplatin and thiotepa; CTT: carboplatin and thiotepa plus topotecan; FU: followup; MA: myeloablative chemotherapy; N/A: not applicable; PB: peripheral blood; PD: progressive disease; SC: stem cells; SD: stable disease; UA: details of dose unavailable.

TABLE 3: Therapy following ASCT and outcomes.

Pt#	Time to radiotherapy after ASCT (weeks)	Treatment at relapse	OS (months) after ASCT	EFS (months) after ASCT
		First complete remission before ASCT		
1	No radiotherapy	None	5.3	1.4
2	12	N/A	239.1	239.1
3	10	Irinotecan/temozolomide; cyclophosphamide/vinorelbine; sunitinib; bevacizumab	48.4	13.7
4	15	Oral etoposide	30.1	13.2
5	12	Unknown	51.1	21.4
6	12	None	26.7	16.5
7	12	N/A	196.0	196.0
8	No radiotherapy	Paclitaxel, thiotepa	14.3	8.4
		Persistent but chemosensitive disease before ASCT		
9	21	Vincristine, cyclophosphamide, dactinomycin	15.3	5.2
10	11	Palliative radiotherapy; oral etoposide	18.7	12.4
11	13	None	12.0	9.7
12	6	Exatecan	39.5	19.1
13	11	N/A	18.6	8.2 (developed secondary AML)
14	13	Temozolomide	23.8	16.4
15	13	Irinotecan, cisplatin; thalidomide; palliative radiotherapy	80.5	25.3
16	34	Vinorelbine	9.6	3.1
		Relapse before ASCT		
17	12	N/A	39.7	12.1 (developed secondary AML)
18	12	Oral etoposide, vinorelbine, cisplatin, topotecan	23.2	8.7
19	14	None	10.1	7.1

AML: Acute myeloid leukemia; ASCT: autologous stem cell transplant; EFS: event-free survival; N/A: not applicable; OS: overall survival.

cell dose was 4.1 (range 2.1–17.5) × 10^6 CD34+ cells/kg. All patients were engrafted (defined as an absolute neutrophil count >500/μL) at a median of 11 ± 3 (range 6–23) days following ASCT. Median time to platelet recovery (defined as transfusion-independent platelet count >20,000/μL) was 15 ± 15 (range 9–51) days (Table 2).

3.4. Acute Toxicities. There were no treatment-related mortalities. As expected, all patients experienced grade 4 myelosuppression. Toxicities are described in Table 2 and include grades 3 and 4 mucositis (n = 8 and n = 1, resp.), grade 3 diarrhea (n = 3), grades 3 and 4 hyperbilirubinemia (n = 4 and n = 2, resp.), grade 3 and grade 4 sepsis (n = 1 and n = 2, resp.), grade 3 and grade 4 hemorrhagic cystitis (n = 2 and n = 1 resp.), grade 3 vomiting (n = 3), and grade 3 hypertension (n = 1). One patient, with moderate hearing loss prior to ASCT progressed to a grade 4 hearing loss. Median time to discharge from hospital was 21 ± 6 (range 15–37) days, at which point all toxicities except for hearing loss had reverted to < grade 3.

3.5. Responses and Post-ASCT Therapy. Response was evaluated in 9/10 patients with measurable disease prior to ASCT. Seven had SD, one had a mixed response, and one had PD. 17 patients received 3000 cGy whole abdominopelvic radiotherapy (RT) with boosts to the tumor bed sites, as well as sites of bulk metastatic disease, at a median of 12 (range: 6 to 34) weeks following ASCT (Table 3). Two patients were treated with additional therapy following ASCT, one with anti-GD2 anti-idiotypic vaccine A1G4 (#14) and another with irinotecan followed by oral etoposide (#15); both patients died of PD.

3.6. Survival. Fifteen patients developed PD at a median of 12.8 (range 3.1–25.3) months after ASCT, one of whom (#1) died from complications of PD and sepsis 5 months later. Two patients (#13 and #17 Table 3) developed secondary acute myeloid leukemia (AML), 8 and 12 months after ASCT, and succumbed to this disease at 19 and 40 months after ASCT, respectively. Median time to death after relapse or development of AML was 12.4 months. Ten patients received

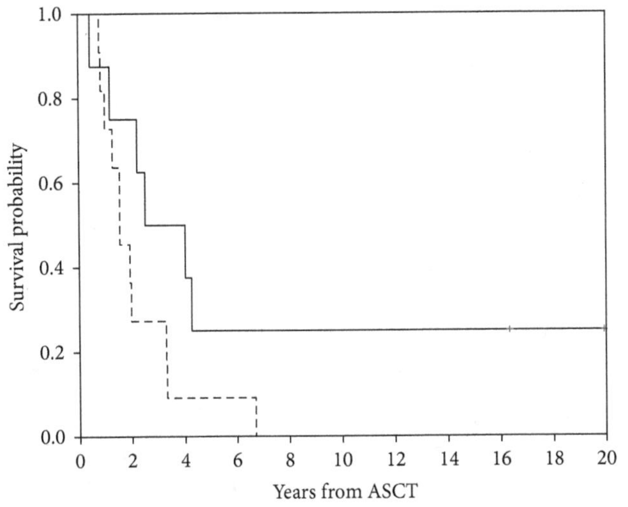

FIGURE 1: Overall survival probabilities of patients in first complete remission (—) prior to autologous stem cell transplant (ASCT) compared to all other patients (- - -).

various additional therapies following disease progression, which are detailed in Table 3. Two patients, neither of whom received any systemic therapy after ASCT, are currently alive without evidence of disease, 196 and 239 months after ASCT. Three-year event-free (EFS) and overall survival (OS) were 11 ± 7% and 26±10%, respectively, while 5-year EFS and OS were 11 ± 7% and 16 ± 8%, respectively. Median EFS and OS for patients in CR prior to ASCT were 13.7 ± 2.3 months and 30.1 ± 15.3 months from ASCT, respectively, while for those patients with measurable disease prior to ASCT EFS and OS were 9.1 ± 2.1 months and 18.7 ± 4.3 months, respectively. OS probability was higher for patients treated in the first CR compared to all other patients though this did not reach statistical significance ($p = 0.07$ for OS; $p = 0.14$ for EFS) in this small group of patients (Figure 1).

4. Discussion

The long-term prognosis for patients with DSRCT has essentially remained unchanged since the disease was first described as a distinct entity 25 years ago. Our group was the first to report responses to high-dose, alkylator-based chemotherapy, which has become the backbone of induction therapy for DSCRT [17]. However, responses were incomplete and aggressive debulking surgery to remove bulky residual disease is almost always necessary to try to achieve remission. In a retrospective analysis of a relatively large number of patients with DSRCT treated at MSKCC, multimodality therapy including high-dose alkylator chemotherapy in combination with aggressive surgical resection and radiotherapy resulted in improvement in intermediate-term (3 years) OS from 27% prior to the use of multimodal therapy to 55% after multimodal therapy was introduced [19]. Similar poor outcomes have been reported by other investigators treating patients with heterogeneous approaches without ASCT [20].

The rationale for the use of ASCT was to further escalate the doses of chemotherapy to overcome potential chemoresistance in disease that is regressing or has been rendered to a minimal state with induction chemotherapy and surgery in an effort to improve long-term outcomes. The toxicities of the chosen chemotherapeutic agents at high doses were primarily hematologic which could be overcome with ASCT. In our initial report, intermediate-term outcomes in patients treated with P6 induction followed by ASCT appeared to be favorable with 2 patients surviving disease-free 13 and 34 months from diagnosis [17]. However, as we now report on the data from a larger group of patients studied prospectively with longer followup, ASCT failed to improve outcomes, as patients treated with ASCT had a long-term survival of only 11%. Other investigators have made similar observations. A retrospective analysis by the Center for International Blood and Marrow Transplant Research of 36 patients with DSRCT treated in multiple centers with a variety of conditioning regimens revealed 3-year DFS of 23% [21]. Bertuzzi et al. reported on a cohort of 10 adult patients prospectively treated with high-dose melphalan plus mitoxantrone or thiotepa and found no improvements in overall survival [22]. Alternative approaches using sequential and multiple ASCTs administered earlier in the course of therapy were associated with equally poor outcomes [23]. Additional evidence of lack of effectiveness of ASCT was the poor response to the regimens used in our study with only a minor response noted in one patient. Moreover, the toxicity of ASCT was significant. Although there was no treatment-related mortality, the incidence of severe mucositis and hepatotoxicity was high. The apparently high incidence of secondary AML (2/19 patients) is likely a statistical anomaly related to the small number of patients undergoing ASCT.

Optimal "consolidation" therapy for patients whose disease burden has been significantly reduced remains to be determined. Based on our experience, ASCT appears to be ineffective in preventing relapse or progression for this group of patients even when post-ASCT whole abdominal radiotherapy is administered. Other options that could be considered for remission consolidation include conventional chemotherapy combinations such as irinotecan plus temozolomide [24, 25], vinorelbine, and low-dose cyclophosphamide [26]. Improvements in external beam radiotherapy using intensity-modulated approaches have significantly reduced radiation-related toxicity, but their efficacy in preventing relapse remains to be evaluated [27].

Directly targeting the peritoneal compartment, the site of relapse or progression in most patients with DSRCT might improve the outcome by eradicating minimal residual disease that is refractory or inaccessible to systemic chemotherapy. Such a strategy has shown to be of benefit for patients with ovarian carcinoma, another malignancy that involves the peritoneum [28] and for patients with malignant ascites [29]. Two such compartmental approaches are currently being studied in patients with DSRCT in early-phase trials. Intraperitoneal anti-B7H3 radioimmunotherapy with the radioiodinated monoclonal antibody 8H9 (NCT01099644) appears to be well tolerated with encouraging initial results in patients treated without measurable disease after surgery

[30, 31]. Similar preliminary results have also been reported with hyperthermic intraperitoneal chemotherapy with cisplatin administered after tumor resection (NCT01277744) [32, 33]. However, the contribution of these interventions in preventing recurrence in patients who have been rendered into a state of minimal disease by surgery will be difficult to evaluate since objective responses cannot be measured.

Understanding the genomic aberrations and pathway abnormalities in DSRCT will be critical to the design of effective therapy. WT1 is a potential target for T-cell, natural killer cell or antibody-mediated immunotherapy. A number of downstream targets of the EWS-WT1 fusion protein such as insulin-like growth factor receptor [34] and platelet derived growth factor-A [35] are involved in growth factor signaling and could be inhibited with therapeutic benefit. Additionally, vascular endothelial growth factor- (VEGF-) A and VEGF receptor-2 are overexpressed in DSRCT [25] and the mTOR pathway is believed to be constitutively activated [36]. To exploit the vascular nature of DSRCT and this differential overexpression of VEGF-A and VEGF receptor-2, bevacizumab is being added to conventional chemotherapy (irinotecan/temozolomide + P6 protocol) in a trial for the upfront treatment of these patients (NCT01189643). Other agents being evaluated for activity in DSRCT include antitype-1 insulin-like growth factor receptor antibodies [37] and multiple tyrosine kinase inhibitors [38–41]. MTOR-inhibitors were found to downregulate the expression of the EWS/WT1 transcript and increase the Bax/BcL-xL ratio resulting in increased tumor cell death [42, 43]. Another potentially targetable aberration that appears unique to DSRCT is the equilibrative nucleoside transporter 4 (ENT4). ENT4 is a pH-dependent adenosine transporter that is directly activated by EWS/WT1 and highly expressed in primary tumors and cell lines, making it an attractive therapeutic target. It remains to be seen whether targeting any of these pathways, alone or in combination [44], has the potential to make a significant impact on patient outcomes.

Ours is the largest prospective study of myeloablative chemotherapy and ASCT in patients with DSRCT. While it supports the feasibility and tolerability of ASCT in patients with DSRCT after induction chemotherapy and surgery, it fails to demonstrate any clear benefit for ASCT in improving outcomes. A continued emphasis will need to be placed on developing and investigating novel approaches and therapies. The recent production of a panel of DSRCT cell lines might accelerate preclinical research in experimental therapeutics for this rare but lethal malignancy [45].

References

[1] W. L. Gerald and J. Rosai, "Case 2. Desmoplastic small cell tumor with divergent differentiation," *Pediatric Pathology*, vol. 9, no. 2, pp. 177–183, 1989.

[2] W. L. Gerald, H. K. Miller, H. Battifora, M. Miettinen, E. G. Silva, and J. Rosai, "Intra-abdominal desmoplastic small round-cell tumor. Report of 19 cases of a distinctive type of high-grade polyphenotypic malignancy affecting young individuals," *The American Journal of Surgical Pathology*, vol. 15, no. 6, pp. 499–513, 1991.

[3] V. Parkash, W. L. Gerald, A. Parma, M. Miettinen, and J. Rosai, "Desmoplastic small round cell tumor of the pleura," *The American Journal of Surgical Pathology*, vol. 19, no. 6, pp. 659–665, 1995.

[4] O. W. Cummings, T. M. Ulbright, R. H. Young, A. P. Dei Tos, C. D. M. Fletcher, and M. T. Hull, "Desmoplastic small round cell tumors of the paratesticular region: a report of six cases," *The American Journal of Surgical Pathology*, vol. 21, no. 2, pp. 219–225, 1997.

[5] M. Yoon, K. Desai, R. Fulton et al., "Desmoplastic small round cell tumor: a potentially lethal neoplasm manifesting in the orbit with associated visual symptoms," *Archives of Ophthalmology*, vol. 123, no. 4, pp. 565–567, 2005.

[6] A. Murphy, R. L. Stallings, J. Howard et al., "Primary desmoplastic small round cell tumor of bone: report of a case with cytogenetic confirmation," *Cancer Genetics and Cytogenetics*, vol. 156, no. 2, pp. 167–171, 2005.

[7] M.-C. Su, Y.-M. Jeng, and Y.-C. Chu, "Desmoplastic small round cell tumor of the kidney," *The American Journal of Surgical Pathology*, vol. 28, no. 10, pp. 1379–1383, 2004.

[8] S. Syed, A. K. Haque, H. K. Hawkins, P. H. B. Sorensen, and D. F. Cowan, "Desmoplastic small round cell tumor of the lung," *Archives of Pathology and Laboratory Medicine*, vol. 126, no. 10, pp. 1226–1228, 2002.

[9] R. H. Young, J. H. Eichhorn, G. R. Dickersin, and R. E. Scully, "Ovarian involvement by the intra-abdominal desmoplastic small round cell tumor with divergent differentiation: a report of three cases," *Human Pathology*, vol. 23, no. 4, pp. 454–464, 1992.

[10] V. Adsay, J. Cheng, E. Athanasian, W. Gerald, and J. Rosai, "Primary desmoplastic small cell tumor of soft tissues and bone of the hand," *The American Journal of Surgical Pathology*, vol. 23, no. 11, pp. 1408–1413, 1999.

[11] N. A. Mihok and I. Cha, "Desmoplastic small round cell tumor presenting as a neck mass: a case report," *Diagnostic Cytopathology*, vol. 25, no. 1, pp. 68–72, 2001.

[12] W. L. Gerald, M. Ladanyi, E. de Alava et al., "Clinical, pathologic, and molecular spectrum of tumors associated with t(11;22)(p13;q12): desmoplastic small round-cell tumor and its variants," *Journal of Clinical Oncology*, vol. 16, no. 9, pp. 3028–3036, 1998.

[13] N. G. Ordóñez, "Desmoplastic small round cell tumor: II: an ultrastructural and immunohistochemical study with emphasis on new immunohistochemical markers," *The American Journal of Surgical Pathology*, vol. 22, no. 11, pp. 1314–1327, 1998.

[14] J. R. Sawyer, A. F. Tryka, and J. M. Lewis, "A novel reciprocal chromosome translocation t(11;22)(p13;q12) in an intraabdominal desmoplastic small round-cell tumor," *The American Journal of Surgical Pathology*, vol. 16, no. 4, pp. 411–416, 1992.

[15] M. Ladanyi and W. Gerald, "Fusion of the EWS and WT1 genes in the desmoplastic small round cell tumor," *Cancer Research*, vol. 54, no. 11, pp. 2837–2840, 1994.

[16] W. L. Gerald and D. A. Haber, "The EWS-WT1 gene fusion in desmoplastic small round cell tumor," *Seminars in Cancer Biology*, vol. 15, no. 3, pp. 197–205, 2005.

[17] B. H. Kushner, M. P. LaQuaglia, N. Wollner et al., "Desmoplastic small round-cell tumor: prolonged progression-free survival with aggressive multimodality therapy," *Journal of Clinical Oncology*, vol. 14, no. 5, pp. 1526–1531, 1996.

[18] A. H. Calvert, D. R. Newell, L. A. Gumbrell et al., "Carboplatin dosage: prospective evaluation of a simple formula based on renal function," *Journal of Clinical Oncology*, vol. 7, no. 11, pp. 1748–1756, 1989.

[19] D. R. Lal, W. T. Su, S. L. Wolden, K. C. Loh, S. Modak, and M. P. La Quaglia, "Results of multimodal treatment for desmoplastic small round cell tumors," *Journal of Pediatric Surgery*, vol. 40, no. 1, pp. 251–255, 2005.

[20] P. Philippe-Chomette, N. Kabbara, N. Andre et al., "Desmoplastic small round cell tumors with EWS-WT1 fusion transcript in children and young adults," *Pediatric Blood and Cancer*, vol. 58, no. 6, pp. 891–897, 2012.

[21] R. J. Cook, Z. Wang, M. Arora et al., "Clinical outcomes of patients with desmoplastic small round cell tumor of the peritoneum undergoing autologous HCT: a CIBMTR retrospective analysis," *Bone Marrow Transplantation*, vol. 47, no. 11, pp. 1455–1458, 2012.

[22] A. Bertuzzi, L. Castagna, V. Quagliuolo et al., "Prospective study of high-dose chemotherapy and autologous peripheral stem cell transplantation in adult patients with advanced desmoplastic small round-cell tumour," *British Journal of Cancer*, vol. 89, no. 7, pp. 1159–1161, 2003.

[23] G. Bisogno, A. Ferrari, A. Rosolen et al., "Sequential intensified chemotherapy with stem cell rescue for children and adolescents with desmoplastic small round-cell tumor," *Bone Marrow Transplantation*, vol. 45, no. 5, pp. 907–911, 2010.

[24] P. M. Rosoff and S. Bayliff, "Successful clinical response to irinotecan in desmoplastic round blue cell tumor," *Medical and Pediatric Oncology*, vol. 33, no. 5, pp. 500–503, 1999.

[25] H. D. Magnan, A. T. Chou, M. P. La Quaglia, W. Gerald, M. Ladanyi, and M. S. Merchant, "Elevated expression of VEGFR-2 and VEGFA in desmoplastic small round cell tumor (DSRCT) and activity of bevacizumab and irinotecan in a xenograft model of DSRCT," *Journal of Clinical Oncology*, vol. 27, supplement 15, 2009.

[26] A. Ferrari, F. Grosso, S. Stacchiotti et al., "Response to vinorelbine and low-dose cyclophosphamide chemotherapy in two patients with desmoplastic small round cell tumor," *Pediatric Blood & Cancer*, vol. 49, no. 6, pp. 864–866, 2007.

[27] N. B. Desai, N. F. Stein, M. P. Laquaglia et al., "Reduced toxicity with intensity modulated radiation therapy (IMRT) for desmoplastic small round cell tumor (DSRCT): an update on the whole abdominopelvic radiation therapy (WAP-RT) experience," *International Journal of Radiation Oncology Biology Physics*, vol. 85, no. 1, pp. e67–e72, 2013.

[28] A. Fagotti, B. Costantini, M. Petrillo et al., "Cytoreductive surgery plus HIPEC in platinum-sensitive recurrent ovarian cancer patients: a case-control study on survival in patients with two year follow-up," *Gynecologic Oncology*, vol. 127, no. 3, pp. 502–505, 2012.

[29] M. Jäger, A. Schoberth, P. Ruf et al., "Immunomonitoring results of a phase II/III study of malignant ascites patients treated with the trifunctional antibody catumaxomab (anti-EpCAM x anti-CD3)," *Cancer Research*, vol. 72, no. 1, pp. 24–32, 2012.

[30] S. Modak, W. Gerald, and N.-K. V. Cheung, "Disialoganglioside G_{D2} and a novel tumor antigen: potential targets for immunotherapy of desmoplastic small round cell tumor," *Medical and Pediatric Oncology*, vol. 39, no. 6, pp. 547–551, 2002.

[31] S. Modak, J. A. Carrasquillo, M. P. La Quaglia et al., "Intraperitoneal radioimmunotherapy for desmoplastic small round cell tumor," *Journal of Clinical Oncology*, vol. 30, supplement, abstract TPS9595, 2012.

[32] S. Msika, E. Gruden, S. Sarnacki et al., "Cytoreductive surgery associated to hyperthermic intraperitoneal chemoperfusion for desmoplastic round small cell tumor with peritoneal carcinomatosis in young patients," *Journal of Pediatric Surgery*, vol. 45, no. 8, pp. 1617–1621, 2010.

[33] A. Hayes-Jordan, H. Green, N. Fitzgerald, L. Xiao, and P. Anderson, "Novel treatment for desmoplastic small round cell tumor: hyperthermic intraperitoneal perfusion," *Journal of Pediatric Surgery*, vol. 45, no. 5, pp. 1000–1006, 2010.

[34] E. Karnieli, H. Werner, F. J. Rauscher III, L. E. Benjamin, and D. Leroith, "The IGF-I receptor gene promoter is a molecular target for the Ewing's sarcoma-Wilms' tumor 1 fusion protein," *The Journal of Biological Chemistry*, vol. 271, no. 32, pp. 19304–19309, 1996.

[35] S. Lee Bong, K. A. Kolquist, K. Nichols et al., "The EWS-WT1 translocation product induces PDGFA in desmoplastic small round-cell tumour," *Nature Genetics*, vol. 17, no. 3, pp. 309–313, 1997.

[36] V. Subbiah, R. E. Brown, Y. Jiang et al., "Morphoproteomic profiling of the mammalian target of rapamycin (mTOR) signaling pathway in desmoplastic small round cell tumor (EWS/WT1), Ewing's sarcoma (EWS/FLI1) and Wilms' tumor(WT1)," *PLoS ONE*, vol. 8, no. 7, Article ID e68985, 2013.

[37] W. D. Tap, G. Demetri, P. Barnette et al., "Phase II study of ganitumab, a fully human anti-type-1 insulin-like growth factor receptor antibody, in patients with metastatic Ewing family tumors or desmoplastic small round cell tumors," *Journal of Clinical Oncology*, vol. 30, no. 15, pp. 1849–1856, 2012.

[38] J. Chao, G. T. Budd, P. Chu et al., "Phase II clinical trial of imatinib mesylate in therapy of KIT and/or PDGFRalpha-expressing Ewing sarcoma family of tumors and desmoplastic small round cell tumors," *Anticancer Research*, vol. 30, no. 2, pp. 547–552, 2010.

[39] A. Italiano, M. Kind, A. Cioffi, R. G. Maki, and B. Bui, "Clinical activity of sunitinib in patients with advanced desmoplastic round cell tumor: a case series," *Targeted Oncology*, vol. 8, no. 3, pp. 211–213, 2013.

[40] J. L. Glade Bender, A. Lee, J. M. Reid et al., "Phase I pharmacokinetic and pharmacodynamic study of pazopanib in children with soft tissue sarcoma and other refractory solid tumors: a children's oncology group phase I consortium report," *Journal of Clinical Oncology*, vol. 31, no. 24, pp. 3034–3043, 2013.

[41] A. Frezza, C. Benson, I. R. Judson et al., "Pazopanib in advanced desmoplastic small round cell tumours: a multi-institutional experience," *Clinical Sarcoma Research*, vol. 4, no. 1, article 7, 2014.

[42] A. M. J. Thijs, W. T. A. van der Graaf, and C. M. L. van Herpen, "Temsirolimus for metastatic desmoplastic small round cell tumor," *Pediatric Blood & Cancer*, vol. 55, no. 7, pp. 1431–1432, 2010.

[43] O. M. Tirado, S. Mateo-Lozano, and V. Notario, "Rapamycin induces apoptosis of JN-DSRCT-1 cells by increasing the Bax : Bcl-xL ratio through concurrent mechanisms dependent and independent of its mTOR inhibitory activity," *Oncogene*, vol. 24, no. 20, pp. 3348–3357, 2005.

[44] G. K. Schwartz, W. D. Tap, L.-X. Qin et al., "Cixutumumab and temsirolimus for patients with bone and soft-tissue sarcoma: a multicentre, open-label, phase 2 trial," *The Lancet Oncology*, vol. 14, no. 4, pp. 371–382, 2013.

[45] C. S. A. Markides, D. R. Coil, L. H. Luong et al., "Desmoplastic small round cell tumor (DSRCT) xenografts and tissue culture lines: establishment and initial characterization," *Oncology Letters*, vol. 5, no. 5, pp. 1453–1456, 2013.

15

Synovial Chondrosarcoma Arising in Synovial Chondromatosis

Scott Evans, Michele Boffano, Samena Chaudhry, Lee Jeys, and Robert Grimer

Royal Orthopaedic Hospital, Birmingham B31 2AP, UK

Correspondence should be addressed to Scott Evans; drscottevans@yahoo.co.uk

Academic Editor: Jos Bramer

Primary synovial chondromatosis (SC) is a rare proliferative disorder that causes pain, swelling, and restriction of movement to the joints it affects. The disease frequently runs a protracted course, often requiring multiple surgical procedures to obtain some control. Few reports exist detailing the natural history of SC, although malignant transformation to synovial chondrosarcoma (CHS) is recognized to be a rare event. The aim of our study was to review a large orthopaedic oncology database in order to evaluate the incidence of CHS arising from SC. We identified 78 patients who have presented to our centre with primary synovial chondromatosis (SC). Of those patients, 5 went on to develop malignant change. This represents a 6.4% incidence of developing synovial chondrosarcoma (CHS) within preexisting primary synovial chondromatosis. The patients had a mean age of 28 years at first diagnosis with synovial chondromatosis with the median time from original diagnosis to malignant transformation being 20 years (range 2.7–39 yrs).

1. Introduction

Synovial chondromatosis is a rare proliferative, metaplastic disorder of the synovium [1]. The disease was first described by Leannac in 1813 [2]; however, its current description was not applied until 1958 by Jaffe [3]. The exact prevalence of primary synovial chondromatosis (SC) is unknown but it usually affects the third to fifth decades of life [4], with men being affected two to four times more frequently than women [5]. The knee is the most commonly affected large joint followed by hip, shoulder, elbow, ankle, and wrist [6]. Patient's clinical symptoms typically include pain, swelling, and restricted joint movement [7]. The symptoms are often insidious at disease onset and are gradually progressive, although rare spontaneous regression has been reported [8]. Patients often have a protracted length of symptoms prior to diagnosis, with an average of 5 years [9, 10].

Three phases of SC have been described [11]; phase 1 active intrasynovial disease with nodules but no calcifications/intraarticular bodies; phase 2 synovitis with osteochondral nodules in the synovial membrane and loose bodies within the joint; phase 3 multiple loose bodies remain but synovitis is quiescent. This highlights the importance of correlating histological and radiological findings to correctly diagnose the benign entity.

Malignant transformation of primary synovial chondromatosis to synovial chondrosarcoma is recognized to be a rare event with reports estimating the incidence to be in the range of 1–5% [12–14].

The aim of our study was to use a large database of patients with orthopaedic oncology to evaluate the incidence of chondrosarcoma arising from primary synovial chondrosarcoma and to review the time taken for the benign entity to transform into its malignant counterpart.

2. Materials and Methods

We conducted a retrospective search of a prospective tumour database to identify all patients treated at our unit with the diagnosis of primary synovial chondromatosis (SC). The diagnosis was made under the auspices of a supraregional multidisciplinary bone tumour unit. Patient demographics were recorded along with the site of primary disease. From this initial search, details of those patients who subsequently developed synovial chondrosarcoma (CHS) were collected.

Table 1: Details of the patients, their tumours, and the outcome.

Case	Age at diagnosis with SC (years)	Site	Treatment(s) for SC	Time to malignant change (years)	Malignancy	Surgical management of chondrosarcoma	Mets	Outcome
1	23	Hip	3 debridements	2.7	Grade I CHS	Hindquarter amputation	—	Alive 13 yrs postoperatively
2	48	Hip	(i) Initially symptomatic (ii) THR 11 yrs after initial diagnosis	11.3	Dedifferentiated chondrosar-coma (osteosarcoma)	Debulking	At presentation (lung)	Died 3 yrs postoperatively
3	25	Hip	(i) 2 arthroscopies (ii) 1 hip resurfacing 17 yrs after diagnosis	20	Grade II CHS	Debulking	At presentation (lung)	Died 4 yrs postoperatively
4	25	Hip	(i) Multiple debridements (ii) THR 2005 (iii) Large recurrence 5 years after THR	39	Grade I CHS	Hindquarter amputation	—	Alive 9 months postoperatively
5	19	Knee	(i) Multiple arthroscopies (ii) TKR aged 55	38.5	Grade II CHS	Above knee amputation	Lung—34 months after amputation	Died 4 yrs postoperatively

3. Results

A search of our database, which holds prospectively gathered data on over 30,000 patients including over 3800 primary bone sarcomas, identified 78 patients with SC. All had been diagnosed following analysis of their radiological and histological findings between 1980 and 2011. There were 33 females (42.3%) and 45 males (57.7%) with a mean age at presentation with SC of 28 years. The primary site of SC was the knee in 30 patients, hip in 22, hand in 7, shoulder in 6, elbow in 5, foot in 5, wrist in 2, and the ankle in 1.

The median time from original diagnosis with SC to malignant transformation was 20 years (range 2.5–39 years). All patients had undergone multiple procedures in an attempt to control their SC prior to the diagnosis of malignancy. All cases of CHS were diagnosed after careful discussion at a multidisciplinary team meeting involving orthopaedic oncologist, histopathologist, and radiologist (Table 1).

One of the main problems in diagnosing malignancy in SC is that biopsies are often not helpful and clinical features often suggest malignancy more than histology. In two patients (case 1 + 4), repeated biopsy demonstrated benign disease, whilst their imaging studies revealed likely extensive primary synovial chondromatosis. However, it was clear from the patients' level of nonmechanical pain in combination with the rapid and repeated progression of their tumours after debulking that they had aggressive disease. The patients were included in a pragmatic discussion and the decision was made to perform hind-quarter amputation. In both cases, the actual diagnosis of malignancy was only confirmed when the whole tumour had been sampled (see Figures 1 and 2).

Two cases (patients 2 and 3) had large tumours with lung metastases by the time of diagnosis and therefore were treated symptomatically. Both patients subsequently died with chest metastases 3 and 4 years, respectively, after diagnosis. Our one patient with CHS affecting the knee (case 5) underwent an above knee amputation as limb salvage was not possible. Histology revealed a grade II synovial chondrosarcoma. He developed lung metastases 34 months postoperatively and subsequently died 4 years after the amputation.

As with other chondrsarcomas, radio/chemotherapy are not typically effective treatments and, therefore, our cases did not receive adjuvant therapy. In summary, 78 patients were identified with SC, with 5 developing CHS. This represents transformation to malignancy in 6.4% of cases. Furthermore, it is apparent from performing Kaplan-Meier survival analysis that the risk of malignant transformation increases as time elapses (see Figure 3).

4. Discussion

Primary synovial chondromatosis is a rare disease. Its true incidence is unknown. The incidence of chondrosarcoma in England is however known and is reported to be 1.8/million population per year [15]. Our unit has treated 800 patients with a chondrosarcoma in the same time period as we treated these 78 primary synovial chondromatosis patients. This would suggest that for every 800 chondrosarcomas diagnosed, 5 originated in synovial chondromatosis; that is, 0.6% of chondrosarcomas are linked to primary synovial chondromatosis. As the incidence of chondrosarcoma in England is known, we would expect to see approximately 95 new cases of chondrosarcoma every year. Therefore, every year, 0.57 cases of chondrosarcomas are associated with preexisting synovial chondromatosis; that is, every 1.7 years (20.4 months), 1 new case of chondrosarcoma can be attributed to primary synovial chondromatosis.

Even though our unit is a supra-regional referral unit, it is unlikely that we were referred all patients with synovial chondromatosis over this time period. If we had been then the incidence of primary synovial chondromatosis would be 78/5

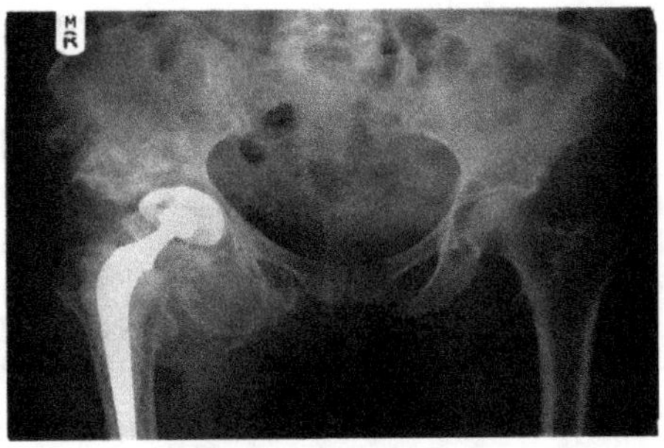

FIGURE 1: Plain X-ray of case 4 preoperatively.

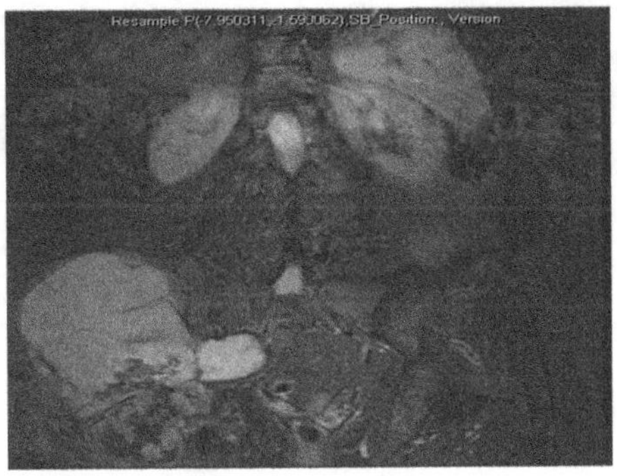

FIGURE 2: STIR MRI of case 4 preoperatively.

of that of chondrosarcoma in primary synovial chondromatosis; that is, 0.06/million per yr, suggesting that there may be 10 new cases of primary synovial chondromatosis diagnosed a year in England. We know no way of confirming this.

Although primary synovial chondromatosis can be locally aggressive with a tendency to recur, it has no metastatic potential. The treatment for symptomatic primary synovial chondromatosis consists of removal of the cartilaginous bodies with or without partial synovectomy. In contrast, chondrosarcoma is a malignant condition requiring more invasive surgery in the form of wide or radical resection or amputation [16] and has a reported incidence of metastases of up to 29% [17, 18].

Clearly because of the differences in prognosis and treatment, it is vitally important to distinguish the benign primary synovial chondromatosis from the malignant chondrosarcoma. In practice, this can be difficult as both conditions have similar patterns of disease presentation with pain, swelling, and restricted joint movement. Numerous authors have found clinical and radiological criteria unhelpful to differentiate between the two disease processes as there is often significant overlap with no definitive features to separate the two [1, 14, 18–20].

Histologically primary synovial chondromatosis reveals lobules of hyaline cartilage that are often hypercellular with atypical histological features, including multinucleation, nuclear crowding, nuclear enlargement, and hyperchromasia with mild myxoid changes often with a variable degree of synovial proliferation or hyperplasia [21]. These atypical features could suggest a malignant neoplasm (grade I or II chondrosarcoma) to the less experienced pathologist when

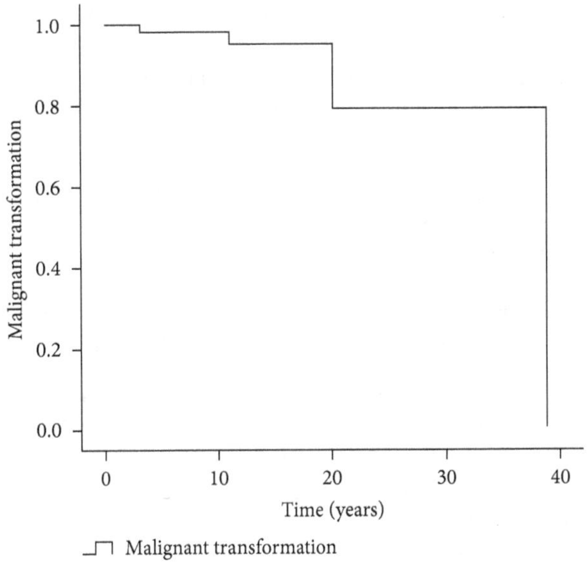

FIGURE 3: Kaplan-Meier survival (malignant transformation = endpoint).

actually they are typical of benign primary synovial chondromatosis [22–24]. Immunohistochemical markers to reliably differentiate between primary synovial chondromatosis and low grade chondrosarcoma would be of great value but, to date, only preliminary studies have been performed [25] with no definitive immunostaining technique being identified as the gold-standard.

The local recurrence of primary synovial chondromatosis has been reported to be as high as 23% [14] despite adequate surgical debridement. The difficulty lies with identifying those recurrences that are benign.

In conclusion, we view multiple recurrences with the development of marrow invasion as highly suspicious of malignant transformation. From our study, it is clear that not all patients with primary synovial chondromatosis require long-term surveillance to monitor for the development of malignant change; however, we recommend that any rapid deterioration in the patient's clinical course, including worsening pain or aggressive recurrence, should be regarded as suspicious and treated at, or referred appropriately to, a tertiary hospital familiar with managing these often complex cases.

References

[1] B. Wittkop, A. M. Davies, and D. C. Mangham, "Primary synovial chondromatosis and synovial chondrosarcoma," *European Radiology*, vol. 12, no. 8, pp. 2112–2119, 2002.

[2] J. M. Crotty, J. U. V. Monu, and T. L. Pope Jr., "Synovial osteochondromatosis," *Radiologic Clinics of North America*, vol. 34, no. 2, pp. 327–342, 1996.

[3] H. L. Jaffe, *Tumours and Tumourous Conditions of the Bones and Joints*, Kimpton, London, UK, 1958.

[4] "Synovial chondromatosis," in *Pathophysiology of Orthopaedic Diseases*, H. J. Mankin, Ed., pp. 53–58, The American Academy of Orthopaedic Surgeons, Rosemont, Ill, USA, 2006.

[5] M. D. Darfam and B. Czerniak, "Synovial lesions," in *Bone Tumours*, pp. 1041–1086, Mosby, St. Louis, Mo, USA, 1998.

[6] G. Hermann, M. J. Klein, I. F. Abdelwahab, and S. Kenan, "Synovial chondrosarcoma arising in synovial chondromatosis of the right hip," *Skeletal Radiology*, vol. 26, no. 6, pp. 366–369, 1997.

[7] F. P. Murphy, D. C. Dahlin, and C. R. Sullivan, "Articular synovial chondromatosis," *The Journal of Bone and Joint Surgery. American*, vol. 44, pp. 77–86, 1962.

[8] S. H. Butt, T. Muthukumar, V. N. Cassar-Pullicino, and D. C. Mangham, "Primary synovial osteochondromatosis presenting as constrictive capsulitis," *Skeletal Radiology*, vol. 34, no. 11, pp. 707–713, 2005.

[9] B. Tins and V. Cassar-Pullicino, "Synovial osteochondromatosis in hereditary arthro-ophthalmopathy (Wagner-Stickler syndrome)," *Skeletal Radiology*, vol. 32, no. 5, pp. 302–305, 2003.

[10] A. Trias and O. Quintana, "Synovial chondrometaplasia: review of world literature and a study of 18 Canadian cases," *Canadian Journal of Surgery*, vol. 19, no. 2, pp. 151–158, 1976.

[11] J. W. Milgram, "Synovial osteochondromatosis: a histopathological study of thirty cases," *The Journal of Bone and Joint Surgery. American*, vol. 59, no. 6, pp. 792–801, 1977.

[12] A. K. Bhadra, R. Pollock, R. P. Tirabosco et al., "Primary tumours of the synovium: a report of four cases of malignant tumour," *The Journal of Bone and Joint Surgery. British*, vol. 89, no. 11, pp. 1504–1508, 2007.

[13] R. I. Davis, A. Hamilton, and J. D. Biggart, "Primary synovial chondromatosis: a clinicopathologic review and assessment of malignant potential," *Human Pathology*, vol. 29, no. 7, pp. 683–688, 1998.

[14] M. D. Murphy, J. A. Vidal, J. C. Famburg-Smith, and D. A. Gajenski, "Imaging of synovial chondromatosis with radiologic-pathologic correlation," *Radiographics*, vol. 27, pp. 1465–1468, 2007.

[15] http://www.ncin.org.uk/publications/data_briefings/bone_sarcomas_incidence_and_survival.

[16] L. D. Rybak, L. Khaldi, J. Wittig, and G. C. Steiner, "Primary synovial chondrosarcoma of the hip joint in a 45-year-old male: case report and literature review," *Skeletal Radiology*, vol. 40, no. 10, pp. 1375–1381, 2011.

[17] D. A. Campanacci, D. Matera, A. Franchi, and R. Capanna, "Synovial chondrosarcoma of the hip: report of two cases and literature review," *La Chirurgia Degli Organi di Movimento*, vol. 92, no. 3, pp. 139–144, 2008.

[18] E. E. Zamora, A. Mansor, D. Vanel et al., "Synovial chondrosarcoma: a report of two cases and literature review," *European Journal of Radiology*, vol. 72, no. 1, pp. 38–43, 2009.

[19] F. Bertoni, K. K. Unni, J. W. Beabout, and F. H. Sim, "Chondrosarcoma of the synovium," *Cancer*, vol. 67, pp. 155–162, 1991.

[20] W. K. Taconis, R. O. van der Heul, and A. M. M. Taminiau, "Synovial chondrosarcoma: report of a case and review of the literature," *Skeletal Radiology*, vol. 26, no. 11, pp. 682–685, 1997.

[21] M. V. Miller, A. Kind, and F. Mertens, "Synovial chondromatosis," in *Pathology and Genetics of Tumours of Soft Tissue and Bone*, C. D. M. Fletcher, K. K. Unni, and F. Mertens, Eds., p. 246, IARC Press, Lyon, France, 2002.

[22] D. Resnik, "Tumours and tumour-like lesions of soft tissues," in *Diagnosis of Bone and Joint Disorders*, pp. 4204–4273, Saunders, Philadelphia, Pa, USA, 4th edition, 2002.

[23] K. K. Unni, C. Y. Inwards, J. A. Bridge, L. G. Kindbolm, and L. E. Wold, "Synovial tumours," in *Tumours of the Bone and Joints*, pp. 386–432, ARP Press, Silver Spring, Md, USA, 4th edition, 2005.

[24] S. W. Weiss and J. R. Goldblum, "Cartilagenous soft tissue tumours," in *Enzinger and Weiss' Soft Tissue Tumours*, pp. 1368–1388, Mosby, Philadelphia, Pa, USA, 4th edition, 2001.

[25] B. L. Sperling, S. Angel, G. Stoneham, V. Chow, A. Mcfadden, and R. Chibbar, "Synovial chondromatosis and chondrosarcoma: a diagnostic dilemma," *Sarcoma*, vol. 7, no. 2, pp. 69–73, 2003.

16

Adult versus Pediatric Neuroblastoma: The M.D. Anderson Cancer Center Experience

Henry J. Conter,[1] Vancheswaran Gopalakrishnan,[1] Vinod Ravi,[2] Joann L. Ater,[3] Shreyaskumar Patel,[2] and Dejka M. Araujo[2]

[1] *Division of Cancer Medicine, M.D. Anderson Cancer Center, 1400 Holcombe Boulevard, Unit 463, Houston, TX 77030, USA*
[2] *Department of Sarcoma Medical Oncology, M.D. Anderson Cancer Center, 1400 Holcombe Boulevard, Unit 463, Houston, TX 77030, USA*
[3] *Department of Pediatrics Patient Care, M.D. Anderson Cancer Center, 1400 Holcombe Boulevard, Unit 463, Houston, TX 77030, USA*

Correspondence should be addressed to Henry J. Conter; hconter@gmail.com

Academic Editor: Andreas Leithner

Background. Staging and treatment of adult neuroblastoma has yet to be formalized. We sought to determine the utility of the pediatric classification system in adults and determine the efficacy of different treatment modalities. *Methods.* Medical records of 118 adults (patients >17 years old) and 112 pediatric patients (ages 2–17), who were treated for neuroblastoma at M.D. Anderson Cancer Center from January 1994 to September 2012, were reviewed. International neuroblastoma risk group (INRG) variables were abstracted. The primary outcome of interest was actuarial progression-free survival. *Results.* Median age of pediatric patients was 5 years (range 3–16) and 47 years (range 18–82) for adult patients. There were no differences in PFS or OS between stage-matched risk categories between pediatric and adult patients (L1-$P = 0.40$, L2-$P = 0.54$, and M-$P = 0.73$). In the treatment of L1 disease, median PFS for adults treated with surgery and radiation was 11.1 months compared with single modality local treatment ± chemotherapy (6.4 and 5.1 months, resp.; $P = 0.07$). Median PFS in L2 adult patients was 5.2 months with local therapy and 4 months with the addition of chemotherapy ($P = 0.23$). *Conclusions.* Adult and pediatric patients with neuroblastoma achieve similar survival outcomes. INRG classification should be employed to stratify adult neuroblastoma patients and help select treatment.

1. Introduction

Neuroblastoma arises from primitive sympathetic neural cells primarily in the adrenal medulla and also in the paraspinal sympathetic ganglia in the neck, chest, abdomen, or pelvis [1]. Although neuroblastoma currently represents 7% of all childhood malignancies or roughly 1 case per 100,000 children per year, only 1 case per 10 million adults per year is diagnosed in adulthood [2–4]. Because of the rarity of adult neuroblastoma, staging systems and risk assessment tools have been developed using primarily pediatric data [5]. Clinically relevant pediatric factors that influence survival in children include stage, age, histology, tumor grade, MYCN oncogene status, chromosome 11q status, and DNA ploidy. These factors are currently part of the international neuroblastoma risk assessment system [6].

Whereas 5-year survival approaches 85% for infants diagnosed with neuroblastoma, adult overall survival at 5 years is 36% [4]. Long-term survival in adults has been reported even in the presence of multiple recurrences [7]. Up to 1/3 of adult patients are diagnosed with metastatic disease at presentation. In the metastatic setting, prognosis between adults and children appears comparable. However, at earlier stages, the prognosis of adults is worse than that of comparable pediatric patients. Adult patients have been reported to have a high incidence of unfavorable histologies [8] but a lower incidence of MYCN amplification [9, 10], which usually correlates with a better prognosis.

No standard therapy exists for adults with neuroblastoma, but all adult patients can be considered at high risk of death from disease regardless of stage [11]. Dose intense cytotoxic chemotherapy has been shown to produce greater response rates and progression-free survival, compared to standard chemotherapy [12, 13]. Commonly used agents include cisplatin, cyclophosphamide, ifosfamide, topotecan, etoposide, doxorubicin, and vincristine. High-dose chemotherapy and autologous stem-cell rescue (HDCSR) have been shown to improve event-free and overall survival in high-risk pediatric patients, based on a meta-analysis of 3 randomized controlled trials including 739 patients [14]. External beam radiation may also play a role in the management of high-risk neuroblastoma, especially in the setting of residual disease after surgery [15]. However, adult patients may have poorer tolerance to high intensity therapy regimens compared to children. For patients with metastatic neuroblastoma, radiation therapy can be an effective treatment modality when local control is required but may hinder attempts at gross total resection of the tumor [16].

Although there has been a trend to improved prognosis of patients over the last three decades [4], only 3 adult case series since 1997, totaling 93 patients, have been published [8–10]. We sought to improve on the volume of the literature on this subject by reviewing the M.D. Anderson Cancer Center experience of treating adult patients with neuroblastoma and comparing outcomes to their pediatric counterparts.

2. Methods

2.1. Study Protocol. Patients were identified by query of the University of Texas M.D. Anderson Cancer Center's (MDACC) institutional database from its inception in January 1994 until the date of search, September 21, 2012. All patients diagnosed by histology with neuroblastoma or ganglioneuroblastoma were eligible for inclusion into the study. However, patients who were 2 years of age or younger at diagnosis were excluded from analysis to limit the effect of spontaneous regression [17]. Adults were defined by convention by being diagnosed after the age of 17. The institutional database routinely captures demographic, histologic, location of the primary tumor, SEER stage, and vital statistic information on all patients seen at MDACC. Data were collected from the database using a standardized form. Additional information concerning the international neuroblastoma risk group (INRG) staging [5] and classification [6] was extracted directly from individual patient charts. To accomplish this, histologic category, grade of tumor differentiation, MYCN, 11q aberration, and ploidy information were obtained. Classification of L1 versus L2 disease was accomplished by review of the staging radiology reports: one or more reported image-defined risk factor indicated L2 disease. Clinical notes were also reviewed for staging. Where there was disagreement between radiology and the clinical note, the patient was classified as per the more advanced stage. Treatment was categorized as surgery, radiation, chemotherapy, or high-dose chemotherapy with hematopoietic stem cell rescue (HDCSR). Therapy was further classified by its intent and the line of treatment.

2.2. Statistical Analysis. The primary point of interest was the patients' age category, pediatric or adult, grouped by INRG classification. The primary outcome of interest was overall survival from the date of diagnosis. Secondary outcomes of interest included the effect of (neo) adjuvant radiation and chemotherapy on progression-free survival (PFS) and overall survival (OS) for stage L1 and L2 adult patients. We also examined the effect of chemotherapy choice on PFS and OS for adult patients with stage M disease. Categorical variables were compared using the Chi-squared test or the two-sided Fisher exact test. Actuarial survival was estimated using the Kaplain-Meier method and compared using the log-rank test. All statistical tests were two-sided with a $P < 0.05$ considered to be statistically significant.

3. Results

3.1. Patients. Querying the University of Texas M.D. Anderson Cancer Center's institutional database yielded 230 patients with a diagnosis of neuroblastoma or ganglioneuroblastoma. Of these, 112 patients were diagnosed before the age of 18 and were considered pediatric patients, leaving 118 adults (Table 1). The median follow-up of living pediatric patients was 6 months and 33 months for adult patients. The longest surviving pediatric patient remains living after 18 years since the date of diagnosis and the longest surviving adult has surpassed 17 years. Of the adult patients, 101 (85%) patients had localized disease, compared with 36 (33%) of pediatric patients. 78 (77%) adult patients with localized disease presented with a head and neck primary. Complete risk stratification of L1 and L2 stage adult patients was not possible: no adult patients had undergone molecular or genetic analysis of their tumors. Stage-for-stage, the category of therapies employed was comparable (Table 2). Chemotherapy agents employed included topoisomerase II inhibitors (doxorubicin and etoposide), alkylating agents (cyclophosphamide, dacarbazine, ifosfamide, melphalan, and thiotepa), platinum analogs (cisplatin, carboplatin, and oxaliplatin), spindle-cell modifiers (paclitaxel and vincristine), topoisomerase I inhibitors (topotecan), vascular endothelial growth factor small-molecule inhibitors (vandetanib and sunitinib), and immunomodulatory agents (lenalidomide and retinoid therapy) in varying combinations and dosing schedules across all stages of disease. Common regimens are listed in Table 3.

3.2. Outcomes. The median overall survival of adult patients was 18.1 years, 9.8 years, and 1.6 years for stages L1, L2, and M, respectively (Figure 1). Adults with L1 disease experienced an actuarial OS of 94%, 90%, and 69% at years 3, 5, and 10, respectively. The cohort who presented with L2 disease had an actuarial OS of 83% at 3 years, 73% at 5 years, and 41% at 10 years. Adults with M disease experienced an actuarial OS of 68%, 33%, and 13% at years 1, 2 and 5, respectively. For all stage-matched categories, the prognosis of adult neuroblastoma patients were not statistically different compared to pediatric neuroblastoma patients (L1-P = 0.40, L2-P = 0.54, and M-P = 0.73). For adult patients with L1 disease,

TABLE 1: Patient characteristics by stage of disease.

	Adult (%)	Pediatric (%)
Stage: L1	**57 (48)**	**24 (22%)**
Median age (range)	48 (18–77)	5.5 (3–15)
Histology		
Ganglioneuroblastoma	6 (11)	6 (25)
Neuroblastoma	51 (89)	18 (75)
Primary location		
Bones, skeletal system	1 (2)	1 (4)
Central nervous system	1 (2)	1 (4)
Chest cavity viscera	2 (4)	4 (17)
Head and neck	46 (81)	3 (12)
Soft tissue	2 (4)	8 (33)
Urinary tract	5 (9)	7 (29)
Stage: L2	**44 (37)**	**12 (11)**
Median age (range)	51.5 (20–81)	5.5 (3–10)
Histology		
Ganglioneuroblastoma	2 (5)	3 (25)
Neuroblastoma	42 (95)	9 (75)
Primary location		
Central nervous system	3 (7)	2 (17)
Chest cavity viscera	2 (5)	1 (8)
Head and neck	32 (73)	1 (8)
Soft tissue	3 (7)	5 (42)
Urinary tract	4 (9)	3 (25)
Stage: M	**17 (14)**	**74 (67)**
Median age (range)	29 (19–75)	5 (3–16)
Histology		
Ganglioneuroblastoma	1 (16)	4 (5)
Neuroblastoma	16 (94)	70 (95)
Primary location		
Abdominal cavity viscera	2 (12)	1 (1)
Central nervous system	0	1 (1)
Chest cavity viscera	1 (6)	5 (7)
Male genital system	1 (6)	0
Head and neck	4 (24)	2 (3)
Metastatic cancer	1 (6)	1 (1)
Soft tissue	4 (24)	25 (34)
Genitourinary tract*	4 (24)	39 (53)

*Includes adrenal primary.

TABLE 2: Treatment by stage of disease.

	Adult (%)	Pediatric (%)	P value
Stage: L1	**57 (48)**	**24 (22)**	
Surgery	56 (99)	22 (92)	0.19
Radiation	31 (54)	9 (38)	0.17
Chemotherapy	3 (5)	8 (33)	0.003
HDCSR	2 (4)	5 (21)	0.02
Stage: L2	**44 (37)**	**12 (11)**	
Surgery	37 (81)	10 (83)	0.95
Radiation	32 (73)	5 (42)	0.05
Chemotherapy	21 (48)	8 (67)	0.25
HDCSR	1 (2)	1 (8)	0.35
Stage: M	**17 (14)**	**74 (67)**	
Surgery	12 (71)	58 (76)	0.62
Radiation	6 (35)	54 (71)	0.008
Chemotherapy	15 (88)	73 (96)	0.22
HDCSR	1 (7)	45 (61)	0.001

TABLE 3: First chemotherapy regimens employed in adult neuroblastoma.

First line chemotherapy regimen	N
Cisplatin and etoposide alternating cyclophosphamide/vincristine/carboplatin	15
Cisplatin and etoposide (+paclitaxel)	10 (+2)
Vincristine and cyclophosphamide + cisplatin/dacarbazine/adriamycin	6
Ifosfamide, carboplatin, and etoposide	3
Irinotecan and/or temozolomide	3
Ifosfamide, adriamycin, and vincristine	2

the combination of surgery and radiation demonstrated a trend ($P = 0.07$) toward improved PFS (median = 11.1 months), compared with surgery or radiation alone (median = 6.4), or local therapy with chemotherapy (median = 5.1) (Figure 2). Similarly, there was no statistical difference ($P = 0.11$) in overall survival amongst patients who received surgery or radiation (median = 9.5 years), surgery and radiotherapy (median = 18.6 years), or local therapy and chemotherapy (median = 9.3 years). For adult neuroblastoma patients with L2, local therapy with surgery and radiation resulted in a median PFS of 5.2 months. The addition of chemotherapy was not associated with an increased PFS (median = 4 months; $P = 0.23$) (Figure 3). As a result of the potential for successful salvage local therapy, the median OS for local therapy and local therapy with chemotherapy was 9.6 years and 8.5 years, respectively ($P = 0.24$).

Over the study period, 17 (14%) adult patients presented with untreated M-stage disease. Conversely, 74 (67%) of the pediatric patients presented to our center with high-risk M-stage disease. The most common chemotherapy regimens employed in this population were cisplatin and etoposide alternating with carboplatin, vincristine, and cyclophosphamide ($n = 5$, 29%); vincristine and cyclophosphamide alternating with cisplatin, doxorubicin, and dacarbazine ($n = 4$, 24%); cisplatin and etoposide only ($n = 3$, 18%); irinotecan ± temozolomide ($n = 2$, 12%). Only 1 adult M-stage patient was treated with HDCSR. Combining the entire cohort of M-stage adult ($n = 1$) and M-stage pediatric ($n = 45$) patients, patients treated with HDCSR ($n = 46$, 51%) achieved a median PFS of 1.47 years and a median OS of 2.25 years compared with a PFS of 1.48 years and an OS of 1.67 years for patients who did not undergo HDCSR ($P = 0.18$, $P = 0.38$, resp.) (Figure 4).

4. Discussion

Neuroblastoma may be rare in adults, but improving our empirical understanding of this disease will help guide future directions. To our knowledge, this is the largest cohorts of adult patients to be examined. Unfortunately, we were unable

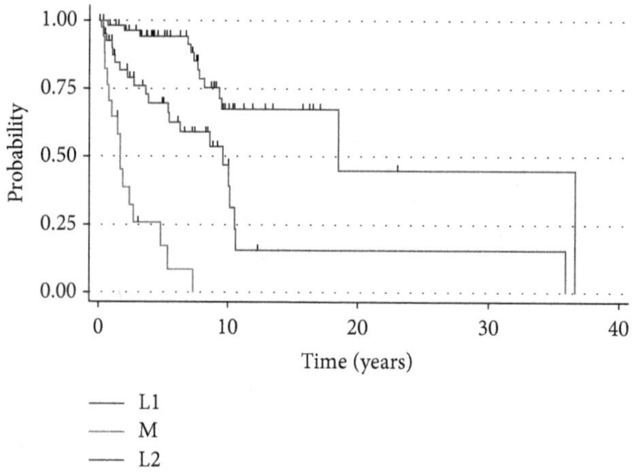

FIGURE 1: Overall survival of adult neuroblastoma patients by stage of disease. $P < 0.001$.

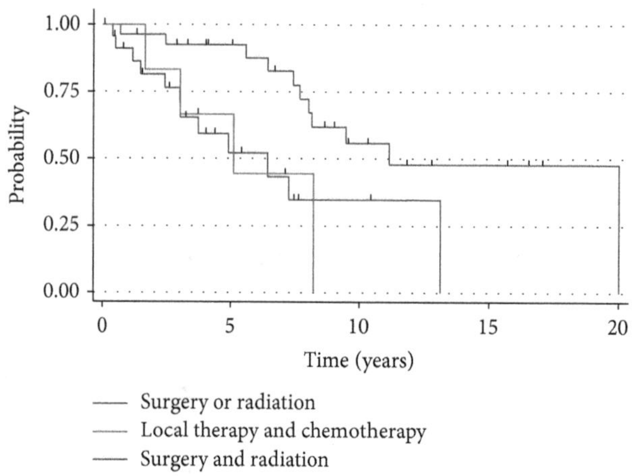

FIGURE 2: Progression-free survival for adults with L1 stage neuroblastoma. $P = 0.07$.

to properly risk-stratify early stage adult patients because of the absence of any molecular or genetic information and tissue for further analysis was not available, making comparison between patients 18 and over and under 18 years of age with L1 or L2 disease difficult. Moreover, the small number of early stage pediatric patients and similarly small number of late-stage adult patients further compromise accurate comparisons. Lastly, since we were unable to rereview all imaging with a dedicated radiologist, some early-stage patients may be misclassified despite best practice to minimize such an error.

For adult patients with L1 disease, combined surgical resection and radiotherapy seems likely to offer better PFS and OS than surgical resection alone, despite the likely scenario that patients who received combined local therapy would have more clinically concerning disease. Conversely, chemotherapy did not seem to offer any additional benefit. Similarly, almost all adult patients with L2 disease received combined surgical resection and radiotherapy, but chemotherapy was not associated with any improvement in outcomes.

Although previous studies have concluded that adult neuroblastoma has a poorer prognosis than its pediatric variant, we were unable to demonstrate a similar result. Although patients under the age of 18 years have been shown to have a better prognosis, we are unable to conclude that there is a difference in prognosis between patients younger than 18 and those 18 and older. Though, without complete staging, a conclusive result is hard to reach. We recommend that all patients of any age be risk-stratified according to the INRG risk assessment system to allow for proper determination of risk. At this time, we are unable to conclude that adult and pediatric patients have a clinically different clinical course, when stage-matched for stage, and so adult patients should be allowed entry onto protocols designed for neuroblastoma patients age > 18 months so that prospective data can be adequately and practically developed. Certainly when enrolling such patients, it would be reasonable to ensure that age is properly balanced between trial arms in the same way that patients older than 65 or 70 are managed in adult clinical trials. Subgroup analysis of such trials would allow for prospective data to be developed on whether there are real

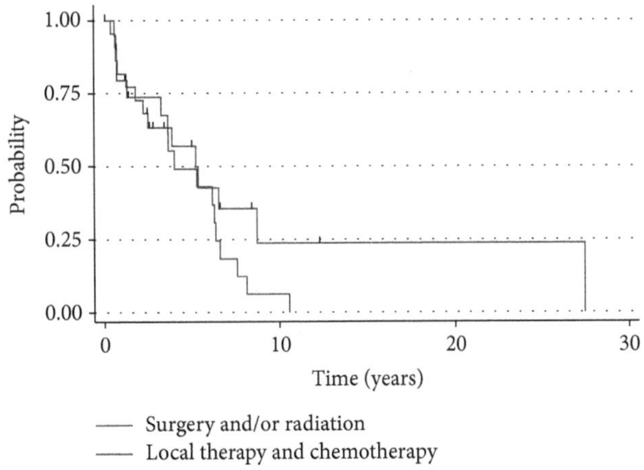

FIGURE 3: Progression-free survival for adults with L2 stage neuroblastoma. $P = 0.23$.

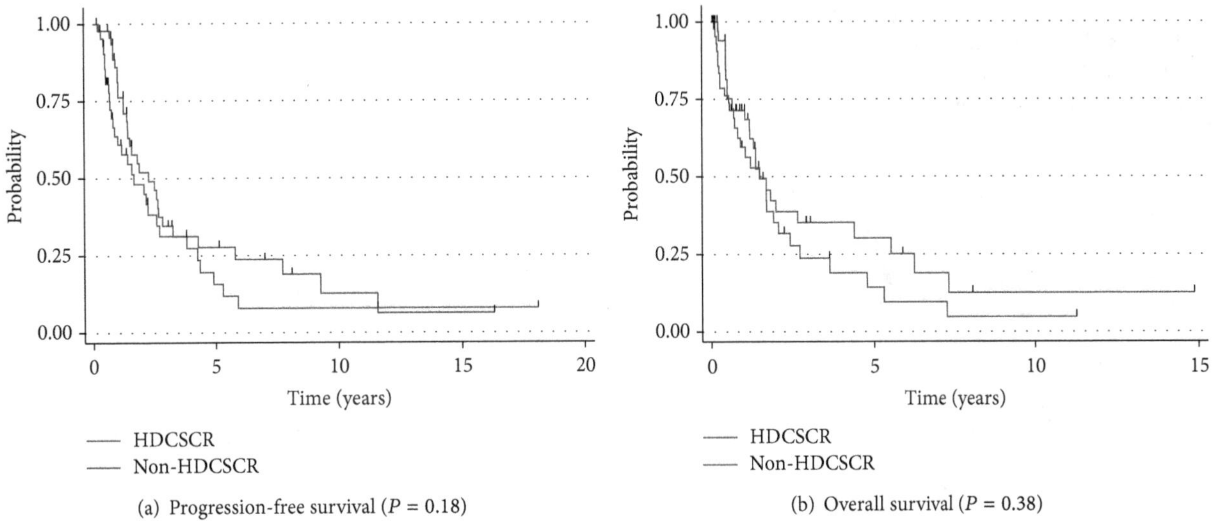

FIGURE 4: Survival of patients treated with HDCSR or non-HDCSR containing regimens.

differences between adult tumor biology and the host system and whether traditionally developed pediatric regimens are reasonable for use in adult patients.

The only difference that we can observe from our data set between adult and pediatric patients is the level of enthusiasm for HDCSR. In our whole cohort, we were unable to demonstrate any benefit from such aggressive therapy. High level evidence exists for its use in the pediatric population, but, without the achievement of complete remission of metastatic neuroblastoma, we would be less eager to recommend such therapy for adults.

In summary, adult and pediatric neuroblastoma may be clinically similar diseases and we should begin accumulating evidence as if this were so.

Conflict of Interests

The authors declare that there is no conflict of interests regarding the publication of this paper.

References

[1] G. M. Brodeur, "Neuroblastoma: biological insights into a clinical enigma," *Nature Reviews Cancer*, vol. 3, no. 3, pp. 203–216, 2003.

[2] R. Siegel, D. Naishadham, and A. Jemal, "Cancer statistics, 2012," *CA: A Cancer Journal for Clinicians*, vol. 62, no. 1, pp. 10–29, 2012.

[3] M. H. Hsieh, M. V. Meng, T. J. Walsh, K. K. Matthay, and L. S. Baskin, "Increasing incidence of neuroblastoma and potentially higher associated mortality of children from nonmetropolitan areas: analysis of the surveillance, epidemiology, and end results database," *Journal of Pediatric Hematology/Oncology*, vol. 31, no. 12, pp. 942–946, 2009.

[4] N. Esiashvili, M. Goodman, K. Ward, R. B. Marcus Jr., and P. A. Johnstone, "Neuroblastoma in adults: incidence and survival analysis based on SEER data," *Pediatric Blood and Cancer*, vol. 49, no. 1, pp. 41–46, 2007.

[5] T. Monclair, G. M. Brodeur, P. F. Ambros et al., "The international neuroblastoma risk group (INRG) staging system: an

INRG task force report," *Journal of Clinical Oncology*, vol. 27, no. 2, pp. 298–303, 2009.

[6] S. L. Cohn, A. D. Pearson, W. B. London et al., "The international neuroblastoma risk group (INRG) classification system: an INRG task force report," *Journal of Clinical Oncology*, vol. 27, no. 2, pp. 289–297, 2009.

[7] L. Venat-Bouvet, V. Le Brun-Ly, J. Martin, O. Gasnier, S. Falkowsky, and N. Tubiana-Mathieu, "Long-term survival in adult neuroblastoma with multiple recurrences," *Case Reports in Oncology*, vol. 3, no. 1, pp. 45–48, 2010.

[8] B. H. Kushner, K. Kramer, M. P. LaQuaglia, S. Modak, and N. V. Cheung, "Neuroblastoma in adolescents and adults: the memorial sloan-kettering experience," *Medical and Pediatric Oncology*, vol. 41, no. 6, pp. 508–515, 2003.

[9] L. M. Franks, A. Bollen, R. C. Seeger, D. O. Stram, and K. K. Matthay, "Neuroblastoma in adults and adolescents: an indolent course with poor survival," *Cancer*, vol. 79, no. 10, pp. 2028–2035, 1997.

[10] M. Conte, S. Parodi, B. de Bernardi et al., "Neuroblastoma in adolescents: the Italian experience," *Cancer*, vol. 106, no. 6, pp. 1409–1417, 2006.

[11] J. M. Maris, "Recent advances in neuroblastoma," *The New England Journal of Medicine*, vol. 362, no. 23, pp. 2202–2211, 2010.

[12] N. V. Cheung and G. Heller, "Chemotherapy dose intensity correlates strongly with response, median survival, and median progression-free survival in metastatic neuroblastoma," *Journal of Clinical Oncology*, vol. 9, no. 6, pp. 1050–1058, 1991.

[13] A. D. Pearson, C. R. Pinkerton, I. J. Lewis et al., "High-dose rapid and standard induction chemotherapy for patients aged over 1 year with stage 4 neuroblastoma: a randomised trial," *The Lancet Oncology*, vol. 9, no. 3, pp. 247–256, 2008.

[14] B. Yalcin, L. C. Kremer, H. N. Caron, and E. C. van Dalen, "High-dose chemotherapy and autologous haematopoietic stem cell rescue for children with high-risk neuroblastoma," *Cochrane Database of Systematic Reviews*, vol. 8, Article ID CD006301, 2013.

[15] D. A. Haas-Kogan, P. S. Swift, M. Selch et al., "Impact of radiotherapy for high-risk neuroblastoma: a children's cancer group study," *International Journal of Radiation Oncology, Biology Physics*, vol. 56, no. 1, pp. 28–39, 2003.

[16] J. R. Robbins, M. J. Krasin, A. S. Pai Panandiker et al., "Radiation therapy as part of local control of metastatic neuroblastoma: the St Jude children's research hospital experience," *Journal of Pediatric Surgery*, vol. 45, no. 4, pp. 678–686, 2010.

[17] B. Hero, T. Simon, R. Spitz et al., "Localized infant neuroblastomas often show spontaneous regression: results of the prospective trials NB95-S and NB97," *Journal of Clinical Oncology*, vol. 26, no. 9, pp. 1504–1510, 2008.

17

Can Experienced Observers Differentiate between Lipoma and Well-Differentiated Liposarcoma using Only MRI?

Patrick W. O'Donnell,[1] Anthony M. Griffin,[2] William C. Eward,[3] Amir Sternheim,[2] Lawrence M. White,[2] Jay S. Wunder,[2] and Peter C. Ferguson[2]

[1] *Department of Orthopaedic Surgery, Markey Cancer Center, University of Kentucky, 740 S. Limestone Avenue, Lexington, KY 40536, USA*
[2] *Department of Orthopaedic Surgery, Mount Sinai Hospital, Toronto, ON, Canada M5G 1X5*
[3] *Department of Orthopaedic Surgery, Duke Cancer Center, Duke University, Durham, NC 27710, USA*

Correspondence should be addressed to Patrick W. O'Donnell; patrick.odonnell@uky.edu

Academic Editor: Cyril Fisher

Well-differentiated liposarcoma represents a radiographic diagnostic dilemma. To determine the accuracy, interrater reliability, and relationship of stranding, nodularity, and size in the MRI differentiation of lipoma and well-differentiated liposarcoma, MRI scans of 60 patients with large (>5 cm), deep, pathologically proven lipomas or well-differentiated liposarcomas were examined by 10 observers with subspecialty training blinded to diagnosis. Observers indicated whether the amount of stranding, nodularity, and size of each tumor suggested a benign or malignant diagnosis and rendered a diagnosis of lipoma or well-differentiated liposarcoma. The accuracy, reliability, and relationship of stranding, nodularity, and size to diagnosis were calculated for all samples. 69% of reader MRI diagnoses agreed with final pathology diagnosis (95% CI 65–73%). Readers tended to err choosing a diagnosis of liposarcoma, correctly identifying lipomas in 63% of cases (95% CI 58–69%) and liposarcomas in 75% of cases (95% CI 69–80%). Assessment of the relationship of stranding, nodularity, and size to correct diagnosis showed that the presence of each was associated with a decreased likelihood of a lipoma pathological diagnosis ($P < 0.01$). While the radiographic diagnosis of lipoma or well-differentiated liposarcoma cannot be made with 100% certainty, experienced observers have a 69% chance of rendering a correct diagnosis.

1. Introduction

Well-differentiated liposarcoma presents a diagnostic dilemma to the treatment team due to the inaccuracy of biopsy and the difficulty in differentiating these low-grade tumors from benign lipomas on imaging alone [1–4]. This difficulty in diagnosis can lead to patient worry, delays in diagnosis, and a considerable risk for local recurrence with inappropriate surgical resection. As well-differentiated liposarcomas show low to no metastatic potential, with appropriate excision, low rates of recurrence can be expected [5–8].

MRI serves as an excellent modality to discern certain soft tissue tumors like lipomas given their specific imaging characteristics [1, 3]. Low-grade fatty tumors represent a radiographic spectrum from innocent appearing homogeneous lesions, isointense to subcutaneous adipose tissue on all sequences to the more ominous appearing lesions with heterogeneity (Figures 1 and 2). The ideal treatment situation for these low-grade fatty tumors would be one where the pathological diagnosis would correspond perfectly with the imaging characteristics. However, this pathological to radiological correlation does not occur in the majority of cases (Figures 1 and 2) [2, 5, 9]. As such, musculoskeletal radiologists and orthopaedic oncologists have evolved to include well-differentiated liposarcoma on the radiographic differential of suspicious fatty lesions.

Several authors have evaluated the sensitivity and specificity of specific MRI sequences in the diagnosis of well-differentiate liposarcoma; however, the diagnostic reliability between specialties (musculoskeletal radiology and orthopaedic oncology) has not been well characterized [1–4, 10]. In addition, specific variables that may portend an elevated likelihood of well-differentiated liposarcoma (stranding, nodularity, and size) have been discussed in the literature extensively, without agreement among the experts [1–4, 10].

The purpose of this study was therefore to evaluate the accuracy, reliability, and association between the variables of size, stranding, and nodularity in the diagnosis of lipoma versus well-differentiated liposarcoma based on MRI imaging alone. In addition, the accuracy and reliability of trained musculoskeletal radiologists and orthopaedic oncologists in the radiographic diagnosis of these tumors were assessed to see if any differences existed between specialties. Our hypothesis was that experienced readers in both specialties blinded to diagnosis would be unable to differentiate between a series of fatty lesions and that the variables of size, nodularity, and stranding would show no predictive association with these diagnoses. If true, this study would support the argument to treat all low-grade fatty lesions with marginal excision regardless of the MRI interpretation or concern regarding variables of size, nodularity, or stranding.

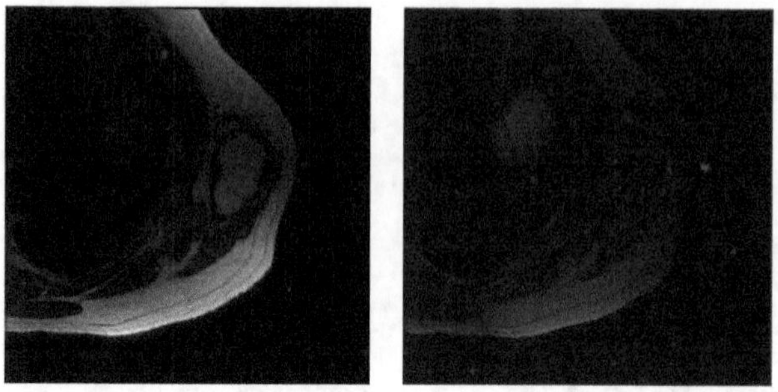

Figure 1: Axial T1 and T2 MRIs of a patient with a fatty tumor. Despite the benign appearance of this tumor radiographically, final pathological review confirmed a diagnosis of low-grade liposarcoma.

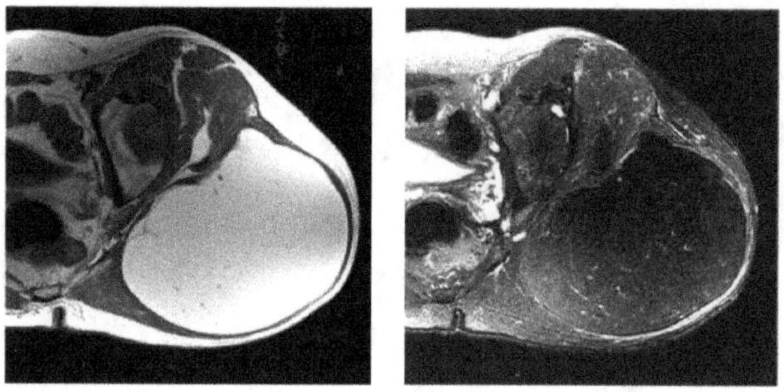

Figure 2: Axial T1 and T2 MRIs of a patient with a large fatty tumor in the buttock. Despite the large size and intratumoral stranding/nodularity, final pathological review confirmed a diagnosis of lipoma.

2. Materials and Methods

After research ethics board approval, MRI scans of 60 patients with large (>5 cm in greatest dimension), deep, pathologically proven lipomas (31 patients) or well-differentiated liposarcomas (29 patients) were identified from a prospectively collected database. Pathological review and diagnosis were made by one of three pathologists with subspeciality training in musculoskeletal oncology and sarcoma pathology following WHO criteria for the classification of sarcoma. Informed consent was obtained from all research subjects as a part of their enrolment into this database. Patient MRI scans were retrospectively examined by 10 observers with subspecialty training in musculoskeletal radiology or orthopaedic oncology, blinded to diagnosis. There were 2 attending staff physicians and 3 fellows from each orthopaedic oncology and musculoskeletal radiology who participated.

After reviewing each patient MRI on a PACS viewing module, observers indicated whether the amount of stranding, nodularity, and size of each tumor was concerning for well-differentiated liposarcoma and rendered a diagnosis of lipoma or well-differentiated liposarcoma. To simulate a clinical scenario, each reader was given the ability to use whatever image sequences available for diagnostic purposes (see later). Stranding (Figure 3) was defined as linear tissue heterogeneity present within the mass, and nodularity (Figure 4) was defined as intralesional tissue heterogeneity that was not linear. The concerning size variable was left to the individual readers discretion for interpretation; however, all tumors were greater than 5 cm in greatest dimension as mentioned above. All variables were categorical and recorded as either "yes" or "no" for the measurements of concerning size, nodularity, and stranding and whether the reader was concerned about a diagnosis of well-differentiated liposarcoma, based on these individual variables. For example, while all lesions were >5 cm, each reader had to independently determine whether the size of the lesion, amount of stranding, or nodularity were concerning for a liposarcoma diagnosis. Diagnosis categorical variables of "lipoma" or "well-differentiated liposarcoma" were also recorded for each tumor.

As the variables of size, stranding, and nodularity are used clinically by radiologists without standardization criteria to interpret such images and render a diagnosis, these variables were intentionally not standardized for individual readers for the purpose of this study. This was done to simulate a clinical scenario and therefore better evaluate the ability of readers to render a correct diagnosis and to determine the reliability and validity of reader diagnoses towards these tumors.

All imaging was performed with 1.5-T MRI system (Signa, GE Medical System, Milwaukee, WI) using a surface coil or body coil depending on the anatomic location. Specific imaging protocols included at least two planes of T1-weighted images (TR 500 ms/TE 10 ms) and fast spin echo T2-weighted images (TR 4800 ms/TE 100 ms) with selective fat saturation. STIR sequences (inversion time 110–150 msec) were also occasionally available. In all of the cases reviewed, either T2W fast spin echo imaging with spectral fat suppression or STIR imaging was performed. Imaging sequences used by readers of this study for diagnostic purposes were performed without contrast agents.

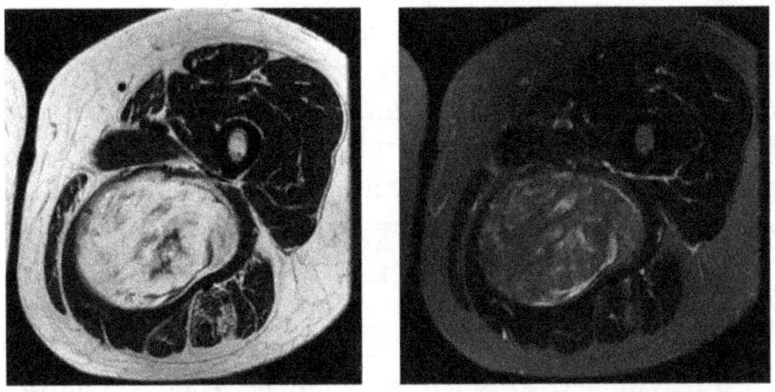

FIGURE 3: Axial T1 and T2 MRIs showing intralesional stranding in a fatty tumor. Final pathological review confirmed a diagnosis of low-grade liposarcoma.

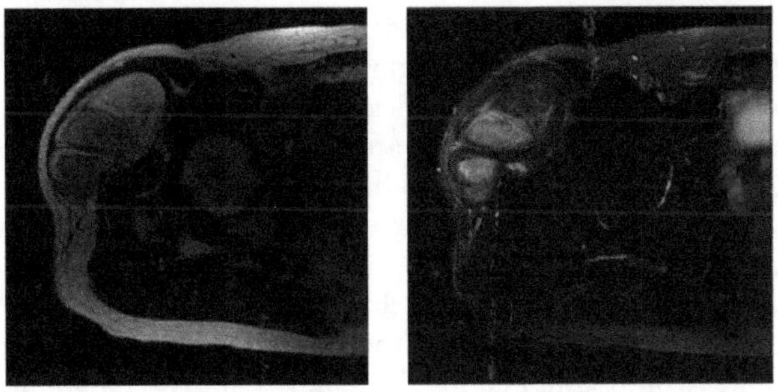

FIGURE 4: Axial T1 and T2 MRIs showing intralesional nodularity in a fatty tumor. Final pathological review confirmed a diagnosis of low-grade liposarcoma.

Kappa statistics along with 95% confidence limits were used to determine the reliability of each categorical measurement [11]. The interobserver reliability was evaluated by determining the agreement among the observers. P values for comparison to "no agreement" were generated from an exact test [12]. All P values were two-sided and any P-values less than 0.05 were considered statistically significant. Sixty MRI studies resulted in 95% power of 0.8 based on a type I error of 5%. Data analysis was performed using SAS version 9.2 computer software.

3. Results

3.1. Accuracy. 413/600 (69%) reader diagnoses agreed with the final pathological diagnosis. The 95% confidence limits for the accuracy percentage were (65%–73%). If the pathology diagnosis was lipoma, readers correctly identified lipoma in 196/310 (63%) cases (95% CI 58%-69%). If the pathology diagnosis was well-differentiated liposarcoma, readers correctly identified liposarcoma in 217/290 (75%) cases (95% CI 69%-80%). All readers chose liposarcoma more frequently than lipoma. There was no difference regarding diagnostic accuracy when compared between the specialties of orthopaedic oncology and musculoskeletal radiology (average 68%, 95% CI 63%–74% versus 69%, 95% CI 64%–75%, resp.). Attending physicians had a slightly high rate of diagnostic accuracy when compared to fellows (average 71%, 95% CI 70%–72% versus 67%, 95% CI 61%–73%, resp.).

TABLE 1: The interrater reliability for diagnosis and each of the categorical variables of stranding, nodularity, and size.

Measure	Kappa estimate	95% CI	Raw proportion of matching responses
Diagnosis	0.63	(0.61, 0.65)	0.82
Stranding	0.17	(0.14, 0.19)	0.76
Nodularity	0.41	(0.39, 0.43)	0.72
Size	0.11	(0.09, 0.13)	0.68

TABLE 2: The relationships of stranding and nodularity to the diagnosis of liposarcoma.

Stranding	Nodularity	% Reader liposarcoma	% True liposarcoma
Yes	Yes	217/228 (95%)	145/228 (64%)
Yes	No	95/268 (35%)	108/268 (40%)
No	Yes	6/11 (55%)	5/11 (45%)
No	No	13/93 (14%)	32/93 (34%)

TABLE 3: The relationship of concerning size to the diagnosis of liposarcoma.

Size	% Reader liposarcoma	% True liposarcoma
Yes	103/138 (75%)	83/138 (60%)
No	228/462 (49%)	207/462 (45%)

3.2. Reliability. Table 1 shows the interrater reliability for diagnosis and each of the categorical variables of stranding, nodularity, and size. Interrater reliability for diagnosis showed "substantial" agreement with a kappa estimate of 0.63 (95% CI 0.61–0.65). Interrater reliability showed only "slight" agreement for stranding and size but "moderate" agreement for nodularity (kappa estimates 0.17, 0.11, and 0.41; (95% CI 0.14–0.19, 0.09–0.13, 0.39–0.43, resp.).

3.3. Relationship of Stranding, Nodularity, and Size to Diagnosis. Tables 2 and 3 show the relationships of stranding, nodularity, and size to the diagnosis of liposarcoma. Positive reader responses for stranding and nodularity were associated with an increased likelihood of liposarcoma diagnosis ($P < 0.01$). Although this combination had a higher probability of a true liposarcoma diagnosis, readers overdiagnosed liposarcoma by a large margin in this instance. The inverse is true if readers choose "no" for both stranding and nodularity, which was associated with a lipoma diagnosis. A positive response for size was also associated with increased likelihood of a liposarcoma diagnosis ($P < 0.01$), although the misdiagnosis gap was not as large as for stranding/nodularity, as readers were overall more likely to choose a diagnosis of liposarcoma. There was no difference regarding interpretation of these categorical variables or their relationship towards the ultimate diagnosis when compared between specialties.

4. Discussion

Well-differentiated liposarcomas are low-grade fatty tumors with negligible metastatic potential and less than 10% chance of local recurrence even after positive margin excision [7, 8, 13]. Well-differentiated liposarcomas do however represent a diagnostic dilemma given the difficulty discerning well-differentiated liposarcoma from lipoma on imaging and problems associated with sampling error during biopsy [2]. Due to poor understanding of the biology of well-differentiated liposarcomas or radiologic phrases like "liposarcoma cannot be ruled out, referral to orthopaedic oncologist is recommended," these tumors are the cause of unnecessary referral to tertiary sarcoma centers and more importantly patient worry. As such, a standardized approach to the radiographic evaluation and treatment of these lesions would be beneficial to both patients and the physicians who care for them.

The goal of this study was to determine whether experienced observers in musculoskeletal radiology and orthopaedic oncology could differentiate between lipomas and well-differentiated liposarcomas on imaging alone and to determine the relative association of variables such as stranding, nodularity, and size to this diagnosis. Our hypothesis was that even experienced observers would be unable to differentiate between lipomas and well-differentiated liposarcomas. Therefore, if treating physicians were unable to accurately diagnose these tumors on imaging or via biopsy, an argument suggesting that all symptomatic low-grade fatty lesions may be treated with marginal excision could be supported. While the results presented here are better than chance alone, they do reaffirm that a definitive diagnosis cannot be made on imaging alone until better imaging criteria are identified.

We also present data here that supports several other variables surrounding the radiographic diagnosis of low-grade fatty lesions. First, there is a substantial interrater reliability based on kappa statistics towards making the radiographic diagnosis. These data are based on a high number of readers and the categorical variables of "lipoma" versus "liposarcoma." In addition, the relative accuracy of observers from musculoskeletal radiology and orthopaedic oncology with various levels of training (fellow versus staff) was not statistically different. Finally, the variables of size, nodularity, and stranding did show an association with the diagnosis of well-differentiated liposarcoma and as such based on these data should continue to be used in the radiographic interpretation of these tumors.

Other authors have evaluated the utility of MRI in the differentiation of well-differentiated liposarcoma from lipoma and determined the value of fluid-sensitive imaging sequences in making this distinction [2, 3, 10]. Doyle et al. evaluated the observer performance using T1-weighted spin echo and fluid-sensitive MRI sequences [1]. They found sensitivity over 94% for T1-weighted images and 100% for fluid-sensitive sequences. Specificities however for these same imaging sequences were 76% and 64% for the T1-weighted sequences and 70% and 73% for the fluid-sensitive images. The interobserver agreement was rated as "good" based on kappa statistics. This study however only had two observers, both radiologists, and a small representative number of well-differentiated liposarcomas in the study design (18 of 51 tumors). In addition, these authors attempted to correlate the radiographic findings with pathological variables like fibrosis, stranding, and nodularity; however, they were unable to make associations between these pathological variables and the observed radiographic parameters. As such, Doyle et al. question the diagnostic importance of nodularity, stranding, and size in the differentiation of lipomas from well-differentiated liposarcomas on imaging alone. Our data however suggests that the variables of nodularity, stranding, and size do show association with the correct radiographic diagnosis and therefore should continue to be used despite the poor correlation to pathological variables. One key point in the differentiation between the presented data and that of Doyle et al. is that the histological variable of fibrosis may not correlate with the radiographic viable of stranding. As those authors did not specifically map this fibrosis within the pathological specimen to areas specified on the MRI, we question the validity of the author's conclusions.

The accuracy of diagnosis presented here (69%) is lower than that documented in previous reports [1–3]. In one such report, Gaskin and Helms retrospectively reviewed 126 lesions and determined the sensitivity, specificity, and accuracy of MRI in making the distinction between lipoma, lipoma variants, and well-differentiated liposarcoma [10]. They reported an overall accuracy in their study of 83%; however, there are several differences between that study and data presented here. Gaskin and Helms selected cases through a radiological database search by identification of key phrases (such as "lipo-" or "fat") in the radiological report. Only after selection of 126 cases which other radiologists had been confident enough to use such terms were the pathological diagnoses reviewed. This method of case inclusion represents a selection bias given the prior documentation by reading radiologists of the terms "lipo-" or "fat." Lesions with concerning heterogeneity, nodularity, or stranding in which the MRI evaluation suggested a more aggressive diagnosis than a lipomatous or fatty tumor would be excluded using this method of selection. Given the heterogeneity of fatty tumors and the fact that the pathological diagnosis is the most valid, our presented accuracy may be appropriate. The second difference between the study by Gaskin and Helms was that only 64 of 126 tumors were resected at their tertiary institution and available for review by their trained musculoskeletal pathologist. Again, given the heterogeneity within the diagnosis of well-differentiated liposarcoma and the specific diagnostic criteria surrounding this diagnosis, the presented radiological accuracy in that study may not be truly representative of all low-grade fatty lesions [9].

Data presented here suggests that the variables of size, nodularity, and stranding show an association with the ultimate pathological diagnosis and as such should continue to be used in the radiographic interpretation [2]. It has been our experience that size is the variable most often used by referral centers or radiologists to suggest a diagnosis of well-differentiated liposarcoma but the variable least used by our treatment team in making the ultimate decision a MRI diagnosis. Obviously size does matter given the association between concerning size and the pathological diagnosis of well-differentiated liposarcoma [2]. While the association of size to the diagnosis of well-differentiated liposarcoma was not as strong as the variables of stranding and nodularity (Figures 3 and 4), all these represent variables that need to be considered when rendering an ultimate radiographic impression.

Recently, the identification and gene amplification of the MDM2 gene have been identified to supplement the pathological diagnosis of liposarcoma [14, 15]. Unfortunately, the majority of the patients utilized in this study did not have MDM2 FISH for the pathological diagnosis. For the majority of patients in this study, the pathological analysis and diagnosis were made without usage of MDM2 gene amplification. This represents a limitation to this study. For this study, pathological review and diagnosis were made by one of three pathologists with subspeciality training in musculoskeletal oncology and sarcoma pathology following WHO criteria for the classification of sarcoma.

At tertiary referral sarcoma centers, where the treatment team understands the low metastatic potential of these lesions and the appropriateness of a marginal excision, the inability to differentiate these lesions on MRI alone does not represent a major treatment dilemma, as symptomatic tumors require marginal excision without adjuvant treatment [5, 6, 16]. On the contrary, at smaller centers with less experience in musculoskeletal oncology or the specific biology of well-differentiated liposarcoma, statements such as "liposarcoma cannot be excluded," or "referral to sarcoma center is necessary," are all too common. Phrases such as these lead to patient worry and unnecessary referral. It has been proposed to characterize all such lesions as "low-grade fatty tumors" which at worst represent well-differentiated liposarcomas. Then, with an understanding of the low metastatic risk and appropriate management of these tumors, treating physicians could more appropriately counsel patients and avoid unnecessary referral.

5. Conclusion

Experienced observers in musculoskeletal radiology and orthopaedic oncology can differentiate between lipomas and well-differentiated liposarcomas in 69% of cases. This level of accuracy needs to be improved upon with accepted and validated mechanisms to differentiate between these two entities. The variables of nodularity, stranding, and relative size do show an association with the diagnosis of well-differentiated liposarcoma and therefore should continue to be used in the radiographic impression. A better understanding of the biology of well-differentiated liposarcomas, appropriate treatment, and risk of local recurrence/overall survival related to this diagnosis is important to appropriately counsel patients and avoid unnecessary referral.

Acknowledgments

The authors would like to thank the participant readers involved in data collection for this study: Drs. Mia Mattar, Grainne Murphy, Roger Chou, and Ali Naraghi. This study could not have been conducted without their involvement.

References

[1] A. J. Doyle, A. K. Pang, M. V. Miller, and J. G. French, "Magnetic resonance imaging of lipoma and atypical lipomatous tumour/well-differentiated liposarcoma: observer performance using T1-weighted and fluid-sensitive MRI," *Journal of Medical Imaging and Radiation Oncology*, vol. 52, no. 1, pp. 44–48, 2008.

[2] F. El Ouni, H. Jemni, A. Trabelsi et al., "Liposarcoma of the extremities: MR imaging features and their correlation with pathologic data," *Orthopaedics & Traumatology, Surgery & Research*, vol. 96, no. 8, pp. 876–883, 2010.

[3] Y. M. Lee, H. W. Chung, M. J. Shin et al., "Musculoskeletal magnetic resonance imaging suggesting the possibility of liposarcoma: correlation between radiologists' certainty of diagnosis and pathology results," *Journal of Computer Assisted Tomography*, vol. 35, no. 4, pp. 512–516, 2011.

[4] K. N. O'Regan, J. Jagannathan, K. Krajewski et al., "Imaging of liposarcoma: classification, patterns of tumor recurrence, and response to treatment," *American Journal of Roentgenology*, vol. 197, no. 1, pp. W37–W43, 2011.

[5] V. Billing, F. Mertens, H. A. Domanski, and A. Rydholm, "Deep-seated ordinary and atypical lipomas : histopathology, cytogenetics, clinical features, and outcome in 215 tumours of the extremity and trunk wall," *Journal of Bone and Joint Surgery B*, vol. 90, no. 7, pp. 929–933, 2008.

[6] H. S. Kim, J. Lee, S. Y. Yi et al., "Liposarcoma: exploration of clinical prognostic factors for risk based stratification of therapy," *BMC Cancer*, vol. 9, article 205, 2009.

[7] T. D. Rozental, L. D. Khoury, R. Donthineni-Rao, and R. D. Lackman, "Atypical lipomatous masses of the extremities: outcome of surgical treatment," *Clinical Orthopaedics and Related Research*, no. 398, pp. 203–211, 2002.

[8] C. A. Smith, S. R. Martinez, W. H. Tseng et al., "Predicting survival for well-differentiated liposarcoma: the importance of tumor location," *Journal of Surgical Research*, vol. 175, no. 1, pp. 12–17, 2012.

[9] A. P. Dei Tos, "Liposarcoma: new entities and evolving concepts," *Annals of Diagnostic Pathology*, vol. 4, no. 4, pp. 252–266, 2000.

[10] C. M. Gaskin and C. A. Helms, "Lipomas, lipoma variants, and well-differentiated liposarcomas (atypical lipomas): results of MRI evaluations of 126 consecutive fatty masses," *American Journal of Roentgenology*, vol. 182, no. 3, pp. 733–739, 2004.

[11] J. Cohen, "A coefficient of agreement for nominal scales," *Educational and Psychological Measurement*, vol. 20, pp. 37–46, 1960.

[12] D. J. Solomon, "The rating reliability calculator," *BMC Medical Research Methodology*, vol. 4, article 11, 2004.

[13] C. H. Gerrand, J. S. Wunder, R. A. Kandel et al., "Classification of positive margins after resection of soft-tissue sarcoma of the limb predicts the risk of local recurrence," *Journal of Bone and Joint Surgery B*, vol. 83, no. 8, pp. 1149–1155, 2001.

[14] M. Brisson, T. Kashima, D. Delaney et al., "MRI characteristics of lipoma and atypical lipomatous tumor/well-differentiated

liposarcoma: retrospective comparison with histology and MDM2 gene amplification," *Skeletal Radiology*, vol. 42, no. 5, pp. 635–647, 2013.

[15] K. Thway, R. Flora, C. Shah, D. Olmos, and C. Fisher, "Diagnostic utility of p16, CDK4, and MDM2 as an immunohistochemical panel in distinguishing well-differentiated and dedifferentiated liposarcomas from other adipocytic tumors," *American Journal of Surgical Pathology*, vol. 36, no. 3, pp. 462–469, 2012.

[16] R. Grimer, I. Judson, D. Peake, and B. Seddon, "Guidelines for the management of soft tissue sarcomas," *Sarcoma*, vol. 2010, Article ID 506182, 15 pages, 2010.

18

Cross-Cultural Adaptation, Translation, and Validation of the Toronto Extremity Salvage Score for Extremity Bone and Soft Tissue Tumor Patients in Netherlands

Julie J. Willeumier, C. W. P. G. van der Wal, Robert J. P. van der Wal, P. D. S. Dijkstra, Thea P. M. Vliet Vlieland, and Michiel A. J. van de Sande

Department of Orthopaedic Surgery, Leiden University Medical Center, Leiden, Netherlands

Correspondence should be addressed to Julie J. Willeumier; j.j.willeumier@lumc.nl

Academic Editor: Akira Kawai

Purpose. The aim of this study was to translate and culturally adapt the Toronto Extremity Salvage Score (TESS) to Dutch and to validate the translated version. *Methods.* The TESS lower and upper extremity versions (LE and UE) were translated to Dutch according to international guidelines. The translated version was validated in 98 patients with surgically treated bone or soft tissue tumors of the LE or UE. To assess test-retest reliability, participants were asked to fill in a second questionnaire after one week. Construct validity was determined by computing Spearman rank correlations with the Short Form- (SF-) 36. *Results.* The internal consistency (0.957 and 0.938 for LE and UE, resp.) and test-retest reliability (intraclass correlation coefficients 0.963 and 0.969 for LE and UE, resp.) were good for both questionnaires. The Dutch LE and UE TESS versions correlated most strongly with the SF-36 physical function dimension (r = 0.737 for LE, 0.726 for UE) and the physical component summary score (r = 0.811 and 0.797 for LE and UE). *Interpretation.* The Dutch TESS questionnaire for lower and upper extremities is a consistent, reliable, and valid instrument to measure patient-reported physical function in surgically treated patients with a soft tissue or bone tumor.

1. Introduction

The preferred treatment of bone and soft tissue tumors of the extremities is limb-sparing surgery. Measuring physical function after surgery is of the utmost importance to determine the success of treatment and to improve patient care. Patient-reported outcome measures enable the surgeon and the patient to objectively evaluate the patient's pain and function in order to optimize clinical care.

The Toronto Extremity Salvage Score (TESS) [1] is a valid and reliable disease-specific measure developed to evaluate physical disability in patients treated for extremity sarcoma. Different questionnaires are available for the upper and lower extremities. The TESS was originally developed in English and has currently been translated and validated in five other languages (Japanese [2, 3], Korean [4], Chinese [5], Danish [6], and Portuguese [7]).

While the TESS is commonly used in the Netherlands, it has not been translated or validated for use in the Dutch language using standardized and methodologically sound procedures. The current study aims to translate and culturally adapt the TESS (for upper and lower extremities) to Dutch and to validate the translated version among patients with surgically treated bone or soft tissue tumors of the extremities.

2. Methods

This research was reviewed and approved by the Medical Ethical Committee of the Leiden University Medical Center. A waiver for informed consent was provided based on the law for medical research on humans in the Netherlands (April 2016; P16.060).

2.1. Translation and Cross-Cultural Adaptation. The methodology used for translation and adaptation concerns a well-established process, based on published guidelines for the cross-cultural adaptation of self-reported measures by Beaton et al. [8] and Guillemin et al. [9]. During the course of translation, adaptation, and validation the TESS questionnaires for the lower extremity (LE) and upper extremity (UE) were handled separately. Forward translation from the English TESS into Dutch was performed by three bilingual translators, with Dutch as mother tongue (JJW, CWPGvdW, and JB). One of these translators (JB) was unaware of the concepts addressed and without a medical background. This led to a first Dutch consensus version. Two independent, bilingual translators with English as mother tongue and without medical background subsequently translated the Dutch version back to English (MH, TT). The expert committee, compromising a methodologist (TVV), the principal investigator (MAJvdS), and four translators (JJW, CWPGvdW, JB, and TT) reviewed all versions and components of the original questionnaire and the translations to reach consensus on the final wording to be used in the Dutch version of the TESS.

2.2. Patients. Consecutive eligible patients who visited the outpatient clinic between July and September 2016 (regarding LE) or February 2017 (regarding UE) for follow-up of previous surgery for bone or soft tissue tumors of the extremities were invited to complete the translated and adapted TESS. Eligible patients were identified by checking the electronic medical records of patients scheduled for follow-up. Inclusion criteria were (i) being 18 or older, (ii) a minimum of 3 months since surgical treatment for an aggressive benign or malignant bone tumor or soft tissue sarcoma, and (iii) no sign of local or systemic recurrent disease. Patients with whom communication was impaired or who could not complete questionnaires unaided were not asked to complete the questionnaires. Baseline characteristics of the participating patients, including age, gender, primary tumor, location of primary tumor, and time since primary surgery were collected.

2.3. Instruments. The TESS is a self-administered questionnaire that includes 30 items regarding activity limitations in daily life, such as restrictions in body movement, mobility, self-care, and performance of daily tasks and routine. The degree of physical disability is rated from 0 (not possible) to 5 (without any problem). The raw score is converted to a score ranging from 0 to 100 points, with higher scores indicating less functional limitations. Patients are able to answer questions concerning activities they do not perform in daily life with "not applicable." These questions are deducted from the calculation of the total score.

The SF-36 is a widely used questionnaire to survey health-related quality of life [10]. The SF-36 has been validated for the Dutch population [11] and is administered as part of standard-care protocol in our hospital. The questionnaire measures eight dimensions of health and reports a score (from 0 (worst) to 100 (best)) for each category [10]. The scores from the eight categories can also be grouped into two summary scores: the physical and mental component summary scores (PCS and MCS). These summary scores were standardized using normative data from the Dutch general population with a mean score of 50 and standard deviation of 10 [11]. The scores give an indication of the functioning of the patient population in comparison with the general population.

2.4. Assessments. Eligible patients were invited to participate in the study by a research assistant when presenting at the outpatient clinic. The questionnaires were provided on paper. The first questionnaire was to be completed while waiting for the outpatient appointment. The second questionnaire (with a stamped return envelope) was handed out at the outpatient clinic together with the first questionnaire and patients were asked to complete the questionnaire one week later at home and send return by post. The questionnaires were paired by a code, to enable test-retest analysis.

Once patients agreed to participate in the study and their name was recorded. Patient identifying information was however not coupled to the questionnaire number, thus ensuring anonymity of the questionnaire.

2.5. Analyses. Prior to analysis, patients who answered 80% or more of the questions of the first TESS questionnaire with "not applicable" were excluded. For calculation of mean scores and analyses of difficult or "not applicable" questions, the first completed questionnaire of each patient was used.

2.6. Reliability. Internal consistency measures the homogeneity of all parts of the instrument, and was evaluated by means of calculation of Cronbach's alpha [12]. Cronbach's alpha provides a measurement of the strength of the relationship among the items of the questionnaire, with a value of >0.80 generally being considered as acceptable for scaling of the measure [13]. Test-retest variability concerns the ability of an instrument to create reproducible results when no real change has occurred for a subject. For this purpose, the intraclass correlation coefficient (ICC) was estimated between the responses to the first (test) and the second (retest) questionnaire for each item and for the total score. Bland-Altman plots were computed to visualize the absolute differences between the two assessments against the mean of the two tests to show the limits of agreement [14].

2.7. Validity. Construct validity measures the extent to which the scores of an instrument relate to other widely accepted measures of the same construct. For this study, construct validity of the TESS was determined by calculating the Spearman rank correlation coefficient between the TESS and the SF-36 dimension and summary scale scores.

All statistical analyses were performed with IBM SPSS version 23.0 (Armonk, NY, USA). The strength of agreement for the correlation coefficients and the ICC was defined as strong (≥0.70), moderate (>0.50 to <0.70), and weak (≤0.50) [15]. A p value of <0.05 was considered statistically significant.

3. Results

3.1. Translation Process. The translators and expert committee encountered no major linguistic or cross-cultural challenges during the translation and cross-cultural adaptation phase of the TESS-LE and TESS-UE questionnaires. The translation and adaptation process finally resulted in a Dutch

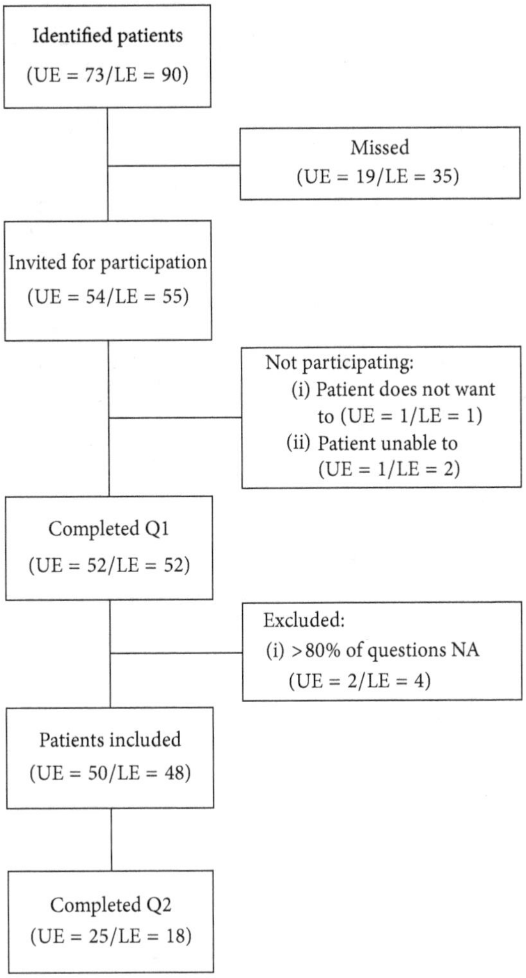

Figure 1: Flowchart of participating patients.

Table 1: Patient and tumor characteristics of patients with benign and malignant bone and soft tissue tumors who completed the TESS questionnaire.

	TESS LE	TESS UE
N	50	48
Age: mean (range)	48.9 (18.6–74.9)	48.5 (18.1–83.8)
Gender: % male	47	52
Time since surgery in years: mean (range)	3.5 (0.03–18.8)	3.0 (0.03–17.8)
Location n (%)		
Shoulder	0	1 (2)
Humerus	0	21 (44)
Upper arm (soft tissue)	0	6 (13)
Radius	0	2 (4)
Metacarpals	0	9 (19)
Digits	0	7 (15)
Femur	22 (44)	0
Upper leg (soft tissue)	1 (2)	0
Knee	2 (4)	0
Tibia	12 (24)	0
Fibula	1 (2)	0
Lower leg (soft tissue)	3 (6)	0
Foot	2 (4)	0
Missing data[a]	7 (14)	2 (4)
Primary tumor n (%)		
Atypical cartilaginous tumor	10 (20)	22 (46)
Chondrosarcoma grade 2/3	5 (10)	4 (8)
Osteosarcoma	6 (12)	3 (6)
Soft tissue sarcoma	4 (8)	5 (10)
(Tenosynovial) Giant cell tumor	6 (12)	2 (4)
Osteochondroma	2 (4)	0
Fibromatosis	1 (2)	1 (2)
Cartilaginous tumour, benign	2 (2)	2 (4)
Bone other, malignant	2 (4)	1 (2)
Soft tissue other, benign	2 (4)	3 (6)
Bone other, benign	3 (6)	3 (6)
Missing data[a]	7 (14)	2 (4)

[a]Baseline characteristics were unavailable for 11 patients (7 LE and 2 UE) because they had not been recorded correctly.

3.2. Patients. Ninety-eight patients (49% male) with a mean age of 48.7 years (range 18.1–83.8) were included (Figure 1). The characteristics of the patients and their TESS and SF-36 scores are presented in Tables 1 and 2.

3.3. Dutch TESS-LE and UE Questionnaire Results. Overall, the mean score of the TESS questionnaire was 77.5 (standard deviation (SD) 19.8) for the lower extremities and 90.2 (SD 14.9) for the upper extremities (Table 2). Getting up from kneeling was regarded the most difficult of all activities (mean score 3.21) in the LE questionnaire. Lifting a box to an overhead shelf was regarded the most difficult of all activities (mean score 3.94) in the UE questionnaire. Five patients (10.0%) scored a maximum score (100) on the TESS-LE, versus 19 patients (39.6%) on the TESS-UE. On the TESS-LE patients answered a median of 1 question with "not applicable" (range 0–17 questions). The questions concerning getting in and out of bath (n = 11, 22%), driving a car (n = 9, 18%), and sexual activities (n = 9, 18%) were most frequently answered as "not applicable." Regarding the TESS-UE, the median number of questions answered with with "not applicable" was 0 (range 0–7 questions). The most common "not applicable" UE-activities were those about working the usual number of hours (n = 5, 10%) and tying a tie or bow at the neck of a blouse (n = 5, 10%).

3.4. Reliability. The internal consistency was good with Cronbach's alpha of R = 0.957 for the TESS-LE and R = 0.938 for the TESS-UE. The Spearman rank correlation coefficients

Table 2: Mean and median scores of TESS and SF-36 for the lower and upper extremities.

	Lower extremity		Upper extremity	
	Mean (SD)	Median (range)	Mean (SD)	Median (range)
TESS	77.5 (19.8)	80.2 (13.3–100)	90.2 (14.9)	96.3 (21.6–100)
SF-36				
Physical functioning	60.5 (26.2)	65.0 (10.0–100.0)	80.4 (22.4)	85.0 (10.0–100.0)
Role limitations: physical	47.5 (43.2)	25.0 (0.0–100.0)	62.0 (42.5)	75.0 (0.0–100.0)
Social functioning	72.8 (25.3)	75.0 (0.0–100.0)	82.8 (22.6)	87.5 (12.5–100.0)
Role limitations: emotional	82.7 (33.8)	100.0 (0.0–100.0)	80.6 (36.2)	100.0 (0.0–100.0)
Mental health	72.9 (19.8)	80.0 (28.0–96.0)	78.2 (18.1)	80.0 (36.0–100.0)
Vitality	61.5 (22.6)	65.0 (15.0–100.0)	62.5 (22.3)	70.0 (15.0–100.0)
Bodily pain	62.1 (27.3)	57.1 (0.0–100.0)	72.9 (26.2)	73.5 (0.0–100.0)
General health perceptions	60.8 (25.5)	67.0 (10.0–100.0)	62.7 (19.9)	65.0 (15.0–100.0)
Physical component score	40.5 (11.2)	39.0 (16.5–58.6)	46.7 (9.9)	48.4 (23.4–61.9)
Mental component score	50.6 (10.9)	54.2 (14.0–67.9)	50.2 (9.8)	53.7 (20.5–62.8)

Table 3: Construct validity. Spearman rank correlations of the TESS (upper and lower extremities) with the SF-36 dimensions.

Spearman	Lower extremity	Upper extremity
Physical functioning	0.737	0.726
Role limitations: physical	0.766	0.766
Social functioning	0.810	0.585
Role limitations: emotional	0.511	0.525
Mental health	0.505	0.383
Vitality	0.704	0.586
Bodily pain	0.777	0.766
General health perceptions	0.540	0.465
Physical component score	0.811	0.797
Mental component score	0.429	0.347

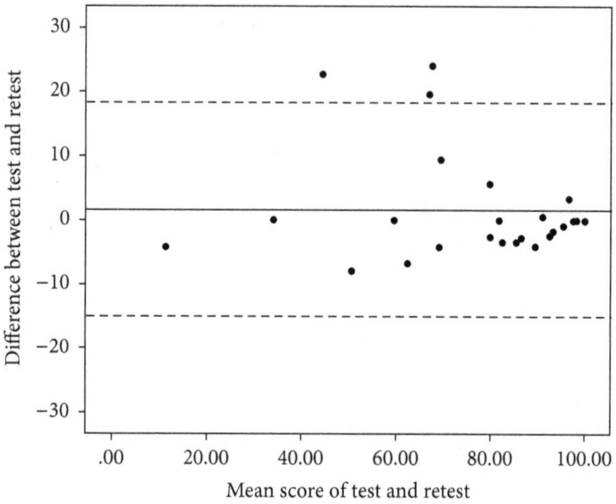

Figure 2: Bland-Altman plot of the test-retest reliability of the Dutch TESS-LE. The solid line shows the mean difference of the two tests (1.65) and the dashed lines show the 95% limits of agreement (−15.11; 18.41).

between one item and the total score (excluding that item) ranged from 0.955–0.958 per item for the TESS-LE and from 0.933–0.939 per item for the TESS-UE.

Twenty-five and eighteen of the LE (50%) and UE patients (38%) completed the "retest" questionnaire, respectively. The test-retest reliability was strong with ICC's of 0.963 (95% confidence interval (CI) 0.916–0.984) and 0.969 (95% CI 0.914–0.989) for the TESS-LE and TESS-UE, respectively. The Bland-Altman plots for both questionnaires showed there were no signs of systematic bias (Figures 2 and 3). The mean difference between the first and second questionnaire was 1.65 (SD 8.55) for the TESS-LE and −1.01 (SD 3.51) for the TESS-UE.

3.5. Validity. The mean scores for the eight SF-36 dimensions of the patients in the study and the physical and mental component scores (PSC/MSC) are shown in Table 2. The correlation was strong between the TESS-LE and the SF-36 dimensions physical functioning, role physical, social functioning, vitality, bodily pain, and PSC (Table 3). There was a moderate correlation between the TESS-LE and the SF-36 dimensions role emotional, mental health, and general health perceptions. The correlation with the MSC was poor. For the TESS-UE the dimensions physical functioning, role physical, bodily pain, and PSC strongly correlated, while the correlation was moderate for the dimensions social functioning, role emotional, and vitality. Mental health, general health perceptions, and MSC were poorly correlated.

4. Discussion

The TESS questionnaires for both the lower and upper extremities (LE and UE) are commonly used patient-reported outcome measures for functioning after the treatment of bone or soft tissue tumors in the Netherlands. However, there is currently no validated Dutch version. This study translated and culturally adapted a Dutch variant of both versions (LE and UE) of the TESS questionnaire.

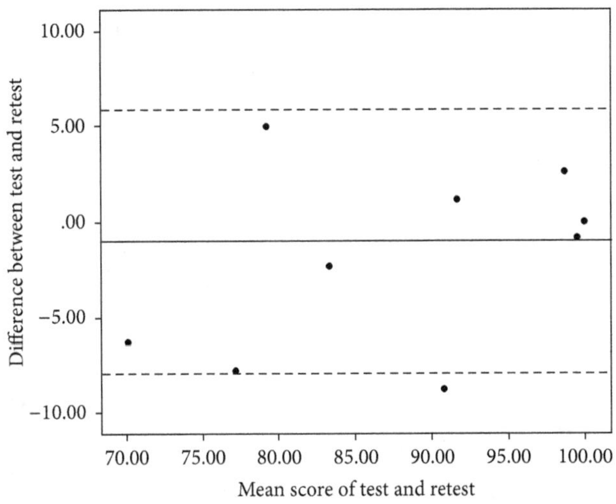

FIGURE 3: Bland-Altman plot of the test-retest reliability of the Dutch TESS-UE. The solid line shows the mean difference of the two tests (−1.01) and the dashed lines show the 95% limits of agreement (−7.89; 5.86). The dot with 0 difference between test and retest and a 100 mean score represents ten patients.

The cultural adaptation was limited to a minimum, which might be due to the similarities regarding the performance of daily activities between the Canadian and the Dutch societies.

Six questionnaires were excluded from the analysis because too many (>80%) questions had been answered with "not applicable." For both the LE and UE versions, there was one questionnaire that was completely answered with "not applicable," of which no score could be computed. In the other four questionnaires, the number of "not applicable" answers ranged from 24 to 29. Although the summary score excludes the "not applicable" answers, a score based on only one or several items did not appear trustworthy to the authors. In the original TESS publication, no advice is given as to dealing with such outcomes neither do previous articles validating the TESS questionnaire report of questionnaires with this amount of "not applicable" answers. Reasons for the high incidence of "incomplete" questionnaires are unclear; however, the TESS was the second questionnaire to fill in, after the SF-36, and it is possible that patients ran out of patience after the first 36 questions.

The internal consistencies and test-retest reliabilities of the Dutch TESS-LE and TESS-UE were comparable with the original version of the TESS [1] and with other translated and validated versions [3–6]. As in all other versions, the test-retest reliability of the UE version was slightly higher than the LE version.

In the TESS-UE 19 patients (39.6%) scored the maximum score. This ceiling effect reduces the possibility of measuring improvement and makes discrimination in patients who are doing well difficult. In the validation of the Japanese translation of the LE-TESS a ceiling effect for 17% of the participants was registered. None of the other translation and validation studies report the presence of absence of a ceiling effect. Therefore, it is difficult to place the current result in context; was the testing group too good or is the TESS-UE really not sensitive enough to discriminate patients with good function of the upper extremity? It is however important to take this result into account when interpreting questionnaire results of individual patients with a good function.

While the original [1] and most other language versions [3–5] test the validity with the MusculoSkeletal Tumor Society (MSTS) score [16], this study tested the validity with the SF-36. The SF-36 was used as comparison with the TESS because it is standard procedure for patients to fill out the questionnaire at the outpatient clinic. Moreover, as opposed to the MSTS questionnaire which is designed as a physician-reported outcome measure, the SF-36 is designed as patient-reported outcome. From that point of view, the SF-36 is suitable to compare with the TESS, which is also patient reported. An additional comparison with the MSTS questionnaire would have brought further information, because that is a disease-specific questionnaire, but this was not possible because the MSTS questionnaire is not regularly completed by the physicians in the outpatient clinic. The correlation between the Dutch TESS (both LE and UE) and SF-36 was strong in the expected dimensions: physical component summary, physical functioning, role physical, and bodily pain. In both questionnaires the correlation with the mental component summary was poor, as was to be expected because the TESS is developed to measure physical functioning only.

This study is limited by several factors. Although the total population is sufficiently large, the subpopulations for the lower and upper extremities are small. The number of patients included in the current study was based on previous studies validating the TESS. The TESS was validated in other languages in cohorts ranging from 22 to 126 patients; thus a total of 98 patients in the current study seems reasonable. The TESS-LE was previously tested in cohorts ranging from 16 to 102 (mean 60, median 48) [3–6], so the LE cohort in this study was of average size. The TESS-UE has been validated in four other languages with small cohorts (6, 23, 43, and 56 patients). The current validation in 48 patients is thus one of the larger cohorts.

The proportion of patients returning the second questionnaire ranged between 38% and 50% which left a small group for the test-retest validity. There are no clear reasons why the return-rate was low. However, as the second questionnaire had to be filled in from home and sent by post, it is conceivable that people simply forgot. It would have been interesting to analyze whether there was a selection in the patients returning the second questionnaire. However, due to the anonymity of the questionnaires, this could not be retrieved.

The comprehension of the questions was not tested in separate questions. However, patients received verbal instructions to report any unclear questions or issues concerning the interpretation of questions to the researcher handing out the questionnaires at the outpatient clinic. Although some patients commented on the amount of questions, no issues were raised concerning the content or meaning of the questions.

The study did not test the Dutch responsiveness to the questionnaire. For use in clinical practice, especially for follow-up in the direct postoperative phase, it would have been useful to know the ability of the questionnaire to accurately detect change when this occurs. However, to test the reliability in the current validation study the population of interest was the group that was longer postoperatively and with a stable situation.

To conclude, the Dutch TESS questionnaire for UE and LE is a reliable and valid instrument to measure patient-reported physical function for patients undergoing limb salvage surgery for benign and malignant bone and soft tissue tumors. The Dutch version of the TESS can be used for future cross-cultural international studies of orthopedic oncology.

Authors' Contributions

Conceptualization/methodology were done by Julie J. Willeumier, Thea P. M. Vliet Vlieland, and Michiel A. J. van de Sande. Investigation was done by Julie J. Willeumier and C. W. P. G. van der Wal. Formal analysis was done by Julie J. Willeumier and Thea P. M. Vliet Vlieland. Resources were provided by Julie J. Willeumier, C. W. P. G. van der Wal, Robert J. P. van der Wal, P. D. S. Dijkstra, and Michiel A. J. van de Sande. Supervision was done by Thea P. M. Vliet Vlieland and Michiel A. J. van de Sande. Writing and original draft were done by Julie J. Willeumier and Thea P. M. Vliet Vlieland. Writing, review, and editing were done by Julie J. Willeumier, C. W. P. G. van der Wal, Robert J. P. van der Wal, P. D. S. Dijkstra, Thea P. M. Vliet Vlieland, and Michiel A. J. van de Sande.

Acknowledgments

The authors would like to thank Jim Bijwaard, Marieke Hampshire, and Trudy Tax for their contribution to the translation process.

References

[1] A. M. Davis, J. G. Wright, J. I. Williams, C. Bombardier, A. Griffin, and R. S. Bell, "Development of a measure of physical function for patients with bone and soft tissue sarcoma," *Quality of Life Research*, vol. 5, no. 5, pp. 508–516, 1996.

[2] T. Akiyama, K. Uehara, K. Ogura et al., "Cross-cultural adaptation and validation of the Japanese version of the Toronto Extremity Salvage Score (TESS) for patients with malignant musculoskeletal tumors in the upper extremities," *Journal of Orthopaedic Science*, vol. 22, no. 1, pp. 127–132, 2017.

[3] K. Ogura, K. Uehara, T. Akiyama et al., "Cross-cultural adaptation and validation of the Japanese version of the Toronto Extremity Salvage Score (TESS) for patients with malignant musculoskeletal tumors in the lower extremities," *Journal of Orthopaedic Science*, vol. 20, no. 6, pp. 1098–1105, 2015.

[4] H.-S. Kim, J. Yun, S. Kang, and I. Han, "Cross-cultural adaptation and validation of the korean toronto extremity salvage score for extremity sarcoma," *Journal of Surgical Oncology*, vol. 112, no. 1, pp. 93–97, 2015.

[5] L. Xu, M. Sun, W. Sun, X. Qin, Z. Zhu, and S. Wang, "Cross-cultural adaptation and validation of the chinese version of toronto extremity salvage score for patients with extremity sarcoma," *SpringerPlus*, vol. 5, no. 1, article 1118, 2016.

musculoskeletal tumors in the lower extremities," *Journal of Orthopaedic Science*, vol. 20, no. 6, pp. 1098–1105, 2015.

[4] H.-S. Kim, J. Yun, S. Kang, and I. Han, "Cross-cultural adaptation and validation of the korean toronto extremity salvage score for extremity sarcoma," *Journal of Surgical Oncology*, vol. 112, no. 1, pp. 93–97, 2015.

[5] L. Xu, M. Sun, W. Sun, X. Qin, Z. Zhu, and S. Wang, "Cross-cultural adaptation and validation of the chinese version of toronto extremity salvage score for patients with extremity sarcoma," *SpringerPlus*, vol. 5, no. 1, article 1118, 2016.

[6] C. Sæbye, A. Safwat, A. K. Kaa, N. A. Pedersen, and J. Keller, "Validation of a danish version of the toronto extremity salvage score questionnaire for patients with sarcoma in the extremities," *Danish medical journal*, vol. 61, no. 1, p. A4734, 2014.

[7] D. Saraiva, B. De Camargo, and A. M. Davis, "Cultural adaptation, translation and validation of a functional outcome questionnaire (TESS) to Portuguese with application to patients with lower extremity osteosarcoma," *Pediatric Blood and Cancer*, vol. 50, no. 5, pp. 1039–1042, 2008.

[8] D. E. Beaton, C. Bombardier, F. Guillemin, and M. B. Ferraz, "Guidelines for the process of cross-cultural adaptation of self-report measures," *Spine*, vol. 25, no. 24, pp. 3186–3191, 2000.

[9] F. Guillemin, C. Bombardier, and D. Beaton, "Cross-cultural adaptation of health-related quality of life measures: Literature review and proposed guidelines," *Journal of Clinical Epidemiology*, vol. 46, no. 12, pp. 1417–1432, 1993.

[10] J. E. Brazier, R. Harper, and N. M. B. Jones, "Validating the SF-36 health survey questionnaire: new outcome measure for primary care," *The British Medical Journal*, vol. 305, no. 6846, pp. 160–164, 1992.

[11] N. K. Aaronson, M. Muller, P. D. A. Cohen et al., "Translation, validation, and norming of the dutch language version of the SF-36 health survey in community and chronic disease populations," *Journal of Clinical Epidemiology*, vol. 51, no. 11, pp. 1055–1068, 1998.

[12] L. J. Cronbach, "Coefficient alpha and the internal structure of tests," *Psychometrika*, vol. 16, no. 3, pp. 297–334, 1951.

[13] J. Nunnally, *Psychometric Theory*, edMcGraw-Hill, New York, NY, USA, 2nd edition, 1978.

[14] J. M. Bland and D. G. Altman, "Measuring agreement in method comparison studies," *Statistical Methods in Medical Research*, vol. 8, no. 2, pp. 135–160, 1999.

[15] C. B. Terwee, S. D. M. Bot, M. R. de Boer et al., "Quality criteria were proposed for measurement properties of health status questionnaires," *Journal of Clinical Epidemiology*, vol. 60, no. 1, pp. 34–42, 2007.

[16] S. S. Enneking WF and MA. Goodman, "A system for the surgical staging of musculoskeletal sarcoma," *Clinical Orthopaedics and Related Research*, vol. 150, pp. 106–120, 1980.

19

Giant Cell Tumor: A Rare Condition in the Immature Skeleton—A Retrospective Study of Symptoms, Treatment, and Outcome in 16 Children

Thale M. Asp Strøm,[1] Anette Torød Skeie,[2] Ingvild Koren Lobmaier,[3] and Olga Zaikova[1]

[1]*Department of Orthopedic Surgery, The Norwegian Radium Hospital, Oslo University Hospital, Oslo, Norway*
[2]*Department of Radiology, The Norwegian Radium Hospital, Oslo University Hospital, Oslo, Norway*
[3]*Department of Pathology, The Norwegian Radium Hospital, Oslo University Hospital, Oslo, Norway*

Correspondence should be addressed to Thale M. Asp Strøm; b21562@ous-hf.no

Academic Editor: Ajay Puri

Background. Pediatric giant cell tumor (GCT) of bone is rare and the course of the disease in the immature skeleton is sparsely described. We performed a retrospective study addressing symptoms, treatment, and outcome in children with GCT. *Methods.* Review of medical records and images of patients with GCT. Patients were detected from our hospital prospective database and those with open epiphyseal cartilages were included. *Results.* 16 children (75% girls) from 6 to 15 years old were identified. Eight lesions (50%) were in long bones and 4 (25%) in flat bones. One lesion appeared to be purely epiphyseal. All patients had pain as the initial symptom. Local recurrence developed in 2 patients. 14 of 16 patients returned to normal activity with no sequelae. One patient developed anisomelia after surgery. *Conclusions.* The biological tumor behavior in children does not seem to differ from what is reported in adults. Lesions in flat bones are very unusual, but our data alone do not provide enough evidence to conclude that this is more common in the immature skeleton. Literature review showed only one previous case report describing a purely epiphyseal GCT. Intralesional curettage is appropriate treatment and gives good functional results with acceptable recurrence rates.

1. Introduction

Giant cell tumor (GCT) of bone is one of the most common benign bone tumors accounting for 22% of benign bone tumors and 4–7% of all primary bone tumors [1, 2].

GCT is a benign but locally aggressive tumor and may even metastasize to the lungs. Rarely it presents as a malignant GCT.

Macroscopically the tumor tissue is soft, friable, and dark chocolate colored; however the color and consistency can vary greatly. Cystic portions may be present (Figure 1) and are sometimes so prominent that the lesion could be mistaken for an aneurysmal bone cyst (ABC) [2–4].

It is characterized microscopically by numerous multinucleated giant cells, which accounts for its name (Figures 2(a) and 2(b)). GCT typically presents as a lytic lesion in the epiphyseal/metaphyseal part of the long bones in an adult between 15 and 40 years of age, with peak incidence in the third decade of life [1–3, 5].

The gold standard for treating these tumors is surgery with intralesional curettage, the aim being local control without sacrificing function. Reported local recurrence rates vary between 14% and 25% in modern literature [6–8].

The lesion is exceptionally rare in children and, as a consequence, there is limited literature documenting the course of the disease in the immature skeleton. Picci et al. [9] presented a case series of 6 children from the Tumor Center in Bologna in 1983. Puri et al. [10] screened their database at Tata Memorial Hospital in Mumbai in 2007 and found 17 patients. These case series document the course of the disease compared with its adult form. Additional two articles from Schütte and Taconis in 1993 [11] and Kransdorf et al. in 1992 [12] describe GCT in younger patients, but mostly covering the radiological presentation.

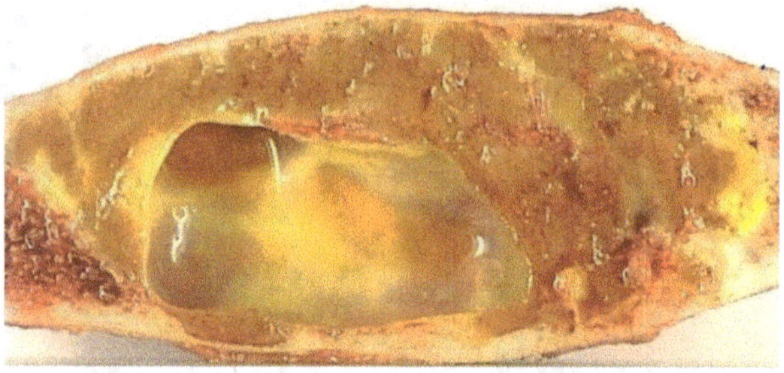

FIGURE 1: Giant cell tumor (GCT) in fibula with secondary aneurysmal bone cyst. Treated with wide resection.

To further our knowledge about this unusual subset of patients we performed a retrospective study addressing symptoms, treatment, and outcome in children with GCT of bone.

2. Materials and Methods

Patients with GCT of bone who were diagnosed and treated at our hospital between 1984 and 2015 were identified from our prospective database (Table 1). As skeletal immaturity can be difficult to ascertain without targeted radiographs with this in mind, we chose to include only patients under 16 years of age. We then excluded anyone among these who still appeared to have closed epiphyseal cartilages.

The patients' records were studied for clinical data, comorbidity, heredity, blood work, diagnostic method, pulmonary metastasis, multicentricity, operative methods, complications, and follow-up results.

A radiologist specialized in the field of musculoskeletal tumors (ATS) reviewed all the patients' radiological images.

A pathologist specialized in the field of mesenchymal tumors (IKL) reviewed the histological slides from all the lesions.

All included patients or their guardians have signed informed consent forms. The study has been approved by a personal data protection official at our institution.

3. Results

154 patients with GCT of bone treated at our hospital in the period 1984 to 2015 were detected. 137 (89%) were older than 15 years at the time of diagnosis and were excluded. One girl of 15 had closed epiphyseal cartilages on her radiographs and was also excluded.

The study population consisted of 12 girls and 4 boys, that is, 75% female predominance. The age range of the included patients was 6 to 15 years.

Lesions around the knee were the most common (25%) and there were 8 lesions in long tubular bones. One lesion seems to have been purely epiphyseal at the time of presentation and then progressed into the metaphysis with time (Figures 3(a) and 3(b)). Further patient and tumor characteristics are presented in Table 1.

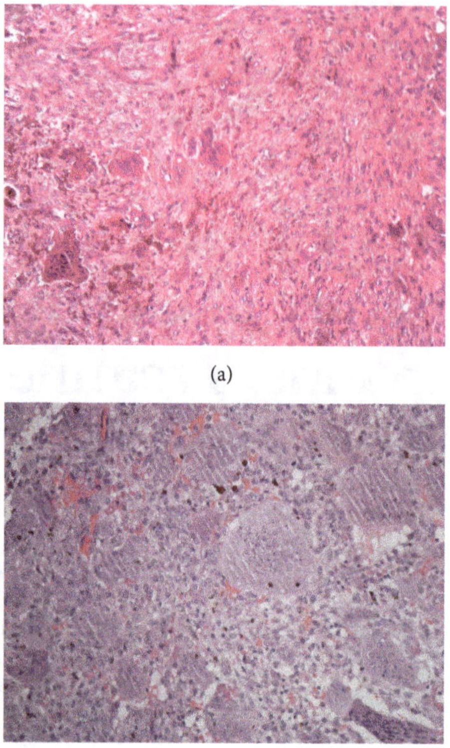

(a)

(b)

FIGURE 2: (a) Characteristic histology of giant cell tumor: mononuclear cells with round to oval nuclei interspersed with numerous multinucleated giant cells. (b) Larger magnification of a typical multinucleated giant cell.

All the patients presented with pain of varying degree. Some experienced pain only during activity. 12 of the patients also had swelling at the initial examination and 4 had reduced range of motion in the adjacent joint. One of the sacral lesions was associated with hip-pain, reduced muscle strength, and muscle atrophy in the ipsilateral lower extremity. Two had frank pathologic fractures and one had a hairline fracture. The duration of symptoms averaged 6 and 4 months (1–48).

Only one patient did not have a biopsy prior to surgery and this was because the lesion was largely cystic and did not present any tissue available for biopsy. The postoperative histology showed benign GCT in 13 of the lesions; 3 had benign GCT with a secondary ABC (Figure 1).

Histologically the tumors showed a variation of features within the normal histological appearance of giant cell tumors (Figures 2(a) and 2(b)): mononuclear cells with round to oval nuclei and eosinophilic, indistinct cytoplasm with some areas with spindle cell appearance. The giant cells had the same nuclear morphology and were partly evenly distributed throughout the tumor, partly in clusters.

Plain chest X-ray or chest CT were obtained of 15 of the 16 patients prior to surgery and there were none presenting with pulmonary metastasis.

One patient had multicentric GCT with two metachronous lesions, one in the proximal tibia and one in the cuneiform bone in the same extremity 15 years later. The

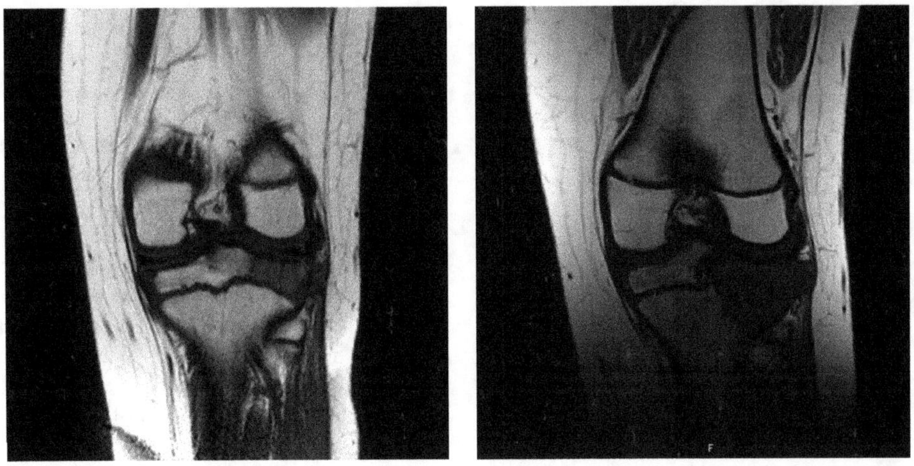

(a) (b)

FIGURE 3: (a) MRI of a purely epiphyseal giant cell tumor in a proximal tibia. (b) 9 months later the lesion had progressed to include the metaphysis as well.

TABLE 1: Patient characteristics.

	Sex	Age at diagnosis (years)	Symptom duration (months)	Affected bone	Localization in bone	Type of operation/reconstruction	Recurrence	Multicentric disease	Follow-up time (months)
Patient 1	M	14	1	Tibia	P-MD	Curettage + cement	–	–	119
Patient 2	F	14	6	Tibia	P-EM	Curettage + cement	–	+	220
Patient 3	F	12	48	Fibula	P-MD	Excision	–	–	50
Patient 4	F	15	2	Tibia	D-M	Curettage + cement	–	–	48
Patient 5	F	6	1	Fibula	D-MD	Curettage + cement	+	–	81
Patient 6	F	9	1	Tibia	P-E	Curettage + cement	–	–	72
Patient 7	F	15	5	Fibula	D-MD	Curettage + autograft	–	–	50
Patient 8	M	15	6	Radius	D-EMD	Curettage + allograft	+	–	35
Patient 9	F	10	4	Sacrum	P	Curettage + cement	–	–	90
Patient 10	F	4	2	Clavicle	P	Curettage + cement	–	–	52
Patient 11	M	6	2	Clavicle	D	Curettage + cement	–	–	59
Patient 12	F	8	5	Sacrum	P	Curettage	–	–	47
Patient 13	F	10	1	Clavicle	D	Curettage + cement	–	–	50
Patient 14	F	8	12	3.metatarsal		Curettage + allograft	–	–	28
Patient 15	M	9	2	Scapula		Curettage	–	–	19
Patient 16	F	10	6	3.metatarsal		Curettage	–		17

Male (M), female (F), proximal (P), distal (D), epiphyseal (E), metaphyseal (M), and diaphyseal (D).

initial lesion was extensive and complicated by fractures before and after surgery. It was initially treated with curettage and cementing. The second lesion was treated with excision and arthrodesis with autograft.

All lesions except one were treated with intralesional curettage. In 5 of these 15 patients some form of adjuvant was used: phenol in 2, high-speed bur in 2, and Pulsavac (high-pressure irrigation with NaCl) in 1. Further treatment details are described in Table 1.

The patients in this material have a follow-up period ranging from 17 to 240 months. 14 of 16 patients returned to normal preoperative level of activity with no sequelae at last follow-up. The patient with a sacral lesion associated with reduced strength and muscle atrophy preoperatively developed contracture of the Achilles tendon. The patient with an extensive proximal tibial lesion and multicentric disease has a varus knee with medial arthrosis as an adult. One of the metatarsal lesions ended up with a shorter 3.metatarsal bone, but unaffected function. One patient had a proximal tibial lesion that crossed the epiphyseal cartilage as a 9-year-old (Figures 3(a) and 3(b)). Consequently an epiphysiodesis of the remaining epiphyseal cartilage was done to prevent an angular deformity. The patient then developed a limb-length inequality which was treated with shortening

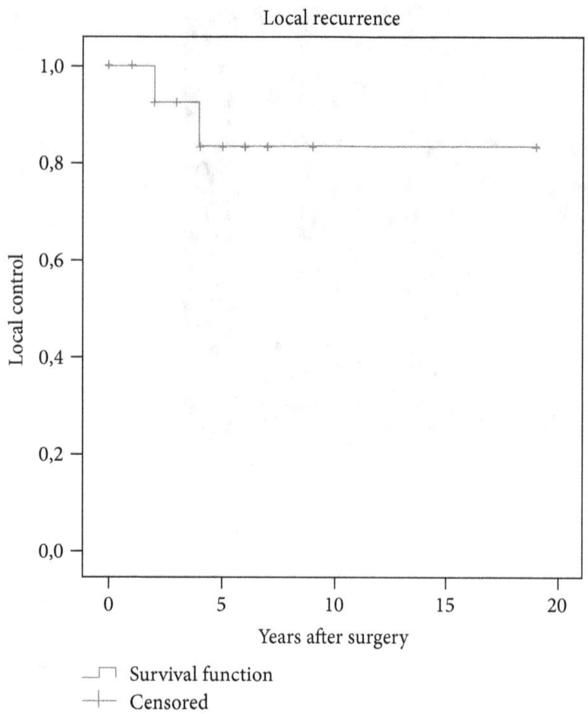

FIGURE 4: Kaplan-Meier cumulative survival curves for all patients under 16 years of age with giant cell tumor of bone (GCT) diagnosed and treated at our institution between 1984 and 2015.

osteotomies on the contralateral side. The patient had an unaffected function at last follow-up.

Local recurrence developed in 2 patients (Figure 4). One case in the distal fibula treated with curettage and cement initially developed a recurrence after 4 months. The other in the distal radius, treated with curettage and allograft initially, developed a recurrence after 14 months. Both reoperations were done with recurettage and cementing. They both remain disease-free at 8 and 2,5 years, respectively, after the initial surgery.

One of the patients with a sacral lesion had to have a reoperation less than 1 month after the initial surgery, but this was a complicated case in a difficult location around the S1 nerve root and it was regarded as residual tumor and not a local recurrence.

4. Discussion

Previously reported incidence of GCT in the immature skeleton varies between 0,5% and 10,6% [1, 2, 9–12]. We showed an incidence of 10,4% of lesions in the immature skeleton from our total of 154 patients with GCT of bone in the selected period.

Some studies suggest a slight female predilection for GCT [2, 3, 5], but others have found no difference between the genders [1, 4]. Dahlin et al found 56% females in the adult population with GCT in the Mayo Clinic files, but 72% in patients under 20 years of age [13]. Interestingly numerous publications have shown a larger female predominance (60–82%) in the younger age groups [9–11]. Kransdorf et al. [12] had 58% male patients, but they included patients up to 19 years of age.

In our material we had 75% girls in the group under 16 years and 72% if we considered patients up to 18 years of age. This seems in accordance with existing literature.

The anatomical region reported as most commonly affected is around the knee. 46–58% of the lesions occur here with the distal femur being the most frequent single location. Other fairly common locations are the distal radius, the proximal femur, the sacrum, and the proximal humerus. 90% are found in the long bones. The small bones of the hands and feet, the vertebrae, the pelvis, and the skull are rarely involved [1–3, 5].

Picci et al. [9] reported 6 children; all with lesions around the knee joint. Other publications regarding children report 22–53% of lesions occur around the knee [10–12]. Kransdorf et al. [12] found the majority (34%) of lesions in the small bones of the hands and feet. It is now commonly accepted that GCT and "giant cell reparative granuloma/giant cell lesion of the small bones" are two distinct entities. The latter is more common in the first and second decades of life and are associated with a very good prognosis [2, 4, 14]. However Kransdorf et al. [12] state that in their opinion there is no cause for such a redefinition because the foci of fibrous proliferation and/or osseous differentiation may also be seen in GCT elsewhere in the skeleton. It is important to note that some authors on the other hand do not include giant cell reparative granulomas in their material on GCT. At our institution there was no prior tradition for differentiating between these two entities.

We report 5 lesions (29%) around the knee which makes this the most common anatomical region in accordance with other publications. The 3 clavicular lesions and 1 in scapula are interesting as the flat bones are hardly ever affected. Puri et al. [10] found one clavicular lesion among the children in their material, and there are some existing case reports [15, 16]. Most of the larger materials contain none [1–3, 5]. There is not enough evidence to conclude that this is more common in the immature skeleton from our small case series alone.

The localization within the bone is a point of special interest with regard to lesions in the immature skeleton. The typical GCT in an adult occurs at the end of a long bone with a metaphyseoepiphyseal location. The tumor very often extends to the subchondral bone or even to the articular cartilage and will in time often involve all/most of the epiphysis [2–4]. Lesions involving the metaphysis or the diaphysis without epiphyseal involvement are exceptionally rare. Historically the GCT was thought to occur in the epiphyseal part of the bone and then extend to the metaphysis [3, 13, 17]. However it became evident from isolated case reports and examples reported in larger series [3, 13, 18] that purely metaphyseal lesions were more common in young patients, often before closure of the epiphyseal cartilage.

Campanacci et al. [1] found one diaphyseal and two metaphyseal lesions among 209 patients with GCT. They go on to say that cases with the tumor restricted exclusively to the epiphysis or apophysis were not known. They consequently advanced the hypothesis that GCT arise in the metaphysis and secondarily invade the epiphysis or apophysis. However, as early as 1952 Dr. Johnson, a pathologist in Washington, published a paper called "A General Theory of Bone Tumors" [19] where he looked at the functional and chemical kinship between different types of bone tumors. He stated that when the very small and presumably early tumors of each category are analyzed, it becomes apparent that there are preferential sites of origin within each bone. As an example he mentions GCTs, which when discovered while they are still small or before the epiphyseal plate closes are always located in the metaphysis.

Several studies have supported the view that a metaphyseal origin is likely. Rietveld et al. [17] looked at 233 cases in 1981 and found that the lesion could occasionally be shown to be restricted to the metaphysis; none were situated exclusively in an epiphysis. The materials published on young patients reinforce this view by showing a very high incidence of purely metaphyseal/predominantly metaphyseal lesions [9, 11, 12, 18]. The lesion is capable of crossing the epiphyseal cartilage [10], but epiphyseal involvement in young patients increases with increasing age [11].

Of our 8 lesions in long tubular bones, 7 involved the metaphysis and only 3 involved the epiphysis. We were surprised to find a lesion that appeared to be purely epiphyseal and then progressed to the metaphysis (Figures 3(a) and 3(b)). Only one previous case report describing a purely epiphyseal GCT was located after literature review so this is clearly unusual [20]. We do however have plain X-rays, CT scans, and MRI images of the early lesion and they all fail to show convincing metaphyseal involvement.

Our findings support a much higher incidence of metaphyseal or predominantly metaphyseal lesions in children.

Pain of variable degree is reported as the predominant symptom in the literature, at onset often only during activity and then more constant as the lesion progresses. More than three-quarters of patients have noted swelling of the affected region. Less common symptoms include weakness, limitation of adjacent joint motion, and pathologic fracture [2–4]. The clinical symptoms of the children in our study were no different from what is reported in the adult population.

Approximately 1% of patients with GCT have multiple synchronous or metachronous lesions. This has been shown to occur more frequently in younger patients [21]. One of our 16 children had multicentric GCT.

Pediatric GCTs have been treated in the same manner as in the adult patients, with curettage being the treatment of choice. We usually fill the cavity with cement, autograft, or banked allograft when the cavity is of some size and in a region which will be submitted to weight-bearing.

The Scandinavian Sarcoma Group Study from 2006 concluded that a local recurrence after curettage and cementing can generally be treated with further curettage and cementing with only a minor risk of increased morbidity, thus giving no incentive for more extensive and disabling surgery to avoid recurrence [8].

In modern literature the recurrence rate after curettage is 14–25% [6–8]. In younger patients it has been reported between 8% and 20% [9–11]. A local recurrence developed in 2 of 16 patients (13%) in our cohort (Figure 4). However for 4 of the 16 patients the follow-up period was less than 4 years.

In spite of being a rare condition in the immature skeleton, GCT should be considered as a differential diagnosis in children with pain. The biological behavior of the tumor in children does not seem to differ significantly from what is reported in adults. Intralesional curettage is appropriate treatment and gives a good functional result with acceptable recurrence rate. 87% had no functional sequelae after surgery at the last follow-up, but one patient needed two additional surgical procedures to achieve a good functional result.

Disclosure

Level of evidence is Level IV, case series.

Competing Interests

The authors declare that there is no conflict of interests regarding the publication of this paper.

Authors' Contributions

Thale M. Asp Strøm collected and analyzed the data and prepared the manuscript. Anette Torød Skeie reviewed all the patients' radiological images. Ingvild Koren Lobmaier reviewed the histological slides from all the lesions. Olga Zaikova supervised the study.

Acknowledgments

The authors thank Trine Thoresen for her help with data collection and Heidi Buvarp Dyrop for advice and IT support. They are also grateful to Nils Jørgen Strøm and Joachim Thorkildsen for linguistic revision.

References

[1] M. Campanacci, A. Giunti, and R. Olmi, "Metaphyseal and diaphyseal localization of giant cell tumors," *La Chirurgia Degli Organi di Movimento*, vol. 62, no. 1, pp. 29–34, 1975.

[2] K. K. Unni and C. Y. Inwards, *Dahlin's Bone Tumors: General Aspects and Data on 10,165 Cases*, Lippincott Williams and Wilkins, 2010.

[3] R. R. Goldenberg, C. J. Campbell, and M. Bonfiglio, "Giant-cell tumor of bone. An analysis of two hundred and eighteen cases," *The Journal of Bone & Joint Surgery—American Volume*, vol. 52, no. 4, pp. 619–664, 1970.

[4] R. E. Turcotte, "Giant cell tumor of bone," *Orthopedic Clinics of North America*, vol. 37, no. 1, pp. 35–51, 2006.

[5] H. L. Jaffe, *Tumors and Tumorous Conditions of the Bones and Joints*, Lea and Febiger, Philadelphia, Pa, USA, 1958.

[6] R. J. O'Donnell, D. S. Springfield, H. K. Motwani, J. E. Ready, M. C. Gebhardt, and H. J. Mankin, "Recurrence of giant-cell tumors of the long bones after curettage and packing with cement," *The Journal of Bone & Joint Surgery—American Volume*, vol. 76, no. 12, pp. 1827–1833, 1994.

[7] R. E. Turcotte, J. S. Wunder, M. H. Isler et al., "Giant cell tumor of long bone: a Canadian Sarcoma Group study," *Clinical Orthopaedics and Related Research*, no. 397, pp. 248–258, 2002.

[8] F. Vult von Steyern, H. C. F. Bauer, C. Trovik et al., "Treatment of local recurrences of giant cell tumour in long bones after curettage and cementing. A Scandinavian Sarcoma Group study," *The Journal of Bone and Joint Surgery. British Volume*, vol. 88, no. 4, pp. 531–535, 2006.

[9] P. Picci, M. Manfrini, V. Zucchi et al., "Giant-cell tumor of bone in skeletally immature patients," *The Journal of Bone & Joint Surgery—American Volume*, vol. 65, no. 4, pp. 486–490, 1983.

[10] A. Puri, M. G. Agarwal, M. Shah, N. A. Jambhekar, C. Anchan, and S. Behle, "Giant cell tumor of bone in children and adolescents," *Journal of Pediatric Orthopaedics*, vol. 27, no. 6, pp. 635–639, 2007.

[11] H. E. Schütte and W. K. Taconis, "Giant cell tumor in children and adolescents," *Skeletal Radiology*, vol. 22, no. 3, pp. 173–176, 1993.

[12] M. J. Kransdorf, D. E. Sweet, P. C. Buetow, M. A. I. Giudici, and R. P. Moser Jr., "Giant cell tumor in skeletally immature patients," *Radiology*, vol. 184, no. 1, pp. 233–237, 1992.

[13] D. C. Dahlin, R. E. Cupps, and E. W. Johnson Jr., "Giant-cell tumor: a study of 195 cases," *Cancer*, vol. 25, no. 5, pp. 1061–1070, 1970.

[14] C. D. M. Fletcher, J. A. Bridge, P. C. W. Hogendoorn, and F. Mertens, *WHO Classification of Tumours of Soft Tissue and Bone*, WHO Press, Lyon, France, 4th edition, 2013.

[15] S. Nagano, T. Tsuchimochi, M. Yokouchi et al., "Giant cell tumor of the clavicle: report of a case in a rare location with consideration of surgical method," *BMC Musculoskeletal Disorders*, vol. 16, article 142, 2015.

[16] V. Vaibhav, D. Kumar, and S. Singh, "Giant cell tumour of clavicle," *Scientific Journal of Medical Science*, vol. 3, no. 7, pp. 352–356, 2014.

[17] L. A. C. Rietveld, J. D. Mulder, G. Brutel de la Riviere, and T. G. van Rijssel, "Giant cell tumour: metaphyseal or epiphyseal origin?" *Diagnostic Imaging*, vol. 50, no. 6, pp. 289–293, 1981.

[18] J. S. Fain, K. K. Unni, J. W. Beabout, and M. G. Rock, "Nonepiphyseal giant cell tumor of the long bones. Clinical, radiologic, and pathologic study," *Cancer*, vol. 71, no. 11, pp. 3514–3519, 1993.

[19] L. C. Johnson, "A general theory of bone tumors," in *The Bulletin New York Pathological Society*, pp. 164–171, 1952.

[20] A. Gandhe, A. Sankhe, G. Aeron, and A. Joshi, "Epiphyseal giant cell tumour in an immature skeleton," *The British Journal of Radiology*, vol. 81, no. 963, pp. e75–e78, 2008.

[21] B. Hoch, C. Inwards, M. Sundaram, and A. E. Rosenberg, "Multicentric giant cell tumor of bone: clinicopathologic analysis of thirty cases," *Journal of Bone and Joint Surgery—Series A*, vol. 88, no. 9, pp. 1998–2008, 2006.

20

Treatment of Recurrent or Metastatic Uterine Adenosarcoma

Michael J. Nathenson,[1] Anthony P. Conley,[2] Heather Lin,[3] Nicole Fleming,[4] and Vinod Ravi[2]

[1]*Dana-Farber Cancer Institute, 450 Brookline Ave., Boston, MA 02215, USA*
[2]*Department of Sarcoma Medical Oncology, The University of Texas MD Anderson Cancer Center, 1515 Holcombe Blvd Unit 450, Houston, TX 77030, USA*
[3]*Department of Biostatistics, The University of Texas MD Anderson Cancer Center, 1515 Holcombe Blvd Unit 450, Houston, TX 77030, USA*
[4]*Department of Gynecologic Oncology and Reproductive Medicine, The University of Texas MD Anderson Cancer Center, 1515 Holcombe Blvd Unit 450, Houston, TX 77030, USA*

Correspondence should be addressed to Michael J. Nathenson; michaelj_nathenson@dfci.harvard.edu

Academic Editor: Quincy Chu

Purpose. This study retrospectively evaluated overall survival (OS) by treatment of recurrent or metastatic uterine adenosarcoma including surgery, radiation, chemotherapy, and hormonal therapy and evaluated OS and progression-free survival (PFS) after 1st line systemic chemotherapy. *Methods.* 78 patients with recurrent or metastatic adenosarcoma comprised the study population. The Kaplan-Meier method was used to estimate OS and PFS. The log-rank test was performed to test the difference in survival between groups. *Results.* Median OS from diagnosis of recurrent or metastatic disease was 1.8 yrs. OS was influenced by pathology on recurrence, $p = 0.035$. Median OS differed by surgery for 1st recurrence 26.3 months versus 15.1 months. OS was not influenced by chemotherapy, $p = 0.58$, palliative radiation, $p = 0.58$, or hormonal therapy, $p = 0.15$. The response rate (CR + PR) per RECIST 1.1 for chemotherapy was 31.2% for doxorubicin-based regimens and 14.3% for gemcitabine/docetaxel. OS since 1st line chemotherapy was not significantly different among chemotherapy regimens. However, the median PFS was superior for doxorubicin/ifosfamide (15.4 months) compared to gemcitabine/docetaxel (5.0 months), platinum-based regimens (5.7 mo), or other doxorubicin-based regimens (6.5 months). *Conclusion.* These results suggest that surgery is an important treatment modality for recurrent or metastatic uterine adenosarcoma, and the most effective chemotherapeutics are doxorubicin/ifosfamide and gemcitabine/docetaxel.

1. Introduction

Uterine adenosarcoma is an extremely rare subtype of uterine sarcoma, which represents only 5.5 to 9% of all uterine sarcomas [1, 2]. Uterine adenosarcoma was first described by Dr. Phillip B. Clement and Dr. Robert E. Scully in 1974 [3]. This tumor is composed of a malignant mesenchymal component and a benign epithelial component [4, 5]. This biphasic cellular differentiation is characteristic of adenosarcomas and required for the diagnosis of this tumor. Adenosarcomas can arise from the uterus but have also been noted to arise from the ovaries, vagina, cervix, and pelvis usually in the setting of prior endometriosis [6–9].

There is a specific FIGO uterine adenosarcoma staging system which divides between stage Ia, Ib, and Ic by the presence and extent of myometrial invasion [10]. The majority of adenosarcoma patients (70 to 80%) will present with stage I disease [11–13]. Despite this, many patients, even with stage I disease, will develop recurrent or metastatic disease. Survival varies with the presence and extent of myometrial invasion and sarcomatous overgrowth [12–15].

Unfortunately, given the rarity of adenosarcoma, there are limited data to guide treatment decisions in the recurrent or metastatic setting. There is no standard treatment for recurrent or metastatic disease, though surgery is often preformed [12]. A recent review suggests that uterine adenosarcomas can respond to doxorubicin/ifosfamide and gemcitabine/docetaxel chemotherapy [16]. Furthermore, the role of hormonal therapy in recurrent or metastatic disease is limited to case reports and case series.

The purpose of this study was to examine the role of surgery, radiation, and hormonal therapy in the recurrent or metastatic setting. Furthermore, this is the first study to report response rates, overall survival, and progression-free survival of adenosarcoma patients treated with chemotherapy for recurrent or metastatic disease.

2. Patients and Methods

With approval by the MD Anderson Cancer Center Institutional Review Board, a search was conducted of the Institutional Tumor Registry. Seventy-eight patients treated at the MD Anderson Cancer Center from August 1982 to December 2014 with recurrent or metastatic uterine or extrauterine adenosarcoma were identified. The diagnosis of uterine adenosarcoma was confirmed by MD Anderson sarcoma or gynecologic pathologists. Demographic, clinicopathologic, and treatment characteristics were abstracted from the patients' medical records. Then, a deidentified database was constructed of all adenosarcoma patients. The stage was assigned using the International Federation of Gynecology and Obstetrics 2009 uterine adenosarcoma staging system [10].

Patients' demographic and clinical characteristics were analyzed, with categorical variables summarized in frequency tables while continuous variables summarized using mean (±S.D.) and median (range). The product limit method of Kaplan and Meier was used to estimate overall survival (OS) and progression-free survival (PFS) [17]. OS was determined from the date of first recurrent or metastatic disease diagnosis to the date of death or date of last contact. OS since the start of chemotherapy for recurrent or metastatic disease was determined from the date of initiation of 1st line chemotherapy for recurrent or metastatic disease to the date of death or date of last contact. Progression-free survival was determined from the date of initiation of chemotherapy for recurrent or metastatic disease to the date of progression or death. Complete response (CR), partial response (PR), stable disease (SD), or progressive disease (PD) were determined by RECIST 1.1 [18]. The log-rank test was performed to test the difference in survival between groups [19]. Regression analyses of survival data utilized the Cox proportional hazards model [20].

3. Results

3.1. Patient Characteristics. Seventy-eight patients with recurrent or metastatic uterine or extrauterine adenosarcoma who received treatment at the MD Anderson Cancer Center were identified from a retrospective review of the Institutional Tumor Registry and were included in this study. The median follow-up time since recurrent or metastatic disease was 8.2 years. The demographic and clinical characteristics for all patients included in this study are summarized in Table 1. The median age at diagnosis was 55 years (range 27 to 79 years). The majority of patients were Caucasian (80.8%). The most common presenting symptom was abnormal uterine bleeding (44.9%), and the second most common presenting symptom was pelvic pain (16.7%). Thirty-nine patients had stage I primary tumor (50.1%). Thirty-six patients had stage II–IV primary tumor (46.2%). The primary tumor location was the uterine corpus in the majority of patients (74.4%). At last follow-up, 24 patients were alive, and 54 have died. Local recurrences occurred within the abdomen and pelvis in seventy-two patients, and sixteen patients developed distant metastasis. Patients who had local and distant recurrences commonly developed the local recurrence first. Sites of distant disease included the lung (14 pts), bone (4 pts), liver (3 pts), brain (1 pt), and subcutaneous tissue (4 pts).

3.2. Treatment Characteristics for Recurrent or Metastatic Disease. Treatment on recurrence varied greatly and was influenced by the location and extent of recurrence. Table 2 describes the treatments that patients received on 1st and 2nd recurrence including surgery, palliative radiation, chemotherapy, and hormonal therapy. First-line chemotherapy for recurrent or metastatic disease was given to 59 patients, at 1st recurrence in 40 pts, at 2nd recurrence in 10 pts, at 3rd recurrence in 2 pts, and at 4th recurrence in 2 pts. Three additional patients had residual disease after primary treatment, and upon progression, they received 1st line chemotherapy (Table 2). One patient had 7 prior surgeries and hormonal therapy prior to receiving chemotherapy, and another patient received chemotherapy for 1st recurrence, though documentation regarding the specific chemotherapy regimen was lacking. The specific chemotherapy regimens utilized greatly differed as well. Table 2 lists the specific chemotherapy regimens that patients received for 1st, 2nd, and 3rd line chemotherapy, as well as the number of patients that received surgery, radiation therapy, or hormonal therapy either before or after their chemotherapy as part of their treatment for recurrent or metastatic disease.

3.3. Pathology on Recurrence. On recurrence, 58 patients had a biopsy available for review: high-grade sarcoma in 36 patients and mixed epithelial and mesenchymal components in 22 patients. Median overall survival differed by the pathology of recurrence. Patients with high-grade sarcoma on recurrence had a median overall survival of 17.6 months versus 33.5 months in patients with mixed histology, $p = 0.035$, HR = 0.47 (95% CI 0.23–0.96) (Figure 1(a) and Table 3).

3.4. Surgery for Recurrent or Metastatic Disease. Forty-five patients underwent surgery for recurrence or metastatic disease.

Forty-one patients underwent resection of recurrence within the abdomen and pelvis. Twenty-five patients underwent one resection, eight patients had two resections, four patients had three resections, three patients had four resections, and one patient had nine resections. Four patients underwent thoracotomies for resection of metastatic disease to the lung. Median overall survival was improved in those patients who underwent resection for recurrent or

Table 1: Patient characteristics.

Variable	Patients with recurrence, no. of patients (%)
Age, median (range)	55 years (27 to 79 years)
Race	
Caucasian	63 (80.8%)
African American	10 (12.8%)
Hispanic	5 (6.4%)
ECOG performance status	
0	17 (21.8%)
1	30 (38.5%)
Unknown	31 (39.7%)
Presenting symptoms	
Abnormal uterine bleeding	35 (44.9%)
Pelvic pain	13 (16.7%)
Incidental finding	4 (5.1%)
Other	6 (7.7%)
Unknown	20 (25.6%)
Size, median (range)	7.1 cm (0.4 to 25 cm)
≤5 cm	14 (17.9%)
>5 cm	36 (46.2%)
Unknown	28 (35.9%)
Myometrial invasion	
No myometrial invasion	12 (15.4%)
≤½ of myometrium	26 (33.3%)
>½ of myometrium	8 (10.3%)
Unknown	32 (41.0%)
Sarcomatous overgrowth	
Absent	15 (19.2%)
Present	58 (74.4%)
Unknown	5 (6.4%)
Lymph node involvement	
None	34 (43.6%)
Present	1 (1.3%)
No lymph node sampling	39 (50.0%)
Unknown	4 (5.1%)
Uterine adenosarcoma FIGO stage at diagnosis	
Ia	7 (9.0%)
Ib	19 (24.4%)
Ic	4 (5.1%)
I (nos.)	9 (11.6%)
IIa	7 (9.0%)
IIb	12 (15.4%)
IIIa	7 (9.0%)
IIIb	4 (5.1%)
IIIc	1 (1.3%)
IVa	4 (5.1%)
IVb	1 (1.3%)
Unknown	3 (3.8%)

Table 1: Continued.

Variable	Patients with recurrence, no. of patients (%)
Tumor location	
Uterine corpus	58 (74.4%)
Ovary	5 (6.4%)
Cervix	2 (2.6%)
Pelvic primary	11 (14.1%)
Vagina	1 (1.3%)
Unknown	1 (1.3%)
Initial treatment strategy	
Surgery alone	45 (57.7%)
Surgery + radiation (adjuvant or neoadjuvant)	22 (28.2%)
Surgery + chemotherapy (adjuvant or neoadjuvant)	6 (7.7%)
Surgery + radiation + chemotherapy	4 (5.1%)
Surgery + hormonal therapy	1 (1.3%)
Bilateral salpingo-oophorectomy	
Yes	55 (70.5%)
No	13 (16.7%)
History of prior BSO	9 (11.5%)
Unknown	1 (1.3%)
Lymphadenectomy	
Yes	31 (39.7%)
No	43 (55.1%)
Unknown	4 (5.1%)
Vital status	
Alive	24 (30.8%)
Dead	54 (69.2%)
Recurrence	
Any recurrence	78
Local (abdomen/pelvis)	61 (78.2%)
Local and distant	11 (14.1%)
Distant	5 (6.4%)
Unknown	1 (1.3%)
Median follow-up	8.2 years

This table described patient demographics (age and race), presenting symptoms, performance status, tumor pathologic characteristics (size, myometrial invasion, sarcomatous overgrowth, and lymph node involvement), tumor stage, tumor location, initial treatments (surgery, radiation, chemotherapy, BSO, and lymphadenectomy), vital status (alive versus dead), and recurrence location for patients with recurrence.

metastatic disease, for 1st recurrence 26.3 months versus 15.1 months, $p = 0.54$ (Figure 1(b) and Table 3).

3.5. Chemotherapy for Recurrent or Metastatic Disease

3.5.1. Response Rates. Of the fifty-nine patients that received 1st line chemotherapy for recurrent or metastatic disease, 9 received chemotherapy after surgical resection to obtain no evidence of disease, so response rate per RECIST 1.1 could not

TABLE 2: Treatment characteristics on recurrence with 1st, 2nd, and 3rd line chemotherapy for recurrent or metastatic disease.

Treatment on 1st recurrence	
Surgery alone	13 (16.7%)
Surgery + radiation	8 (10.3%)
Radiation alone	1 (1.3%)
Surgery + chemotherapy	19 (24.3%)
Chemotherapy alone	18 (23.1%)
Surgery + chemotherapy + radiation	5 (6.4%)
Chemotherapy + radiation	1 (1.3%)
Hormonal therapy alone	3 (3.8%)
None	1 (1.3%)
Unknown	9 (11.6%)
Treatment on 2nd recurrence	
Surgery alone	11 (14.1%)
Surgery + radiation	2 (2.6%)
Surgery + chemotherapy	6 (7.7%)
Chemotherapy alone	11 (14.1%)
Chemotherapy + radiation	2 (2.6%)
Unknown	17 (21.8%)
Did not obtain NED after 1st recurrence	29 (37.2%)
1st line chemotherapy additional treatments	
Chemotherapy alone	30 (50.9%)
Chemotherapy + surgery	20 (33.9%)
Chemotherapy + radiation	2 (3.4%)
Chemotherapy + radiation + surgery	4 (6.8%)
Chemotherapy + hormonal therapy	1 (1.7%)
Chemotherapy + surgery + hormonal therapy	2 (3.4%)
Chemotherapy given for residual disease after initial treatment	3 (5.1%)
Chemotherapy given for 1st recurrence	40 (67.8%)
Chemotherapy given for 2nd recurrence	10 (16.9%)
Chemotherapy given for 3rd recurrence	2 (3.4%)
Chemotherapy given for 4th recurrence	2 (3.4%)
Chemotherapy given for >4th recurrence	1 (1.7%)
Recurrence chemotherapy given for unknown	1 (1.7%)
1st line chemotherapy regimens	
Doxorubicin based	28 (47.5%)
Doxorubicin alone⁺	4
AI (doxorubicin/ifosfamide)	9
VAI (vincristine/doxorubicin/ifosfamide)	1
ADIC (doxorubicin/dacarbazine)	3
MAID (doxorubicin/ifosfamide/dacarbazine)	1
Other doxorubicin based*	10
Gemcitabine/docetaxel	14 (23.7%)
Platinum based**	12 (20.3%)
Other (ifosfamide/paclitaxel (2), paclitaxel, gemcitabine)	4 (6.8%)
Unknown	1 (1.7%)
2nd line chemotherapy regimens	
Doxorubicin based	6 (25.0%)
Doxorubicin alone⁺	3
AI (doxorubicin/ifosfamide)	3
Gemcitabine/docetaxel	9 (37.5%)
Platinum based (cisplatin/ifosfamide in one patient)***	4 (16.7%)
Other (ifosfamide, paclitaxel, paclitaxel/bevacizumab, irinotecan/dacarbazine, trabectedin)	5 (20.8%)
3rd line chemotherapy regimens	
Doxorubicin based	4 (36.4%)
Doxorubicin alone	2
AI (doxorubicin/ifosfamide)	1
ADIC (doxorubicin/dacarbazine)	1
Platinum based****	2 (18.2%)
Other (ifosfamide (2), paclitaxel, I/E⁺⁺, TMZ⁺⁺⁺)	5 (45.5%)

Chemotherapy dosing: gemcitabine 675 to 900 mg/m^2, docetaxel 75 to 100 mg/m^2, vincristine 2 mg, doxorubicin 60 to 75 mg/m^2, ifosfamide 7.5 to 10 gm/m^2, and dacarbazine 750 to 1000 mg/m^2; *doxorubicin/cyclophosphamide/cisplatin (1), low-dose doxorubicin/ifosfamide (50 mg/m^2, 2.4 gm/m^2) (1), doxorubicin/cisplatin (1), vincristine/doxorubicin/cyclophosphamide (1), doxorubicin/cisplatin/paclitaxel (1), doxorubicin/dacarbazine/cyclophosphamide (3), doxorubicin/carboplatin (1), and vincristine/doxorubicin/cyclophosphamide/dacarbazine (1); **carboplatin/docetaxel (2), bleomycin/etoposide/cisplatin (2), carboplatin/paclitaxel (4), cisplatin with weekly radiation (2), carboplatin/paclitaxel/bevacizumab (1), and carboplatin/cyclophosphamide (1); ***carboplatin/docetaxel (1), carboplatin/paclitaxel (1), cisplatin/ifosfamide (1), and carboplatin/gemcitabine (1); ****carboplatin/gemcitabine (1) and cisplatin/gemcitabine (1); ⁺one patient had liposomal doxorubicin; ⁺⁺ifosfamide/etoposide; ⁺⁺⁺temozolomide.

be calculated. Four patients received only 1 cycle of chemotherapy and were excluded. Imaging was not accessible for review in another twenty-five patients. Twenty-one patients with chemotherapy for 1st line recurrent or metastatic disease were evaluable for response per RECIST 1.1 (Table 4). The complete response (CR) + partial response (PR) rate for doxorubicin-based 1st line chemotherapy was 40% versus 25% for gemcitabine/docetaxel. Another 14 patients received 2nd or 3rd line chemotherapy and were evaluable for response per RECIST 1.1. The CR + PR rate for doxorubicin-based 1st, 2nd, and 3rd line chemotherapy was 31.2% versus 14.3% for gemcitabine/docetaxel (Table 3). The majority of the responses with doxorubicin-based regimens were seen in patients receiving the combination of doxorubicin and ifosfamide (4/5 pts) or doxorubicin and dacarbazine (1/5 pts). The rate of CR + PR + stable disease (SD) was 87.5% for doxorubicin-based regimens and only 42.9% for gemcitabine/docetaxel. Only five patients with a platinum-based regimen were evaluable for RECIST 1.1, 80% had SD, and the one patient with a partial response, also, received ifosfamide.

3.6. Survival Analysis

3.6.1. Overall Survival and Progression-Free Survival. The median overall survival after 1st recurrence was 1.8 yrs. Table 3 shows the median overall survival and progression-free survival from the beginning of 1st line chemotherapy for patients receiving 1st line chemotherapy for recurrent or metastatic disease. Thirty-seven patients were evaluable for time-to-event outcomes. Nine patients received only one cycle of chemotherapy and were excluded from these

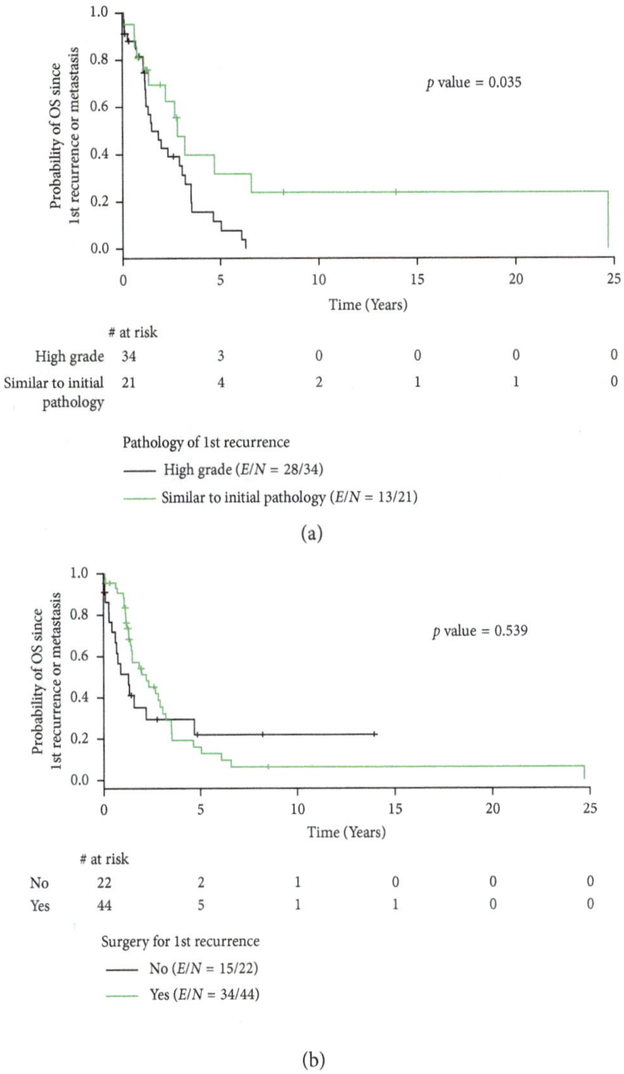

FIGURE 1: (a). Overall survival by pathology on recurrence. (b) Overall survival by surgery on recurrence.

analyses. The median overall survival from the beginning of 1st line chemotherapy was 16.6 months. Median overall survival differed by the chemotherapy regimen (Figure 2(a)). Median overall survival was worse for all doxorubicin-based regimens, 14.9 months, when compared to gemcitabine/docetaxel, 24.9 months, or platinum-based chemotherapy, 24.3 months. The median overall survival for doxorubicin/ifosfamide (AI) was 22.5 months, not statistically different from gemcitabine/docetaxel ($p = 0.99$) or platinum-based regimens (0.49). The median overall survival for doxorubicin-based regimens, other than AI, was 13.1 months. Additionally, patients who received AI had improved PFS (15.4 months) compared to other doxorubicin-based regimens (6.5 months), gemcitabine/docetaxel (5.0 mo), and platinum-based regimens (5.7 months) (Figure 2(b)). This difference trended toward statistical significance when comparing AI to other doxorubicin-based regimens $p = 0.083$ or to platinum-based regimens $p = 0.06$.

Patients were analyzed for other factors which may have influenced the effectiveness of their chemotherapeutic regimens, such as chemotherapy dosing, # of chemotherapy cycles, presence of sarcomatous overgrowth (SO), point in their disease course when they received chemotherapy, and time to recurrence prior to initiation of chemotherapy, a potential indicator of the aggressiveness of their disease. Patients did not significantly differ in terms of chemotherapy dosing, # of chemotherapy cycles, presence of SO, or point in their disease course when they received chemotherapy. The median time to recurrence prior to initiation of 1st line chemotherapy was 10.1 months for all doxorubicin-based regimens, 12.9 months for AI, 9.6 months for other doxorubicin-based regimens, 8.1 months for platinum-based regimens, and 21.7 months for gemcitabine/docetaxel, indicating a possible physician bias for treating patients with doxorubicin-based regimens in patients with quicker relapses, so more aggressive disease.

3.7. Hormonal Therapy for Recurrent or Metastatic Disease. Twenty-eight patients received hormonal therapy at some point during their treatment course. Seven patients received more than 1 line of hormonal therapy. Initial hormonal therapies included GnRH agonists (leuprolide, 9 pts), progesterones (megestrol acetate, 7 pts), SERMs (tamoxifen 3 pts and raloxifene 1 pt), and aromatase inhibitors (anastrozole 3 pts and letrozole 1 pt). The medial overall survival for patients with recurrent disease who received hormonal therapy was 34.7 months compared to 17.6 months, a trend toward improved outcomes that was not statistically significant, $p = 0.15$.

Out of these twenty-eight patients, there were four that derived several years of benefit from hormonal therapy. Two patients treated with leuprolide had disease control for >2 years. Their tumors were not stained for the estrogen receptor (ER) or progesterone receptor (PR). A third patient was placed on leuprolide after surgical resection with the development of progression after two years. This patient was then placed on megestrol acetate without response and then on anastrozole with a complete response lasting for eight years. This patient developed a 2nd malignancy. She was taken off anastrozole at the time of surgery for her cholangiocarcinoma. Shortly after completing adjuvant chemotherapy for her cholangiocarcinoma, she developed recurrence of her adenosarcoma, biopsy proven. She was placed back on anastrozole with response lasting for another five years. More recently, she developed progression and is now on systemic chemotherapy with trabectedin. This patient's tumor stained for ER 80% and PR 40%. The mesenchymal portion of her initial tumor was described as endometrial stromal sarcoma, though she did have sarcomatous overgrowth noted as well. A fourth elderly patient with locally advanced unresectable disease was treated with leuprolide and carboplatin for seven cycles leading to a partial response. Her leuprolide was continued after chemotherapy resulting in a complete response after five years with resolution of her pelvic mass and remaining subcentimeter pelvic lymphadenopathy. She continued leuprolide for 14 years, at which point her leuprolide was stopped. She then developed radiographic recurrence within the abdomen and was restarted on leuprolide with stable

Table 3: Treatment outcomes on recurrence with chemotherapy for recurrent or metastatic disease.

	Median survival	p value	HR	95% CI
OS by pathology on recurrence				
High-grade sarcomatous component only	17.6 mo			
Similar to initial pathology	33.5 mo	0.035	0.47	0.23–0.96
1st line chemotherapy				
OS				
All patients	16.6 mo	—		
Doxorubicin-based regimen	14.9 mo	—		
Doxorubicin/ifosfamide	22.5 mo	ref		
Other doxorubicin-based regimens	13.1 mo	0.18	2.18	0.69–6.88
Gemcitabine/docetaxel	24.9 mo	0.99	0.99	0.30–3.38
Platinum-based regimen	24.3 mo	0.49	0.60	0.14–2.53
PFS				
All patients	7.0 mo	—		
Doxorubicin-based regimen	8.5 mo	—		
Doxorubicin/ifosfamide	15.4 mo	ref		
Other doxorubicin-based regimens	6.5 mo	0.083	2.65	0.88–7.98
Gemcitabine/docetaxel	5.0 mo	0.27	1.87	0.62–5.63
Platinum-based regimen	5.7 mo	0.06	3.08	0.95–9.93
1st line chemotherapy additional treatments				
OS				
Surgery	21.6 mo			
No surgery	11.9 mo	0.12	1.36	0.73–2.53
PFS				
Surgery	12.0 mo			
No surgery	3.6 mo	0.02	2.04	1.10–3.77
OS by hormonal therapy for patients with recurrence				
Received hormonal therapy	34.7 mo			
No hormonal therapy	17.6 mo	0.15	1.58	0.85–2.95
OS therapy for 1st recurrence	21.8 mo			
Surgery	26.3 mo			
No surgery	15.1 mo	0.54	1.21	0.66–2.24
Radiation	16.5 mo			
No radiation	23.4 mo	0.58	0.83	0.42–1.63
Chemotherapy	18.6 mo			
No chemotherapy	27.6 mo	0.58	0.85	0.47–1.53
Chemotherapy + surgery	23.4 mo			
No chemotherapy + surgery	16.5 mo	0.97	1.01	0.55–1.85

OS, overall survival; PFS, progression-free survival; TTP, time to progression.

disease until her death at age 95. The ER/PR status and SO status of her tumor are unknown.

4. Discussion

In this study, we report the largest single-institution experience with recurrent or metastatic uterine and extrauterine adenosarcoma. There is no standard treatment for patients with local recurrence or metastatic uterine adenosarcoma. Treatment options include surgery, radiation, chemotherapy, and hormonal therapy. This study is the first to show that the pathology on recurrence influences outcomes. Specifically, those patients that present with a recurrence that is purely high-grade sarcoma have significantly worse outcomes than those patients who present with a recurrent tumor with mixed epithelial and mesenchymal components. This may represent selective clonal evolution of these tumors such that patients with a recurrence of pure high-grade sarcoma have a more clinically aggressive course.

The majority of uterine adenosarcomas recur locally, suggesting that resection of a local recurrence may improve overall survival and time to next recurrence. Previous reports have indicated a benefit for secondary cytoreduction of recurrent adenosarcoma in terms of overall survival and

Table 4: Response rates with chemotherapy for recurrent or metastatic disease.

	1st line chemotherapy	All lines of chemotherapy (1, 2, 3)
Doxorubicin-based regimens		
CR	2 (20%)	3 (18.7%) (AI (2), ADIC)
PR	2 (20%)	2 (12.5%) (AI, VAI)
(CR + PR)	4 (40%)	5 (31.2%)
SD	5 (50%)	9 (56.3%) (AI (4), ADIC, Dox (3), CyA)
(CR + PR + SD)	9 (90%)	14 (87.5%)
PD	1 (10%)	2 (12.5%) (AI, Dox)
Total patients	10	16
Gemcitabine/docetaxel		
CR	1 (12.5%)	1 (7.1%)
PR	1 (12.5%)	1 (7.1%)
(CR + PR)	2 (25%)	2 (14.3%)
SD	3 (37.5%)	6 (42.9%)
(CR + PR + SD)	5 (62.5%)	8 (57.1%)
PD	3 (37.5%)	6 (42.9%)
Total patients	8	14
Platinum-based regimens		
CR	0	0
PR	0	1 (20%) (Cis/Ifos)
(CR + PR)	0	1 (20%)
SD	3 (100%)	4 (80%) (Cis/Gem, Cis + XRT, carbo/taxol (2))
(CR + PR + SD)	3 (100%)	5 (100%)
PD	0	0
Total patients	3	5

CR, complete response; PR, partial response; SD, stable disease; PD, progressive disease; AI, doxorubicin/ifosfamide; ADIC, doxorubicin/dacarbazine; VAI, vincristine/doxorubicin/ifosfamide; Dox, doxorubicin; CyA, doxorubicin/cyclophosphamide; Cis, cisplatin; Ifos, ifosfamide; Gem, gemcitabine; carbo, carboplatin; XRT, radiation; taxol, paclitaxel.

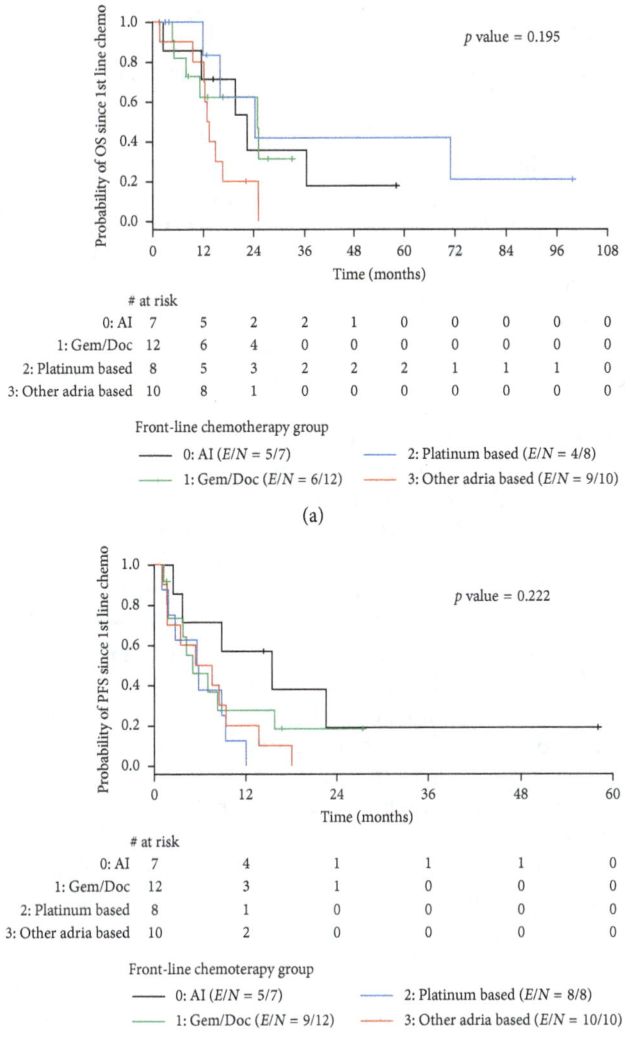

Figure 2: (a) and (b) Overall survival and progression-free survival for 1st line chemotherapy for recurrent or metastatic disease.

time to next recurrence [12, 21]. Our study shows an improvement in overall survival for those patients that underwent surgery for 1st recurrence, though this was not statistically significant. There is a selection bias in this result, in that patients able to undergo surgery likely had better functional status at the time of surgery, less medical comorbidities, and recurrence amenable to surgical resection. However, given the improvement in overall survival, it may be worth considering surgical resection of a recurrence, for those patients amenable to surgery.

This is the first retrospective report to examine the use of systemic chemotherapy in a large population of recurrent uterine adenosarcoma. Case reports and case series have described responses in adenosarcoma with the use of doxorubicin-based regimens [21–26], gemcitabine/docetaxel [21, 27], trabectedin [28], or platinum-based regimens [21]. This report shows that active agents in uterine adenosarcoma are doxorubicin/ifosfamide (AI), doxorubicin/dacarbazine (ADIC), and gemcitabine/docetaxel. The most effective agents for adenosarcoma in terms of response per RECIST 1.1 were the combination of doxorubicin and ifosfamide. All three are reasonable chemotherapeutic choices for recurrent or metastatic uterine adenosarcoma. The dosing of chemotherapy in this retrospective study varied greatly; however, the patients that received gemcitabine/docetaxel received 675 to 900 mg/m^2 of gemcitabine and 75 to 100 mg/m^2 of docetaxel; the patients that received doxorubicin-based regimens received 60 to 75 mg/m^2 of doxorubicin, 7.5 to 10 gm/m^2 of ifosfamide, and 750 to 1000 mg/m^2 of dacarbazine. This is standard sarcoma chemotherapy dosing.

The OS after 1st line chemotherapy for recurrent or metastatic disease was not statistically different between AI, gem/doc, or platinum-based regimens. However, OS may be affected by subsequent therapies such as surgery, hormonal therapy, or further chemotherapy. Additionally, there was a trend toward worse survival for patients that received other doxorubicin-based regimens excluding AI, suggesting that ifosfamide is required to obtain the higher response rate and clinical benefit. However, whether this effective is limited to ifosfamide alone or a result of synergy between doxorubicin/ifosfamide, as noted in soft tissue sarcomas, is undetermined [29].

PFS may be a better measure of benefit from systemic chemotherapy. Patients who received AI had the longest PFS (15.4 months), with a trend toward statistical significance when compared to patients who received doxorubicin alone or in combination with a 2nd agent or platinum-based regimens. If the goal of therapy is to produce reduction in tumor size prior to surgical resection of recurrent disease, AI chemotherapy may have advantages over gemcitabine/docetaxel. If patients are older with poor function status and multiple medical comorbidities, they are not a doxorubicin/ifosfamide candidate; then gemcitabine/docetaxel may be the preferred regimen. Cisplatin- and carboplatin-based regimens appear to be the least effective in uterine adenosarcomas and should not be recommended for treatment of recurrent or metastatic disease. Further study is required to evaluate the role of trabectedin in the treatment of uterine adenosarcomas.

It should be noted that there was likely a physician bias in choosing treatment with doxorubicin-based regimens over gemcitabine/docetaxel. There was a shorter median time to recurrence prior to the start of 1st line chemotherapy with AI (12.9 months) or other doxorubicin-based regimens (9.6 months) compared to gemcitabine/docetaxel (21.7 months), indicating that physicians were more likely to treat with doxorubicin-based regimens than with gemcitabine/docetaxel for patients that had quicker relapses, or more aggressive disease. This suggests a benefit of doxorubicin/ifosfamide over gemcitabine/docetaxel in the treatment of uterine adenosarcomas, despite similar median OS, as patients with more aggressive disease would be expected to have worse survival.

Evidence for the use of hormonal therapy in uterine adenosarcoma is even more limited than evidence for the use of chemotherapy. Case reports or case series have noted responses to hormonal therapy lasting 10 months to 7 years [12, 30–33]. Agents used include GnRH agonists, progesterones, selective estrogen receptor modulators, or aromatase inhibitors. Responses have been occasionally correlated with the presence of estrogen receptor (ER) and progesterone receptor (PR) staining. Loss of ER and PR expressions has been associated with sarcomatous overgrowth [34]. Furthermore, loss of response to hormonal therapy was associated with reduced ER/PR expression in one case report [33]. This suggests ER and PR as possible predictors of response to hormonal therapy in uterine adenosarcomas, though this has not been studied in a systematic manner. In this study, the majority of patients (86%) did not receive benefit from hormonal therapy, though there were 4 patients that derived benefit in terms of stable disease and improved survival from leuprolide or anastrozole for 2 to 15 years, suggesting that select patients may have a benefit from hormonally targeted therapy. Unfortunately, we are currently unable to determine which patients will receive such a large benefit from hormonal therapy.

This study is limited by its retrospective nature and small sample size, though this is the largest single-institution recurrent or metastatic uterine or extrauterine adenosarcoma series to date. Overall, uterine adenosarcoma is a rare disease with limited evidence-based data to determine treatment recommendations. Treatment of recurrence or metastatic disease can consist of surgery, chemotherapy, preferable with doxorubicin/ifosfamide or gemcitabine/docetaxel, or hormonal therapy in select patients.

Acknowledgments

This study was funded by the WWWW Foundation, Inc. (QuadW), and Amschwand Sarcoma Cancer Foundation.

References

[1] V. M. Abeler, O. Royne, S. Thoresen, H. E. Danielsen, J. M. Nesland, and G. B. Kristensen, "Uterine sarcomas in Norway. A histopathological and prognostic survey of a total population from 1970 to 2000 including 419 patients," *Histopathology*, vol. 54, no. 3, pp. 355–364, 2009.

[2] V. Benito, A. Lubrano, O. Arencibia et al., "Clinicopathologic analysis of uterine sarcomas from a single institution in the Canary Islands," *International Journal of Gynaecology and Obstetrics*, vol. 107, no. 1, pp. 44–49, 2009.

[3] P. B. Clement and R. E. Scully, "Müllerian adenosarcoma of the uterus. A clinicopathologic analysis of ten cases of a distinctive type of Müllerian mixed tumor," *Cancer*, vol. 34, no. 4, pp. 1138–1149, 1974.

[4] P. B. Clement and R. E. Scully, "Müllerian adenosarcoma of the uterus: a clinicopathologic analysis of 100 cases with a review of the literature," *Human Pathology*, vol. 21, no. 4, pp. 363–381, 1990.

[5] T. Kaku, S. G. Silverberg, F. J. Major, A. Miller, B. Fetter, and J. A. Blessing, "Adenosarcoma of the uterus: a gynecologic oncology group clinicopathologic study of 31 cases," *International Journal of Gynecological Pathology*, vol. 11, no. 2, pp. 75–88, 1992.

[6] J. H. Eichhorn, R. H. Young, P. B. Clement, and R. E. Scully, "Mesodermal (müllerian) adenosarcoma of the ovary: a clinicopathologic analysis of 40 cases and a review of the literature," *American Journal of Surgical Pathology*, vol. 26, no. 10, pp. 1243–1258, 2002.

[7] M. W. Jones and M. Lefkowitz, "Adenosarcoma of the uterine cervix: a clinicopathological study of 12 cases," *International Journal of Gynecological Pathology*, vol. 14, no. 3, pp. 223–229, 1995.

[8] Y. Wang, Y. W. Huang, and Y. F. Li, "Primary vaginal sarcoma: experience of a regional cancer center in China," *Journal of Obstetrics and Gynaecology Research*, vol. 41, no. 9, pp. 1463–1468, 2015.

[9] P. B. Clement and R. E. Scully, "Extrauterine mesodermal (müllerian) adenosarcoma: a clinicopathologic analysis of five cases," *American Journal of Clinical Pathology*, vol. 69, no. 3, pp. 276–283, 1978.

[10] J. Prat, "FIGO staging for uterine sarcomas," *International Journal of Gynecology and Obstetrics*, vol. 104, no. 3, pp. 177-178, 2009.

[11] S. E. Brooks, M. Zhan, T. Cote, and C. R. Baquet, "Surveillance, epidemiology, and end results analysis of 2677 cases of uterine sarcoma 1989–1999," *Gynecologic Oncology*, vol. 93, no. 1, pp. 204–208, 2004.

[12] A. Carroll, P. T. Ramirez, S. N. Westin et al., "Uterine adenosarcoma: an analysis on management, outcomes, and

risk factors for recurrence," *Gynecologic Oncology*, vol. 135, no. 3, pp. 455–461, 2014.

[13] B. Bernard, B. A. Clarke, J. I. Malowany et al., "Uterine adenosarcomas: a dual-institution update on staging, prognosis and survival," *Gynecologic Oncology*, vol. 131, no. 3, pp. 634–639, 2013.

[14] R. Arend, M. Bagaria, S. N. Lewin et al., "Long-term outcome and natural history of uterine adenosarcomas," *Gynecologic Oncology*, vol. 119, no. 2, pp. 305–308, 2010.

[15] R. Blom and C. Guerrieri, "Adenosarcoma of the uterus: a clinicopathologic, DNA flow cytometric, p53 and mdm-2 analysis of 11 cases," *International Journal of Gynecological Cancer*, vol. 9, no. 1, pp. 37–43, 1999.

[16] M. J. Nathenson, V. Ravi, N. Fleming, W.-L. Wang, and A. Conley, "Uterine adenosarcoma: a review," *Current Oncology Reports*, vol. 18, no. 11, p. 68, 2016.

[17] E. L. Kaplan and P. Meier, "Nonparametric estimator from incomplete observations," *Journal of the American Statistical Association*, vol. 53, no. 282, pp. 457–481, 1958.

[18] E. A. Eisenhauer, P. Therasse, J. Bogaerts et al., "New response evaluation criteria in solid tumours: revised RECIST guideline (version 1.1)," *European Journal of Cancer*, vol. 45, no. 2, pp. 228–247, 2009.

[19] N. Mantel, "Evaluation of survival data and two new rank order statistics arising in its consideration," *Cancer Chemotherapy Reports*, vol. 50, no. 3, pp. 163–170, 1966.

[20] D. R. Cox, "Regression models and life tables (with discussion)," *Journal of the Royal Statistical Society: Series B*, vol. 34, no. 2, pp. 187–220, 1972.

[21] E. J. Tanner, T. Toussaint, M. M. Leitao Jr. et al., "Management of uterine adenosarcomas with and without sarcomatous overgrowth," *Gynecologic Oncology*, vol. 129, no. 1, pp. 140–144, 2013.

[22] W. Yamagami, N. Susumu, T. Ninomiya et al., "A retrospective study on combination therapy with ifosfamide, adriamycin and cisplatin for progressive or recurrent uterine sarcoma," *Molecular and Clinical Oncology*, vol. 2, pp. 591–595, 2014.

[23] M. G. del Carmen, D. Lovett, and A. Goodman, "A case of müllerian adenosarcoma of the uterus treated with liposomal doxorubicin," *Gynecologic Oncology*, vol. 88, no. 3, pp. 456–458, 2003.

[24] M. Maeda, S. Mabuchi, Y. Matsumoto et al., "Activity of pegylated liposomal doxorubicin for extragenital müllerian adenosarcoma with sarcomatous overgrowth: a case report and a review of the literature," *European Journal of Gynaecological Oncology*, vol. 32, no. 5, pp. 542–546, 2011.

[25] G. S. Huang, R. C. Arend, A. Sakaris, T. M. Hebert, and G. L. Goldberg, "Extragenital adenosarcoma: a case report, review of the literature, and management discussion," *Gynecologic Oncology*, vol. 115, no. 3, pp. 472–475, 2009.

[26] L. D. Roman, M. F. Mitchell, C. Tornos, A. Glover, and J. J. Kavanagh, "Dedifferentiated extrauterine adenosarcoma responsive to chemotherapy," *Gynecologic Oncology*, vol. 49, no. 3, pp. 389–394, 1993.

[27] C. F. Verschraegen, H. Arias-Pulido, S. J. Lee et al., "Phase IB study of the combination of docetaxel, gemcitabine, and bevacizumab in patients with advanced or recurrent soft tissue sarcoma: the Axtell regimen," *Annals of Oncology*, vol. 23, no. 3, pp. 785–790, 2012.

[28] B. A. Schroeder, E. T. Rodler, E. T. Loggers, S. M. Pollack, and R. L. Jones, "Clinical benefit of trabectedin in uterine adenosarcoma," *Medical Oncology*, vol. 30, no. 2, p. 501, 2013.

[29] J. H. Edmonson, L. M. Ryan, R. H. Blum et al., "Randomized comparison of doxorubicin alone versus ifosfamide plus doxorubicin or mitomycin, doxorubicin, and cisplatin against advanced soft tissue sarcomas," *Journal of Clinical Oncology*, vol. 11, no. 7, pp. 1269–1275, 1993.

[30] B. J. Hines, R. F. Porges, K. Mittal et al., "Use of medroxyprogesterone acetate in the treatment of müllerian adenosarcoma: a case report," *Gynecologic Oncology*, vol. 85, no. 1, pp. 192–195, 2002.

[31] SJ. Lee, JH. Bae, DC. Kim, J. S. Park, and S. E. Namkoong, "Oral progesterone treatment in a young woman with müllerian adenosarcoma whose ovary was preserved: a case report," *International Journal of Gynecological Cancer*, vol. 20, no. 7, pp. 1222–1224, 2010.

[32] T. J. Gruber, A. J. Fabiano, G. Deeb, S. B. Lele, and R. A. Fenstermaker, "Intracranial meningiomas in patients with uterine sarcoma treated with long-term megestrol acetate therapy," *World Neurosurgery*, vol. 76, no. 5, pp. 477.e16–477.e20, 2011.

[33] N. Tasaka, K. Matsumoto, T. Satoh et al., "Therapeutic effect of dienogest on adenosarcoma arising from endometriosis: a case report," *SpringerPlus*, vol. 2, no. 1, p. 618, 2013.

[34] R. A. Soslow, A. Ali, and E. Oliva, "Müllerian adenosarcomas: an immunophenotypic analysis of 35 cases," *American Journal of Surgical Pathology*, vol. 32, no. 7, pp. 1013–1021, 2008.

21

Multiple Soft Tissue Sarcomas in a Single Patient: An International Multicentre Review

Johnathan R. Lex,[1] Ahmed Aoude,[2] Jonathan D. Stevenson,[3] Jay S. Wunder,[4] Scott Evans,[3] Peter C. Ferguson,[4] Nikolaos A. Stavropoulos,[2] Lee Jeys,[3,5] Krista Goulding,[2] and Robert E. Turcotte[2]

[1]*University of Birmingham, Birmingham B15 2TT, UK*
[2]*McGill University Health Centre, Montreal, QC, Canada H4A 3J1*
[3]*Royal Orthopaedic Hospital, Birmingham B31 2AP, UK*
[4]*University of Toronto Musculoskeletal Oncology Unit, Mount Sinai Hospital, Toronto, ON, Canada M5G 1X5*
[5]*School of Life and Health Sciences, Aston University, Birmingham B4 7ET, UK*

Correspondence should be addressed to Robert E. Turcotte; robert.turcotte@muhc.mcgill.ca

Academic Editor: Antoine Italiano

Developing multiple soft tissue sarcomas (STSs) is a rare process, sparsely reported in the literature to date. Little is known about the pattern of disease development or outcomes in these patients. Patients were identified from three tertiary orthopaedic oncology centres in Canada and the UK. Patients who developed multiple extremity STSs were collated retrospectively from prospective oncology databases. A literature review using MEDLINE was also performed. Six patients were identified in the case series from these three institutions, and five studies were identified from the literature review. Overall, 17 patients were identified with a median age of 51 years (range: 19 to 77). The prevalence of this manifestation in STS patients is 1 in 1225. The median disease-free interval between diagnoses was 2.3 years (range: 0 to 19 years). Most patients developed the secondary STS in a metachronous pattern, the remaining, synchronously. The median survival after the first sarcoma was 6 years, and it was 1.6 years after the second sarcoma. The 5-year overall survival rate was 83.3% and 50% following the first and second STS diagnoses, respectively. A diagnosis of two STSs does not confer a worse prognosis than the diagnosis of a single STS. Developing a second STS is a rare event with no identifiable histological pattern of occurrence. Presentation in a metachronous pattern is more common. A high degree of vigilance is required in patients with a previous STS both to detect both local recurrence and to identify new masses remote from the previous STS site. Acquiring an early histological diagnosis should be attempted.

1. Introduction

Soft tissue sarcoma (STS) is a general term assigned to a group of rare malignant tumours arising from a mesenchymal stem cell. The term "sarcoma" encompasses approximately 100 different histological subtypes of tumour as per the latest World Health Organization Classification of Tumours of Soft Tissue and Bone (4th edition) [1]. STS accounts for less than 1% of all malignant neoplasms in adults and around 4–8% in children [2]. Prognosis for sarcomas has improved, on average the 5-year overall survival rate being around 60% [3]. However, this figure varies widely depending on the tumour grade, size, stage at diagnosis, depth, location, and histological subtype [4]. The most commonly used staging system for STS (the American Joint Committee on Cancer [5]) uses the first three listed prognostic factors when calculating the stage of a sarcoma.

Commonly, the primary complaint of a patient presenting with a suspected soft tissue sarcoma is the presence of an enlarging, painless mass. Detailed evaluation of the mass and its association with surrounding structures is crucial [6]. Certain types of STSs (synovial sarcoma,

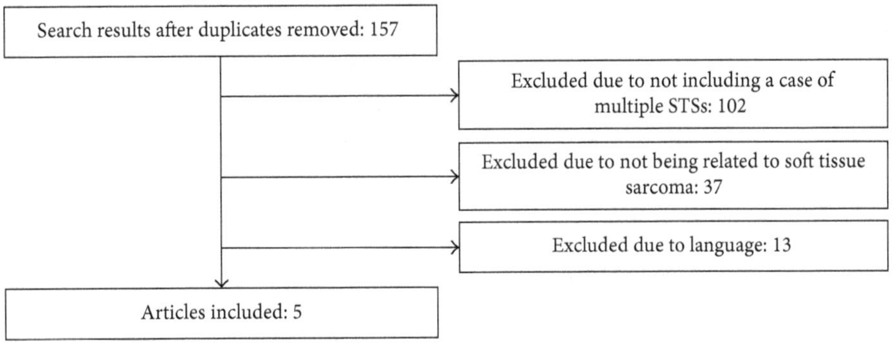

FIGURE 1: Results of the literature search.

epithelioid sarcoma, clear-cell sarcoma, rhabdomyosarcoma, and angiosarcoma) have a tendency to spread via the lymphatic system, thereby warranting palpation of local lymphatics for other masses [7]. However, it is not currently considered routine practice to screen for a second primary soft tissue mass on an initial evaluation for sarcoma.

Although uncommon, patients with STS have an increased risk of developing a second primary neoplasm (carcinoma), even when excluding known syndromic associations such as Li–Fraumeni syndrome and neurofibromatosis [8, 9]. Outside of these syndromes, there have been very few reports on patients developing multiple STSs. Furthermore, there are no reports on how the development of multiple STSs correlates with patient survival. This study aims to elucidate the impact of a diagnosis of multiple STSs on survival and whether there are any associated chronological or histological disease patterns.

2. Methods

2.1. Patient Identification. Two tertiary sarcoma centres in Canada and one in the United Kingdom collaborated in this study. A retrospective review from 1997 to July 2017 was conducted using the prospectively collated oncology databases at each centre. Electronic notes were searched using a combination of the following terms: "sarcoma," "multiple," "new," "different," "synchronous," and "metachronous." A list of patients was generated when the database notes indicated the possibility of a second primary soft tissue sarcoma. Patients with two or more histologically confirmed extremity STSs were manually identified. Clinical information including the patient demographics, pathologic diagnosis, tumour site, operation, and survival outcomes were gathered from clinical notes. Diagnoses were made by specialized musculoskeletal pathologists at the three centres. No minimum follow-up criteria were assigned in order to maximize inclusion.

In most cases, access to both STS specimens was available to allow direct comparison for accurate histological diagnosis and to distinguish this from a distant soft tissue metastasis of the original primary sarcoma or a radiation-induced sarcoma. Cahan's criteria were used to discern a second primary sarcoma from an iatrogenic sarcoma secondary to radiation, which are a latency period of at least 2 years, the tumour must arise in the direct region of previous radiation, and the sarcoma must be histologically different from the previously radiated lesion [10].

2.2. Literature Review. A search was conducted using the MEDLINE OVID interface from 1946 to July 2017. The search strategy used was [Sarcoma OR ST neoplasm] AND [synchronous OR metachronous]. Inclusion criteria included English, human studies with one or more of the subjects with multiple sarcomas. This yielded 157 results, of which five papers were identified that met the inclusion criteria (Figure 1). Manual searching through reference lists was also conducted.

Patients identified in our case series and in the literature review with desmoid tumours, Kaposi sarcoma, and gastrointestinal stromal tumours (GISTs) were excluded from the study due to their unique disease pattern which differs from that of other STSs.

3. Results

3.1. Case Series. Six patients were identified to meet the study inclusion criteria after detailed interrogation of the databases from the three tertiary orthopaedic oncology centres. Amongst all patients with STS at these centres ($n = 7351$), this amounted to a prevalence of 0.08%. The median age of the patients in our series was 54.5 years (range: 28 to 67). Five (83.3%) of the patients were male, and the other was female. The median interval between the diagnosis of the primary and secondary sarcomas was 2.7 years (range: 0.1 to 4.6 years).

Four (66.7%) patients developed sarcomas in a metachronous pattern. The diagnosis interval for the remaining two patients was 1 and 5 months. Although both primary tumours were not diagnosed at the same time, the interval is short enough to be considered a synchronous pattern. Four patients developed their second STS on the ipsilateral side to the first, three of which occurred in different areas of the same limb, while the fourth patient's first STS occurred in the hand followed by one in the lower limb. Liposarcoma was the most common diagnosis, followed by undifferentiated pleomorphic sarcoma (Table 1).

The median time from first sarcoma diagnosis to last follow-up was 7.7 years (range: 0.8 to 12.9). Five (83.3%) patients were alive with no evidence of disease at last follow-

TABLE 1: Case series: patient demographics and outcomes.

Patient	Age	Gender	First tumour type	Location	Second tumour type	Location	Radiotherapy (1st or 2nd)	Time between diagnoses (months)	Diagnosis to last f/u (months)	Status at last f/u
1	28	M	Pseudomyogenic hemangioendothelioma	R 5th metatarsal	Myxoid liposarcoma	R popliteal	Yes (2)	1	6	NED
2	60	M	Pleomorphic liposarcoma	L groin	Epitheliod hemangioendothelioma	L thigh and calf	Yes (1)	28	32	NED
3	67	F	Fibrosarcoma	R forearm	Undifferentiated pleomorphic sarcoma	L buttock	Yes (1)	41	137	NED
4	49	M	Epithelioid sarcoma	L thumb	Myxoid liposarcoma	L popliteal	Yes (2)	5	125	NED
5	67	M	Undifferentiated pleomorphic sarcoma	R calf	Malignant solitary fibrous tumour	R ankle	Yes (2)	55	155	Deceased
6	38	M	Malignant solitary fibrous tumour	L thigh	Undifferentiated pleomorphic sarcoma	R chest wall	Yes (1 + 2)	36	60	NED

M = male; F = female; R = right; L = left; 1 = radiotherapy for the first sarcoma; 2 = radiotherapy for the second sarcoma; NED = no evidence of disease; f/u = follow-up.

up. One patient developed a local recurrence 33 months after resection of their second sarcoma; however, this was resected, and the patient remained free of disease before dying 7 years later with no evidence of sarcoma recurrence. Two patients developed metastasis amenable to complete metastasectomy at 2 and 60 months after the first and second STS excision, respectively. Following metastasectomy, these patients had no evidence of disease at 10.1 and 3.2 years of follow-up.

All patients were managed under the care of a sarcoma multidisciplinary team (MDT), with treatment following international guidelines active at the time. One patient was treated with radiotherapy for both sarcomas, while five patients received radiation for only one of their two sarcomas. Of the patients who underwent radiotherapy for only one sarcoma, two received it for the first sarcoma and three for the second sarcoma. No patients received adjuvant chemotherapy treatment.

Postoperative surveillance comprised clinical examination for evidence of local and regional recurrence with subsequent magnetic resonance imaging (MRI) based on concerning clinical findings and chest radiography with subsequent computerized tomography (CT) to confirm metastasis based on abnormal radiographs. Follow-up occurred at 3-month intervals for the first 2 years, 6-month intervals until 5 years, and annually until 10 years following resection as per international guidelines [11].

3.2. Literature Review. Five patient series were identified that included patients with multiple different histologically confirmed STSs [8, 9, 12–14]. Two of the articles were case reports, and three were case series. From these five articles, 17 additional patients were identified. However, seven patients did not meet our inclusion criteria and were therefore excluded. Six patients were excluded from the study by Grobmyer et al. since the diagnoses include GIST or malignant mixed Mullerian tumour. One patient was excluded from the study by Merimsky et al. due to the possibility of the second sarcoma being radiation-induced [8, 9].

3.3. Combination of Case Series and Literature Review Cases. Combining data from our current case series and patients selected from the other five series equated to a total of 17 patients with a median age of 51 years (range: 19 to 77) including 9 males and 6 females (two patients' sex were not reported). The median interval between the first and second STS diagnoses was 2.3 years (range: 0 to 19). This included 6 (35.3%) synchronous manifestations of multiple sarcomas and 11 patients (64.7%) that developed distinct tumours in a metachronous pattern. The most common diagnosis was undifferentiated pleomorphic sarcoma ($n = 8$, 23.5%) followed by liposarcoma ($n = 6$, 17.6%) and leiomyosarcoma ($n = 5$, 14.7%). From available data, 7 (53.8%) patients' second tumours arose on the contralateral side and 6 (46.2%) on the ipsilateral side. Overall, tumours presented as high grade (grade 3) in 57.1% of cases, intermediate grade (grade 2) in 28.6% of cases, and low grade (grade 1) in 14.3% of cases (Tables 1 and 2).

The median time from first tumour diagnosis to death or last follow-up was 6 years (range: 0.2 to 26). The 5-year overall survival rate was 83.3%. Median survival time from the second sarcoma diagnosis was 1.6 years (range: 0 to 19) with a 5-year disease-free survival rate of 50%. Overall, six patients were deceased, and 11 were alive with no evidence of disease at last follow-up.

One series which included four patients did not report information on adjuvant therapy [8]. From the available information pertaining to the other 14 patients, adjuvant or neoadjuvant radiotherapy was utilized in 12 patients (85.7%). Three patients were treated with chemotherapy.

4. Discussion

A case series of 6 patients and literature review of 11 patients were conducted on multiple primary STSs occurring in individual patients. The aim of the study was to determine the impact developing a second primary STS had on overall survival and whether there are any predictable histological or chronological patterns to disease presentation. We hoped to better enable clinicians to provide a prognosis when faced with these patients as well as to advise on routine STS follow-up. The prognosis in these patients was found to be poor relative to patients with one STS diagnosis, and no predictable patterns of disease presentation were identified.

There are many possible explanations for the development of multiple sarcomas in a single patient. One possibility is that these patients may have a genetic predisposition to malignant mesenchymal disease that is currently not described. Alternatively, general risk factors for malignancy may have been the underlying cause such as immunocompromise or exposure to carcinogens, either environmental or iatrogenic. These factors have been associated with the formation of cancers [15–17], although uncommonly associated with STS. Many other possibilities can be hypothesized but are difficult to identify due to the rarity of the disease.

The median survival time from the first STS diagnosis was 6 years; however, it was only 1.6 years after the second STS diagnosis. The 5-year disease-free survival was 83.3% and 50%, after the first and second STS diagnoses, respectively. The American Cancer Society reported the mean 5-year survival rate of STS as 64% in 2017 [3]. In our review, the survival rate following the first STS diagnosis compares favourably. However, the 5-year survivorship of 50% following the second STS diagnosis is lower relative to the reported mean. This may be due to the morbidity associated with having a second tumour or the complications associated with additional treatment. However, these survival rates may have been negatively affected by a number of confounding factors, such as the short length of follow-up, the second STS diagnosis representing soft tissue metastases of the primary STS rather than a new primary, or because patients in one of the identified studies generally doing poorly [9]. Isolating patients from our case series, there was no evidence of multiple STSs conferring a poorer prognosis, as five of six patients had no evidence of disease at last follow-up with the other patient dying of unrelated causes.

Table 2: Literature review: patient demographics and outcomes by the study [8, 9, 12–14].

Study	Patient	Age	Gender	First tumour type	Location	Second tumour type	Location	Adjuvant treatment	Time between diagnosis (years)	Diagnosis to last f/u (years)
Schiffman [12]	1	26	M	Synovial sarcoma	L knee	Epithelioid sarcoma	L knee	CTx and RTx	7	26 (DOD)
Merimsky et al. [9]	2	—	—	Meningioma	Frontal lobe	Liposarcoma	Thigh	RTx and CTx	15	16.6 (NED)
	3	—	—	Undifferentiated pleomorphic sarcoma	Thigh	Undifferentiated pleomorphic sarcoma	Buttock	None	19	20.5 (NED)
Grobmyer et al. [8]	4	77	M	Dedifferentiated liposarcoma	Extremity	Solitary fibrous tumour	—	—	0	1 (NED)
	5	51	F	Well-differentiated liposarcoma	Extremity	Leiomyosarcoma	Retroperitoneum	—	0	0.16 (NED)
	6	56	F	Dermatofibrosarcoma protuberans	Extremity	Solitary fibrous tumour	Spine	—	0.5	0.5 (NED)
Daigeler et al. [13]	7	—	F	Leiomyosarcoma	R thigh	Leiomyosarcoma	L thigh	RTx	1.3	1.9 (DOD)
	8	—	M	Undifferentiated pleomorphic sarcoma	L thigh	Undifferentiated pleomorphic sarcoma	R thigh/groin	RTx	0.3	3.1 (DOD)
	9	—	M	Clear-cell sarcoma	R elbow	Clear-cell sarcoma	L elbow	RTx and CTx	9.5	11 (DOD)
	10	—	F	Leiomyosarcoma	L shin	Leiomyosarcoma	R calf	—	5.5	7.5 (DOD)
Scepanovic et al. [14]	11	19	F	Undifferentiated pleomorphic sarcoma	R shoulder	Undifferentiated pleomorphic sarcoma	L shoulder	RTx	1.5	6 (NED)

M = male; F = female; R = right; L = left; CTx = chemotherapy; RTx = radiotherapy; DOD = dead of disease; NED = no evidence of disease; f/u = follow-up.

Using available data, it is difficult to determine whether the length of the latent period between the STS diagnoses correlates with survival. However, we could anticipate an improved prognosis following the second STS if this tumour arises whilst patients are still being followed-up at a sarcoma centre for their first STS.

The prevalence of a patient with one STS developing a second STS is low, 0.082% or 1 in 1225. Grobmyer et al. were also able to determine the incidence of developing two STSs. They reported that, in a patient previously diagnosed with STS, the incidence of a second primary sarcoma was 1 per 2500 population, or 12.5 times greater than the standard incidence of STS [8]. Therefore, although still a relatively unusual event, the higher incidence in primary sarcoma patients needs to be kept in mind when following up these patients [18, 19].

No identifiable patterns were identified in terms of distinct STS subtypes presenting together in the same patient. The type of sarcoma that arises secondarily appears to be random, independent of the first sarcoma diagnosis. The time used to define synchronous development was 6 months or less between diagnoses. This cutoff time was chosen as it would be too narrow of an interval to develop two individual primaries meaning that the second tumour likely went unrecognized previously. The median time between sarcoma diagnoses was 2.3 years. Approximately one-third of patients developed the second sarcoma in a synchronous pattern, while in two-thirds, the second sarcoma developed metachronously. Therefore, more attention should be paid to identifying a second STS in patients during the postoperative follow-up period. Over recent years, there has been an increase in the use of whole-body staging studies, such as fluorodeoxyglucose positron emission tomography (FDG-PET) or whole body MRI. This may lead to an earlier detection of a second primary tumour in those patients who are undergoing staging at the initial diagnosis but also have a synchronous second primary STS. However, the cost and availability associated with the routine use of these tests need to be considered in light of the rarity of a diagnosis of a second soft tissue sarcoma.

The occurrence of a second STS in the same patient is very rare, and therefore, no change to the management of new patients or patient follow-up is recommended. During follow-up visits for a primary STS, a short screening phrase such as "Have you noticed any new lumps or bumps?" is recommended to raise attention to any newly developing masses. Any second mass a patient develops should not be presumed to be the same disease, and new histological diagnosis should be made. Therefore, we recommend reimaging, restaging, and a biopsy to help diagnose new disease, including radiation-induced tumours, from recurrence or metastasis [18]. In fact, new disease should always be suspected. Merimsky et al. noticed that the risk of developing a secondary neoplasm in patients with STS is significantly greater than that in the general population, 7.5% compared to 1% [9]. Therefore, thorough screening for new STSs or other neoplasms should be considered for patients with new symptoms at follow-up since they are at increased risk.

Unfortunately, several limitations to interpreting these figures exist including the short follow-up period of many patients. Only 12 of the 17 patients had follow-up to five years after diagnosis of their first sarcoma. As well, all patients from one series had very short survival after the second STS diagnosis, which may have skewed the results [9]. Another limitation includes the limited number of patients, hand-selected from observational data potentially introducing selection bias. Although all histologies were reviewed by a specialist musculoskeletal pathologist, they were not reviewed by the same pathologist, which may have slightly altered certain diagnoses. There were six cases identified in the literature review with the same histological diagnosis for the first and second sarcomas. Although reported as different sarcomas, we are uncertain as to whether these cases truly represent multiple distinct STSs or soft tissue metastases of previous sarcomas. Genetic testing was not routinely conducted; however, this could be considered for future studies. Although these limitations are recognized, this study helps to clarify this rare manifestation.

Further research is recommended as current available evidence is limited. Larger series of other orthopaedic oncology centres' experience and more case reports are encouraged to increase the amount of described information. This will hopefully help to uncover any patterns of disease occurrence which may lead to identifying risk factors or certain genetic predispositions.

5. Conclusion

In conclusion, this study aimed to help define the pattern of disease and outcomes in patients with nonsyndromic, non-radiation-induced multiple extremity STSs. The incidence of this scenario is very low, and more reports are encouraged. This study was unable to definitively demonstrate that patient prognosis with multiple STSs is poor relative to those diagnosed with a single sarcoma. A high index of suspicion should be maintained to detect a second STS in patients with a current or previous primary STS as they are at an increased risk compared to the general population. Our results demonstrate that majority of patients with multiple STSs present in a metachronous pattern of disease and require routine long-term screening. Management of the second sarcoma should continue in line with internationally recognized guidelines. The recommendations for practice include thorough screening for any new symptoms as well as ensuring a second histological diagnosis is made in the setting of a new mass.

References

[1] V. Y. Jo and C. D. Fletcher, "WHO classification of soft tissue tumours: an update based on the 2013 (4th) edition," *Pathology*, vol. 46, no. 2, pp. 95–104, 2014.

[2] F. Ducimetiere, A. Lurkin, D. Ranchère-Vince et al., "Incidence of sarcoma histotypes and molecular subtypes in

a prospective epidemiological study with central pathology review and molecular testing," *PloS One*, vol. 6, no. 8, article e20294, 2011.

[3] American Cancer Society, *Cancer Facts & Figures*, American Cancer Society, Atlanta, Georgia, 2017.

[4] R. Grimer, I. Judson, D. Peake, and B. Seddon, "Guidelines for the management of soft tissue sarcomas," *Sarcoma*, vol. 2010, Article ID 506182, 15 pages, 2010.

[5] J. S. Wunder, J. H. Healey, A. M. Davis, and M. F. Brennan, "A comparison of staging systems for localized extremity soft tissue sarcoma," *Cancer*, vol. 88, no. 12, pp. 2721–2730, 2000.

[6] E. M. Ramu, M. T. Houdek, C. E. Isaac, C. I. Dickie, P. C. Ferguson, and J. S. Wunder, "Management of soft-tissue sarcomas; treatment strategies, staging, and outcomes," *SICOT Journal*, vol. 3, no. 20, 2017.

[7] S. Riad, A. M. Griffin, B. Liberman et al., "Lymph node metastasis in soft tissue sarcoma in an extremity," *Clinical Orthopaedics and Related Research*, vol. 426, pp. 129–134, 2004.

[8] S. R. Grobmyer, N. Luther, C. Antonescu, S. Singer, and M. Brennan, "Multiple primary soft tissue sarcomas," *Cancer*, vol. 101, no. 11, pp. 2633–2635, 2004.

[9] O. Merimsky, Y. Kollender, J. Issakov et al., "Multiple primary malignancies in association with soft tissue sarcomas," *Cancer*, vol. 91, no. 7, pp. 1363–1371, 2001.

[10] W. G. Cahan, H. Q. Woodard, N. L. Higinbotham, F. W. Stewart, and B. L. Coley, "Sarcoma arising in irradiated bone; report of 11 cases," *Cancer*, vol. 1, no. 1, pp. 3–29, 1948.

[11] The ESMO/European Sarcoma Network Working Group, "Soft tissue and visceral sarcomas: ESMO Clinical Practice Guidelines," *Annals of Oncology*, vol. 25, no. 3, pp. iii102–iii112, 2014.

[12] R. Schiffman, "Epithelioid sarcoma and synovial sarcoma in the same knee," *Cancer*, vol. 45, no. 1, pp. 158–166, 2001.

[13] A. Daigeler, M. Lehnhardt, A. Sebastian et al., "Metachronous bilateral soft tissue sarcoma of the extremities," *Langenbeck's Archives of Surgery*, vol. 393, no. 2, pp. 207–212, 2008.

[14] D. Scepanovic, A. Masarykova, M. Pobijakova, A. Hanicova, and M. Fekete, "Multiple metachronous malignant fibrous histiocytomas of the upper limbs–a case report," *Klinicka Onkologie*, vol. 27, no. 6, pp. 438–441, 2014.

[15] E. S. Gilbert, "Ionizing radiation and cancer risks: what have we learned from epidemiology?," *International Journal of Radiation Biology*, vol. 85, no. 6, pp. 467–482, 2009.

[16] A. E. Grulich, M. T. van Leeuwen, M. O. Falster, and C. M. Vajdic, "Incidence of cancers in people with HIV/AIDS compared with immunosuppressed transplant recipients: a meta-analysis," *The Lancet*, vol. 370, no. 9581, pp. 59–67, 2007.

[17] S. R. Patel, "Radiation-induced sarcoma," *Current Treatment Options in Oncology*, vol. 1, no. 3, pp. 258–261, 2000.

[18] P. G. Casali, J. Y. Blay, and ESMO/CONTICANET/EUROBONET Consensus Panel of experts, "Soft tissue sarcomas: ESMO Clinical Practice Guidelines for diagnosis, treatment and follow-up," *Annals of Oncology*, vol. 21, no. 5, pp. 198–203, 2010.

[19] M. A. Clark, C. Fisher, I. Judson, and J. M. Thomas, "Soft-tissue sarcomas in adults," *New England Journal of Medicine*, vol. 353, no. 7, pp. 701–711, 2005.

22

High-Dose Chemotherapy with Stem Cell Rescue in Desmoplastic Small Round Cell Tumor

Kayleen Bailey,[1] **Michael Roth**,[2] **Daniel Weiser**,[3] **and Jonathan Gill**[2]

[1]*Division of Pediatric Hematology Oncology, Memorial Sloan Kettering Cancer Center, New York Presbyterian Hospital Cornell, New York, NY, USA*
[2]*Division of Pediatrics, University of Texas MD Anderson Cancer Center, Houston, TX, USA*
[3]*Division of Pediatric Hematology, Oncology, Marrow and Blood Cell Transplantation, The Children's Hospital at Montefiore, Bronx, NY, USA*

Correspondence should be addressed to Jonathan Gill; jbgill@mdanderson.org

Academic Editor: C. Verhoef

Purpose. Desmoplastic small round cell tumor (DSRCT) is a rare cancer that predominantly affects males averaging 21 years of age at the time of diagnosis. We describe four cases from our institution and place them within the context of a comprehensive review of the literature. *Patients and Methods.* Study population included any patient who received treatment at Children's Hospital at Montefiore (CHAM) with histologic diagnosis of DSRCT. A search of the electronic databases PubMed, Cochrane Central Register of Controlled Trials, MEDLINE, and EMBASE for the terms "desmoplastic" AND "small" AND "round" AND "cell" AND "tumor" was performed. *Results.* One CHAM patient died of disease at 39 months, one patient has relapsed disease at 40 months, and two patients have no evidence of disease at 60 and 91 months. In the literature review, the 3-year OS was 36% and 5-year OS was 13%. There was a statistically significant difference in OS between no transplant and SCT in remission ($p = 0.004$); however, there was no difference between no transplant and SCT not in remission ($p = 0.23$). *Conclusion.* Given the poor prognosis in DSRCT, this study supports further prospective research into the possible benefit of consolidation of autologous SCT in patients with DSRCT who are in remission, with the alternative inference that these patients in remission may fare well without SCT. Our retrospective review of the literature does not support SCT for patients who are not in remission.

1. Introduction

Desmoplastic small round cell tumor (DSRCT) is a rare cancer which predominantly affects males averaging 21 years of age at the time of diagnosis [1]. Since its first description in 1991, approximately 500 cases have been published worldwide [2, 3]. Depending on the size of the tumor, patients can present with a range of symptoms: nausea, emesis, abdominal pain or distention, constipation, bowel obstruction, and acute renal failure. DSRCT has been described histologically as clusters of small round blue cells with polyphenotypic differentiation within a desmoplastic framework [4]. Because it contains epithelial, neural, and mesenchymal features, the tumor stains positive for desmin, keratin, vimentin, and epithelial membrane antigen. DSRCT is characterized by the fusion of the Wilms tumor (*WT1*) gene and the Ewing sarcoma (*EWS*) gene to form the t(11;22)(p13;q12) fusion, resulting in the upregulation of growth factors on the *EWS* gene and loss of tumor suppressor function of *WT1* [5]. The *EWS/WT1* fusion gene can be identified utilizing polymerase chain reaction (PCR) or fluorescent in situ hybridization (FISH), which proves especially helpful in diagnosing extra-abdominal tumors (that have been previously identified in pleural, intrathoracic, posterior cranial fossa, soft tissue, bones, ovarian, and sinonasal spaces) [6].

Published studies have varied widely with regard to the type and sequence of treatment regimens utilized (i.e., chemotherapy, surgery, radiation, and stem cell transplant (SCT)). Overall survival (OS) rates range from 26 to 64% at 3 years and 10 to 33% at 5 years [7–13]. Median OS range from 13 to 60 months [7–13]. DSRCT has demonstrated to be both alkylator-sensitive and dose-responsive to chemotherapeutic agents. Most institutions tend to use a treatment protocol similar to that of Ewing sarcoma due to the similarities observed in genetics, age, gender, and primitive appearance of neoplastic cells. The addition of whole abdominopelvic radiation (WAP) to multimodal therapy has resulted in median survival of 37.7 and 48 months; one study found postoperative WAP to be predictive of improvement in 3-year OS [14, 15]. Published studies differ in definitions of aggressive surgery, for example, removal of >90% of the tumor, all visible tumors, or leaving no more than 2 cm of tumor. Regardless, it has been shown that more complete surgery results in statistically significant prolonged OS, 49 months versus 12 months ($p = 0.004$) [9]. Recent studies indicate promising survival statistics when cytoreductive surgery is used in combination with hyperthermic intraperitoneal chemotherapy (HiPEC), an emerging treatment modality in various peritoneal sarcomatosis such as DSRCT, rhabdomyosarcoma, leiomyosarcoma, gastrointestinal stromal tumors (GISTs), and liposarcoma [3, 16]. A phase 2 trial of complete resection, HiPEC, and WAP had 3-year overall survival of 79% [17].

Perhaps as a consequence of the dearth of research involving DSRCT, there has not been a validated method of stratifying patients into different risks and/or prognostication categories. One example of prognostic indicator is that, the presence of extra-abdominal metastases may portend a poor prognosis with median OS of 40 months without metastasis and 16 months with metastasis ($p = 0.21$) [16]. Bertuzzi et al. identified several factors associated with disease recurrence including "metastatic disease to sites other than lung, tumor volume >100 mL, axial site involvement, lack of response to first-line therapy, and relapsed disease" [18]. Such heterogeneity in the available literature necessitates a further exploration of the outcomes of recently published high-intensity treatment regimens consisting of chemotherapy, radiation, surgical excision, and SCT.

Since 1996, the Children's Hospital at Montefiore (CHAM) has utilized a standard DSRCT treatment regimen that begins with a four-pronged approach of surgery, P6 chemotherapy (an intense alkylator-based induction regimen), and SCT, which is later followed by WAP. We performed a comprehensive review of the literature to help further elucidate the current landscape of DSRCT treatment.

2. Materials and Methods

2.1. Objectives. The primary objective of this study was to compare the outcome of SCT patients with that of non-SCT patients in the literature. We hypothesized that SCT would prolong OS when compared to regimens without SCT. Secondary objectives included adding cases of patients with DSRCT treated at CHAM from 1996 to 2013 to the literature and confirming published prognostic indicators.

2.2. Case Studies. Study population included any patient who received treatment at CHAM with histologic diagnosis of DSRCT. Data were collected on patients' treatment regimens, disease-free survival (DFS) rate, and OS rate. All pediatric and adult patients with DSRCT who present to any Montefiore-associated hospital are treated by the Pediatric Oncology Division at CHAM. The electronic medical record at CHAM was searched using the Clinical Looking Glass tool for all patients with a diagnosis of DSRCT. The study was approved by the Institutional Review Board at Montefiore.

Inclusion criteria consisted of those patients with histologically confirmed diagnosis of DSRCT who received ≥1 treatment at CHAM between the years 1996 and 2013. These treatments included debulking surgery (removal of >90% of tumor), cytoreductive surgery (resection of tumor to a visible size of <1.0 cm), SCT, abdominal radiation, chemotherapy (neoadjuvant or adjuvant), and immunotherapy.

Those patients who only presented to CHAM for consultation but were not treated within our institution were excluded. Additionally, those patients who had <6 months of follow-up time were not included in the study.

2.3. Literature Review. A search of the electronic databases PubMed, Cochrane Central Register of Controlled Trials (CENTRAL), MEDLINE, and EMBASE for the terms "desmoplastic" AND "small" AND "round" AND "cell" AND "tumor" was performed. Additionally, the bibliographies of the chosen articles were hand-searched in an effort to capture any additional published and unpublished trials.

Published reports of 1-2 cases were felt to represent a positive publication bias; thus, a study was only included if it included ≥3 cases of histologically confirmed DSRCT. Studies that contained general descriptions of patient populations but did not individually identify patients and their respective disease course (namely, last known event and time to last known event) were excluded. Any publications from the same institution were compared to ensure that each patient was represented only once; if a patient's demographics were similar to those of another patient, then the older data were excluded for that patient.

2.4. Statistical Analysis. Data were collected from the electronic medical records at CHAM. Potential confounders to the success of SCT included the presence of extra-abdominal metastasis and the extent of surgery (cytoreductive versus debulking), which have previously been published in the literature as having statistically significant prognostic implications. Patient demographics were tabulated using mean, median, and mode for continuous variables and percentages for categorical variables. The statistical methods used to evaluate the study objectives included Kaplan–Meier to estimate survival and log-rank to compare OS and DFS. OS was calculated as date of diagnosis to date of death or last follow-up.

3. Results and Discussion

3.1. Case Studies. For the four CHAM patients, the average follow-up was 58 months. One patient died of disease at 39 months after diagnosis, one patient remains alive with relapsed disease at 40 months, and two patients have no evidence of disease at 60 and 91 months. An overview of these patients' treatment courses can be seen in Table 1.

Patient #1 initially presented with decreased appetite, worsening asthma, weight gain, and left-sided pain. Computed tomography (CT) scan was concerning for an ovarian tumor. An oophorectomy revealed DSRCT. The patient underwent P6 chemotherapy (consisting of alternating cycles of cyclophosphamide, doxorubicin, and vincristine with ifosfamide and etoposide), debulking surgery, consolidation therapy with high-dose chemotherapy, autologous SCT, and WAP. The patient is alive and disease free at 91 months.

Patient #2 presented with bright red blood per rectum with a normal colonoscopy, followed by abdominal pain and vomiting. CT scan revealed abdominal masses in the right lower quadrant and another mass in the perirectal area. CT-guided biopsy provided a diagnosis of DSRCT. The patient's treatment course consisted of P6 chemotherapy, debulking surgery, SCT, and partial course of radiation. The patient's course was complicated by colonic perforation with hemicolectomy and ostomy placement, followed by bowel reanastamosis with wound infection. The patient relapsed at 32 months after diagnosis and is currently still alive receiving treatment at 48 months after diagnosis.

Patient #3's course began with P6 chemotherapy. Tumor resection included distal pancreatectomy, splenectomy, and transverse colon resection with colonic anastamosis. The patient then underwent SCT followed by radiation. The course was complicated by surgical evacuation of an abdominal hematoma. The patient was alive and disease free at 60 months after diagnosis.

Patient #4 had unilateral ear pain followed by development of stiff neck. Magnetic resonance imaging (MRI) was done showing inflammation of the spine; at the same time, a chest X-ray (CXR) showed a lesion in the spine. CT abdomen/pelvis showed a right kidney mass, and a bone scan was positive in the sternum, spine, and head. Bone marrow biopsy showed DSRCT. Treatment began with P6 chemotherapy, followed by tumor resection with radical nephrectomy and retroperitoneal lymph node dissection. The patient then underwent autologous SCT and radiation. The patient relapsed 20 months after diagnosis. The patient eventually passed away from metastatic disease approximately 30 months after completing treatment.

3.2. Literature Review

3.2.1. Demographics. The systematic review of the literature revealed 512 publications in the literature (Supplementary Figure S1). A total of 492 publications were excluded for lack of OS data ($n = 7$), non-DSRCT diagnosis ($n = 231$), ≤2 patients ($n = 249$), or a single-agent study ($n = 5$), which left a remainder of 20 published papers; these included 279 patients in the literature including the patients treated at CHAM (Supplemental Table S1). Within that population, 23 were omitted for lack of OS data ($n = 17$), initial misdiagnosis ($n = 2$), palliative treatment only ($n = 2$), and suspected overlap with other patients ($n = 2$). A total of 256 patients were available for our statistical analysis (Table 2).

The median age was 18.3 years (range 2–64 years) with 86% male patients and 13% female patients. With regard to the primary site of disease, 77% (198) had primary abdominal/pelvic site and 9% (24) had nonabdominal/pelvic site, while 13% (34) were unknown. Liver metastasis was present in 126 (49%) patients. There was reported extra-abdominal metastasis in 62 patients (24%), while 55% did not have extra-abdominal metastasis. The remainder of the patients did not have this information available in the publication.

Of the 256 patients, 71 patients (28%) had SCT as part of their treatment regimen. Of the 71 patients who underwent SCT, 23 (32%) were not in remission, 13 (18%) were in remission, and 35 (49%) had unknown status at time of remission. There were 86 (34%) patients who had radiation and 167 (65%) patients who did not undergo radiation. Sixteen patients (6%) underwent HiPEC, while 202 (78%) did not. The remaining patients did not have this information clearly stated in the publication. Within the various treatment regimens, 130 (51%) patients received doxorubicin and 15 (6%) had regimens that did not contain doxorubicin. The other patients' chemotherapy regimens were not clearly defined whether they contained doxorubicin. As part of their chemotherapy regimen, 55% of patients received an alkylating agent, and 1% reported no alkylating agent; the remainder of the patients did not have this number reported. The number of total treatments (e.g., chemotherapy, radiation, SCT, surgery, or HiPEC) per patient was reported as 0 (3.5%), 1 (20%), 2 (34%), 3 (25%), and 4-5 (14%). For surgical excision, 22% were reported as complete and 15% were reported as incomplete. Surgical information was not available for the remainder of the patients.

3.2.2. Outcomes. For all patients, the 3-year OS was 36% and 5-year OS was 13% (Table 3). There was not enough information in the literature to calculate DFS for patients, as most studies reported OS only.

3.2.3. Treatment. A Kaplany–Meier curve of the OS of 256 patients whose information was available for our statistical analysis is shown in Figure 1(a). Figure 1(a). Those with SCT ($n = 71$) had an improved OS compared to those with no SCT ($n = 185$, $p = 0.02$; Figure 1(b)). There was a statistically significant difference in OS between no transplant ($n = 185$), SCT in remission ($n = 13$), and SCT not in remission ($n = 13$, $p = 0.007$) (Figure 1(c)), as well as between no transplant ($n = 185$) and SCT in remission ($n = 14$, $p = 0.004$) seen in Supplementary Figure 2A. No difference was seen in comparing no transplant ($n = 185$) with transplant not in remission ($n = 23$, $p = 0.07$) (Supplementary Figure 2B). Finally, there was no difference between SCT not in remission ($n = 22$) and transplant in remission ($n = 14$, $p = 0.07$) (Supplementary Figure 2C).

Patients who underwent more thorough surgical excision had improved OS compared to those who underwent incomplete or no surgery ($p = 0.02$) (Figure 2(a)). Radiation also improved OS ($p < 0.0001$) (Figure 2(b)). HiPEC therapy did not provide a statistically significant improvement in OS

Table 1: Patients with desmoplastic small round cell tumor treated at Children's Hospital at Montefiore.

Patient	Age at diagnosis	Gender	Date of diagnosis	Date of relapse	Date of last follow-up	Status at last follow-up	Months to last follow-up	1st treatment	2nd treatment	3rd treatment	4th treatment	5th treatment
1	16	Female	5/8/2008		12/8/2015	Alive, disease free	91	Oophorectomy	P6 chemotherapy	Surgery at MSKCC	SCT	Total abdominal radiation
2	21	Male	9/24/2012	6/1/2015	9/24/2016	Alive, relapsed	40	Resection of abdominal tumor	P6 chemotherapy	Surgery at MSKCC	SCT	Partial course of radiation
3	11	Male	11/16/2010		11/16/2015	Alive, disease free	60	Vincristine, dactinomycin, cyclophosphamide	Tumor resection	SCT	Radiation	
4	19	Male	1/9/2008	9/28/2009	4/27/2011	Death from metastatic disease	39	P6 chemotherapy	Tumor resection	SCT	Radiation	

MSKCC: Memorial Sloan Kettering Cancer Center; SCT: stem cell transplant.

TABLE 2: Demographics of patients with desmoplastic small round cell tumor treated at Children's Hospital at Montefiore and in literature review.

All patients		
Median age at diagnosis	18.3 years	
Overall survival	3 years, 36%	5 years, 13%
Category	*N*	*Percentage*
Female	34	13
Male	220	86
Unknown	2	1
Primary abdominal/pelvic disease	198	77
Primary nonabdominal disease	24	9
Unknown	34	13
Liver metastasis	126	49
No liver metastasis	54	21
Unknown	76	30
Extra-abdominal metastasis	62	24
No extra-abdominal metastasis	142	55
Unknown	52	20
SCT	71	28
SCT not in remission	23	
SCT in remission	13	
SCT unknown remission	35	
No SCT	185	72
Radiation	86	34
No radiation	167	65
Unknown	3	1
HiPEC	16	6
No HiPEC	202	79
Unknown	38	15
Doxorubicin	130	51
No doxorubicin	15	6
Unknown	111	43
Alkylating agent	134	52
Alkylating-like agent	8	3
No alkyating agent	3	1
Unknown	111	43
0 treatment	9	4
1 treatment	52	20
2 treatments	87	34
3 treatments	65	25
4–5 treatments	38	15
Unknown	4	2
Complete surgical excision (2,3,4)	56	22
Incomplete surgical excision (0,1)	39	15
Unknown	161	63

SCT: stem cell transplant; HiPEC: hyperthermic intraperitoneal chemotherapy.

($p = 0.08$) (Figure 2(c)). Chemotherapy did demonstrate an improved OS ($p = 0.004$) (Figure 2(d)), though using a regimen with doxorubicin did not ($p = 0.12$) (Supplementary Figure 3A). Finally, those who underwent surgery and radiation had an improved OS compared to either treatment alone or neither treatment ($p < 0.001$) (Figure 2(e)).

3.2.4. Prognostic Indicators. Several prognostic indicators were compared to those previously reported in the literature. We found that the presence of primary disease outside of the abdomen had an improved OS ($p < 0.03$), as seen in Figure 3(a). We also found that those who had extra-abdominal metastasis or liver metastasis did not have a statistically significant worsening of their OS versus patients without those characteristics ($p = 0.22$ and $p = 0.57$, resp.; Figures 3(b) and 3(c)).

4. Conclusions

Our review of over 250 patients in the literature with DSRCT demonstrates that treatment with SCT in remission, complete surgical resection, and radiation had statistically significantly improved OS at 3 and 5 years, compared to the patients who were not in remission at the time of SCT, incomplete or no surgical resection, and no radiation, respectively. The results of this study postulate that more aggressive multimodal treatment (consisting of extensive surgical resection, chemotherapy, and/or radiation) that achieves remission, followed by SCT, could result in improved long-term outcomes for these patients. A prospective study would be required to accurately assess whether SCT in this patient population is necessary; patients with DSRCT in remission may fare as well without a SCT.

The last major published review of the DSRCT literature by Kretschmar et al. in 1996 included 101 patients, for which median survival was 17 months (range 3–72 months) with only two patients disease free beyond 2 years at 40 and 48 months [1]. Our large-scale review contributes to the literature in that it represents more current treatment regimens and improved OS compared to the prior time period.

Multimodal aggressive treatment portends a survival advantage in our study and may benefit from further prospective evaluation. A previous publication showed that chemotherapy, surgery, and radiation therapy together produced a 55% OS at 3 years versus 27% if one of these therapeutic modalities was missing [13]. In another study, there was a median survival of 34 months in patients who had complete surgical resection with systemic chemotherapy versus 14 months for chemotherapy alone [19].

Since those who were in remission at the time of SCT fared the best, SCT may be a possible consideration for those who respond to first-line chemotherapy. A previous study by Fraser et al. published data on SCT in a variety of patients, including four patients with DSRCT [20]. When these patients were in complete remission, the 3-year OS was 76% as compared to 27% for those in partial remission ($p = 0.08$). Thus, SCT may be most beneficial in a select group of DSRCT that has no evidence of disease.

We investigated prognostic indicators that were previously published in the literature. In our study, we demonstrate that the presence of primary disease outside of the abdomen had an improved OS compared to intra-abdominal disease, which has not been previously reported. This may be due to the containment of the tumor allowing for complete surgical resection, as in testicular disease. Those who had extra-abdominal metastasis or liver metastasis showed no worsening in OS, which was different from previously published studies [6, 14]. This distinction may be attributable to differences in treatment with more patients receiving multimodal therapy.

In addition, the efficacies of other treatment options (surgery, chemotherapy, and radiation) were investigated.

TABLE 3: Overall survival for all patients, patients with stem cell transplant, patients with stem cell transplant not in remission, patients with stem cell transplant in remission, and patients with no stem cell transplant.

	3-year overall survival	5-year overall survival
All	36%	13%
SCT[ab]	45%	17%
SCT not in remission[b]	38%	15%
SCT in remission[bc]	71%	37%
No SCT[ac]	30%	11%

SCT: stem cell transplant. [a]SCT versus no SCT ($p = 0.02$); [b]SCT versus SCT not in remission versus SCT in remission ($p = 0.007$); [c]SCT in remission versus no SCT ($p = 0.004$). The remainder of p values were not significant.

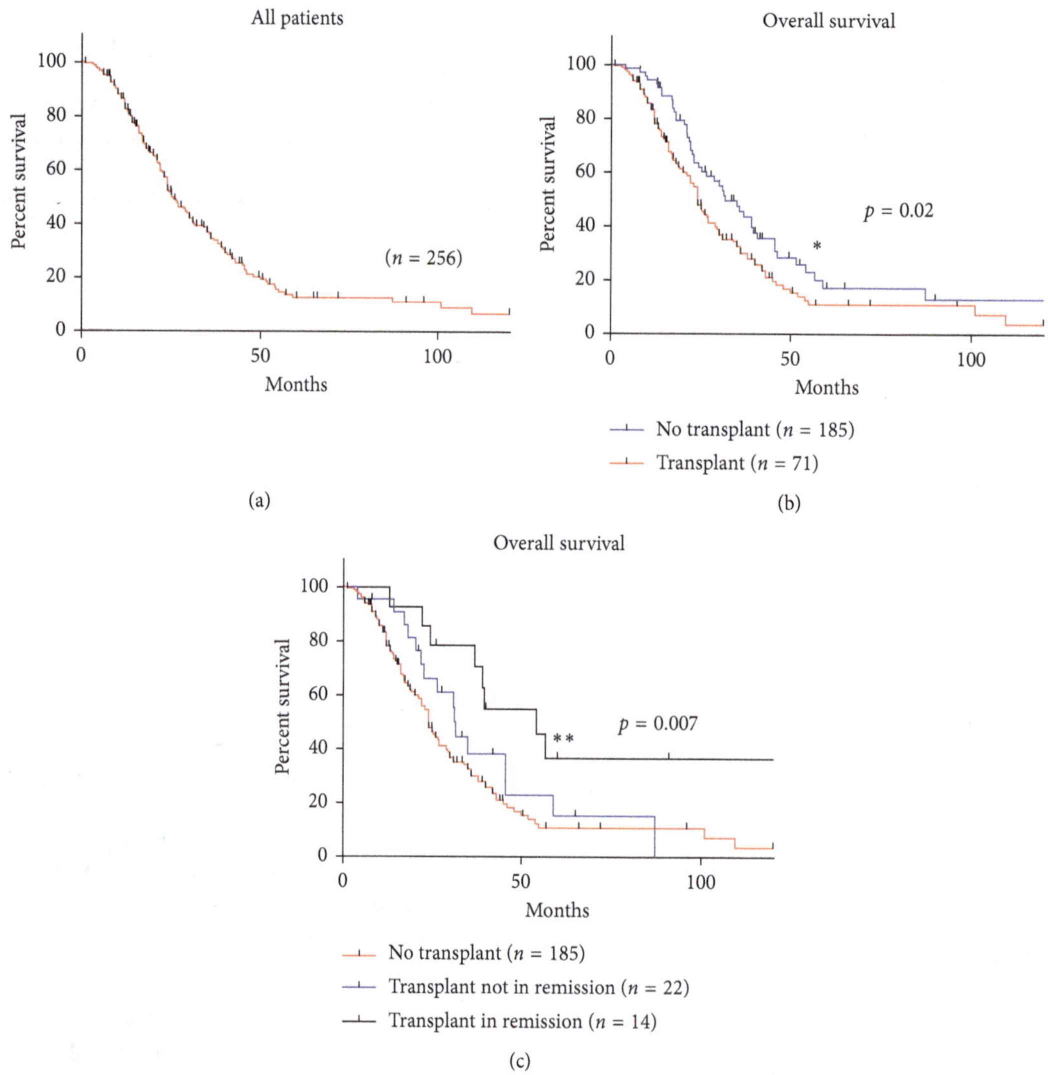

FIGURE 1: (a) The Kaplan–Meier curve of all patients included in the data analysis. (b) The Kaplan–Meier curve of patients who did not receive a stem cell transplant and patients who received a stem cell transplant. (c) The Kaplan–Meier curve of patients who did not receive a stem cell transplant, patients who received a stem cell transplant not in remission, and patients who received a stem cell transplant in remission.

In one study, incomplete cytoreduction was associated with no patient surviving >15 months [21]. Lal et al. demonstrated the necessity for completeness of surgical excision. While patients who underwent gross tumor resection had an OS of 58% at 3 years, there was 0% OS in patients where visible deposits remained [13]. Our study also indicated that more complete surgical excision results in improved overall outcome, thus substantiating that having tumor burden amenable to complete resection improved survival.

Due to the heterogeneity of treatment in the literature, we did not find statistically significant advantages in using

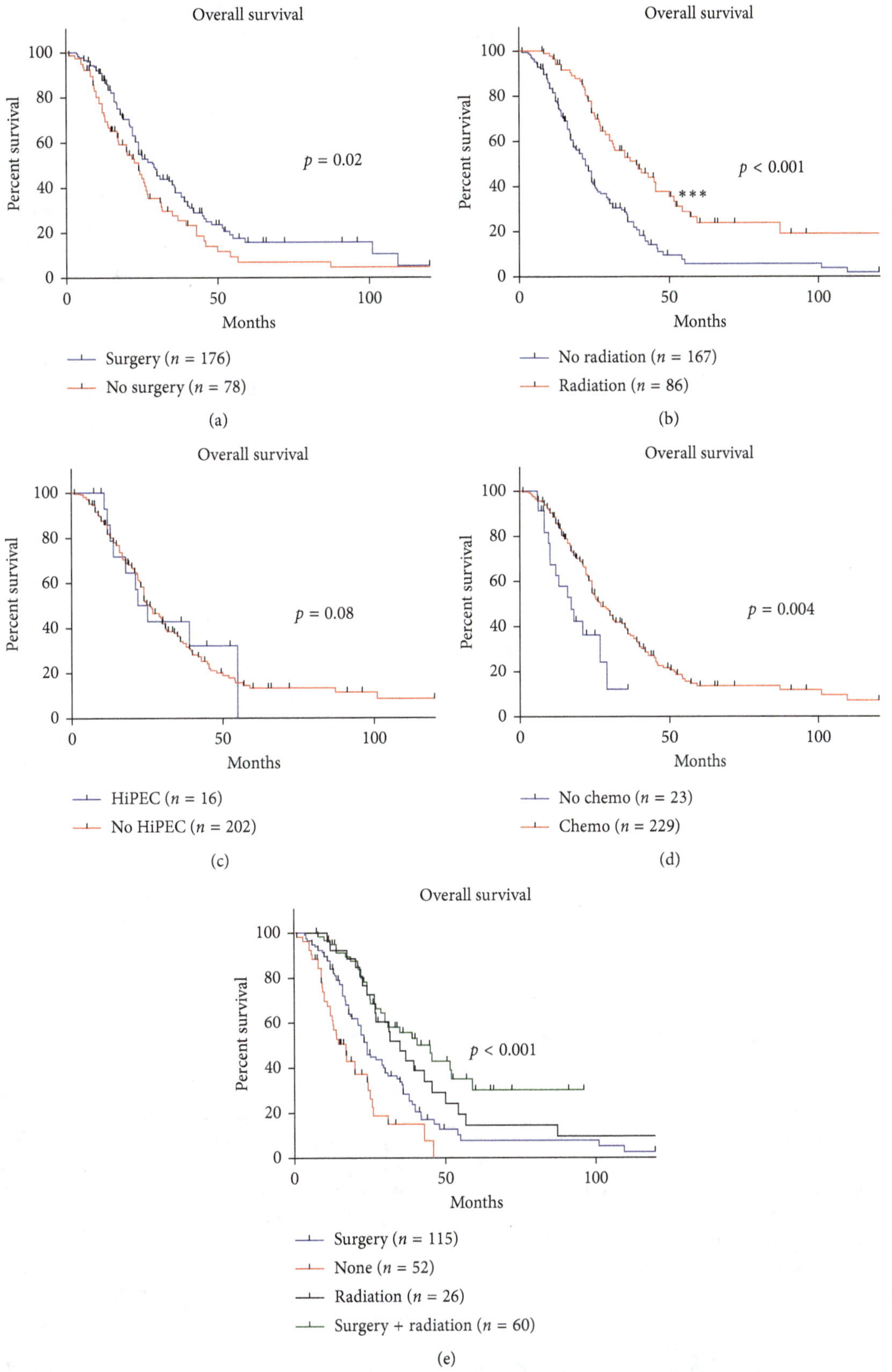

FIGURE 2: (a) The Kaplan–Meier curve of patients who had surgery and patients who did not have surgery. (b) The Kaplan–Meier curve of patients who did not receive radiation and patients who received radiation. (c) The Kaplan–Meier curve of patients who received hyperthermic intraperitoneal chemotherapy and patients who did not receive hyperthermic intraperitoneal chemotherapy. (d) The Kaplan–Meier curve of patients who received chemotherapy and patients who did not receive chemotherapy. (e) The Kaplan–Meier curve of patients who received surgery, patients who received radiation, patients who received radiation and surgery, and patients who did not receive radiation or surgery. HiPEC = hyperthermic intraperitoneal chemotherapy; chemo = chemotherapy.

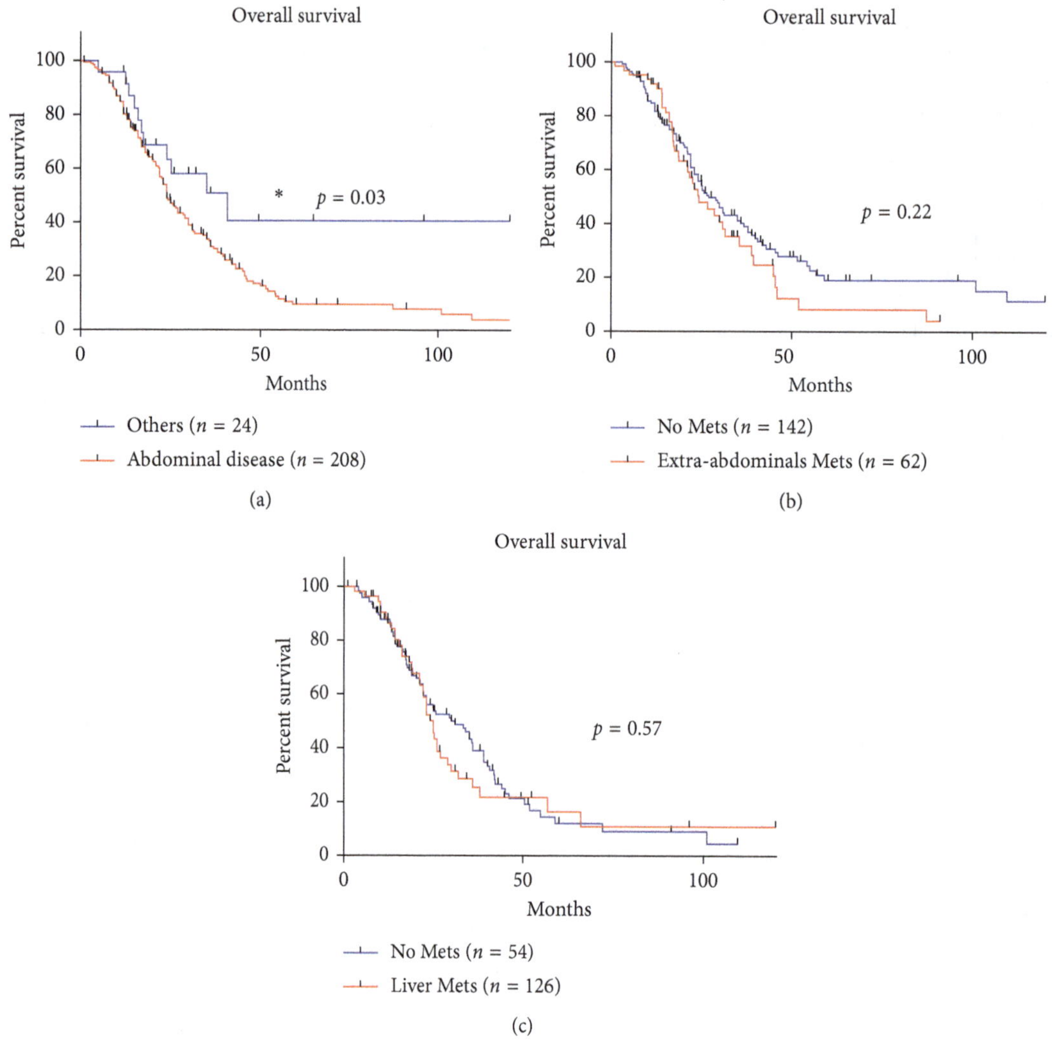

FIGURE 3: (a) The Kaplan–Meier curve of patients whose primary site of disease was in the abdomen and patients whose primary site of disease was outside of the abdomen. (b) The Kaplan–Meier curve of patients who had extra-abdominal metastasis at time of diagnosis and patients who did not have extra-abdominal metastasis at time of diagnosis. (c) The Kaplan–Meier curve of patients who had liver metastasis at time of diagnosis and patients who did not have liver metastasis at time of diagnosis. Mets = metastasis.

a doxorubicin-containing chemotherapy regimen or HiPEC. Like HiPEC, radiotherapy is generally indicated for local disease confined to the abdomen; thus, it would not be feasible for patients with larger tumor burden [22]. Patients in our study who underwent radiation as part of multimodal therapy had improved OS. This finding may be biased by selection of only those patients with minimal tumor burden or functional status to be able to tolerate the treatment.

There are several limitations to our study. Studies that did not report individual patient outcomes or grouped DSRCT with other soft tissue sarcomas (STSs) were excluded. Our results are similar to those of studies consisting of aggregated DSRCT data in the literature. For example, a study conducted by Zhang et al. analyzed a cohort of 48 patients with DSRCT and found median overall survival of 24 months; the variables associated with improved OS included "surgery, effective debulking surgery, chemotherapy, and any two or more combined therapeutics" ($p < 0.05$). There was also a Cochrane Review that examined SCT in nonrhabdomyosarcoma STS, within which 27 patients carried a diagnosis of DSRCT [9, 23]. The graph of OS of the 27 patients with DSRCT appeared similar to the graph of the 80 total patients, but there was no direct statistical comparison. A randomized control trial (RCT), which included multiple STS histologies, did not show a significant difference in OS between the SCT and non-SCT groups; the authors concluded that there was some evidence that there might not be improved survival after SCT [24]. Another RCT by Bui-Nguyen et al. had 87 STS patients, 2 of which had DSRCT. In their population, patients who had achieved a complete response prior to SCT had a longer OS compared to all patients. However, the findings of these studies are difficult to extrapolate as they involve multiple histologies with variable chemosensitivity.

Other limitations of this study are consistent with the methodologies of a literature review and the potential for reporting bias. We were unable to complete a multivariate analysis, systematic review, or meta-analysis due to our limited number of patients and lack of published details on individual patients; conclusions that could be reached from these analyses are beyond the scope of this article. Future analyses would benefit from a centralized registry of DSRCT patients to aggregate individual patient data. Treatment regimens varied widely among the included patient population. A total of 26 different chemotherapy regimens are represented in this review. Furthermore, the order of all treatment regimens (chemotherapy, radiation, surgery, and SCT) amongst all studies was not uniform. Lastly, the review of the literature cannot always discern the tolerability of the treatment. As such, variability in the treatment may reflect toxicity rather than differences in the planned treatment.

This review of the literature supports additional investigation of SCT as part of the multimodal treatment for patients who are able to achieve remission. Further research is warranted to validate these findings in this narrow population. Complete resection (and by extension, likely more limited disease) has consistently been reported to be most important facet of multimodal treatment. Likewise, the role of HiPEC in a select group of DSRCT may need to be further explored. Given the poor prognosis, there are several ongoing clinical trials investigating other agents, such as Irinotecan, Temozolomide and Bevacizumab in Combination with Existing High Dose Alkylator Based Chemotherapy and Phase I Trial of Intraperitoneal Radioimmunotherapy with ^{131}I-8H9 [25, 26]. Shukla et al. found no consistent targetable mutations found in DSRCT samples using Sequenom analysis, but perhaps whole genome sequencing may lead to identification of other potential targets of transcriptional dysregulation [27]. Further research targeting the *EWS/WT1* translocation (as currently being explored in early phase trials of the Ewing sarcoma) may provide promise in this difficult to treat disease.

Abbreviations

DSRCT: Desmoplastic small round cell tumor
OS: Overall survival
SCT: Stem cell transplant
CHAM: Children's Hospital at Montefiore
WAP: Whole abdominopelvic radiation
WT1: Wilms' tumor gene
EWS: Ewing's sarcoma gene
HiPEC: Hyperthermic intraperitoneal chemotherapy
GIST: Gastrointestinal stromal tumor
MRI: Magnetic resonance imaging
CT: Computed tomography
CXR: Chest X-ray
STS: Soft tissue sarcoma
RCT: Randomized control trial
PCI: Peritoneal cancer index
Mets: Metastasis
PCR: Polymerase chain reaction
FISH: Fluorescent in situ hybridization.

Conflicts of Interest

The authors disclose no conflicts of interest.

Acknowledgments

The authors would like to acknowledge the Memorial Sloan Kettering Cancer Center Support Grant (P30CA008748).

References

[1] C. S. Kretschmar, C. Colbach, I. Bhan, and T. M. Crombleholme, "Desmoplastic small cell tumor: a report of three cases and a review of the literature," *Journal of Pediatric Hematology/Oncology*, vol. 18, no. 3, pp. 293–298, 1996.

[2] W. L. Gerald, H. K. Miller, H. Battifora, M. Miettinen, E. G. Silva, and J. Rosai, "Intra-abdominal desmoplastic small round-cell tumor. Report of 19 cases of a distinctive type of high-grade polyphenotypic malignancy affecting young individuals," *American Journal of Surgical Pathology*, vol. 15, no. 6, pp. 499–513, 1991.

[3] A. Gil, A. Gomez Portilla, E. A. Brun, and P. H. Sugarbaker, "Clinical perspective on desmoplastic small round-cell tumor," *Oncology*, vol. 67, no. 3-4, pp. 231–242, 2004.

[4] N. G. Ordóñez, A. K. El-Naggar, J. Y. Ro, E. G. Silva, and B. Mackay, "Intra-abdominal desmoplastic small cell tumor: a light microscopic, immunocytochemical, ultrastructural, and flow cytometric study," *Human Pathology*, vol. 24, no. 8, pp. 850–865, 1993.

[5] M. Ladanyi and W. Gerald, "Fusion of the EWS and WT1 genes in the desmoplastic small round cell tumor," *Cancer Research*, vol. 54, no. 11, pp. 2837–2840, 1994.

[6] Y. Tang, H. Song, Y. Bao, and Y. Zhi, "Multimodal treatment of abdominal and pelvic desmoplastic small round cell tumor with relative good prognosis," *International Journal of Surgery*, vol. 16, pp. 49–54, 2015.

[7] C. K. Lettieri, P. Garcia-Filion, and P. Hingorani, "Incidence and outcomes of desmoplastic small round cell tumor: results from the surveillance, epidemiology, and end results database," *Journal of Cancer Epidemiology*, vol. 2014, Article ID 680126, 5 pages, 2014.

[8] E. M. Osborne, T. M. Briere, A. Hayes-Jordan et al., "Survival and toxicity following sequential multimodality treatment including whole abdominopelvic radiotherapy for patients with desmoplastic small round cell tumor," *Radiotherapy and Oncology*, vol. 119, no. 1, pp. 40–44, 2016.

[9] J. Zhang, H. Xu, F. Ren, Y. Yang, B. Chen, and F. Zhang, "Analysis of clinicopathological features and prognostic factors of desmoplastic small round cell tumor," *Pathology and Oncology Research*, vol. 20, no. 1, pp. 161–168, 2014.

[10] L. Mingo, F. Seguel, and V. Rollán, "Intraabdominal desmoplastic small round cell tumour," *Pediatric Surgery International*, vol. 21, no. 4, pp. 279–281, 2005.

[11] C. J. Forlenza, B. H. Kushner, N. Kernan et al., "Myeloablative chemotherapy with autologous stem cell transplant for desmoplastic small round cell tumor," *Sarcoma*, vol. 2015, Article ID 269197, 9 pages, 2015.

[12] B. H. Kushner, M. P. LaQuaglia, N. Wollner et al., "Desmoplastic small round-cell tumor: prolonged progression-free survival with aggressive multimodality therapy," *Journal of Clinical Oncology*, vol. 14, no. 5, pp. 1526–1531, 1996.

[13] D. R. Lal, W. T. Su, S. L. Wolden, K. C. Loh, S. Modak, and M. P. La Quaglia, "Results of multimodal treatment for desmoplastic small round cell tumors," *Journal of Pediatric Surgery*, vol. 40, no. 1, pp. 251–255, 2005.

[14] C. Honoré, K. Amroun, L. Vilcot et al., "Abdominal desmoplastic small round cell tumor: multimodal treatment combining chemotherapy, surgery, and radiotherapy is the best option," *Annals of Surgical Oncology*, vol. 22, no. 2, pp. 1073–1079, 2014.

[15] K. A. Goodman, S. L. Wolden, M. P. La Quaglia, and B. H. Kushner, "Whole abdominopelvic radiotherapy for desmoplastic small round-cell tumor," *International Journal of Radiation Oncology*Biology*Physics*, vol. 54, no. 1, pp. 170–176, 2002.

[16] A. Hayes-Jordan, H. Green, N. Fitzgerald, L. Xiao, and P. Anderson, "Novel treatment for desmoplastic small round cell tumor: hyperthermic intraperitoneal perfusion," *Journal of Pediatric Surgery*, vol. 45, no. 5, pp. 1000–1006, 2010.

[17] A. A. Hayes-Jordan, B. A. Coakley, H. L. Green et al., "Desmoplastic small round cell tumor treated with cytoreductive surgery and hyperthermic intraperitoneal chemotherapy: results of a phase 2 trial," *Annals of Surgical Oncology*, vol. 25, no. 4, pp. 872–877, 2018.

[18] A. Bertuzzi, L. Castagna, A. Nozza et al., "High-dose chemotherapy in poor-prognosis adult small round-cell tumors: clinical and molecular results from a prospective study," *Journal of Clinical Oncology*, vol. 20, no. 8, pp. 2181–2188, 2002.

[19] I. Hassan, R. Shyyan, J. H. Donohue et al., "Intraabdominal desmoplastic small round cell tumors: a diagnostic and therapeutic challenge," *Cancer*, vol. 104, no. 6, pp. 1264–1270, 2005.

[20] C. J. Fraser, B. J. Weigel, J. P. Perentesis et al., "Autologous stem cell transplantation for high-risk Ewing's sarcoma and other pediatric solid tumors," *Bone Marrow Transplantation*, vol. 37, no. 2, pp. 175–181, 2006.

[21] A. Hayes-Jordan and P. M. Anderson, "The diagnosis and management of desmoplastic small round cell tumor: a review," *Current Opinion in Oncology*, vol. 23, no. 4, pp. 385–389, 2011.

[22] M. P. Quaglia and M. F. Brennan, "The clinical approach to desmoplastic small round cell tumor," *Surgical Oncology*, vol. 9, no. 2, pp. 77–81, 2000.

[23] F. Peinemann, L. A. Smith, and C. Bartel, "Autologous hematopoietic stem cell transplantation following high dose chemotherapy for non-rhabdomyosarcoma soft tissue sarcomas," *Cochrane Database of Systematic Reviews*, vol. 2013, no. 8, p. CD008216, 2013.

[24] B. Bui-Nguyen, I. Ray-Coquard, C. Chevreau et al., "High-dose chemotherapy consolidation for chemosensitive advanced soft tissue sarcoma patients: an open-label, randomized controlled trial," *Annals of Oncology*, vol. 23, no. 3, pp. 777–784, 2012.

[25] Irinotecan, Temozolomide and Bevacizumab in Combination with Existing High Dose Alkylator Based Chemotherapy for Treatment of Newly Diagnosed Patients with Desmoplastic Small Round Cell Tumor, https://ClinicalTrials.gov/show/NCT01189643, 2010.

[26] Intraperitoneal Radioimmunotherapy with 131I-8H9 for Patients with Desmoplastic Small Round Cell Tumors and Other Solid Tumors Involving the Peritoneum, https://ClinicalTrials.gov/show/NCT01099644, 2010.

[27] N. Shukla, N. Ameur, I. Yilmaz et al., "Oncogene mutation profiling of pediatric solid tumors reveals significant subsets of embryonal rhabdomyosarcoma and neuroblastoma with mutated genes in growth signaling pathways," *Clinical Cancer Research*, vol. 18, no. 3, pp. 748–757, 2012.

23

Molecular Targets and Emerging Therapeutic Options for Uterine Leiomyosarcoma

Heather Miller,[1] Chiemeka Ike,[2] Jennifer Parma,[2] Ramya P. Masand,[3] Claire M. Mach,[1,2] and Matthew L. Anderson[1,3,4]

[1]*Department of Obstetrics & Gynecology, Baylor College of Medicine, Houston, TX 77030, USA*
[2]*College of Pharmacy, University of Houston, Houston, TX 77030, USA*
[3]*Department of Pathology & Immunology, Baylor College of Medicine, Houston, TX 77030, USA*
[4]*Dan L Duncan Cancer Center, Baylor College of Medicine, Houston, TX 77030, USA*

Correspondence should be addressed to Matthew L. Anderson; matthew@bcm.edu

Academic Editor: Chandrajit Premanand Raut

Uterine leiomyosarcoma (uLMS) is an aggressive malignancy characterized by its early metastasis, high rates of recurrence, and poor prognosis. Multiple obstacles complicate the clinical management of uLMS. These include the fact that most uLMS are typically identified only after a woman has undergone hysterectomy or myomectomy, the limited efficacy of adjuvant therapy for early stage disease, and the poor response of metastatic disease to current treatments. Here, we discuss recent insights into the molecular basis of uLMS and discuss emerging options for its clinical management. Particular attention is given to the biologic basis of these strategies with the goal of understanding the rationale motivating their use.

1. Introduction

Uterine leiomyosarcoma (uLMS) is an aggressive cancer characterized by its poor prognosis and high rates of recurrence [1, 2]. Although fewer than 3,000 women are diagnosed with this disease in the United States each year, uLMS is the most common sarcoma arising in the genital tract of reproductive-aged women [3, 4].

A number of long-standing challenges complicate clinical management of uLMS. Perhaps one of the most important of these challenges is the fact that uLMS are typically diagnosed only after a woman has undergone hysterectomy or myomectomy. This problem occurs for a number of reasons. The most important of these reasons is that strategies used to identify other types of uterine cancer, such as endometrial biopsy, are not useful for diagnosing this disease [5, 6]. Currently, uLMS are diagnosed on the basis of the histologic identification of a high mitotic count (>10 mitotic figures/10 high power fields) and the presence of coagulative tumor necrosis and moderate to severe cytologic atypia [7]. Unfortunately, these features cannot be sufficiently evaluated by small volume core biopsies or needle aspirations to differentiate malignant from nonmalignant myometrial tissue. In addition, symptoms associated with uLMS, such as irregular vaginal bleeding or pelvic pain, are nonspecific and frequently caused by multiple, more common but benign etiologies [8]. A rapidly growing myometrial mass is often presumed to be pathognomonic, although existing data fail to support this belief [9].

Recognizing a clear area of clinical need, investigators have explored the utility of different imaging modalities to distinguish uLMS from benign leiomyomas preoperatively. Although a number of specific radiographic features, such as infiltrative margins, have been associated with uLMS visualized by magnetic resonance imaging (MRI), these features are not found frequently enough to allow routine use of MRI to prospectively distinguish benign from malignant myometrial masses [10]. Furthermore, there are no radiographic features capable of reliably distinguishing uLMS from benign myometrial masses by pelvic ultrasonography, computed tomography (CT), or positron emission tomography (PET).

A second key clinical challenge complicating management of uLMS is the need for effective adjuvant therapy

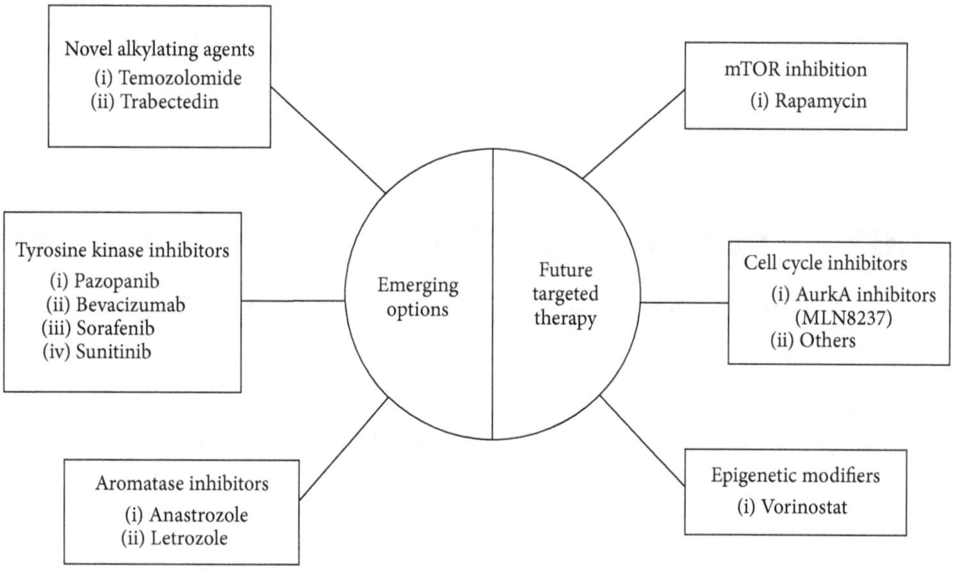

Figure 1: Graphic summary of emerging and potential future targeted therapy for uLMS.

following hysterectomy. Most uLMS (68%) are diagnosed as a solitary mass grossly confined to the uterus, which is defined as stage I disease according to the 2009 revised FIGO criteria [11]. Recurrence rates even for early stage disease are high, ranging from 53 to 71% [12, 13]. As a result, three-year survival for FIGO stage I uLMS is estimated to be only 52% [1]. Unfortunately, surgical staging is largely unable to identify women at risk of experiencing a recurrence of their disease. In the absence of grossly visible metastases, routine pelvic and para-aortic lymphadenectomy identifies microscopic metastases in only 2-3% of cases [14, 15]. Routine oophorectomy similarly fails to provide prognostic insight. In fact, oophorectomy has been associated with worse overall survival, although data addressing this issue remains conflicted [16].

Given the high recurrence rates associated with early stage disease, adjuvant therapy is frequently administered to women who have recently undergone hysterectomy for uLMS. Multiple, early retrospective studies promoted the use of adjuvant radiotherapy to reduce the incidence of disease recurrence [17, 18]. However, at least one recent prospective randomized control trial has failed to demonstrate any improvement in progression-free or overall survival for women with early stage uterine sarcomas including uLMS treated with radiotherapy [1, 19]. As a result, use of adjuvant radiotherapy has largely been abandoned. Several large retrospective studies have suggested that adjuvant chemotherapy may also provide little benefit. The role of adriamycin as adjuvant therapy following surgical management of stage I or II disease has been studied with no difference in PFS or OS observed [20]. More recently, a phase III clinical trial compared the uses of doxorubicin, ifosfamide, and cisplatin as adjuvant therapy with and without radiotherapy for uterine sarcoma. Data from this study revealed a slight increase in 3-year disease-free survival in subjects who received both chemotherapy and radiotherapy [21]. Another phase II clinical trial examined the efficacy of adjuvant gemcitabine and docetaxel in patients with completely resected stage I and II disease. The outcome of this study demonstrated 57% progression-free survival (PFS) at 3 years, which was significantly greater than the 35% PFS observed at 3 years among historical controls [11, 22]. Despite the fact that each of these studies demonstrated modest improvements in PFS associated with the use of adjuvant chemotherapy, none of the regimens studied to date have yet to emerge as a consistent standard.

A final challenge is the treatment of advanced stage and/or recurrent uLMS. Similar to early stage disease, doxorubicin with or without ifosfamide has been historically used as frontline therapy for advanced or recurrent disease. However, response rates to doxorubicin-based strategies range from 15 to 30% [23]. A more recent phase II study has shown that the combination of gemcitabine and docetaxel may be more effective, with response rates reported to be as high as 36% [24, 25]. The use of gemcitabine and docetaxel as first line therapy has been prospectively compared to doxorubicin as part of a phase III randomized trial (GeDDIS) enrolling patients with metastatic soft tissue sarcomas. Although similar progression-free survival rates were observed in both treatment arms, subjects treated with doxorubicin experienced significantly less toxicity. Study investigators concluded that doxorubicin should remain first line treatment for patients with metastatic soft tissue sarcomas [26].

Given these challenges, there is an overwhelming need to develop more effective strategies for the diagnosis and treatment of uLMS. Solutions will be made more difficult by the fact that uLMS now appears to be a unique biologic entity which responds differently to treatments than leiomyosarcomas arising at extrauterine sites [27–30]. Here, we review recent advances in the clinical management of uterine leiomyosarcoma, emphasizing the biologic basis of emerging therapeutic options (Figure 1).

2. Novel Targeted Therapies

2.1. Tyrosine Kinase Inhibitors. Uterine leiomyosarcoma is a highly vascular cancer that expresses significantly greater levels of vascular endothelial growth factor (VEGF) expression than many other tumors [31]. The overexpression of VEGF in uLMS has been shown to correlate with higher tumor grade, disease metastasis, and decreased survival [32, 33]. Although multiple antiangiogenic agents are now available for clinical use, the response of uLMS to many of these agents, such as bevacizumab, has been disappointing [34, 35]. A recent phase III clinical trial compared treatment with gemcitabine plus docetaxel with or without bevacizumab as first line therapy for advanced stage or recurrent uLMS. The results of this study failed to demonstrate any improvement in either progression-free or overall survival for patients who received bevacizumab [35].

More recently, results of randomized clinical trials have shown that a novel multityrosine kinase inhibitor known as pazopanib may be effective in treating soft tissue sarcomas. Pazopanib differs from bevacizumab in that it targets and inhibits not only the inherent tyrosine kinase activity of the VEGF receptor, but also those of the PDGF receptor and stem cell factor receptor (c-kit) [36]. Overexpression of EGFR, PDGFR-α, PDGFR-β, and PDGF-B has been reported to be a feature of uLMS [29]. Furthermore, levels of PDGF-B expression in uLMS specimens from the same study have been shown to correlate with outcome [29]. These observations suggest that the activation of PDGF-regulated pathways plays a particularly important role in promoting the growth and metastasis of uLMS.

Recently, the European Organization for the Research and Treatment of Cancer study concluded a phase III clinical trial entitled PALETTE, which compared pazopanib to placebo as a treatment for soft tissue sarcomas. Patients diagnosed with both uterine and nonuterine leiomyosarcomas were enrolled. In this multicenter, double blind study, patients with progressive disease were randomized to receive either pazopanib 800 mg once daily or placebo. Investigators reported a 3-month increase in progression-free survival for patients who received pazopanib [37].

Regorafenib is a multikinase inhibitor with documented efficacy for the treatment of gastrointestinal stromal tumors. Regorafenib has also recently been studied as a treatment for LMS [38]. A phase II double-blinded, randomized control trial compared regorafenib to placebo in patients with metastatic soft tissue sarcomas previously treated with anthracycline chemotherapy. In the subgroup of LMS patients enrolled in this study, PFS was found to be 4.0 months in patients receiving regorafenib compared to 1.9 months in the placebo arm. The most common adverse events noted were hypertension, skin toxicity, asthenia, and diarrhea [39, 40].

Olaratumab is a human antiplatelet derived growth factor receptor alpha monoclonal antibody that has been shown to have antitumor effects in human sarcoma xenografts [41]. Olaratumab specifically binds PDGFRα and blocks activation of this receptor by PDGF-AA, PDGF-BB, and PDGF-CC. A phase II randomized control trial compared the use of doxorubicin with and without olaratumab in patients with soft tissue sarcoma who had not previously been treated with an anthracycline. Subjects treated with doxorubicin and olaratumab had PFS of 6.6 months compared to 4.1 months with doxorubicin alone. Overall survival was better for subjects treated with the combination of doxorubicin and olaratumab (26.5 months compared to 14.7 months in those treated with doxorubicin alone). Neutropenia, mucositis, nausea, vomiting, and diarrhea each occurred more commonly in those subjects treated with olaratumab [42]. A phase III clinical trial is currently ongoing.

2.2. Antihormonal Agents. Reflecting their origin in the female reproductive tract, gynecologic sarcomas often express receptors for estrogen and progesterone. When examined immunohistochemically, 25–60% of uLMS have been found to express estrogen receptor (ER), while 35–60% of cases express progesterone receptor (PR) [43, 44].

Multiple studies have shown that estrogen and progesterone receptor expression in uLMS correlates with improved prognosis [43, 45, 46]. However, at least one group has suggested that activation of PR may serve to promote the growth of uterine smooth muscle [47]. Transgenic expression of Simian Virus 40 large T antigen driven by the promoter for oviduct-specific glycoprotein has been recently shown to result in the development of leiomyosarcoma [48, 49]. Of note, these transgenic animals develop LMS only under the influence of estrogen. These findings suggest that circulating levels of ligand-specific ER activation play an important role in tumor development.

Options currently available to inhibit activity at both the estrogen (ER) and progesterone (PR) receptors include both direct receptor antagonists as well as aromatase inhibitors. A number of studies have also examined the efficacy of direct ER antagonists such as tamoxifen. However, response to tamoxifen appears quite limited [44]. Aromatase inhibitors are orally available medications that decrease circulating levels of estrogen by targeting the peripheral conversion of testosterone and androstenedione to estrogen in adipose tissue. Retrospective studies have shown objective response rates and improvement in progression-free survival in patients with uLMS treated with aromatase inhibitors such as anastrozole or letrozole [50, 51]. A phase II clinical trial was conducted that examined the effect of letrozole 2.5 mg daily in 27 patients with unresectable uLMS, most of whom had already received cytotoxic treatment. All patients had confirmed ER/PR expression as evidenced by immunohistochemical staining. Stable disease was observed in 54% of patients receiving letrozole, with no evidence of disease progression at 12 weeks for 46% of patients [52].

Given the central role of both ER and PR in regulating the growth and remodeling of uterine smooth muscle, future work aimed at understanding the potential role of targeting steroid hormone receptors and/or their coactivators or corepressors as therapeutic options in uLMS are clearly warranted. Better understanding of the role of ER and PR in this disease may also help to decipher the circumstances under which oophorectomy may benefit the outcome.

2.3. Next Generation Alkylating Agents. As mentioned above, doxorubicin and other alkylating agents have been one of the primary approaches used to treat both metastatic and recurrent uLMS [23, 53]. Over the past 5 years, use of these agents has declined, with clinicians more frequently favoring the use of other regimens. However, recent success with orally available alkylating agents, such as temozolomide, has precipitated renewed interest in their use in the treatment of soft tissue sarcomas [54, 55]. A small retrospective study of 12 women with unresectable disease compared the efficacy of two dosing regimens for temozolomide in uLMS. Response rates appeared higher in patients treated with a bolus regimen (14%) rather than with a continuous dosing regimen (8%) [56]. A recent report has found that O6-methylguanine-DNA methyltransferase (MGMT) gene promoter hypermethylation is associated with response of glioblastoma to temozolomide therapy and may be a key factor determining a response to this agent. In a number of cancers, promoter hypermethylation has been shown to result in decreased expression of MGMT and gene as well as diminished DNA repair activity, rendering cells more susceptible to alkylating agents [57]. Hypermethylation of the MGMT gene promoter has also been observed in uterine sarcomas and thus could serve as a potential marker to identify patients who would benefit from temozolomide use [58, 59].

Trabectedin is another novel alkylating agent that has been recently approved in the United States for use in treating unresectable uLMS that have progressed despite receiving a standard cytotoxic chemotherapy regimen, which included an anthracycline. Trabectedin is a marine-derived alkaloid that interacts with the minor groove of DNA, leading to apoptosis [60]. Studies have examined the use of trabectedin alone and in combination with other chemotherapeutic agents. A phase II study examining the use of trabectedin as a single agent in chemotherapy naïve patients with advanced uLMS reported a 10% partial response rate [61]. However, trabectedin must be continued in absence of progression of disease, as discontinuation of the drug is associated with decreased progression-free survival. Another phase II study examined the efficacy of first line therapy with the combination of trabectedin and doxorubicin and reported a partial response rate of 60% [62]. The role of MGMT promoter hypermethylation in determining clinical responses to trabectedin is not currently known.

2.4. mTOR Inhibition. mTOR is a serine/threonine kinase involved in cell growth, proliferation, survival, and metabolism [63]. mTOR activation has been shown to contribute to uLMS cell growth and cell cycle progression. Specifically, loss of PTEN (phosphatase and tensin homolog) results in AKT-mTOR activation. In transgenic mice, inactivation or loss of PTEN leads to the development of uLMS [64, 65]. Rapamycin blocks the mTOR pathway and has been shown to have antitumor effects in preclinical models and has been shown to inhibit growth and cell cycle progression in uLMS cell lines [66, 67]. In PTEN knockout mice, everolimus, a rapamycin derivative, was shown to decelerate tumor growth [64]. mTOR inhibitors have been used clinically for treatment of soft tissue sarcomas [68]. Additional work is needed to determine the efficacy of mTOR inhibitors in uLMS specifically.

3. Novel Targets with Potential for Future Utility

3.1. Cell Cycle Inhibitors. In contrast to tumors, such as gastrointestinal stromal sarcomas (GIST), leiomyosarcoma regardless of its anatomic origin is considered genetically heterogeneous. This means that dominant driver mutations for uLMS have not been identified. A number of recent studies have examined patterns of gene expression in LMS of both uterine and nonuterine origin. It is clear from this work that the robust overexpression of gene products regulating the G2-M phase of the cell cycle is single predominant feature of these tumors [69, 70]. In one recent study, 26 of the 50 gene products most overexpressed when specimens of uLMS were compared to either healthy myometrium or benign uterine leiomyomas which played a role in regulation of the G2-M checkpoint [70]. Aurora kinase-A (AurkA) is a serine-threonine kinase involved in centrosome function and spindle assembly and has been shown to be highly overexpressed in uLMS. Use of MLN82237, an oral Aurk-A inhibitor, has been found to inhibit growth and metastasis of uLMS both *in vitro* and *in vivo*, using xenograft models [69]. Additional therapeutic benefit was observed when MLN82237 was combined with mTOR inhibition, consistent with AurkA's ability to cross-regulate mTOR pathway activity [67, 71]. A small, phase II clinical trial has examined the efficacy of MLN8237 (alisertib) monotherapy in 21 women with recurrent or persistent uLMS. All subjects in this study had received 1 to 2 prior cytotoxic regimens. Although no objective responses were reported, stable disease was observed in 38% of patients with mean progression-free and overall survival of 1.7 and 14.5 months, respectively [72]. Although the investigators for this trial concluded that alisertib did not demonstrate meaningful clinical activity against uLMS, it is possible that better efficacy will be observed when used in combination with mTOR inhibitors or even other types of cytotoxic or targeted agents.

3.2. Epigenetic Modifiers. Histone deacetylases (HDAC) are enzymes, which regulate patterns of gene expression modulating cell growth and apoptosis by removing acetyl moieties from histones [73, 74]. HDAC expression has been shown to be consistently elevated in endometrial stromal sarcomas [75]. Data has also shown that HDAC inhibitors can enhance chemotherapy-induced apoptosis and reduce sarcoma tumor volume in preclinical models [76]. Vorinostat is an oral HDAC inhibitor that has already been FDA approved for the treatment of cutaneous T cell lymphoma [77]. Studies have shown that vorinostat suppresses tumor growth in uterine sarcoma cells [76]. Given this preclinical data, HDAC inhibitors are being studied for targeted therapy in uterine sarcomas. A phase I trial evaluated the use of a HDAC inhibitor, abexinostat, in combination with doxorubicin for patients with metastatic sarcoma and showed manageable toxicities [78]. Further studies are needed to evaluate the efficacy of HDAC inhibitors in combination with cytotoxic agents and in uLMS specifically.

4. Conclusion

Management options for uLMS have evolved rapidly over the past several years with the advent of specific targeted therapies. These options have given patients new hope for improving their outcome. Given that uLMS likely represents a unique subset, distinct from extrauterine leiomyosarcomas, future therapeutic advances for this aggressive disease will need to consider its unique biologic basis.

Competing Interests

The authors have no conflict of interests to declare.

References

[1] N. S. Reed, C. Mangioni, H. Malmström et al., "Phase III randomised study to evaluate the role of adjuvant pelvic radiotherapy in the treatment of uterine sarcomas stages I and II: an European Organisation for Research and Treatment of Cancer Gynaecological Cancer Group Study (protocol 55874)," *European Journal of Cancer*, vol. 44, no. 6, pp. 808–818, 2008.

[2] F. J. Major, J. A. Blessing, S. G. Silverberg et al., "Prognostic factors in early-stage uterine sarcoma: A Gynecologic Oncology Group study," *Cancer*, vol. 71, no. 4, pp. 1702–1709, 1993.

[3] R. L. Siegel, K. D. Miller, and A. Jemal, "Cancer statistics, 2015," *CA—A Cancer Journal for Clinicians*, vol. 65, no. 1, pp. 5–29, 2015.

[4] S. M. Ueda, D. S. Kapp, M. K. Cheung et al., "Trends in demographic and clinical characteristics in women diagnosed with corpus cancer and their potential impact on the increasing number of deaths," *American Journal of Obstetrics & Gynecology*, vol. 198, no. 2, pp. 218.el–218.e6, 2008.

[5] N. Bansal, T. J. Herzog, W. Burke, C. J. Cohen, and J. D. Wright, "The utility of preoperative endometrial sampling for the detection of uterine sarcomas," *Gynecologic Oncology*, vol. 110, no. 1, pp. 43–48, 2008.

[6] E. M. Hinchcliff, K. M. Esselen, J. C. Watkins et al., "The role of endometrial biopsy in the preoperative detection of uterine leiomyosarcoma," *Journal of Minimally Invasive Gynecology*, vol. 23, no. 4, pp. 567–572, 2016.

[7] S. Chiang and E. Oliva, "Recent developments in uterine mesenchymal neoplasms," *Histopathology*, vol. 62, no. 1, pp. 124–137, 2013.

[8] A. A. Gockley, J. A. Rauh-Hain, and M. G. Del Carmen, "Uterine leiomyosarcoma a review article," *International Journal of Gynecological Cancer*, vol. 24, no. 9, pp. 1538–1542, 2014.

[9] W. H. Parker, Y. S. Fu, and J. S. Berek, "Uterine sarcoma in patients operated on for presumed leiomyoma and rapidly growing leiomyoma," *Obstetrics and Gynecology*, vol. 83, no. 3, pp. 414–418, 1994.

[10] S. H. Tirumani, V. Ojili, A. K. P. Shanbhogue, N. Fasih, J. G. Ryan, and C. Reinhold, "Current concepts in the imaging of uterine sarcoma," *Abdominal Imaging*, vol. 38, no. 2, pp. 397–411, 2013.

[11] M. L. Hensley, O. Zivanovic, M. M. Leitao et al., "Stage-specific outcomes of patients with Uterine leiomyosarcoma: a comparison of the international federation of gynecology and obstetrics and american joint committee on cancer staging systems," *Journal of Clinical Oncology*, vol. 27, no. 12, pp. 2066–2072, 2009.

[12] O. Zivanovic, L. M. Jacks, A. Iasonos et al., "A nomogram to predict postresection 5-year overall survival for patients with uterine leiomyosarcoma," *Cancer*, vol. 118, no. 3, pp. 660–669, 2012.

[13] A. Iasonos, E. Z. Keung, O. Zivanovic et al., "External validation of a prognostic nomogram for overall survival in women with uterine leiomyosarcoma," *Cancer*, vol. 119, no. 10, pp. 1816–1822, 2013.

[14] M. M. Leitao, Y. Sonoda, M. F. Brennan, R. R. Barakat, and D. S. Chi, "Incidence of lymph node and ovarian metastases in leiomyosarcoma of the uterus," *Gynecologic Oncology*, vol. 91, no. 1, pp. 209–212, 2003.

[15] K. Y. Tse, R. Crawford, and H. Y. S. Ngan, "Staging of uterine sarcomas," *Best Practice & Research Clinical Obstetrics & Gynaecology*, vol. 25, no. 6, pp. 733–749, 2011.

[16] D. S. Kapp, J. Y. Shin, and J. K. Chan, "Prognostic factors and survival in 1396 patients with uterine leiomyosarcomas: emphasis on impact of lymphadenectomy and oophorectomy," *Cancer*, vol. 112, no. 4, pp. 820–830, 2008.

[17] P. Wong, K. Han, J. Sykes et al., "Postoperative radiotherapy improves local control and survival in patients with uterine leiomyosarcoma," *Radiation Oncology*, vol. 8, no. 1, article 128, 2013.

[18] S. Sampath, T. E. Schultheiss, J. K. Ryu, and J. Y. C. Wong, "The role of adjuvant radiation in uterine sarcomas," *International Journal of Radiation Oncology* Biology* Physics*, vol. 76, no. 3, pp. 728–734, 2010.

[19] P. Pautier, A. Floquet, L. Gladieff et al., "A randomized clinical trial of adjuvant chemotherapy with doxorubicin, ifosfamide, and cisplatin in localized uterine sarcomas. Results on 81 randomized patients," *European Journal of Cancer*, vol. 47, supplement 2, p. 15, 2011.

[20] G. A. Omura, J. A. Blessing, F. Major et al., "A randomized clinical trial of adjuvant adriamycin in uterine sarcomas: a Gynecologic Oncology Group Study," *Journal of Clinical Oncology*, vol. 3, no. 9, pp. 1240–1245, 1985.

[21] P. Pautier, A. Floquet, L. Gladieff et al., "A randomized clinical trial of adjuvant chemotherapy with doxorubicin, ifosfamide, and cisplatin followed by radiotherapy versus radiotherapy alone in patients with localized uterine sarcomas (SARCGYN study). A study of the French sarcoma group," *Annals of Oncology*, vol. 24, no. 4, Article ID mds545, pp. 1099–1104, 2013.

[22] M. L. Hensley, J. K. Wathen, R. G. Maki et al., "Adjuvant therapy for high-grade, uterus-limited leiomyosarcoma: results of a phase 2 trial (SARC 005)," *Cancer*, vol. 119, no. 8, pp. 1555–1561, 2013.

[23] G. Sutton, J. A. Blessing, and J. H. Malfetano, "Ifosfamide and doxorubicin in the treatment of advanced leiomyosarcomas of the uterus: A Gynecologic Oncology Group study," *Gynecologic Oncology*, vol. 62, no. 2, pp. 226–229, 1996.

[24] M. L. Hensley, J. A. Blessing, R. Mannel, and P. G. Rose, "Fixed-dose rate gemcitabine plus docetaxel as first-line therapy for metastatic uterine leiomyosarcoma: a Gynecologic Oncology Group phase II trial," *Gynecologic Oncology*, vol. 109, no. 3, pp. 329–334, 2008.

[25] R. G. Maki, J. K. Wathen, S. R. Patel et al., "Randomized phase II study of gemcitabine and docetaxel compared with gemcitabine

alone in patients with metastatic soft tissue sarcomas," *Journal of Clinical Oncology*, vol. 25, no. 19, pp. 2755–2763, 2007.

[26] B. Seddon, J. Whelan, S. Strauss et al., "A prospective randomized controlled phase III trial of gemcitabine and docetaxel compared wiht doxorubicin as first-line treatment in previously untreated advanced unresectable or metastatic soft tissue sarcomas," *Journal of Clinical Oncology*, vol. 33, supplement, abstract 10500, 2015.

[27] W. Lamm, C. Natter, S. Schur et al., "Distinctive outcome in patients with non-uterine and uterine leiomyosarcoma," *BMC Cancer*, vol. 14, no. 1, article 981, 2014.

[28] D. J. Worhunsky, M. Gupta, S. Gholami et al., "Leiomyosarcoma: one disease or distinct biologic entities based on site of origin?" *Journal of Surgical Oncology*, vol. 111, no. 7, pp. 808–812, 2015.

[29] K. Lusby, K. B. Savannah, E. G. Demicco et al., "Uterine leiomyosarcoma management, outcome, and associated molecular biomarkers: a single institution's experience," *Annals of Surgical Oncology*, vol. 20, no. 7, pp. 2364–2372, 2013.

[30] X. Guo, V. Y. Jo, A. M. Mills et al., "Clinically relevant molecular subtypes in leiomyosarcoma," *Clinical Cancer Research*, vol. 21, no. 15, pp. 3501–3511, 2015.

[31] S. S. Yoon, N. H. Segal, A. B. Olshen, M. F. Brennan, and S. Singer, "Circulating angiogenic factor levels correlate with extent of disease and risk of recurrence in patients with soft tissue sarcoma," *Annals of Oncology*, vol. 15, no. 8, pp. 1261–1266, 2004.

[32] D. S. McMeekin, M. W. Sill, K. M. Darcy et al., "A phase II trial of thalidomide in patients with refractory leiomyosarcoma of the uterus and correlation with biomarkers of angiogenesis: A Gynecologic Oncology Group Study," *Gynecologic Oncology*, vol. 106, no. 3, pp. 596–603, 2007.

[33] U. Graeven, N. Andre, E. Achilles, C. Zornig, and W. Schmiegel, "Serum levels of vascular endothelial growth factor and basic fibroblast growth factor in patients with soft-tissue sarcoma," *Journal of Cancer Research and Clinical Oncology*, vol. 125, no. 10, pp. 577–581, 1999.

[34] S. Pacey, M. J. Ratain, K. T. Flaherty et al., "Efficacy and safety of sorafenib in a subset of patients with advanced soft tissue sarcoma from a phase II randomized discontinuation trial," *Investigational New Drugs*, vol. 29, no. 3, pp. 481–488, 2011.

[35] M. L. Hensley, A. Miller, D. M. O'Malley et al., "Randomized phase III trial of gemcitabine plus docetaxel plus bevacizumab or placebo as first-line treatment for metastatic uterine leiomyosarcoma: An NRG Oncology/ Gynecologic Oncology Group Study," *Journal of Clinical Oncology*, vol. 33, no. 10, pp. 1180–1185, 2015.

[36] J.-M. Schlaeppi and J. M. Wood, "Targeting vascular endothelial growth factor (VEGF) for anti-tumor therapy, by anti-VEGF neutralizing monoclonal antibodies or by VEGF receptor tyrosine-kinase inhibitors," *Cancer and Metastasis Reviews*, vol. 18, no. 4, pp. 473–481, 1999.

[37] W. T. A. Van Der Graaf, J.-Y. Blay, S. P. Chawla et al., "Pazopanib for metastatic soft-tissue sarcoma (PALETTE): a randomised, double-blind, placebo-controlled phase 3 trial," *The Lancet*, vol. 379, no. 9829, pp. 1879–1886, 2012.

[38] K. A. Lyseng-Williamson, "Regorafenib: a guide to its use in advanced gastrointestinal stromal tumor (GIST) after failure of imatinib and sunitinib," *BioDrugs*, vol. 27, no. 5, pp. 525–531, 2013.

[39] O. Mir, T. Brodowicz, J. Wallet et al., "Activity of regorafenib (RE) in leiomyosarcomas (LMS) and other types of soft-tissue sarcomas (OTS): results of a double-blind, randomized placebo (PL) controlled phase II trial," *Journal of Clinical Oncology*, vol. 33, no. 15, supplement 1, 2015.

[40] T. Brodowicz, B. Liegl-Atzwager, E. Tresch et al., "Study protocol of REGOSARC trial: activity and safety of regorafenib in advanced soft tissue sarcoma: a multinational, randomized, placebo-controlled, phase II trial," *BMC Cancer*, vol. 15, article 127, 2015.

[41] N. Loizos, Y. Xu, J. Huber et al., "Targeting the platelet-derived growth factor receptor α with a neutralizing human monoclonal antibody inhibits the growth of tumor xenografts: implications as a potential therapeutic target," *Molecular Cancer Therapeutics*, vol. 4, no. 3, pp. 369–379, 2005.

[42] W. D. Tap, R. L. Jones, B. A. Van Tine et al., "Olaratumab and doxorubicin versus doxorubicin alone for treatment of soft-tissue sarcoma: an open-label phase 1b and randomised phase 2 trial," *The Lancet*, vol. 388, no. 10043, pp. 488–497, 2016.

[43] K. Bodner, B. Bodner-Adler, O. Kimberger, K. Czerwenka, S. Leodolter, and K. Mayerhofer, "Estrogen and progesterone receptor expression in patients with uterine leiomyosarcoma and correlation with different clinicopathological parameters," *Anticancer Research*, vol. 23, no. 1, pp. 729–732, 2003.

[44] Y. J. Ioffe, A. J. Li, C. S. Walsh et al., "Hormone receptor expression in uterine sarcomas: prognostic and therapeutic roles," *Gynecologic Oncology*, vol. 115, no. 3, pp. 466–471, 2009.

[45] S. E. Akhan, E. Yavuz, A. Tecer et al., "The expression of Ki-67, p53, estrogen and progesterone receptors affecting survival in uterine leiomyosarcomas. A Clinicopathologic Study," *Gynecologic Oncology*, vol. 99, no. 1, pp. 36–42, 2005.

[46] M. M. Leitao Jr., M. L. Hensley, R. R. Barakat et al., "Immunohistochemical expression of estrogen and progesterone receptors and outcomes in patients with newly diagnosed uterine leiomyosarcoma," *Gynecologic Oncology*, vol. 124, no. 3, pp. 558–562, 2012.

[47] J. J. Kim, T. Kurita, and S. E. Bulun, "Progesterone action in endometrial cancer, endometriosis, uterine fibroids, and breast cancer," *Endocrine Reviews*, vol. 34, no. 1, pp. 130–162, 2013.

[48] I. Miyoshi, K. Takahashi, Y. Kon et al., "Mouse transgenic for murine oviduct-specific glycoprotein promoter-driven simian virus 40 large T-antigen: tumor formation and its hormonal regulation," *Molecular Reproduction and Development*, vol. 63, no. 2, pp. 168–176, 2002.

[49] A. M. Friel, W. B. Growdon, C. K. McCann et al., "Mouse models of uterine corpus tumors: clinical significance and utility," *Frontiers in Bioscience*, vol. 2, pp. 882–905, 2010.

[50] R. O'Cearbhaill, Q. Zhou, A. Iasonos et al., "Treatment of advanced uterine leiomyosarcoma with aromatase inhibitors," *Gynecologic Oncology*, vol. 116, no. 3, pp. 424–429, 2010.

[51] E. Thanopoulou, K. Thway, K. Khabra, and I. Judson, "Treatment of hormone positive uterine leiomyosarcoma with aromatase inhibitors," *Clinical Sarcoma Research*, vol. 4, no. 1, article 5, 2014.

[52] S. George, Y. Feng, J. Manola et al., "Phase 2 trial of aromatase inhibition with letrozole in patients with uterine leiomyosarcomas expressing estrogen and/or progesterone receptors," *Cancer*, vol. 120, no. 5, pp. 738–743, 2014.

[53] S. Sleijfer, C. Seynaeve, and J. Verweij, "Using single-agent therapy in adult patients with advanced soft tissue sarcoma can still be considered standard care," *Oncologist*, vol. 10, no. 10, pp. 833–841, 2005.

[54] S. M. Talbot, M. L. Keohan, M. Hesdorffer et al., "A phase II trial of temozolomide in patients with unresectable or metastatic soft tissue sarcoma," *Cancer*, vol. 98, no. 9, pp. 1942–1946, 2003.

[55] P. J. Woll, I. Judson, S. M. Lee et al., "Temozolomide in adult patients with advanced soft tissue sarcoma: a phase II study of the EORTC soft tissue and bone sarcoma group," *European Journal of Cancer*, vol. 35, no. 3, pp. 410–412, 1999.

[56] S. Anderson and C. Aghajanian, "Temozolomide in uterine leiomyosarcomas," *Gynecologic Oncology*, vol. 98, no. 1, pp. 99–103, 2005.

[57] M. E. Hegi, A.-C. Diserens, T. Gorlia et al., "MGMT gene silencing and benefit from temozolomide in glioblastoma," *The New England Journal of Medicine*, vol. 352, no. 10, pp. 997–1003, 2005.

[58] M. Bujko, M. Kowalewska, A. Danska-Bidzinska, E. Bakula-Zalewska, J. A. Siedecki, and M. Bidzinski, "The promoter methylation and expression of the O6-methylguanine-DNA methyltransferase gene in uterine sarcoma and carcinosarcoma," *Oncology Letters*, vol. 4, no. 3, pp. 551–555, 2012.

[59] J. S. Ferriss, K. A. Atkins, J. A. Lachance, S. C. Modesitt, and A. A. Jazaeri, "Temozolomide in advanced and recurrent uterine leiomyosarcoma and correlation with O6-methylguanine DNA methyltransferase expression a case series," *International Journal of Gynecological Cancer*, vol. 20, no. 1, pp. 120–125, 2010.

[60] M. D'Incalci and C. M. Galmarini, "A review of trabectedin (ET-743): a unique mechanism of action," *Molecular Cancer Therapeutics*, vol. 9, no. 8, pp. 2157–2163, 2010.

[61] B. J. Monk, J. A. Blessing, D. G. Street, C. Y. Muller, J. J. Burke, and M. L. Hensley, "A phase II evaluation of trabectedin in the treatment of advanced, persistent, or recurrent uterine leiomyosarcoma: A Gynecologic Oncology Group Study," *Gynecologic Oncology*, vol. 124, no. 1, pp. 48–52, 2012.

[62] P. Pautier, A. Floquet, C. Chevreau et al., "Trabectedin in combination with doxorubicin for first-line treatment of advanced uterine or soft-tissue leiomyosarcoma (LMS-02): a non-randomised, multicentre, phase 2 trial," *The Lancet Oncology*, vol. 16, no. 4, pp. 457–464, 2015.

[63] D. D. Sarbassov, D. A. Guertin, S. M. Ali, and D. M. Sabatini, "Phosphorylation and regulation of Akt/PKB by the rictor-mTOR complex," *Science*, vol. 307, no. 5712, pp. 1098–1101, 2005.

[64] E. Hernando, E. Charytonowicz, M. E. Dudas et al., "The AKT-mTOR pathway plays a critical role in the development of leiomyosarcomas," *Nature Medicine*, vol. 13, no. 6, pp. 748–753, 2007.

[65] T. F. Wong, T. Takeda, B. Li et al., "Curcumin disrupts uterine leiomyosarcoma cells through AKT-mTOR pathway inhibition," *Gynecologic Oncology*, vol. 122, no. 1, pp. 141–148, 2011.

[66] X. Wan and L. J. Helman, "The biology behind mTOR inhibition in sarcoma," *Oncologist*, vol. 12, no. 8, pp. 1007–1018, 2007.

[67] K. J. Brewer Savannah, E. G. Demicco, K. Lusby et al., "Dual targeting of mTOR and Aurora-A kinase for the treatment of uterine leiomyosarcoma," *Clinical Cancer Research*, vol. 18, no. 17, pp. 4633–4645, 2012.

[68] S. Vemulapalli, A. Mita, Y. Alvarado, K. Sankhala, and M. Mita, "The emerging role of mammalian target of rapamycin inhibitors in the treatment of sarcomas," *Targeted Oncology*, vol. 6, no. 1, pp. 29–39, 2011.

[69] W. Shan, P. Y. Akinfenwa, K. B. Savannah et al., "A small-molecule inhibitor targeting the mitotic spindle checkpoint impairs the growth of uterine leiomyosarcoma," *Clinical Cancer Research*, vol. 18, no. 12, pp. 3352–3365, 2012.

[70] J. N. Barlin, Q. C. Zhou, M. M. Leitao et al., "Molecular subtypes of uterine leiomyosarcoma and correlation with clinical outcome," *Neoplasia*, vol. 17, no. 2, pp. 183–189, 2015.

[71] X. Wang, Y.-X. Zhou, W. Qiao et al., "Overexpression of aurora kinase A in mouse mammary epithelium induces genetic instability preceding mammary tumor formation," *Oncogene*, vol. 25, no. 54, pp. 7148–7158, 2006.

[72] D. M. Hyman, M. Sill, J. K. Cho et al., "A phase II study of alisertib (MLN8237) in recurrent or persistent uterine leiomyosarcoma: an NRG Oncology/Gynecologic Oncology Group study (GOG-0231D)," *Journal of Clinical Oncology*, vol. 33, supplement, abstract e16512, 2015, Proceedings of the 2015 ASCO Annual Meeting.

[73] M. Dokmanovic, C. Clarke, and P. A. Marks, "Histone deacetylase inhibitors: overview and perspectives," *Molecular Cancer Research*, vol. 5, no. 10, pp. 981–989, 2007.

[74] W. S. Xu, R. B. Parmigiani, and P. A. Marks, "Histone deacetylase inhibitors: molecular mechanisms of action," *Oncogene*, vol. 26, no. 37, pp. 5541–5552, 2007.

[75] A. Hrzenjak, F. Moinfar, M.-L. Kremser et al., "Valproate inhibition of histone deacetylase 2 affects differentiation and decreases proliferation of endometrial stromal sarcoma cells," *Molecular Cancer Therapeutics*, vol. 5, no. 9, pp. 2203–2210, 2006.

[76] A. Hrzenjak, F. Moinfar, M.-L. Kremser et al., "Histone deacetylase inhibitor vorinostat suppresses the growth of uterine sarcomas in vitro and in vivo," *Molecular Cancer*, vol. 9, article 49, 2010.

[77] M. Duvic and J. Vu, "Vorinostat: a new oral histone deacetylase inhibitor approved for cutaneous T-cell lymphoma," *Expert Opinion on Investigational Drugs*, vol. 16, no. 7, pp. 1111–1120, 2007.

[78] E. Choy, Y. Flamand, S. Balasubramanian et al., "Phase 1 study of oral abexinostat, a histone deacetylase inhibitor, in combination with doxorubicin in patients with metastatic sarcoma," *Cancer*, vol. 121, no. 8, pp. 1223–1230, 2015.

24

Ewing's Sarcoma as a Second Malignancy in Long-Term Survivors of Childhood Hematologic Malignancies

Fabian Wolpert,[1,2] Michael A. Grotzer,[3] Felix Niggli,[3] Dieter Zimmermann,[4] Elisabeth Rushing,[5] and Beata Bode-Lesniewska[4]

[1]*Department of Neurology, University Hospital Zurich, Frauenklinikstrasse 26, 8091 Zurich, Switzerland*
[2]*Department of Medical Oncology, University Hospital Zurich, Rämistrasse 100, 8091 Zurich, Switzerland*
[3]*Department of Pediatric Oncology, University Children's Hospital, Zurich, Steinwiesstrasse 75, 8032 Zurich, Switzerland*
[4]*Institute of Surgical Pathology, University Hospital Zurich, Schmelzbergstrasse 12, 8091 Zurich, Switzerland*
[5]*Department of Neuropathology, University Hospital Zurich, Schmelzbergstrasse 12, 8091 Zurich, Switzerland*

Correspondence should be addressed to Beata Bode-Lesniewska; beata.bode@usz.ch

Academic Editor: Natia Esiashvili

Modern multimodal treatment has significantly increased survival for patients affected by hematologic malignancies, especially in childhood. Following remission, however, the risk of developing a further malignancy is an important issue. The long-term estimated risk of developing a sarcoma as a secondary malignancy is increased severalfold in comparison to the general population. Ewing's sarcoma family encompasses a group of highly aggressive, undifferentiated, intra- and extraosseous, mesenchymal tumors, caused by several types of translocations usually involving the *EWSR1* gene. Translocation associated sarcomas, such as Ewing sarcoma, are only rarely encountered as therapy associated secondary tumors. We describe the clinical course and management of three patients from a single institution with Ewing's sarcoma that followed successfully treated lymphoblastic T-cell leukemia or non-Hodgkin lymphoma. The literature on secondary Ewing's sarcoma is summarized and possible pathogenic mechanisms are critically discussed.

1. Introduction

Modern multimodal treatment strategies have significantly increased the survival of patients affected by hematologic malignancies, including indolent and aggressive forms of lymphoma and leukemia [1, 2]. In long-term survivors of childhood cancer, the risk of a second cancer is an important issue [3]. Standard treatment for newly diagnosed malignancies varies according to the phenotype, the line of differentiation, biological markers, and extent of the disease and comprises various combinations of chemotherapy [4], radiotherapy, targeted therapy with monoclonal antibodies, and stem cell transplantation, all of which have been implicated as risk factors for second malignancies. The most common second cancers reported in this population include cancers of the head and neck, melanoma, lung cancer, colon cancer, bladder cancer, renal cancer, Hodgkin disease, leukemia, and Kaposi sarcoma [5]. Patients who received radiation therapy are more likely to develop sarcomas, breast cancers, and mesothelioma compared with patients who have not received it [5].

Ewing's sarcoma (ES) is an aggressive malignancy occurring as a primary tumor mostly in adolescents and young adults with an incidence of about 1/1 000 000, male to female ratio being 1,5 : 1 [6]. Most cases of ESs (80%) originate in bones, where this entity comprises the second most common primary tumor following osteosarcoma in children and adolescents. Up to 20% of primary ESs are located extraosseously in soft tissues, affecting not only extremities but also various internal organs [7–10]. ESs are characterized at the molecular level by the presence of a balanced translocation between the *EWSR1* gene and a member of the ETS gene family, in at least 80% of cases the partner gene being the *FLI1* gene (translocation t(11;22) (q24;q12) *(EWS-FLI1)*) [11]. This molecular signature and the clinical characteristics of the patients are typical for the peripheral primitive neuroectodermal tumor (PNET) as well. Accordingly, in the current WHO classification [11], PNET once considered a separate entity is now considered to represent part of the histologic spectrum of the "Ewing family of tumors" [6, 12]. The presence of the fusion gene containing the *EWSR1* gene and a member of the ETS family is the most important tumorigenic factor in ES; however, recent genomewide association studies (GWAS) have demonstrated an association of this tumor with the germline background of the affected patients [13]. These studies provide a plausible explanation for the epidemiological finding of a different incidence of ESs across human populations, for example, the significantly higher incidence in patients of Caucasian compared to African origin.

ESs, in contrast to sarcomas with complex karyotypes and without recurring genetic aberrations such as osteosarcoma, have only rarely been reported to occur secondary to cancer therapy, including multimodal therapy for hematologic malignancies [7, 14, 15]. The aim of this study is to analyze three cases of secondary ES in patients from our institutions with T-cell leukemia or non-Hodgkin lymphoma (NHL) as well as summarize documented similar cases from the literature. In addition, the literature review on Ewing's sarcoma as a secondary cancer is summarized and possible pathogenic mechanisms are critically discussed.

2. Materials and Methods

2.1. Patients. Three patients with a diagnosis of a genetically confirmed Ewing sarcoma who were previously treated for leukemia or lymphoma during the period of 1991 to 2014 were identified among 98 Ewing sarcoma patients in the archives of the Institute of Surgical Pathology, University Hospital Zurich, Switzerland. Complete follow-up data were available for all 3 patients, including information regarding tumor site and specific treatment modalities of the primary as well as of the secondary malignancy. The available histopathological slides of all 3 cases were reviewed to confirm the diagnosis of ES. A review of the literature published in PUBMED of previously reported cases of ES following another primary malignancy was performed.

The study has been carried out according to the ethical guidelines of our institution.

2.2. Histology and Immunohistochemistry. Tumor tissue samples were fixed in buffered 4% formalin and embedded in paraffin. 2 μm thick sections were stained with hematoxylin and eosin (H&E) according to standard procedures. Immunohistochemistry (IHC) using the CD99 antibody (dilution 1:25, clone HO36-1.1, Novocastra Lab Ltd) was performed on 2 μm thick paraffin sections, using the Ventana Benchmark XT automated staining system (Ventana Medical Systems, Tucson, Arizona).

2.3. Fluorescence In Situ Hybridization (FISH). Fluorescence in situ hybridization (FISH) studies were performed on formalin-fixed, paraffin-embedded, 4 μm thick tissue sections as described earlier [16]. Dual color break-apart FISH detecting translocations involving the *EWSR1* (22q11) gene was performed using commercial probes (Vysis, Abbott AG, Baar, Switzerland). The SpectrumOrange- and SpectrumGreen-labeled EWSR1 probes covered 500 kb and 1,100 kb proximal and distal to the EWSR1 gene. The fluorescence staining was visualized with an Olympus BX61 microscope (Olympus, Volketswil, Switzerland) equipped with DAPI, SpectrumGreen and SpectrumOrange filters. Images were acquired with a CCD camera and processed with the AnalySIS imaging software (Soft Imagining System, Munster, Germany). For the assessment of *EWSR1* gene rearrangements at least 50 nonoverlapping tumor nuclei were analyzed. If the sample contained at least 25% of split red and green signals, the tumor was regarded as translocation positive. The signal was considered as split, when red and green fluorescent spots were separated by at least twice the distance occupied by a single probe [17].

2.4. RNA Extraction and RT-PCR. To detect EWSR1-FLI1 and EWSR1-ERG fusions transcripts, total RNA was extracted form paraffin-embedded tissue as described earlier [18]. Amplification was done in a GeneAmp PCR System 9700 (Applied Biosystems) using an OneStep RT-PCR Kit (Qiagen). The 25 μL reactions contained 0.4 mM dNTP, 1x OneStep RT-PCR Buffer, 5 μL Q-solution, 1 μL enzyme mix (all from Qiagen), and 8 units of RNase OUT (Life Technologies). The primer pairs were as follows: (A) TCCTACAGCCAA GCTCCAAGTC (EWSR1-Ex7b) and ATTCATGTTGGG-CTTGCTTTTC (FLI1-Ex9); (B) AGAGTAGCTATGGTC-AACAA (EWSR1-Ex7a) and CCCA(TA)GCTCCTCT TCTG (FLI1-Ex6); (C) TCCTACAGCCAAGCTCCAAGTC (EWSR1-Ex7b) and CTCCAGGAGGAACTGCCAAA (ERG-Ex9).

The reverse transcription was done for 30 minutes at 50°C, followed by a PCR activation step for 15 minutes at 95°C and 40 cycles consisting of 1 minute at 94°C, 1 minute at 56°C, and 1 minute at 72°C followed by final extension at 72°C for 10 minutes. RNA-integrity was tested by running ACTB- and IPO8-specific internal control reactions for each sample.

3. Results

3.1. Patients. The basic patient characteristics are summarized in Table 1.

3.1.1. Patient 1. T-cell lymphoblastic non-Hodgkin lymphoma was diagnosed in this male patient at the age of 5 years. He first presented with supraclavicular swelling. Histopathologic examination of the resected lymph node revealed high grade T-cell lymphoblastic non-Hodgkin lymphoma (Figure 1(a); unfortunately, except for the text of the final diagnosis and one H&E slide no further histopathological details are available). Diagnostic workup including chest and abdominal CT scans revealed no further tumor manifestations. He was treated according to the NHL-BFM 90 therapy (Berlin-Frankfurt-Munster), which comprises cyclophosphamide,

Table 1: Clinical data on the patients in the current study.

Pat.	Gender	Age at Dx (T-ALL)	Age at Dx (ES)	Latency (y)	Location of ES	Treatment of the primary hematological malignancy				
						Anthracyclines, TPII-Inh	Vinca	Alkylating agent	Antimetabolite	RT
1	m	5	8	3	Paravertebral (L5)	ADR	None	CPA, IFO	Ara-C	None
2	m	16	21	5	Brain, temporal lobe	DNR	VCR	CPA	MTX, Ara-C, 6-MP, 6-TG	Whole brain (12 Gy)
3	f	9	11	2	Mandible	DNR	VCR	CPA	MTX, Ara-C, 6-MP, 6-TG	Whole body (12 Gy)

DNR, daunorubicin; ADR, doxorubicin; VCR, vincristine; CPA, cyclophosphamide; IFO, ifosfamide; MTX, methotrexate; Ara-C, cytarabine; 6-MP, 6-mercaptopurine; 6-TG, thioguanine; RT, radiotherapy.

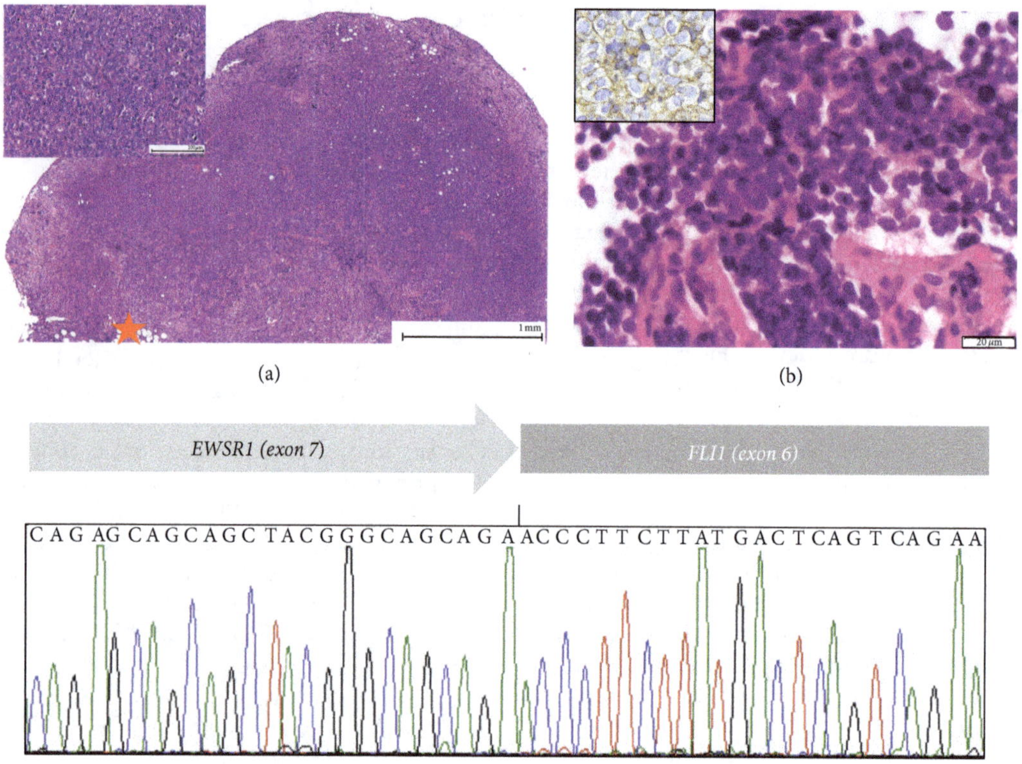

(a) (b) (c)

Figure 1: (a) Biopsy of the cervical mass of patient 1, 3 years prior to current presentation. Diffuse infiltration of the lymph node tissue with effacement of the lymph node architecture and spread to the adjacent adipose tissue (star) by sheets of atypical lymphatic blasts (inset) (H&E; original magnification 400x). (b) Core biopsy of the paravertebral mass of patient 1. Solid small, blue round undifferentiated tumor with strong immunohistochemical membranous expression of CD99 (brown reaction product shown in the inset) (H&E; original magnification 400x). (c) Sanger-sequencing of the RT-PCR amplicon derived from the fusion transcript reveals the most common EWSR1-FLI1 fusion of exon 7 to exon 6, respectively, in the paravertebral tumor tissue of patient 1 confirming the diagnosis of a Ewing sarcoma.

dexamethasone, ifosfamide, methotrexate, cytarabine, prednisolone, etoposide, and cyclophosphamide without radiotherapy. Chemotherapy was completed after 2.5 years in 03/1998. The patient showed complete remission in the comprehensive follow-up investigations that included laboratory testing, CT scan of brain, chest, and abdomen, bone scan, bone marrow biopsy, cardiac scan, and renal scan.

Three years after the first presentation, he developed nocturnal thigh pain. A bone scan showed a large paravertebral (level L5) mass. Chest and thorax CT revealed lun metastases. Biopsy of the paravertebral lesion showed a malignant small, blue, round, cell tumor, histopathologically consistent with ES (Figure 1(b)). The diagnosis was confirmed by RT-PCR demonstrating the t(11;22) translocation with the *EWSR1/FLI1* fusion transcript (Figure 1(c)).

The patient received chemotherapy with vincristine, actinomycin, ifosfamide, adriamycin, carboplatin, epirubicin, and etoposide, based on the CWS-96 protocol (high risk) [19]. Furthermore, he received radiotherapy to the chest and paravertebral region with a cumulative dose of 44.8 Gy. Subsequently, CT scans of the chest, abdomen, and spine revealed complete remission of the pulmonary metastases

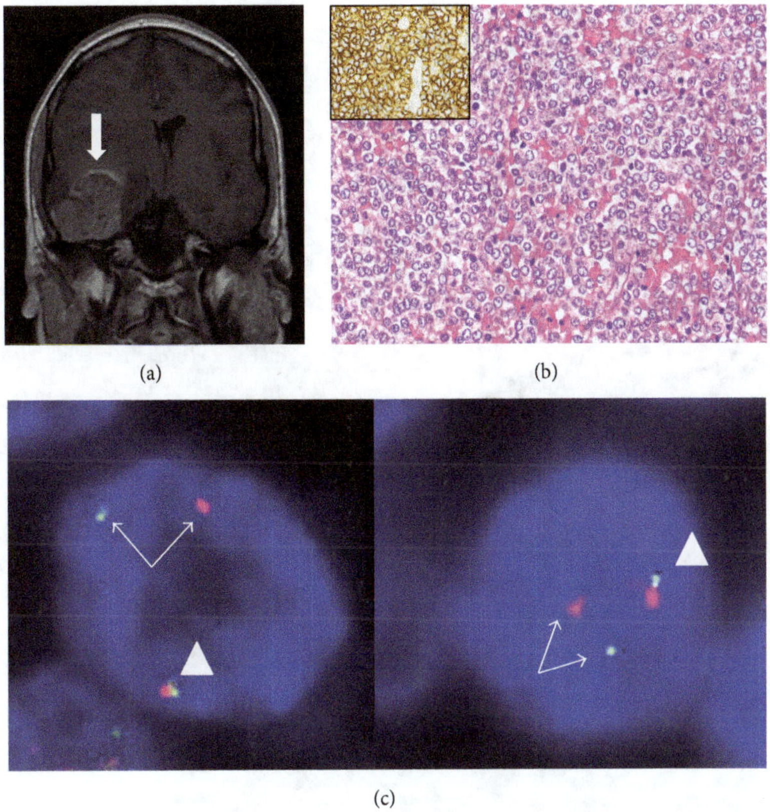

FIGURE 2: (a) Coronary T1 MRI section demonstrating a 4 cm mass (arrow) within the right temporal lobe with middle line shift in patient 2. (b) Biopsy of the intracerebral temporal tumor of patient 2 shows solid small, blue round undifferentiated proliferation with a strong immunohistochemical membranous expression of CD99 (brown reaction product shown in the inset) (H&E; original magnification 200x). (c) Fluorescence in situ hybridization (FISH) of the brain tumor of patient 2, demonstrating the rearrangement of the EWSR1 gene. The nuclei of the tumor cells contain one fused signal (arrow head) and one pair of split green and red signals (arrows).

and size reduction of the left sided paravertebral mass at L4-5 level.

One year later, the patient underwent high dose chemotherapy with busulfan and alkeran and autologous stem cell transplantation. Unfortunately, he developed an infection with an unknown pathogen one month later that proved refractory to antibiotic treatment and he died from acute respiratory distress syndrome.

3.1.2. Patient 2. Acute lymphoblastic T-cell leukemia was diagnosed in this male patient at the age of 16 years. He presented with a mediastinal mass without central nervous system involvement. Bone marrow aspiration showed 95% blasts infiltration: CD3c+; CD3+; CD4+; CD8+; CD7+; CD5+; CD34+; CD56+; CD2+; TDT+; TCR a/b+. The patient underwent chemotherapy with vincristine, daunorubicin, L-asparaginase, methotrexate (MTX), and Ara-C. Dexamethasone and thioguanine were given during induction and reinduction. He received whole brain radiation (cumulative dose 12 Gy) and 4 doses of intrathecal therapy with MTX, prednisolone, and Ara-C. After completion of therapy in 10/2002, the patient showed hematological remission in the follow-up controls.

Five years and 8 months later, the patient presented to the emergency unit with headache and vomiting. MRI imaging revealed a large intracerebral tumor mass (Figure 2(a)). Resection of the tumor revealed a strongly CD99 positive, small, blue, round cell malignant tumor on histopathological examination (Figure 2(b)) that lacked the expression of lymphatic markers. No rearrangement of the TCR-γ gene locus was found on genotyping. The RT-PCR of the fusion products of the two most common Ewing sarcoma translocations t(11;22) *EWSR1/FLI1* and t(21;22) *ESWR1/ERG* was negative; however, FISH analysis revealed the *EWSR1* gene rearrangement (Figure 2(c)), confirming the diagnosis of Ewing sarcoma and suggesting the presence of one of the rare ES translocation types.

Postoperatively, radiotherapy with 54 Gy was applied to the right temporoparietal region over 6 weeks. The patient underwent two cycles of cisplatin and CCNU/lomustine; however, chemotherapy had to be discontinued in 02/2007 due to myelotoxicity. At the most recent follow-up in 7/2015, the patient was alive and doing well under anticonvulsive treatment; however, a small mass was found on control MRI in the right frontal lobe, suggesting a metastasis.

3.1.3. Patient 3. This female patient developed acute T-cell leukemia at the age of 9 years. She initially presented with fatigue accompanied by leukocytosis, mediastinal mass, and hepatosplenomegaly, but without CNS involvement.

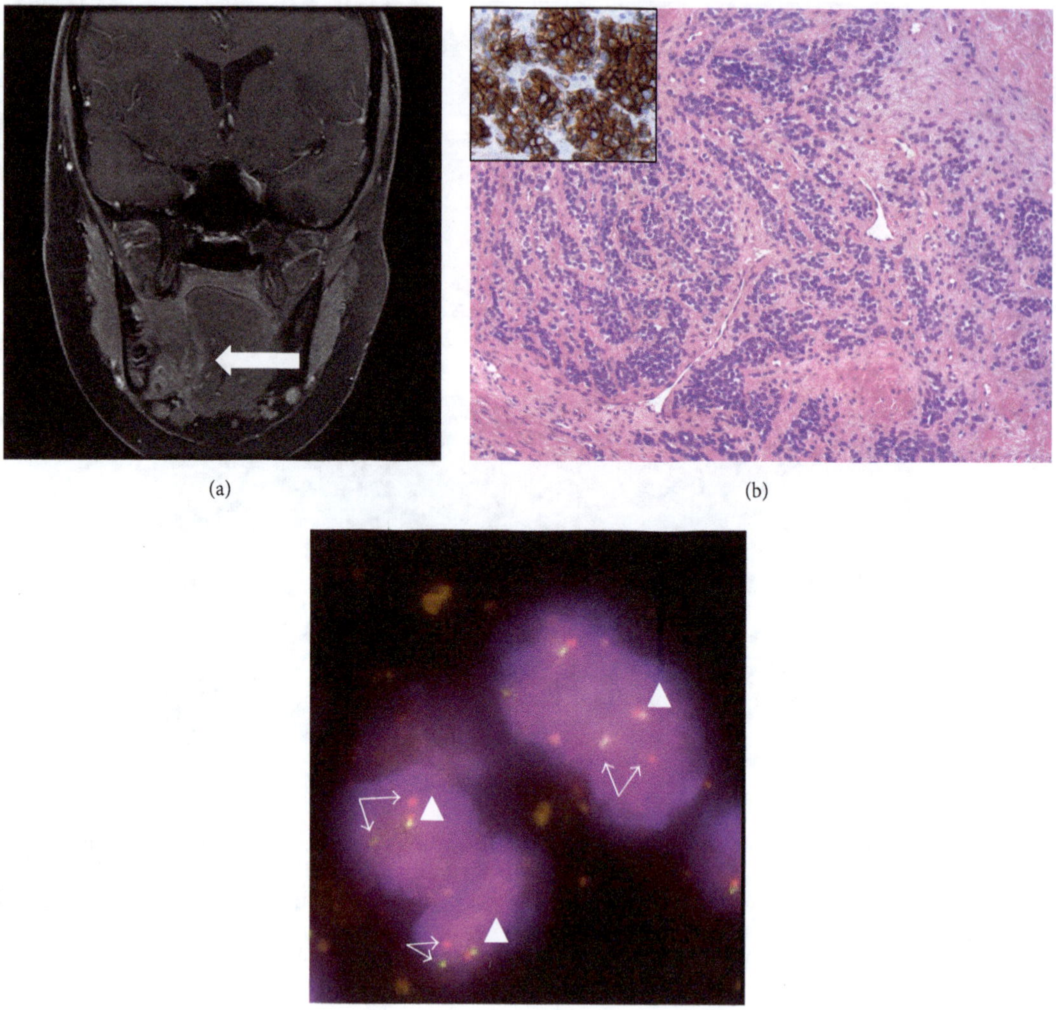

Figure 3: (a) Coronary T1 MRI section demonstrating a large mass (arrow) of the right mandible with infiltration and displacement of the tongue of patient 3. (b) Biopsy of the intraoral mass of patient 3. Diffuse infiltrates of a small, blue round, undifferentiated tumor with strong immunohistochemical membranous expression of CD99 (brown reaction product shown in the inset) (H&E; original magnification 100x). (c) Fluorescence in situ hybridization (FISH) of the jaw tumor of patient 3, demonstrating the rearrangement of the EWSR1 gene. The nuclei of the tumor cells contain one fused signal (arrow head) and one pair of split green and red signals (arrows).

Cytogenetic analysis of the bone marrow aspiration revealed t(1;16), loss of TLX3, and biallelic deletion of 12p. The patient was treated according to the high risk protocol of the ALL-BFM-2000 trial with prednisone, vincristine, daunorubicin, L-asparaginase, cyclophosphamide, high dose methotrexate, cytarabine, mercaptopurine, thioguanine, and etoposide. Due to the risk stratification an allogenic bone marrow transplantation with an unrelated donor had to be performed five months after the presentation. Conditioning regimen included total body irradiation with a cumulative dose of 12 Gy (6 × 2 Gy), etoposide, and antithymocyte globulin Fresenius. A graft versus host disease- (GvHD-) prophylaxis with MTX and cyclosporin A was applied. In the following controls, she showed an enduring remission.

Two years and four months later, the patient reported a swelling in the region of the right 2nd lower molar tooth. MRI of the head (Figure 3(a)) demonstrated a large tumor mass of the right lower jaw that infiltrated the soft tissues of the floor of the mouth and displaced the tongue. Biopsy revealed the diagnosis of Ewing sarcoma with characteristic small, round, and blue cell histology and typical strong and membranous immunohistochemical expression of CD99 protein (Figure 3(b)). This diagnosis was confirmed by the demonstration of the *EWSR1* gene rearrangement on FISH analysis (Figure 3(c)), with the fusion transcript *EWSR1/FLI1* of the diagnostic translocation by RT-PCR (the same type of the translocation as in patient 1) (Figure 1(c)). The patient was then treated according to the Euro-Ewing 99 protocol with vincristine, ifosfamide, doxorubicin, etoposide, actinomycin D, and cyclophosphamide. Local tumor control was achieved with total tumor resection and mandibular reconstruction with a fibula plastic. Unfortunately, local ES recurrence with biopsy confirmation was detected one year later and the patient underwent radiotherapy with a cumulative dose of 54 Gy (30 × 1,8 Gy) accompanied by second-line chemotherapy (cyclophosphamide, topotecan). Bone metastases in the right femur and fibula were first diagnosed in the following year, followed by wide metastatic spread (spine, lung), which prompted renewed chemotherapy with ifosfamide and palliative mediastinal radiotherapy.

3.2. Review of the Literature. There are only few reports on ES as a secondary malignancy (Table 2), mostly comprising single case reports or short series describing ES following treatment for unrelated tumors, such as breast carcinoma [20, 21], retinoblastoma [22, 23], or testicular mixed germ cell tumor [24]. The largest series of secondary ES by Applebaum et al. [25] evaluated data from the Surveillance, Epidemiology, and End Results Program (SEER) database between 1973 and 2008 and found 58 cases of secondary ES, accounting for up to 2.1% of all ES. Only 12.1% of patients received radiation to the ES site, while the frequency of previous chemotherapy is not reported. Interestingly, five further patients were diagnosed with ES concurrent with other tumors and were therefore not included in the study group of "secondary" ES. This study, however, is purely epidemiological, not including reevaluation of the diagnoses or molecular confirmation of ES. The most common group of primary tumors did not comprise further specified carcinomas (41%: 24 of 58), with rare cases of non-ES sarcomas, melanomas, brain tumors, or other neoplasia as a the primary tumor. In 24% (14/58) of cases in this study, hematological malignancies preceded secondary ES, representing the second most common primary malignancy group after carcinomas.

The first case of genetically confirmed ES following a chemotherapy malignancy (ALL) was described in 1984 by Tilly et al. [26], although the first case without genetic documentation was mentioned by Meadows et al. [27] in 1977. According to the review of available literature, 38 cases (including the current study) of secondary ES have been described following the diagnosis of a hematologic malignancy (Table 2); however, confirmatory data on genetic tumor background (karyotype, FISH, and/or RT-PCR) has been provided in only 14 cases [14, 26, 28–33].

The diagnosis of secondary ES followed in 1 to 16 years (mean 6 y) the diagnosis of a hematologic neoplasm, most often an acute lymphoblastic leukemia (46%: 11 of 24 cases with available information), Hodgkin lymphoma, or an aggressive form of non-Hodgkin lymphoma (5 cases (20%) each). There were only two patients with myelogenous neoplasia and 1 with no further specified small cell non-Hodgkin lymphoma. The age of the patients at the first tumor diagnosis ranged from 3 to 22 y (mean 10 y) and at ES diagnosis from 7 to 27 y (mean 16 y), with only one substantially older patient (diagnoses at 57 and 65 y, resp.). All patients with available data received disease specific chemotherapy for their primary malignancy, consisting of a combination of various groups of cytostatic and cytotoxic substances (Table 2) with no obvious causative association. Secondary ES occurred most commonly in the chest wall and long bones (7 cases each) followed by visceral organs (3), pelvis (2), somatic soft tissue (2), and mandible (1).

4. Discussion

Modern multimodal therapy has led to markedly improved long-term survival of cancer patients. Concomitantly, a well-documented increased incidence of malignancies in cancer survivors in comparison to general population has been observed. Most cases of secondary tumors can be attributed to the effects of long-term toxicity of radio- and/or chemotherapy; however, the underlying mechanisms of tumorigenesis in this setting remain unclear. In most instances, nonrandom somatic molecular or chromosomal alterations are thought to be involved in the pathogenesis of secondary tumors. Among sarcomas, most therapy associated tumors belong to the category of tumors showing complex karyotypes with mostly nonrecurring genetic aberrations, including undifferentiated pleomorphic sarcoma, osteosarcoma, or rarely malignant peripheral nerve sheath tumors [41]. Therapy associated angiosarcomas show recurrent amplifications of the c-myc gene [42]. Alternatively, sarcomas with simple karyotypes, carrying specific translocations or point mutations, have only rarely been described in the context of secondary, therapy associated tumors [43]. The underlying pathomechanism of therapy-induced malignancies has been elucidated for only selected secondary tumor entities. For example, secondary leukemia following the use of mitoxantrone as an immune modulating drug in patients with multiple sclerosis has been attributed to inhibition of topoisomerase II (TI-II) [44, 45]. TI-II inhibition has been identified as being crucial in the development of the t(15;17) balanced translocation and generation of the PML-RARalpha fusion transcript characteristic for promyelocytic leukemia [46]. Anthracyclines or other drugs inhibiting TI-II are part of therapeutic regimens for hematologic malignancies (Table 2); however, it remains to be elucidated whether these agents play pathogenetically relevant role in the occurrence of ES as a secondary tumor.

It is well known that immunodeficiency after radio-/chemotherapy and hematopoietic stem cell transplantation are major challenges for survivors of hematological malignancies [47, 48]. Impaired antitumor activity of the innate or adaptive immune system might represent critical factors that predispose to the failure of the system to detect and eliminate newly mutated cells carrying the Ewing sarcoma translocation, thus allowing for the initiation of secondary ES.

Two of the patients described in the current study received radiation therapy, one total body radiation (TBI) and one to the site of the ES occurrence (brain), suggesting a possible role for the radiotherapy in the induction of the subsequent ES. However, among the data in the literature, previous irradiation to the ES site was noted in only 12.1% of the patients in the study of Applebaum et al. [25] and among the cases compiled in Table 2 with available data on the previous radiation, there were some patients with TBI (2 of 7), but also patients with no radiation to the body parts later affected by ES.

The pathogenesis of Ewing sarcoma is strongly linked to the presence of a translocation between the *EWSR1* gene and a member of the ETS gene family [11]. The occurrence of the translocation itself was for a long time considered

TABLE 2: Review of the published cases of the Ewing sarcoma following the therapy of the hematologic malignancy as a primary tumor.

Number	Nr with genetic confirmation (any method)	Reference	Pub year	Age at Dx PT	Age at Dx ES	Latency (y)	Primary cancer	Location ES	Molecular test	Treatment of the primary hematological malignancy						
										Anthracyclines, TopoII-INH	Vinca	Alkylating agent	Antimetabolite	Other drugs	Rth	Additional treatment
1		Meadows et al. [27]	1977			5	ALL	ND	ND							
2	1	Tilly et al. [26]	1984	8	19	11	ALL	Sacrum	Karyotype	DNR	VCR	DTIC		PD	Cranial RT 24 Gy	
3		Anselmo et al. [34]	1994	20	27	7	HL	Chest wall	ND							
4	2	Zoubek et al. [28]	1995	12	20	8	Anaplastic T LCL	Pelvis	Karyotype RT-PCR	VP16		CPA, MEL	MTX, Ara-C		TBI 12 Gy	SCT (auto)
5		Delgado-Chavez et al. [35]	1995	22	26	4	HL	Chest wall	ND							
6	3	Antillon et al. [29]	1997	7	16	9	ALL	Tibia	RT-PCR	DNR	VCR			PD, L-asp		
7		Aparicio et al. [30]	1998	3	15	12	ALL	Ulna	ND	ADR	VCR		6-MP, MTX, Ara-C	L-asp	Cranial RT	
8				11	18	7	AML	Fibula	ND	DNR, ADR, MTZ, VP16			6-MP, 6-TG, Ara-C			
9		Bisogno et al. [31]	2004	4	7	3	HL	Thoracic wall	ND	ADR	VBL	DTIC			RT 20 Gy	
10				7	18	11	CML	Thigh	ND				HU		TBI 9 Gy,	SCT (allo)
11		Suarez et al. [36]	2004	8	9	1	ALL	Chest wall	ND	ARD	VCR	CPA	MTX, 6-MP, Ara-C	PD		
12	4	Kim et al. [32]	2005	3	7	4	ALL	Humerus	Karyotype RT-PCR	ADR	VCR	CPA	6-TG, MTX, Ara-C	PD, L-asp		
13	5			9	12	3	LCL	Rib	FISH	ADR	VCR	CPA		PD	RT 15 Gy	
14	6			8	16	8	ALL	Tibia	RT-PCR	DNR, VP16	VCR	CPA	6-MP, MTX, Ara-C	PD, L-asp		
15	7	Spunt et al. [33]	2006	7	23	16	Small, noncleaved cell lymphoma	Rib	FISH	ADR	VCR	CPA	MTX, Ara-C			
16	8			12	17	5	HL	Chest wall	RT-PCR	ADR, BLE	VBL		MTX	PD		
17		Khadwal et al. [37]	2006	8	10	2	HL	Knee	ND	ADR, BLE	VBL				RT 24 Gy	
18	9	Osone et al. [38]	2007	10	16	6	ALL	Urinary bladder	RT-PCR	ADR	VCR	CPA	MTX, 6-TG	PD, L-asp	none	
19		Renard et al. [39]	2011	7	19	12	ALL	ND	ND	ND	ND	ND	ND	ND	ND	ND
20	10	Lim et al. [40]	2013	20	22	2	Burkitt	Adrenal gland	FISH	ADR	VCR	CPA	MTX, Ara-C	DEXA		
21	11	Hiramoto et al. [14]	2013	57	65	8	B-LCL	Soft tissue back	RT-PCR	DNR	VCR	CPA		PD		GCSF
14 more cases		Applebaum et al. [25]	2013	ND	ND	ND	ND	ND	ND	ND	ND	ND	ND	ND	ND	ND
36	12	Current series	2016	5	8	3	Lymphoblastic lymphoma	Paravertebral	RT-PCR	ADR		CPA, IFO	Ara-C			

TABLE 2: Continued.

Number	Nr with genetic confirmation (any method)	Reference	Pub year	Age at Dx PT	Age at Dx ES	Latency (y)	Primary cancer	Location ES	Molecular test	Treatment of the primary hematological malignancy					Rth	Additional treatment
										Anthracyclines, TopoII-INH	Vinca	Alkylating agent	Antimetabolite	Other drugs		
37	13	Current series	2016	16	21	4	T-ALL	Brain	FISH	DNR	VCR	CPA	MTX, Ara-C, 6-MP, 6-TG		RT 12 Gy	
38	14	Current series	2016	9	11	2	T-ALL	Mandible	FISH, RT-PCR	DNR	VCR	CPA	MTX, Ara-C, 6-MP		TBI RT 12 Gy	

DNR, daunorubicin; VP-16, etoposide; ADR, doxorubicin; ACT, actinomycin D; MTZ, mitoxantrone; BLE, bleomycin; VCR, vincristine; VBL, vinblastine; DTIC, dacarbazine; CPA, cyclophosphamide; MEL, melphalan; IFO, ifosfamide; MTX, methotrexate; Ara-C, cytarabine; 6-MP, 6-mercaptopurine; 6-TG, thioguanine; HU, hydroxyurea; PD, prednisone; L-asp, L-asparaginase; RT, radiotherapy; TBI, total body irradiation; SCT, stem cell transplantation. ND: no data.

to be a random event. In addition, the risk of developing ES has been linked to increased maternal age [44] and there are associations with exposure to environmental toxins [3, 8, 9]. Alternatively, there are striking differences in the incidence ES according to racial background, ES showing significantly higher incidence among Caucasians than in patients of African origin. Recently published observations [13] of a different frequency of SNPs variants of the *EGR2* gene related to Ewing sarcoma susceptibility and may account for this observation, since the frequency of the SNP variant is significantly higher in the non-Africans than in patients of African origin. This important study provides deeper insights into the etiology of the occurrence of this specific translocation associated sarcoma and allows the conclusion that this is not a random disease but rather the expression of a germ line predisposition syndrome, thus accounting for the strong predilection of the Ewing sarcoma to occur in young patients, similar to other genetically linked tumors.

Due to advances in next generation sequencing techniques and the application of powerful computational tools, similar germ line association studies (genomewide association studies, GWAS) are currently possible on large sets of genetic data for many tumor types. Germ line associations of patients with ALL has been recorded for susceptibility, drug response, and toxicities of ALL therapy [49]. Speculatively, as yet not identified common genetic predisposition trait may exist for Ewing sarcoma and some other neoplasia, including hematologic diseases.

Interestingly, in the recent comprehensive study of germ line mutations in the best characterized genes associated with cancer predisposition syndromes in pediatric cancer patients, 5 patients with relevant mutations (3 patients with TP53 gene mutations, one patients with PMS2 gene mutation, and one patient with RET gene mutation) were identified among 46 (10.8%) patients with Ewing sarcoma, frequency of which was higher than in cases of rhabdomyosarcoma (7%, 3/43) [50]. Ewing sarcoma has been rarely reported in well-defined germ line mutation associated syndromes (Cowden syndrome [51], multiple osteochondromatosis [52], and Williams syndrome [15]); however it has never been listed as a syndrome defining entity. Of note, none of the patients in our study had known cancer predisposition syndromes or family history of a recognized risk constellation.

According to Sultan et al. [53], 3% of Ewing sarcoma patients develop secondary tumors (4–9-fold risk compared to the general population, the risk being higher for children). In such cases, therapy associated hematologic neoplasms, radiation associated sarcomas, or carcinomas follow multimodal Ewing sarcoma therapy. The relative risk of developing a second malignancy seems to be higher for Ewing sarcoma patients in comparison to other tumors (except for retinoblastoma and primitive neuroectodermal tumors of the central nervous system), suggesting a relationship of ES to either aggressive chemotherapy or genetic predisposition, which may be augmented by the application of cytostatic and cytotoxic drugs.

In summary, we provide a detailed description of well-documented cases of Ewing sarcoma following a primary hematologic malignancy. Additionally we have reviewed the literature on this association and discussed the possible pathogenetic aspects. As the survival of cancer patients will continue to improve in the future, it is important to understand the risks associated with this success, including the risk of the development of second malignancies, both therapy related and/or linked to the genetic background of the patients.

Competing Interests

The authors declare that they have no competing interests.

Acknowledgments

The authors thank José Alves do Carmo, M.D., and Sara Ismail, M.D. (Department of Hematology and Department of Pathology, Hospital Santa Maria, Centro Hospitalar Lisboa Norte, Lisbon, Portugal), for sharing data.

References

[1] P. C. Nathan, B. Hayes-Lattin, J. J. Sisler, and M. M. Hudson, "Critical issues in transition and survivorship for adolescents and young adults with cancers," *Cancer*, vol. 117, no. 10, pp. 2335–2341, 2011.

[2] A. Kishtagari, M. Tavakkoli, and J. H. Park, "Survivorship in adolescents and young adults," *Acta Haematologica*, vol. 132, no. 3-4, pp. 383–390, 2014.

[3] D. K. Choi, I. Helenowski, and N. Hijiya, "Secondary malignancies in pediatric cancer survivors: perspectives and review of the literature," *International Journal of Cancer*, vol. 135, no. 8, pp. 1764–1773, 2014.

[4] K. Dunleavy, M. Roschewski, and W. H. Wilson, "Precision treatment of distinct molecular subtypes of diffuse large B-cell lymphoma: ascribing treatment based on the molecular phenotype," *Clinical Cancer Research*, vol. 20, no. 20, pp. 5182–5193, 2014.

[5] J. D. Tward, M. M. M. Wendland, D. C. Shrieve, A. Szabo, and D. K. Gaffney, "The risk of secondary malignancies over 30 years after the treatment of non-Hodgkin lymphoma," *Cancer*, vol. 107, no. 1, pp. 108–115, 2006.

[6] N. Esiashvili, M. Goodman, and R. B. Marcus Jr., "Changes in incidence and survival of Ewing sarcoma patients over the past 3 decades: surveillance epidemiology and end results data," *Journal of Pediatric Hematology/Oncology*, vol. 30, no. 6, pp. 425–430, 2008.

[7] M. A. Applebaum, J. Worch, K. K. Matthay et al., "Clinical features and outcomes in patients with extraskeletal Ewing sarcoma," *Cancer*, vol. 117, no. 13, pp. 3027–3032, 2011.

[8] N. J. Balamuth and R. B. Womer, "Ewing's sarcoma," *The Lancet Oncology*, vol. 11, no. 2, pp. 184–192, 2010.

[9] E.-Y. K. Choi, J. M. Gardner, D. R. Lucas, J. B. McHugh, and R. M. Patel, "Ewing sarcoma," *Seminars in Diagnostic Pathology*, vol. 31, no. 1, pp. 39–47, 2014.

[10] G. M. Ibrahim, A. Fallah, M. Shahideh, U. Tabori, and J. T. Rutka, "Primary Ewing's sarcoma affecting the central nervous system: a review and proposed prognostic considerations," *Journal of Clinical Neuroscience*, vol. 19, no. 2, pp. 203–209, 2012.

[11] E. de Alava, L. S. Lessnik, and P. H. Sorensen, "Ewing sarcoma," in *WHO Classification of Tumours of Soft Tissue and Bone*, C. D.

M. Fletcher, J. A. Bridge, P. C. W. Hogendoorn, and F. Mertens, Eds., pp. 305–309, IARC, Lyon, France, 2013.

[12] K. N. Ganjoo and S. Patel, "The treatment outcome for adult patients with Ewing's sarcoma," *Current Oncology Reports*, vol. 15, no. 4, pp. 372–377, 2013.

[13] T. G. P. Grünewald, V. Bernard, P. Gilardi-Hebenstreit et al., "Chimeric EWSR1-FLI1 regulates the Ewing sarcoma susceptibility gene *EGR2* via a GGAA microsatellite," *Nature Genetics*, vol. 47, no. 9, pp. 1073–1078, 2015.

[14] N. Hiramoto, Y. Kobayashi, J. Nomoto et al., "Ewing sarcoma arising after treatment of diffuse large B-cell lymphoma," *Japanese Journal of Clinical Oncology*, vol. 43, no. 4, pp. 417–421, 2013.

[15] N. Vanhapiha, S. Knuutila, K. Vettenranta, and O. Lohi, "Burkitt lymphoma and Ewing sarcoma in a child with Williams syndrome," *Pediatric Blood and Cancer*, vol. 61, no. 10, pp. 1877–1879, 2014.

[16] B. Bode-Lesniewska, J. Hodler, A. von Hochstetter, L. Guillou, U. Exner, and R. Caduff, "Late solitary bone metastasis of a primary pulmonary synovial sarcoma with SYT-SSX1 translocation type: case report with a long follow-up," *Virchows Archiv*, vol. 446, no. 3, pp. 310–315, 2005.

[17] U. Yamaguchi, T. Hasegawa, Y. Morimoto et al., "A practical approach to the clinical diagnosis of Ewing's sarcoma/primitive neuroectodermal tumour and other small round cell tumours sharing EWS rearrangement using new fluorescence in situ hybridisation probes for EWSR1 on formalin fixed, paraffin wax embedded tissue," *Journal of Clinical Pathology*, vol. 58, no. 10, pp. 1051–1056, 2005.

[18] B. Bode, S. Frigerio, S. Behnke et al., "Mutations in the tyrosine kinase domain of the EGFR gene are rare in synovial sarcoma," *Modern Pathology*, vol. 19, no. 4, pp. 541–547, 2006.

[19] D. Modritz, R. Ladenstein, U. Pötschger et al., "Treatment for soft tissue sarcoma in childhood and adolescence. Austrian results within the CWS 96 study," *Wiener Klinische Wochenschrift*, vol. 117, no. 5-6, pp. 196–209, 2005.

[20] J. Zhong, N. Chen, X. Chen et al., "Peripheral primitive neuroectodermal tumor of the kidney in a 51-year-old female following breast cancer: a case report and review of the literature," *Oncology Letters*, vol. 9, no. 1, pp. 108–112, 2015.

[21] M. Cole, S. Parajuli, D. Laske et al., "Peripheral primitive neuroectodermal tumor of the dura in a 51-year-old woman following intensive treatment for breast cancer," *American Journal of Case Reports*, vol. 15, pp. 294–299, 2014.

[22] K. J. Helton, B. D. Fletcher, L. E. Kun, J. J. Jenkins III, and C. B. Pratt, "Bone tumors other than osteosarcoma after retinoblastoma," *Cancer*, vol. 71, no. 9, pp. 2847–2853, 1993.

[23] J. U. Cope, M. Tsokos, and R. W. Miller, "Ewing sarcoma and sinonasal neuroectodermal tumors as second malignant tumors after retinoblastoma and other neoplasms," *Medical and Pediatric Oncology*, vol. 36, no. 2, pp. 290–294, 2001.

[24] S. Tanik, K. Zengin, S. Albayrak, R. Eryilmaz, D. Yilmaz, and N. Pirinççi, "Cutaneous Ewing's sarcoma secondary to chemotherapy given for testis tumor: case report," *International Journal of Surgery Case Reports*, vol. 5, no. 12, pp. 972–974, 2014.

[25] M. A. Applebaum, R. Goldsby, J. Neuhaus, and S. G. DuBois, "Clinical features and outcomes in patients with secondary Ewing sarcoma," *Pediatric Blood and Cancer*, vol. 60, no. 4, pp. 611–615, 2013.

[26] H. Tilly, C. Bastard, B. Chevallier, E. Halkin, and M. Monconduit, "Chromosomal abnormalities in secondary Ewing's sarcoma," *The Lancet*, vol. 324, no. 8406, p. 812, 1984.

[27] A. T. Meadows, G. J. D'Angio, V. Mike et al., "Patterns of second malignant neoplasms in children," *Cancer*, vol. 40, supplement 4, pp. 1903–1911, 1977.

[28] A. Zoubek, I. Simonitsch, E. R. Panzer-Grümayer et al., "Ewing tumor after treatment of Ki-1^+ anaplastic large cell lymphoma Therapy-associated secondary neoplasm or unrelated coincidence?" *Cancer Genetics and Cytogenetics*, vol. 83, no. 1, pp. 5–11, 1995.

[29] F. Antillon, S. C. Kaste, J. J. Jenkins et al., "Primitive neuroectodermal tumor of bone as a second malignant neoplasm in a child previously treated for acute lymphoblastic leukemia," *Journal of Pediatric Hematology/Oncology*, vol. 19, no. 5, pp. 473–476, 1997.

[30] J. Aparicio, A. Segura, J. Montalar, A. Verdeguer, V. Castel, and A. B. Sanchez-Heras, "Letter to the editor: 'secondary cancers after ewing sarcoma and ewing sarcoma as second malignant neoplasm'," *Medical and Pediatric Oncology*, vol. 30, no. 4, pp. 259–260, 1998.

[31] G. Bisogno, G. Sotti, Y. Nowicki et al., "Soft tissue sarcoma as a second malignant neoplasm in the pediatric age group," *Cancer*, vol. 100, no. 8, pp. 1758–1765, 2004.

[32] G. E. Kim, B. Beach, J. M. Gastier-Foster et al., "Ewing sarcoma as a second malignant neoplasm after acute lymphoblastic leukemia," *Pediatric Blood & Cancer*, vol. 45, no. 1, pp. 57–59, 2005.

[33] S. L. Spunt, C. Rodriguez-Galindo, C. E. Fuller et al., "Ewing sarcoma-family tumors that arise after treatment of primary childhood cancer," *Cancer*, vol. 107, no. 1, pp. 201–206, 2006.

[34] A. P. Anselmo, C. Cartoni, A. Pacchiarotti et al., "Peripheral neuroectodermal tumor of the chest (Askin tumor) as secondary neoplasm after Hodgkin's disease: a case report," *Annals of Hematology*, vol. 68, no. 6, pp. 311–313, 1994.

[35] R. Delgado-Chavez, P. Sobrevilla-Calvo, L. Green-Schneewiss, E. Reynoso-Gomez, and L. Quintanilla-Martinez, "Peripheral neuroectodermal tumor of the chest wall in a patient treated for Hodgkin's disease," *Leukemia and Lymphoma*, vol. 17, no. 5-6, pp. 509–513, 1995.

[36] C. R. Suarez, S. J. Bertolone, A. B. Raj, and S. Coventry, "Second malignant neoplasms in childhood acute lymphoblastic leukemia: primitive neuroectodermal tumor of the chest wall with germline p53 mutation as a second malignant neoplasm," *American Journal of Hematology*, vol. 76, no. 1, pp. 52–56, 2004.

[37] A. Khadwal, G. Biswas, B. Arora, P. A. Kurkure, C. Deshmukh, and V. Shetty, "Primitive neuroectodermal tumor (PNET) as second malignancy after treatment of Hodgkin's disease," *Indian Journal of Pediatrics*, vol. 73, no. 5, pp. 437–438, 2006.

[38] S. Osone, H. Hosoi, K. Tanaka et al., "A case of a Ewing sarcoma family tumor in the urinary bladder after treatment for acute lymphoblastic leukemia," *Journal of Pediatric Hematology/Oncology*, vol. 29, no. 12, pp. 841–844, 2007.

[39] M. Renard, S. Suciu, Y. Bertrand et al., "Second neoplasm in children treated in EORTC 58881 trial for acute lymphoblastic malignancies: low incidence of CNS tumours," *Pediatric Blood and Cancer*, vol. 57, no. 1, pp. 119–125, 2011.

[40] S. H. Lim, J. Y. Lee, J. Y. Lee et al., "Unusual presentation of Ewing sarcoma in the adrenal gland: a secondary malignancy from a survivor of Burkitt lymphoma," *Japanese Journal of Clinical Oncology*, vol. 43, no. 6, pp. 676–680, 2013.

[41] T. O. Henderson, J. Whitton, M. Stovall et al., "Secondary sarcomas in childhood cancer survivors: a report from the childhood cancer survivor study," *Journal of the National Cancer Institute*, vol. 99, no. 4, pp. 300–308, 2007.

[42] J. Manner, B. Radlwimmer, P. Hohenberger et al., "MYC high level gene amplification is a distinctive feature of angiosarcomas after irradiation or chronic lymphedema," *The American Journal of Pathology*, vol. 176, no. 1, pp. 34–39, 2010.

[43] J.-F. Egger, J.-M. Coindre, J. Benhattar, P. Coucke, and L. Guillou, "Radiation-associated synovial sarcoma: clinicopathologic and molecular analysis of two cases," *Modern Pathology*, vol. 15, no. 9, pp. 998–1004, 2002.

[44] M. Joannides and D. Grimwade, "Molecular biology of therapy-related leukaemias," *Clinical and Translational Oncology*, vol. 12, no. 1, pp. 8–14, 2010.

[45] J. L. Nitiss, "Targeting DNA topoisomerase II in cancer chemotherapy," *Nature Reviews Cancer*, vol. 9, no. 5, pp. 338–350, 2009.

[46] M. Pendleton, R. H. Lindsey, C. A. Felix, D. Grimwade, and N. Osheroff, "Topoisomerase II and leukemia," *Annals of the New York Academy of Sciences*, vol. 1310, no. 1, pp. 98–110, 2014.

[47] C. N. Duncan, N. S. Majhail, R. Brazauskas et al., "Long-term survival and late effects among one-year survivors of second allogeneic hematopoietic cell transplantation for relapsed acute leukemia and myelodysplastic syndromes," *Biology of Blood and Marrow Transplantation*, vol. 21, no. 1, pp. 151–158, 2015.

[48] W. Leung, G. Neale, F. Behm et al., "Deficient innate immunity, thymopoiesis, and gene expression response to radiation in survivors of childhood acute lymphoblastic leukemia," *Cancer Epidemiology*, vol. 34, no. 3, pp. 303–308, 2010.

[49] T. Moriyama, M. V. Relling, and J. J. Yang, "Inherited genetic variation in childhood acute lymphoblastic leukemia," *Blood*, vol. 125, no. 26, pp. 3988–3995, 2015.

[50] J. Zhang, M. F. Walsh, G. Wu et al., "Germline mutations in predisposition genes in pediatric cancer," *The New England Journal of Medicine*, vol. 373, no. 24, pp. 2336–2346, 2015.

[51] M. C. Chandhanayingyong, N. M. Bernthal, P. Ungarreevittaya, S. D. Nelson, S. P. Chawla, and A. S. Singh, "Ewing sarcoma in a patient with Cowden syndrome," *Journal of the National Comprehensive Cancer Network*, vol. 13, no. 11, pp. 1310–1314, 2015.

[52] P. A. Marrero Barrera and P. V. Marrero Ortiz, "Ewing sarcoma superimposed on a previous osteochondroma in multiple osteochondromatosis," *Orthopedics*, vol. 37, no. 4, pp. e403–e406, 2014.

[53] I. Sultan, R. Rihani, R. Hazin, and C. Rodriguez-Galindo, "Second malignancies in patients with Ewing Sarcoma Family of Tumors: a population-based study," *Acta Oncologica*, vol. 49, no. 2, pp. 237–244, 2010.

25

Surveillance Strategies for Sarcoma: Results of a Survey of Members of the Musculoskeletal Tumor Society

David D. Greenberg and Brooke Crawford

Saint Louis University Hospital, 7th Floor, Desloge Towers, 3635 Vista Avenue, St. Louis, MO 63110, USA

Correspondence should be addressed to Brooke Crawford; crawford.brooke.1227@gmail.com

Academic Editor: John D. Reith

Background. Surveillance is crucial to oncology, yet there is scant evidence to guide strategies. *Purpose.* This survey identified sarcoma surveillance strategies for Musculoskeletal Tumor Society (MSTS) members and rationales behind them. Understanding current practice should facilitate studies to generate evidence-based surveillance protocols. *Methods.* Permission was granted by the Research and Executive Committee of the MSTS to survey members on surveillance strategies. First, the questionnaire requested demographic and clinical practice information. Second, the survey focused on clinicians' specific surveillance soft tissue and bone sarcoma protocols. *Results.* 20 percent of MSTS members completed the survey. The primary rationale for protocols was training continuation, followed by published guidelines, and finally personal interpretation of the literature. 95% of the respondents believe that additional studies regarding appropriate surveillance protocols are needed. 87% reported patient concerns regarding radiation exposure from surveillance imaging. For soft tissue and bone sarcoma local recurrence, responders identified surgical margin, histologic grade, and tumor size as the most important factors. For metastases, important risk factors identified included histologic grade, tumor size, and histologic type. Protocols demonstrated wide variation. *Conclusion.* This survey demonstrates that surveillance strategies utilized by MSTS members are not evidence-based, providing rationale for multi-institutional studies. It also confirms the public health issue of excessive radiation exposure.

1. Introduction

Surveillance to detect local or distant recurrence, identify adverse effects of treatment, and extend disease-free survival is an important component of oncology. Despite the recognized significance, there is a paucity of evidence to guide the intensity of surveillance strategies. The duration of surveillance needs to continue throughout the period of time in which the tumor is likely to recur. This potentially prolonged period creates substantial clinical and fiscal considerations. An ideal surveillance strategy should be easy to implement, accurate, and cost-effective [1].

Prior investigations support the notion that current follow-up strategies vary widely, are controversial and ill-defined, and lack evidence-based guidance [2–5]. Furthermore, the matters of cost and excessive radiation exposure are public health issues gaining national attention. Estimates that 1.5–2% of all cancers in the United States may be attributable to radiation from computed tomography (CT) studies have intensified the concern for unnecessary testing [6].

Surveys of members of the Society of Surgical Oncology (SSO) and United Kingdom (UK) clinicians who manage sarcomas have demonstrated significant variation in surveillance strategies and costs [6, 7]. However, orthopaedic oncologists comprise only 5% of SSO membership and practice patterns in the United States and UK are distinct.

The purpose of this study was to determine the current sarcoma surveillance strategies of members of the Musculoskeletal Tumor Society (MSTS) and the rationale behind them. Greater understanding of the current practice should facilitate future studies to generate the evidence-based surveillance protocols currently lacking.

TABLE 1: The demographic data obtained from the MSTS member respondents.

Specialty (%)	*Orthopaedic surgery*	*General surgery*	*Medical oncology*	*Radiation oncology*	
	38 (100)	0	0	0	
Country of practice (%)	*USA*	*Canada*	*Other*		
	34 (89)	3 (8)	1 (3)		
Age (%)	*<30*	*30–40*	*41–50*	*51–60*	*>60*
	0	22 (58)	7 (18)	7 (18)	2 (5)
Gender (%)	*Male*	*Female*			
	79	21			
Length of career (%)	*0–5*	*6–10*	*11–15*	*16–20*	*>20*
	16 (42)	9 (24)	4 (11)	1 (3)	8 (21)
# ST sarcomas/yr (%)	*<10*	*10–30*	*>30*		
	1 (3)	22 (58)	15 (39)		
# bone sarcomas/yr (%)	*0–5*	*5–10*	*10–20*	*>20*	
	3 (8)	18 (47)	12 (32)	5 (13)	
Multidisciplinary sarcoma team (%)	*Yes*	*No*			
	95	5			

2. Materials and Methods

Permission was granted by the Research and Executive Committee of the MSTS to survey members on their surveillance strategies. All members of the MSTS with a known email address were asked to participate in the survey through the MSTS email list. Qualtrics Survey Software (Qualtrics, LLC; Provo, Utah) was utilized to generate an online survey and a direct link to the survey was emailed to MSTS members.

The survey consisted of three parts. The first portion of the questionnaire requested physician demographic and clinical practice information. Additional questions focused on the rationale for the clinician's surveillance protocol and gauged perception of current surveillance guidelines. Questions regarding clinician and/or patient concerns for radiation exposure were also included in this section. The second part of the survey focused on soft tissue sarcomas (STS). Clinicians were asked to rank factors they considered to increase the risk of local recurrence or distant metastases. Charts were also provided to outline the clinician's specific surveillance protocol for STS. These charts were divided into soft tissue sarcomas believed to be at low or high risk for relapse. The final question in the second part asked whether early detection of metastases leads to improved survival in patients with STS. The third part of the survey was similar to the second but the focus was on bone sarcomas rather than STS. Clinicians were asked to complete this portion of the survey if their surveillance strategy differed for bone and soft tissue sarcomas.

After several email reminders with a survey link were distributed, the survey was closed and the data was analyzed using Qualtrics Survey Software.

3. Results

20 percent (38 of 193) of MSTS members completed the survey. The demographics profile for all respondents is presented in Table 1. The reasoning responders provided for surveillance is depicted in Figure 1. The most common rationale for the specific protocol utilized was continuation of the protocol used during training. The second most important was recommendations from published guidelines (National Comprehensive Cancer Network [NCCN]) followed by personal interpretation of available literature. When asked whether there is a need for additional studies regarding appropriate surveillance protocols, 95% of respondents answered in the affirmative and stated they would be willing to enroll their patients into such trials. Patients may also be interested in surveillance studies as 33 respondents (87%) reported that their patients expressed concern regarding radiation exposure from surveillance imaging. Greater than half of responding physicians (56%) have changed their surveillance protocol in response to these concerns.

In the soft tissue sarcoma section, responders were surveyed regarding their perceived risk factors for relapse. Eight factors were provided for consideration of risk of local recurrence (Figure 2(a)). From the 35 respondents who answered the question, the three factors most commonly selected were surgical margin, histologic grade, and tumor size. Of note, age over 50 years was the factor perceived to be the least significant. In regard to risk of metastatic disease, Figure 2(b) depicts the provided factors. Histologic grade was overwhelmingly chosen as the factor that most significantly increases the risk of metastases (mean ranking of 1.26 out of the eight factors), followed by tumor size and histologic type. Here again, age over 50 years was selected as the least significant. Surgical margin had a mean ranking of 5.34 regarding significance for risk of metastases.

MRI was the modality most frequently utilized for detection of local recurrence of a soft tissue sarcoma. For a STS considered at *low risk* of relapse, an average of 1.68 MRI tests (mode: 2; range: 0–4) were ordered during the first year of surveillance. For soft tissue sarcomas considered *high risk* for recurrence, an average of 2.08 MRI tests (mode: 2; range: 0–4) were ordered during the first year of surveillance. The final

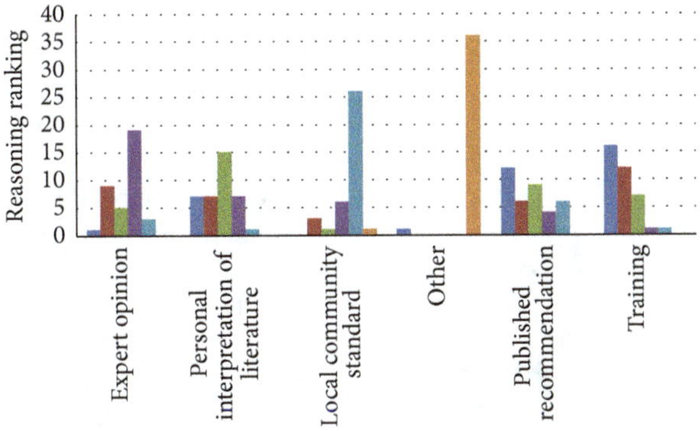

	Expert opinion	Personal interpretation of literature	Local community standard	Other	Published recommendation	Training
1	1	7	0	1	12	16
2	9	7	3	0	6	12
3	5	15	1	0	9	7
4	19	7	6	0	4	1
5	3	1	26	0	6	1
6	0	0	1	36	0	0

FIGURE 1: Reasoning behind surveillance strategies. Respondents numerically ranked reasoning options 1–6, with 1 being the most important reason supporting surveillance protocol. The majority (16 of 36 respondents) ranked continuation of the protocol used during training as the most important reason for current surveillance strategy. For those noting published recommendations, all referenced NCCN guidelines as their resource, with one respondent also referencing COG.

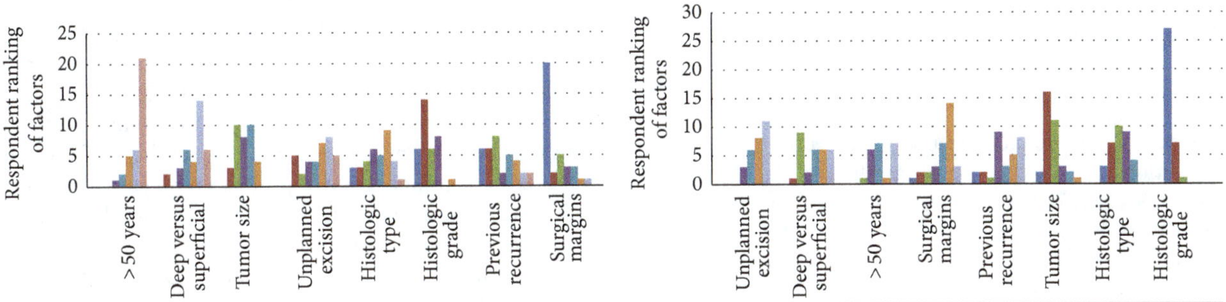

	>50 years	Deep versus superficial	Tumor size	Unplanned excision	Histologic type	Histologic grade	Previous recurrence	Surgical margins
1	0	0	0	0	3	6	6	20
2	0	2	3	5	3	14	6	2
3	0	0	10	2	4	6	8	5
4	1	3	8	4	6	8	2	3
5	2	6	10	4	5	0	5	3
6	5	4	4	7	9	1	4	1
7	6	14	0	8	4	0	2	1
8	21	6	0	5	1	0	2	0

(a) Perceived risk factors for local recurrence

	Unplanned excision	Deep versus superficial	>50 years	Surgical margins	Previous recurrence	Tumor size	Histologic type	Histologic grade
1	0	0	0	1	2	2	3	27
2	0	1	0	2	2	16	7	7
3	0	9	1	2	1	11	10	1
4	3	2	6	3	9	3	9	0
5	6	6	7	7	3	2	4	0
6	8	6	1	14	5	1	0	0
7	11	6	7	3	8	0	0	0

(b) Perceived risk factors for metastases

FIGURE 2: (a) Respondents were asked to rank 8 factors according to contribution to risk of local recurrence. The factor ranked 1 was perceived to most significantly increase risk of local recurrence. Of the 8 factors listed, respondents felt surgical margin was the factor that contributed most to local recurrence (20 ranked it as #1), followed by histologic grade. Age was the factor ranked lowest by survey participants (21 ranked it #8). (b) Respondents were asked to rank 8 factors according to contribution to risk of metastases. The factor ranked 1 was perceived to most significantly increase risk of metastasis. The most important risk factor for metastatic disease was felt to be histologic grade (27 respondents ranked it #1), followed by tumor size and histologic type. Unplanned excision before referral was perceived to contribute the least to subsequent metastatic disease.

question in the soft tissue sarcoma section asked whether early detection of metastases leads to improved survival in patients with STS. Responses were yes (41%), no (27%), or do not know (32%).

Bone sarcoma surveillance was generally similar to the soft tissue sarcoma protocols utilized by the responders of the survey. 34 respondents (92%) reported similar systemic monitoring (one respondent did not complete this section of the survey). X-ray of the primary site was the modality frequently utilized for local imaging for bone sarcomas as opposed to MRI for STS. More respondents felt that early detection of metastases leads to improved survival in patients with bone sarcoma as compared to soft tissue sarcomas (67% yes, 19% no, and 14% do not know).

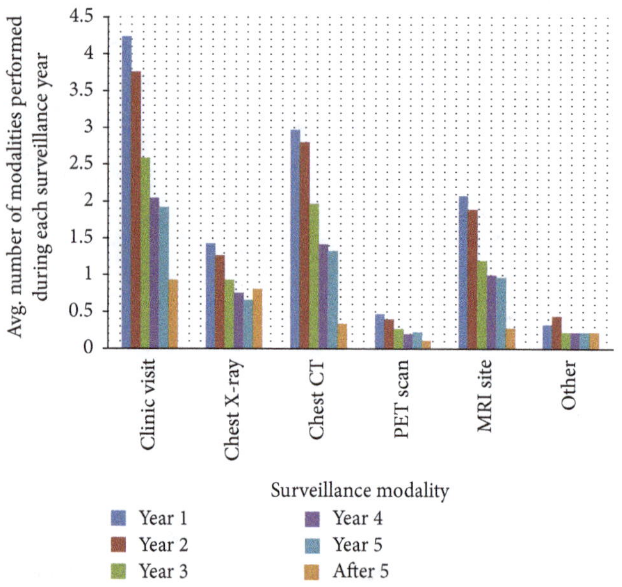

Figure 3: Surveillance protocols. Average surveillance strategies based on 38 respondents depicted as the average number of all modalities performed during each year of surveillance. Chest CT was more common for surveillance as compared to chest X-ray by an approximate 2 : 1 ratio in years 1–3, with reversal in strategy after year 5 with X-ray becoming more common by an 8 : 3 ratio.

The actual surveillance protocols utilized by the respondents demonstrated wide variation during the course of follow-up (Figure 3). In the first year of surveillance, the range of clinic visits for soft tissue sarcoma was 2–12, with 4 visits being the most common pattern. Regarding chest imaging during the first two years of surveillance for STS considered at high risk of local or systemic relapse, the number of chest X-rays ranged from 0 to 13 and the number of chest CT scans ranged from 1 to 8. The most common pattern reported (46% of respondents) was 4 chest CT scans in each of the first two years of surveillance then tapering thereafter. Survey respondents also varied considerably in how long they performed surveillance on STS patients, with 19% following up for a lifetime, 32% following up for 1–5 years, and 43% following up for 5–10 years. With bone sarcomas, first-year surveillance clinic visits ranged from 3 to 6, chest X-rays ranged from 0 to 3, chest CT scans ranged from 1 to 4, and X-ray of the primary site ranged from 3 to 6. 65% of respondents reported following up bone sarcoma patients for life with the remaining 35% selecting 5–10 years.

4. Discussion

Surveillance is an important component of patient care after completion of definitive treatment. The factors to consider when designing a surveillance protocol should include the following: (1) the interval between examinations and duration of testing should be consistent with time of maximal risk of recurrence; (2) tests should focus on the most likely recurrence locations and have high positive and negative predictive values; (3) there should be a possibility of cure, prolongation of life, or palliation; and (4) risk of secondary malignancy should be considered when ordering tests [8]. It is unclear whether all of these goals are achievable for sarcoma, as illustrated by only 41% of respondents to this study believing that early detection of metastases leads to improved survival in patients with STS. However, almost all patients treated for sarcoma undergo some level of surveillance and 95% of those surveyed believe that efforts to achieve these goals need to be evidence-based. The results of this survey demonstrate that current surveillance strategies utilized by members of the MSTS are not guided by high-quality evidence and demonstrate wide variation, with most continuing the protocol taught during fellowship training. The findings lend credence to prior articles that express concerns regarding the quality of evidence underlying surveillance rationale [1, 3, 6, 7].

This survey study is not without limitations. Most concerning is the low percentage of respondents with only 20% of MSTS members completing the survey. This fairly low rate of response generates the potential for significant nonresponse bias. Counteracting this weakness is the fact that the responders were entirely made up of a population previously underrepresented in surveillance surveys. Beitler et al. published results of follow-up strategies of members of the Society of Surgical Oncology [2]; however, orthopaedic oncologists comprised only 5% of the responders. Only 30 of 121 survey respondents were orthopaedic surgeons in a similar follow-up survey in the United Kingdom [7]. One hundred percent of responders in the current survey were orthopaedic surgeons. Furthermore, members of the MSTS represent a significant portion of sarcoma care providers in the United States and surveillance data on this membership has not been previously reported. Another limitation is the generalizability of this data. Current surveillance strategies of MSTS members may not be reflective of sarcoma care nationally or internationally. However, the fact that our survey results are similar to previously reported SSO and UK surveys does support the translatability of the findings.

A key finding in both the current survey and previous sarcoma surveillance surveys is the wide variation among respondents' protocols. This was illustrated most simply in the UK survey by the cost analysis, with low risk trunk/extremity tumor surveillance costs ranging from 372 to 7,852 pounds and high risk tumor surveillance costs ranging from 1,091 to 7,961 pounds [7]. Our survey showed wide ranges in the frequencies of modalities utilized: for example, first-year surveillance clinic visits ranged from 2 to 12, chest radiographs ranged from 0 to 9, and chest CTs ranged from 0 to 4. While these ranges may fall within the current NCCN guidelines for sarcoma follow-up, the cost and radiation exposure differences are substantial.

NCCN guidelines are most commonly utilized by responders of this survey. The NCCN sarcoma follow-up guidelines call for chest radiograph or chest CT every 3–6 months for 2-3 years and then every 6 months for the next 2 years and then annually [1]. This guideline allows for tremendous variation in frequency and modality of chest imaging for sarcoma surveillance, a finding reflected in the results of this survey. As stated above, this variation has important implications regarding not only cost but also radiation exposure for the patient. This survey confirmed that the public health issue of excessive radiation exposure is something patients are aware of [2, 9], with 87% of respondents reporting having patients express concern. The fact that over half of survey respondents have changed their protocol in response is also alarming as reaction to patient anxiety is not better justification for surveillance strategies than the empiric rationale currently utilized.

Puri et al. in a randomized noninferiority trial demonstrated that chest radiography did not lead to worsened survival and was not inferior to chest CT scan in terms of detecting pulmonary metastasis during sarcoma surveillance [5]. Our survey revealed significant utilization of chest CT for pulmonary surveillance, especially during the first two years after treatment. The fiscal and radiation reduction gained by converting from chest CT to chest radiography has been highlighted previously [1, 4, 7]. It is not the intention nor is it within the scope of a survey study to outline an appropriate surveillance strategy for sarcomas. However, this survey does establish that there is interest among respondents in pursuing evidence-based guidelines and willingness to enroll patients in such a trial.

The results of this study illustrate that in general the issues in sarcoma surveillance are not unique to any one subspecialty but rather universal to all clinicians following up sarcoma patients. One key difference was identified specific to orthopaedic oncologists in their surveillance protocols as compared to multispecialty surveys done in the United Kingdom and among SSO members. Chest CT is the surveillance modality most commonly used by the MSTS respondents for the first five years posttreatment. In the UK survey, >85% of those surveyed used chest X-rays as primary imaging for low and high risk trunk or extremity tumors, whereas only 16% used chest CT scans for low grade tumors and 29% used them for high grade tumors [7]. In an SSO survey, Johnson et al. showed that chest X-ray was used more than chest CT across metropolitan areas, in managed care organizations, and by US Census Regions [3]. Neither of these surveys identified differences in practices between specialties treating sarcomas.

Perceived risk factors between MSTS respondents and those surveyed in the United Kingdom were similar, with both groups ranking surgical margin and histologic grade as the most important risk factors for recurrence and histologic grade and tumor size for metastasis. This question was not addressed in the SSO survey.

In conclusion, this study confirms that the wide variation in surveillance practice demonstrated in prior studies also exists among members of the MSTS. High-quality evidence for guidance is currently absent but the need for it is recognized and warranted. Combined, these factors provide sound rationale for a multi-institutional study on appropriate sarcoma surveillance.

Acknowledgments

The authors are grateful to the MSTS for authorization and facilitation of distributing the survey and to the survey respondents for sharing their information.

References

[1] B. P. Whooley, M. M. Mooney, J. F. Gibbs, and W. G. Kraybill, "Effective follow-up strategies in soft tissue sarcoma," *Seminars in Surgical Oncology*, vol. 17, no. 1, pp. 83–87, 1999.

[2] A. L. Beitier, K. S. Virgo, F. E. Johnson, J. F. Gibbs, and W. G. Kraybill, "Current follow-up strategies after potentially curative resection of extremity sarcomas: results of a survey of the members of the society of surgical oncology," *Cancer*, vol. 88, no. 4, pp. 777–785, 2000.

[3] F. E. Johnson, K. Sakata, W. G. Kraybill et al., "Long-term management of patients after potentially curative treatment of extremity soft tissue sarcoma: practice patterns of members of the Society of Surgical Oncology," *Surgical Oncology*, vol. 14, no. 1, pp. 33–40, 2005.

[4] B. J. Miller, E. E. C. Soni, J. D. Reith, C. P. Gibbs, and M. T. Scarborough, "CT scans for pulmonary surveillance may be overused in lower-grade sarcoma," *The Iowa Orthopaedic Journal*, vol. 32, pp. 28–34, 2012.

[5] A. Puri, A. Gulia, R. Hawaldar, P. Ranganathan, and R. A. Badwe, "Does intensity of surveillance affect survival after surgery for sarcomas? Results of a randomized noninferiority trial," *Clinical Orthopaedics and Related Research*, vol. 472, no. 5, pp. 1568–1575, 2014.

[6] D. J. Brenner and E. J. Hall, "Computed tomography—an increasing source of radiation exposure," *The New England Journal of Medicine*, vol. 357, no. 22, pp. 2277–2284, 2007.

[7] C. H. Gerrand, L. J. Billingham, P. J. Woll, and R. J. Grimer, "Follow up after primary treatment of soft tissue sarcoma: a survey of current practice in the United Kingdom," *Sarcoma*, vol. 2007, Article ID 34128, 6 pages, 2007.

[8] B. Crawford and D. Greenberg, *Patient Surveillance after Cancer Treatment: Introduction to Cancer Surveillance Strategies*, Springer, New York, NY, USA, 2013.

[9] Consumer Reports, "The surprising dangers of CT scans and C-rays," 2015, http://www.consumerreports.org/cro/magazine/2015/03/index.htm.

26

Overall Survival and Response to Systemic Therapy in Metastatic Extrauterine Leiomyosarcoma

A. N. Shoushtari,[1,2] J. Landa,[3] D. Kuk,[4] A. Sanchez,[1] B. Lala,[1] N. Schmidt,[1] C. Okoli,[1] P. Chi,[1,2] M. A. Dickson,[1,2] M. M. Gounder,[1,2] M. L. Keohan,[1,2] A. M. Crago,[2,5] W. D. Tap,[1,2] and S. P. D'Angelo[1,2]

[1] *Sarcoma Oncology Service, Department of Medicine, Memorial Sloan Kettering Cancer Center, 1275 York Avenue, New York, NY 10065, USA*

[2] *Weill Cornell Medical College, 1300 York Avenue, New York, NY 10065, USA*

[3] *Department of Radiology, Memorial Sloan Kettering Cancer Center, 1275 York Avenue, New York, NY 10065, USA*

[4] *Department of Epidemiology and Biostatistics, Memorial Sloan Kettering Cancer Center, 1275 York Avenue, New York, NY 10065, USA*

[5] *Department of Surgery, Memorial Sloan Kettering Cancer Center, 1275 York Avenue, New York, NY 10065, USA*

Correspondence should be addressed to S. P. D'Angelo; dangelos@mskcc.org

Academic Editor: Akira Kawai

Background. Leiomyosarcomas (LMS) represent a heterogeneous subset of soft tissue sarcomas. Factors influencing prognosis for patients with metastatic extrauterine LMS (euLMS) are not well described. Limited data are available regarding responses to systemic therapy. *Methods.* We collected clinical and pathologic information for all patients with metastatic euLMS seen at Memorial Sloan Kettering Cancer Center between 1989 and 2012. Objective responses to first-line therapy were analyzed for a subset of patients with available baseline and on-treatment imaging using RECIST 1.1. *Results.* 215 patients with metastatic euLMS had a median overall survival (OS) of 2.6 years from the time of metastasis. Older age, male sex, and ≥3 initial sites of metastasis were associated with worse OS on multivariate analysis. Objective response rate (ORR) in $N = 113$ was 19% overall and 25%, 26%, and 25% for gemcitabine, gemcitabine plus docetaxel, and anthracycline-alkylator combinations. Patients whose tumors objectively responded to first-line therapy had a lower risk of death versus those who did not (Hazard Ratio 0.46; 95% CI: 0.26–0.79, $p = 0.005$). *Conclusions.* Anthracycline- and gemcitabine-based regimens have similar activity in this cohort of euLMS. Prognostic factors for OS include older age, male sex, and ≥3 initial sites.

1. Introduction

Leiomyosarcomas (LMS) are a heterogeneous group of smooth muscle neoplasms that can arise in the uterus, extremity, or other primary sites [1]. Together, LMS comprise the most common single soft tissue sarcoma histology (24% of all soft tissue sarcomas), with an incidence of approximately 1.2 cases per 100,000 person-years [2]. Increasing clinical and genetic data suggest LMS arising from an extrauterine primary site represents a distinct subset of tumors [3–5]. Until the identification of KIT positive tumors, many prior analyses of extrauterine LMS (euLMS) were likely contaminated by unrecognized gastrointestinal stromal tumors, limiting our understanding of this disease entity. A recent single-center, retrospective review of 332 patients with primary euLMS identified size and grade as distinct factors that influenced disease-specific survival [1]. Little is known, however, about factors influencing prognosis for patients with metastatic euLMS. A series of all LMS subtypes included 101 with euLMS and found that the sole factor influencing OS was a shorter interval from diagnosis to metastatic disease [6].

The choice of systemic therapy agents is extrapolated using prospective and retrospective analyses of LMS pooled from uterine and euLMS, most often utilizing gemcitabine with or without docetaxel or doxorubicin with or without an alkylator such as ifosfamide (AIM) [7–9]. Recently, the results of GeDDiS, a randomized Phase 3 trial comparing gemcitabine plus docetaxel with doxorubicin in the front-line setting, were reported in multiple soft tissue sarcoma subtypes, including uterine and euLMS [10]. The primary endpoint of 24-week PFS was identical between arms, 46% each. Two separate, randomized Phase 3 trials identified agents in the second-line setting that provided clinical benefit for patients with any type of LMS. Trabectedin was recently FDA-approved for treatment of LMS previously treated with an anthracycline on the basis of a significant PFS benefit versus dacarbazine (4.3 versus 1.5 months, $p < 0.001$) [11]. Eribulin significantly prolonged OS versus dacarbazine in a cohort of patients with LMS or liposarcoma, although an exploratory subgroup analysis suggested that the majority of benefit was limited to patients with liposarcoma [12]. A prospective study of 2nd-line therapy with gemcitabine or gemcitabine plus docetaxel in euLMS reported a response rate of 14% and 5%, respectively [13].

Response rates to first-line systemic therapy in advanced euLMS have been reported in small retrospective case series utilizing anthracycline- or alkylator-based regimens such as AIM. One series that reported ORR specifically in euLMS included 32 patients who either received doxorubicin or other single-agent alkylators ($n = 19$), ifosfamide ($n = 9$), or AIM ($n = 4$); overall, the pooled ORR was 22% [14]. Another series of 18 patients, the majority of which received doxorubicin ($n = 9$) or epirubicin plus ifosfamide ($n = 6$), reported a response rate of 33% [15].

In euLMS, it is not well described whether the choice of systemic therapy agent is associated with differences in response rate or whether the objective response to first-line systemic therapy influences clinical outcomes. We therefore undertook a retrospective, single-center analysis of patients with advanced euLMS to analyze the association of clinicopathologic factors, first-line systemic therapy agent, and objective response to first-line systemic therapy with survival from the time of metastatic disease.

2. Methods

After institutional IRB approval, patients were identified from a database query who met the following criteria: (1) ≥1 visit at Memorial Sloan Kettering Cancer Center (MSKCC) between 1989 and 2012; (2) a pathologic diagnosis of leiomyosarcoma arising from an extrauterine primary site; and (3) developed metastatic disease at any point from diagnosis to last follow-up visit. Clinicopathologic data included age at first diagnosis, status at presentation (primary versus metastatic), year of development of metastatic disease, time interval between primary and metastatic diseases, sex, depth, grade (utilizing the Fédération Nationale des Centres de Lutte Contre le Cancer (FNCLCC) system), primary tumor size, site, Karnofsky Performance Status (KPS) at time of metastasis, margins, number of metastatic sites at first presentation of advanced disease, presence versus absence of lung or liver metastases, treatment type at first recurrence, and first-line systemic therapy agent. Patients with missing clinicopathologic data were included and data were marked as "unknown" for that specific category.

Treatment type at first recurrence was analyzed only for patients who initially presented with localized disease and characterized as systemic therapy only, local therapy only (surgery, embolization), or combination systemic and local therapy. Systemic therapy agents in this retrospective cohort were up to the discretion of the treating physician and were classified for our analysis as follows: doxorubicin alone, liposomal doxorubicin alone, gemcitabine alone, gemcitabine plus docetaxel, anthracycline-alkylator combinations (doxorubicin, ifosfamide, and mesna [AIM], AIM plus dacarbazine, and doxorubicin plus dacarbazine), tyrosine kinase inhibitors (sunitinib, sorafenib), and other combination or single agents. Patients were considered evaluable for response to first-line therapy if at least 1 CT or MRI was available both before and at least three weeks after initiating first-line therapy. Radiographic responses to first-line systemic therapy were assessed by a radiologist blinded to treatment (JL) using Response Evaluation Criteria in Solid Tumors (RECIST) 1.1, with the exception that repeat assessments to confirm response were not required in this retrospective analysis. Time to treatment failure (TTF) was calculated as start of systemic therapy until date of progressive disease by RECIST 1.1 or new therapy, whichever was first.

Patient demographics are presented by median and range for continuous variables and by frequency and percentage for categorical variables. Overall survival (OS) was calculated from date of development of metastatic disease to date of death or last follow-up. Patients alive at last follow-up were censored. The Kaplan-Meier method, log-rank test, and Cox proportional hazards regression were used for estimation, testing, and regression modeling of overall survival, respectively. For patients with RECIST response data, the relationship between response and OS was evaluated. OS in this subset of patients was calculated from date of start of chemotherapy to date of death or last follow-up. RECIST response was treated as a time dependent covariate in the Cox proportional hazards model. For chemotherapy regimens, time to treatment failure (TTF) is calculated as date from start of chemotherapy to date of progression by RECIST 1.1 or first day of subsequent-line chemotherapy. The Kruskal-Wallis test was used to compare TTF between the different chemotherapy regimens. p values < 0.05 are considered significant. All analysis was done using R version 3.1.1 (https://cran.r-project.org/).

3. Results

3.1. Overall Survival. A total of 215 patients met inclusion criteria. See Table 1 for demographics. Median age was 56 (range: 24–85), and 63% of patients were female. A majority of patients initially presented with localized disease (61%). The median primary tumor size was 9 cm (range: 2–30 cm), and the most common primary site was in the abdomen or retroperitoneum ($n = 151$, 70%). The majority of primary

TABLE 1: Patients' demographics, $n = 215$.

Age (range)	56.4 (23.4–85.4)
Tumor size (range)	9 (2–30)
Number of metastatic sites (range)	2 (1–8)
Presentation status	
Primary disease	132 (61)
Metastatic disease	83 (39)
Gender	
Female	135 (63)
Male	80 (37)
Primary tumor size	
<5 cm	34 (16)
5–10 cm	81 (38)
>10 cm	80 (37)
Unknown primary	10 (5)
Known primary, unknown size	10 (5)
KPS	
60	2 (1)
70	8 (4)
80	46 (21)
90	65 (30)
100	22 (10)
Unknown	72 (33)
Primary site	
A/P or RP	151 (70)
Extremity	45 (21)
Trunk	9 (4)
Unknown primary	10 (5)
Margins	
Negative	95 (44)
Positive	45 (21)
Gross disease	3 (1)
N/A—no surgery	47 (22)
Unknown	25 (12)
Grade	
Low	7 (3)
Intermediate	5 (2)
High	176 (82)
Unknown	27 (14)
Depth	
Superficial	5 (2)
Deep	196 (91)
Unknown	14 (7)
Number of metastatic sites	
<3	144 (67)
≥3	71 (33)
Lung metastases	
No	102 (47)
Yes	113 (53)
Liver metastases	
No	159 (74)
Yes	56 (26)

Numbers may not add to 100 due to rounding. KPS: Karnofsky Performance Status; A/P: abdomen/pelvis, RP: retroperitoneal; and N/A: not applicable.

tumors were high grade ($n = 176$, 82%) and deep ($n = 196$, 91%). For patients diagnosed with localized disease, the median time to developing metastases was 15.8 months (range: 2.1–232 months). The median number of metastatic sites was 2 (range: 1–8). The most common sites of metastatic disease were lung (53%) and liver (26%). KPS at time of metastasis was relatively preserved in this cohort; only 10 of 215 (5%) had KPS of 70 or below (ECOG ≥ 2), and 72 (33%) had an unknown performance status.

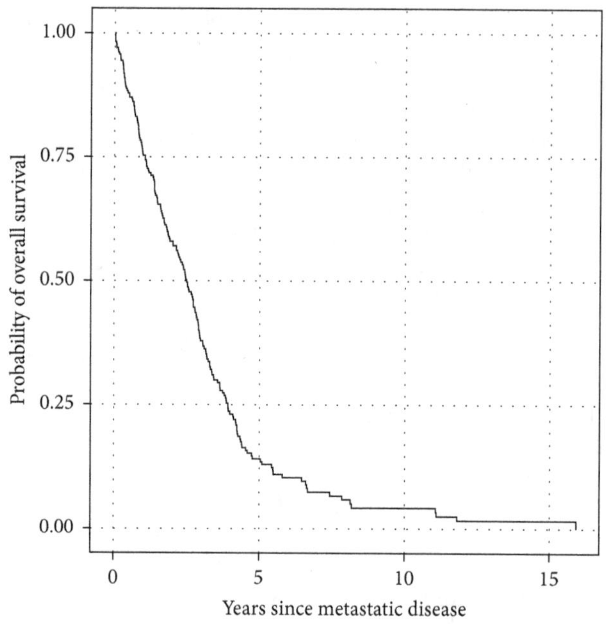

FIGURE 1: Overall survival from date of metastatic disease. Median OS was 2.6 years.

Median follow-up amongst survivors is 14.6 years. There were 190 deaths. Median OS from time of diagnosis of metastatic disease is 2.6 years (Figure 1). On univariate analysis, older age, male sex, shorter interval between primary and metastatic disease, and higher number of initial metastatic sites were significantly associated with an increased risk of death (Table 2). Median OS for patients above versus below the median age of 56 was 2.4 versus 2.8 years ($p = 0.006$); 2.9 versus 2.2 years for females versus males ($p = 0.005$); and 2.0 versus 2.8 years for ≥3 metastatic sites versus 1-2 metastatic sites ($p = 0.002$). On multivariate analysis (Table 3), (Hazard ratio [HR] and 95% confidence interval): older age (HR = 1.36; 1.01–1.84), male sex (HR = 1.42; 1.05–1.92), and higher number of initial metastatic sites (HR = 1.49; 1.10–2.03) remained significant. The time to development of metastatic disease was no longer significant (HR = 0.92; 0.84–1.01). The other variables assessed were not associated with OS from time of development of metastatic disease on univariate analysis.

3.2. First-Line Systemic Therapy. One hundred thirteen patients received first-line systemic therapy agents and were evaluable for objective response. The first-line chemotherapy classes and objective responses are depicted in Figure 2. The objective response rate (ORR) to first-line chemotherapy was 19% overall (21 of 113). The majority of regimens

TABLE 2: Univariate analysis of clinicopathologic features on OS from time of metastasis.

Variable	n	Number of events	Median OS	p value
Time to metastatic disease (years, continuous)	215	190	—	**0.036****
Age				
≤56	104	85	2.79	**0.006**
>56	111	105	2.38	
Primary tumor size				
<5 cm	34	26	2.92	0.711
5–10 cm	81	75	2.54	
>10 cm	80	69	2.69	
Gender				
Female	135	115	2.91	**0.005**
Male	80	75	2.19	
Primary site				
A/P or RP	151	131	2.73	0.097
Extremity	45	40	2.54	
Trunk	9	9	1.74	
Unknown	10	10	2.51	
Margins				
Negative	95	82	2.58	0.801
Positive	48	43	2.9	
Grade				
Low/intermediate	12	11	4.17	0.165
High	176	155	2.54	
Depth				
Superficial	5	4	1.49	0.538
Deep	196	173	2.69	
Number of metastatic sites				
<3	144	125	2.83	**0.002**
≥3	71	65	2.03	
KPS				
≤70	10	9	2.35	0.115
>70	133	116	2.91	
Lung metastases				
No	102	90	2.46	0.586
Yes	113	100	2.71	
Liver metastases				
No	159	143	2.71	0.529
Yes	56	47	2.37	
Treatment for recurrence*				
Chemo only	49	40	2.37	0.077
Local therapy only	33	30	3.06	
Chemo + local treatment	40	35	2.98	
Year of metastatic disease				
Before 2000	51	48	2.23	0.387
2000 and after	164	142	2.71	

*Treatment for recurrence only analyzed in $n = 132$ patients presenting with primary disease. **p value comes from score test. A/P: abdomen/pelvis, RP: retroperitoneal, and chemo: chemotherapy.

Table 3: Multivariate analysis of clinicopathologic features on OS from time of metastasis.

	HR	95% lower	95% upper	p value
Age (>56 versus ≤56)	1.36	1.01	1.84	0.045
Gender (M versus F)	1.42	1.05	1.92	0.023
Number of metastatic sites (≥3 versus <3)	1.49	1.10	2.03	0.011
Time to metastatic disease (cont.)	0.92	0.84	1.01	0.078

Table 4: First-line systemic therapy regimens and median time to treatment failure (TTF).

Systemic therapy	n	Median TTF (months)
Gemcitabine + docetaxel	31	5.2
Gemcitabine	12	4.3
Doxorubicin-alkylator combo	20	3.1
Liposomal doxorubicin	12	2.9
Doxorubicin	6	3.3
Alkylator, single	3	1.8
Tyrosine kinase inhibitors	7	9.3
Other combos	13	7.2
Other single agents	9	1.6

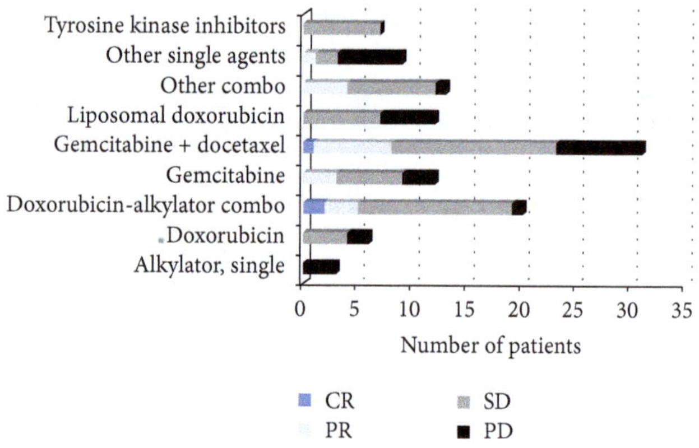

Figure 2: Response to first-line systemic therapy regimens. Objective responses were seen with gemcitabine + docetaxel (8/31, 26%), gemcitabine (3/12, 25%), and doxorubicin-alkylator combinations (5/20, 25%). CR = complete response, PR = partial response, SD = stable disease, and PD = progressive disease.

included either gemcitabine ($n = 47$, 42%) or anthracycline ($n = 42$, 37%). The most common regimens were combined gemcitabine plus docetaxel ($n = 31$, 27%) and combined anthracycline plus alkylator ($n = 20$, 18%). The ORR did not vary significantly between these two groups (26% versus 25%, $p = 1.0$). Objective responses were seen in both combination regimens and with single-agent gemcitabine but not single-agent doxorubicin or liposomal doxorubicin. For a detailed list of all regimens, see Supplemental Table 1 of the Supplementary Material available online at http://dx.doi.org/10.1155/2016/3547497.

When comparing classes of first-line therapy, there were no significant differences in TTF (Table 4). For example, the median TTF for doxorubicin alone, anthracycline plus alkylator combinations, and liposomal doxorubicin was 3.3, 3.1, and 2.9 months, respectively ($p = 0.99$). Gemcitabine plus docetaxel versus gemcitabine alone had a median TTF of 5.2 and 4.3 months, respectively ($p = 0.83$). The difference between gemcitabine plus docetaxel and anthracycline plus alkylator combinations was not statistically significant ($p = 0.95$). The small group of patients receiving TKIs (sorafenib, $n = 6$, sunitinib, $n = 1$) had a median TTF of 9.3 months.

To determine the possible effect of prognostic confounders on patients evaluable for response to first-line systemic therapy, the variables significantly associated with OS on univariate analysis (age, sex, metastasis-free interval, and number of initial metastatic sites) were analyzed by therapy class. Only metastasis-free interval ($p = 0.04$) varied significantly across tumor types (Table 5). The metastasis-free interval was shortest for those treated with anthracycline plus alkylator combinations or gemcitabine plus docetaxel (median 0 and 0.23 years) and longest for the $N = 18$ patients who were treated without systemic therapy (1.5 years). Objective responses to first-line systemic therapy were significantly associated with OS. Patients whose tumors have an objective response had a lower risk of death during follow-up than those who had no objective response (HR: 0.46; 95% CI: 0.26–0.79, $p = 0.005$). There was no significant association of systemic therapy type with OS ($p = 0.40$, data not shown). Of the 113 patients evaluable for response, 10 (9%) received trabectedin after first-line therapy (range: 2nd–9th therapies), and no patients received subsequent eribulin. Overall, 98 of 113 patients received at least 1 subsequent systemic therapy.

4. Discussion

There are relatively little data published regarding factors influencing survival in patients with metastatic extrauterine leiomyosarcoma. This is to our knowledge the largest study of the impact of clinical and pathologic variables on clinical outcomes in advanced euLMS. Median OS was 2.6 years from the time of developing metastatic disease. Independent predictors of improved outcome included younger age, female sex, and 2 or fewer metastatic sites at first presentation of advanced disease. This is consistent with the trend reported in one study of improved PFS and OS with female sex and younger age in patients with euLMS receiving systemic therapy [14]. Although another study of 50 patients with euLMS found no significant association between clinical variables and outcome [15], this may be due to a difference in population. Their study included all patients with euLMS, not just those who developed metastatic disease, and they had a preponderance of smaller primary extremity tumors that were in the minority in this cohort. It is notable that in this cohort, performance status was not associated with outcome, given that this is a well-established prognostic variable in a large analysis of soft tissue sarcomas [16]. Our analysis is limited, however, by the small percentage of those with lower

TABLE 5: Association between clinicopathologic features associated with OS and first-line systemic therapy regimens. The variability of the number of metastatic sites is presented as the 75th percentile to better reflect the true variability rather than displaying the median.

Systemic therapy	Median age (years)	Female : male ratio	Median time to metastases (years)	Number of metastatic sites, 75th percentile*
Gemcitabine + docetaxel	56.5	2.6	0.23	5
Gemcitabine	72	1.3	0.78	2
Doxorubicin-alkylator combo	56.2	1	0	2
Liposomal doxorubicin	66.7	2.9	1.0	3.5
Doxorubicin	58.7	5	0	5
Alkylator, single	65.4	2	0.81	3.5
Tyrosine kinase inhibitors	51.7	1.3	1.1	3.5
Other combos	58.7	1.6	0.56	2
Other single agents	51.8	2.3	1.1	3
None	55.2	1.6	1.5	2
p value	0.20	0.66	0.04	0.10

*Defined as number at which 75% had fewer and 25% had greater metastases.

performance status (<10%) and a relatively high percentage of patients with missing data at the time of metastasis (33%). Our analysis did not demonstrate any association with liver involvement or grade and OS, in contrast to the larger analysis across all sarcoma subtypes [16]. It is not clear whether this is due to an euLMS-specific difference in clinical behavior or whether larger sample sizes are required to appreciate this association.

Our study is the largest to analyze response to first-line systemic therapy in euLMS. The ORR across all chemotherapy types in this study (19%, $n = 113$) is similar to that reported by the Dutch group (22%, $n = 32$) [14]. Both are slightly lower rates than that reported in the smaller Austrian cohort (33%, $n = 18$) [15]. This euLMS cohort includes a large series of patients receiving non-anthracycline-based regimens, including 47 receiving gemcitabine with or without docetaxel and other agents. The response rates of ~25% and median TTF of 4-5 months are comparable to the efficacy seen in randomized trials in uterine LMS, euLMS, and other sarcomas [8, 10, 17]. In this cohort, there was no significant difference in ORR or TTF between gemcitabine with or without docetaxel and anthracycline plus alkylator combinations such as AIM. Notably, patient age and metastasis-free interval were similar between gemcitabine plus docetaxel and anthracycline plus alkylator combinations.

In the first-line GeDDiS trial [10], within the subgroup of all patients with LMS, which included 47 patients with euLMS and 71 with uterine LMS, there was no detectable difference in PFS (HR: 1.12, 95% CI: 0.75–1.66). There was no evidence for subgroup differences between euLMS and uterine LMS (p value for interaction = 0.73), and the euLMS subgroup could not detect a significant difference in PFS when analyzed separately (HR: 1.34, 0.98–1.83). It is also notable that a 25% lower dose of gemcitabine was used in GeDDiS versus the other Phase 2/3 published trials (675 mg/m^2 versus 900 mg/m^2) [8, 17]. Given these data and the results of our cohort, we believe that gemcitabine with or without docetaxel remains a reasonable alternative to doxorubicin in euLMS.

The median TTF in our study for anthracycline-based regimens was approximately 3 months. There was no difference between doxorubicin monotherapy and doxorubicin plus an alkylator. This lack of median TTF benefit with the addition of an alkylator is echoed by the report across all LMS subtypes ($n = 147$) by the French Sarcoma Group [6]. The TTF value in our report is comparable to the median PFS of 3.8 months reported by the Dutch group focused on euLMS [14]. While liposomal doxorubicin did not lead to any responses in this cohort, it was associated with a similar median TTF to doxorubicin of approximately 3 months. Taken together, these data suggest that the addition of ifosfamide or dacarbazine to doxorubicin or liposomal doxorubicin monotherapy may not provide additional benefit, outside of a higher objective response rate [18], to justify the historically higher rate of adverse events of combination cytotoxic therapy.

This retrospective analysis, as with many others investigating sarcoma subtypes, is limited by selection bias and relatively by low numbers for certain classes of chemotherapy. Patients with more clinically aggressive disease may have been more likely to receive combination cytotoxic regimens, while patients with indolent progression may have been more likely to receive single agents such as sorafenib. This is supported by the data suggesting that patients who received gemcitabine plus docetaxel or doxorubicin had a shorter metastasis-free interval than those receiving a tyrosine kinase inhibitor. This may explain the particularly high median TTF of over 9 months in the small multityrosine kinase inhibitor group; interestingly, this value was higher than the median PFS of 3.2 months seen in all patients with LMS treated on a recent Phase 2 study [19]. Regardless, this does provide equipoise for utilizing single agents when deemed clinically feasible. For example, liposomal doxorubicin could be considered an alternative to anthracycline-alkylator combinations in cases where disease stability would suffice. This is consistent with the results of a prior Phase 2 study showing similar efficacy of liposomal doxorubicin and doxorubicin across multiple sarcoma subtypes [20].

The two randomized Phase 3 trials demonstrating clinical benefit for patients with LMS treated with trabectedin [11] and eribulin [12] in the second-line setting raise interesting questions for future study that cannot be answered by our cohort. During the era analyzed in this cohort, trabectedin was not widely available in the US. Only 1 patient received trabectedin as a first-line therapy, and only 10 patients (9%) received it at any time subsequently. No patients received eribulin in our analysis. As a result, our analysis neither is significantly confounded by nor can add significant insight into the activity of these agents. They represent promising cytotoxic therapies for patients with LMS. For example, in a recent Phase 2 study of trabectedin combined with doxorubicin, 24 of 61 evaluable patients (39%) with euLMS had an objective response [21], underscoring the promise of this agent for this sarcoma subtype.

A significant finding in this study is the fact that patients whose tumors had objectively responding disease to the first systemic treatment had better OS than those who had stable or primary progressive disease. This underscores the importance of understanding how to best select therapies that may benefit patients with advanced euLMS. Given that chemotherapy class alone was not associated with survival in this analysis, one particular regimen cannot be uniformly viewed as superior to any other across all patients.

Taken together, this study suggests that more research must be done to understand which genetic and epigenetic factors influence the response of euLMS to cytotoxic therapy. One active area of investigation is the role that the tumor and immunologic microenvironments play in objective responses [22]. Lymphopenia has been identified as a predictor of worse OS in advanced sarcomas [23]. In preclinical models of sarcoma, antitumor efficacy of doxorubicin is linked to the presence of an intact innate immune system that can produce interferon-alpha and induce a "type-1 interferon" response in tumor cells [24]. These investigators then performed a retrospective analysis of patients with high risk breast carcinoma receiving adjuvant anthracycline-based therapy. They identified an improved metastasis-free survival for those with tumors harboring a high rather than low expression of this type-1 interferon signature [24]. Further work is needed to explore the molecular and immunologic heterogeneity of euLMS and the impact of these aberrations on clinical outcomes. This will help "personalize" treatment strategies for these patients that will help them live longer with advanced disease.

5. Conclusions

In the largest cohort to date to analyze outcomes in extrauterine leiomyosarcoma, factors that influenced prognosis from the time of metastatic disease were sex, age, and metastatic disease burden. No significant difference in clinical activity could be detected between anthracycline-based and gemcitabine-based therapies in the first-line setting. Those whose tumors responded to first-line therapy tended to live longer, suggesting that future studies in this sarcoma subtype should focus on understanding the genetic and tumor microenvironmental factors that underlie this heterogeneity.

Disclosure

This work was presented in modified form at the American Society of Clinical Oncology 2015 Annual Meeting.

Competing Interests

The authors declare that they have no competing interests.

Acknowledgments

N. Schmidt and C. Okoli were supported by Grant no. 5R25CA020449. All authors acknowledge the support of the Core Grant (P30 CA008748).

References

[1] R. A. Gladdy, L.-X. Qin, N. Moraco, N. P. Agaram, M. F. Brennan, and S. Singer, "Predictors of survival and recurrence in primary leiomyosarcoma," *Annals of Surgical Oncology*, vol. 20, no. 6, pp. 1851–1857, 2013.

[2] J. R. Toro, L. B. Travis, H. J. Wu, K. Zhu, C. D. M. Fletcher, and S. S. Devesa, "Incidence patterns of soft tissue sarcomas, regardless of primary site, in the surveillance, epidemiology and end results program, 1978–2001: an analysis of 26,758 cases," *International Journal of Cancer*, vol. 119, no. 12, pp. 2922–2930, 2006.

[3] A. Italiano, M. Toulmonde, E. Stoeckle et al., "Clinical outcome of leiomyosarcomas of vascular origin: comparison with leiomyosarcomas of other origin," *Annals of Oncology*, vol. 21, no. 9, pp. 1915–1921, 2010.

[4] K. M. Skubitz and A. P. N. Skubitz, "Differential gene expression in leiomyosarcoma," *Cancer*, vol. 98, no. 5, pp. 1029–1038, 2003.

[5] J. Yang, X. Du, K. Chen et al., "Genetic aberrations in soft tissue leiomyosarcoma," *Cancer Letters*, vol. 275, no. 1, pp. 1–8, 2009.

[6] N. Penel, A. Italiano, N. Isambert, E. Bompas, G. Bousquet, and F. Duffaud, "Factors affecting the outcome of patients with metastatic leiomyosarcoma treated with doxorubicin-containing chemotherapy," *Annals of Oncology*, vol. 21, no. 6, pp. 1361–1365, 2009.

[7] J.-O. Bay, I. Ray-Coquard, J. Fayette et al., "Docetaxel and gemcitabine combination in 133 advanced soft-tissue sarcomas: a retrospective analysis," *International Journal of Cancer*, vol. 119, no. 3, pp. 706–711, 2006.

[8] R. G. Maki, J. K. Wathen, S. R. Patel et al., "Randomized phase II study of gemcitabine and docetaxel compared with gemcitabine alone in patients with metastatic soft tissue sarcomas," *Journal of Clinical Oncology*, vol. 25, no. 19, pp. 2755–2763, 2007.

[9] G. Sutton, J. A. Blessing, and J. H. Malfetano, "Ifosfamide and doxorubicin in the treatment of advanced leiomyosarcomas of the uterus: a Gynecologic Oncology Group study," *Gynecologic Oncology*, vol. 62, no. 2, pp. 226–229, 1996.

[10] B. M. Seddon, J. Whelan, S. J. Strauss et al., "GeDDiS: A prospective randomised controlled phase III trial of gemcitabine and docetaxel compared with doxorubicin as first-line treatment in

previously untreated advanced unresectable or metastatic soft tissue sarcomas (EudraCT 2009-014907-29)," *ASCO Meeting Abstracts*, vol. 33, p. 10500, 2015.

[11] G. D. Demetri, M. von Mehren, R. L. Jones et al., "Efficacy and safety of Trabectedin or Dacarbazine for metastatic Liposarcoma or Leiomyosarcoma after failure of conventional chemotherapy: results of a phase III randomized multicenter clinical trial," *Journal of Clinical Oncology*, vol. 34, no. 8, pp. 786–793, 2016.

[12] P. Schöffski, S. Chawla, R. G. Maki et al., "Eribulin versus dacarbazine in previously treated patients with advanced liposarcoma or leiomyosarcoma: a randomised, open-label, multicentre, phase 3 trial," *The Lancet*, vol. 387, no. 10028, pp. 1629–1637, 2016.

[13] P. Pautier, A. Floquet, N. Penel et al., "Randomized multicenter and stratified phase II study of gemcitabine alone versus gemcitabine and docetaxel in patients with metastatic or relapsed leiomyosarcomas: a Fédération Nationale Des Centres De Lutte Contre le Cancer (FNCLCC) French Sarcoma Group study (TAXOGEM study)," *Oncologist*, vol. 17, no. 9, pp. 1213–1220, 2012.

[14] A. W. Oosten, C. Seynaeve, P. I. M. Schmitz, M. A. Den Bakker, J. Verweij, and S. Sleijfer, "Outcomes of first-line chemotherapy in patients with advanced or metastatic leiomyosarcoma of uterine and non-uterine origin," *Sarcoma*, vol. 2009, Article ID 348910, 6 pages, 2009.

[15] W. Lamm, C. Natter, S. Schur et al., "Distinctive outcome in patients with non-uterine and uterine leiomyosarcoma," *BMC Cancer*, vol. 14, no. 1, article 981, 2014.

[16] M. Van Glabbeke, A. T. van Oosterom, J. W. Oosterhuis et al., "Prognostic factors for the outcome of chemotherapy in advanced soft tissue sarcoma: an analysis of 2,185 patients treated with anthracycline-containing first-line regimens—a European organization for research and treatment of cancer soft tissue and bone sarcoma group study," *Journal of Clinical Oncology*, vol. 17, no. 1, pp. 150–157, 1999.

[17] M. L. Hensley, A. Miller, D. M. O'Malley et al., "Randomized phase III trial of gemcitabine plus docetaxel plus bevacizumab or placebo as first-line treatment for metastatic uterine leiomyosarcoma: an NRG oncology/gynecologic oncology group study," *Journal of Clinical Oncology*, vol. 33, no. 10, pp. 1180–1185, 2015.

[18] I. Judson, J. Verweij, H. Gelderblom et al., "Doxorubicin alone versus intensified doxorubicin plus ifosfamide for first-line treatment of advanced or metastatic soft-tissue sarcoma: a randomised controlled phase 3 trial," *The Lancet Oncology*, vol. 15, no. 4, pp. 415–423, 2014.

[19] R. G. Maki, D. R. D'Adamo, M. L. Keohan et al., "Phase II study of sorafenib in patients with metastatic or recurrent sarcomas," *Journal of Clinical Oncology*, vol. 27, no. 19, pp. 3133–3140, 2009.

[20] I. Judson, J. A. Radford, M. Harris et al., "Randomised phase II trial of pegylated liposomal doxorubicin (DOXIL®/CAELYX®) versus doxorubicin in the treatment of advanced or metastatic soft tissue sarcoma: a study by the EORTC Soft Tissue and Bone Sarcoma Group," *European Journal of Cancer*, vol. 37, no. 7, pp. 870–877, 2001.

[21] P. Pautier, A. Floquet, C. Chevreau et al., "Trabectedin in combination with doxorubicin for first-line treatment of advanced uterine or soft-tissue leiomyosarcoma (LMS-02): a non-randomised, multicentre, phase 2 trial," *The Lancet Oncology*, vol. 16, no. 4, pp. 457–464, 2015.

[22] L. Zitvogel, O. Kepp, and G. Kroemer, "Immune parameters affecting the efficacy of chemotherapeutic regimens," *Nature Reviews Clinical Oncology*, vol. 8, no. 3, pp. 151–160, 2011.

[23] I. Ray-Coquard, C. Cropet, M. Van Glabbeke et al., "Lymphopenia as a prognostic factor for overall survival in advanced carcinomas, sarcomas, and lymphomas," *Cancer Research*, vol. 69, no. 13, pp. 5383–5391, 2009.

[24] A. Sistigu, T. Yamazaki, E. Vacchelli et al., "Cancer cell-autonomous contribution of type I interferon signaling to the efficacy of chemotherapy," *Nature medicine*, vol. 20, no. 11, pp. 1301–1309, 2014.

27

Variations of Surveillance Practice for Patients with Bone Sarcoma: A Survey of Australian Sarcoma Clinicians

Jeremy Lewin,[1,2] Kate Thompson,[1] Susie Bae,[3] Jayesh Desai,[3] Robyn Strong,[4] Denise Caruso,[3] Deborah Howell,[1] Alan Herschtal,[5] Michael Sullivan,[6,7] and Lisa Orme[1,6]

[1] *Victorian Adolescent & Young Adult Cancer Service, Peter MacCallum Cancer Centre, Melbourne, VIC, Australia*
[2] *Adolescent and Young Adult Oncology, Princess Margaret Cancer Centre, Toronto, ON, Canada*
[3] *Australasian Sarcoma Study Group, Melbourne, VIC, Australia*
[4] *Australian and New Zealand Children's Hematology/Oncology Group, Melbourne, VIC, Australia*
[5] *Centre for Biostatistics and Clinical Trials, Peter MacCallum Cancer Centre, Melbourne, VIC, Australia*
[6] *Children's Cancer Centre, Royal Children's Hospital, Melbourne, VIC, Australia*
[7] *Department of Paediatrics, University of Melbourne, Melbourne, VIC, Australia*

Correspondence should be addressed to Jeremy Lewin; jeremy.lewin@uhn.ca

Academic Editor: R. Lor Randall

Introduction. After treatment, bone sarcoma patients carry a high chance of relapse and late effects from multimodal therapy. We hypothesize that significant variation in surveillance practice exists between pediatric medical oncology (PO) and nonpediatric medical oncology (NP) sarcoma disciplines. *Methods.* Australian sarcoma clinicians were approached to do a web based survey that assessed radiologic surveillance (RS) strategies, late toxicity assessment, and posttreatment psychosocial interventions. *Results.* In total, 51 clinicians responded. No differences were identified in local disease RS. In metastatic disease response assessment, 100% of POs (23/23) and 93% of NPs (24/26) conducted CT chest. However, this was more likely to occur for NPs in the context of a CT chest/abdomen/pelvis (NP: 10/26; PO: 1/23; $p = 0.006$). POs were more likely to use CXR for RS ($p = 0.006$). POs showed more prescriptive intensity in assessment of heart function ($p = 0.001$), hearing ($p < 0.001$), and fertility ($p = 0.02$). POs were more likely to deliver written information for health maintenance/treatment summary ($p = 0.04$). The majority of respondents described enquiring about psychosocial aspects of health ($n = 33/37$, 89%), but a routine formal psychosocial screen was only used by 23% ($n = 6/26$). *Conclusion.* There is high variability in bone sarcoma surveillance between PO and NP clinicians. Efforts to harmonize approaches would allow early and late effects recognition/intervention and facilitate improved patient care/transition and research.

1. Background

Sarcomas of the bone are rare primary malignant tumors arising from mesenchymal or neuroectodermal tissue and account for less than 1% of all malignancies [1]. The most common subtypes are osteosarcoma (OS) and Ewing's sarcoma family tumors (ESFT) with an average of 3000 new cases being diagnosed in the United States [2] and 200 cases being diagnosed in Australia each year [3]. Prior to the era of multimodality therapy, bone sarcomas were associated with an 80–90% risk of metastasis with resection alone [4]. However, advances in treatment have led to 5-year overall survival approximating 60–70% [5]. With improving survival, follow-up procedures for patients with bone sarcoma are becoming increasingly important, especially as primary treatment carries significant risks of long-term physical and psychological sequelae.

The aim of surveillance is multifold, including the potential to detect treatable recurrences, manage chronic toxicities, and screen for late effects. However, these benefits need to be tempered with healthcare expenditure concerns [6], anxiety associated with surveillance procedures, and cumulative radiation exposure from surveillance imaging [7]. Systematic, uniform, and sustainable targeted disease surveillance (DS) and long-term follow-up (LTFU) strategies that take these factors into account would allow evaluation and evidence generation regarding best practice in posttreatment follow-up. However, differences in established guidelines (which often do not translate into uniform practice) will potentially lead to significant variation in surveillance approaches. For example, guidelines written by the Children's Oncology Group (COG) [8], National Comprehensive Cancer Network (NCCN) [9], and European Society for Medical Oncology (ESMO) [10], which are all based on consensus opinion, vary slightly with regard to the optimal timing for DS, with pediatric protocols showing more concern for cumulative radiation exposure (Table 1). Thus it is likely that posttreatment surveillance schedules vary in regard to timing of clinical reviews, investigation choice, frequency, and duration, both between and within adult and pediatric sectors.

Previous US and UK based clinician surveys have demonstrated significant variation in follow-up procedures for patients with primarily soft tissue sarcoma [11–13]. This survey of Australian clinicians was undertaken to evaluate variations in bone sarcoma surveillance between exclusively pediatric based medical oncologists and nonexclusively pediatric based specialties (NP) and assist in informing the development of Australian guidelines for DS and LTFU strategies in bone sarcomas.

2. Materials and Methods

2.1. Recruitment of Respondents. As there was no definitive list of Australian clinicians involved in the surveillance of sarcoma patients, an overinclusive population of clinicians was identified via the internal databases of the Australasian Sarcoma Study Group (ASSG) and the Australian and New Zealand Children's Hematology Oncology Group (ANZCHOG). In addition, a manual search was conducted of clinicians involved in the major national sarcoma units. Participants were invited to participate via a web based survey (SurveyMonkey, Palo Alto, USA). Consent was assumed based on return response. The survey was open for a 4-month period between June and September 2015.

2.2. Survey Development. The cross-sectional survey was designed to assess a variety of domains associated with both disease and late effects surveillance of bone sarcoma patients. The complete survey is shown in Supplemental Appendix 1 (see Supplementary Material available online at https://doi.org/10.1155/2017/1837475). The 27 questions were distributed as follows: baseline demographics (e.g., type of practice, age demographic of patients, and case load); approach to end of treatment radiological assessment; approach to disease surveillance after primary treatment; approach to screening for late effects (e.g., blood work, ototoxicity, cardiotoxicity, and fertility); and practice for psychosocial support. Responses were designed based on available international surveillance protocols. In addition, respondents were given the opportunity to add comments in free text boxes to expand on specific details related to their particular practice. Before distribution, the questionnaire was piloted by a small group of clinicians. Reminder emails were sent at 2 time points to maximize the response rate.

2.3. Statistical Analysis. The data collected from SurveyMonkey was exported to the R statistical programming language for analysis [14]. Descriptive statistics were used to summarize characteristics of the respondents. Differences between PO and NPs were tested using Fisher's exact test for categorically valued policies and Wilcoxon's test for ordinal valued policies. Given that not all questions were mandatory, sample size varied according to the particular question. Thus responses have been displayed with the numerator (n) and denominator (N) (largest possible number of available responses). The denominator is reported for each section once, unless it changes. Statistical significance was set at a p value < 0.05 and all p values were 2-sided.

3. Results

3.1. Participants. The survey was sent to Australian clinician memberships of the ASSG ($n = 228$) and ANZCHOG ($n = 129$) database, of which 12 emails were undeliverable. In total, 51 clinicians responded (response rate = 15%). Demographics of the respondents are shown in Table 2. Of the 51 who responded, 23 (45%) were pediatric medical oncologists, 11 (22%) were adult medical oncologists, 9 (18%) were radiation oncologists, and 8 (16%) were surgical oncologists/orthopedic surgeons. The majority of respondents worked primarily in a public general hospital ($n = 35$, 69%). The number of respondents who saw pediatric, adolescent/young adult (AYA, defined as 15–25), and adult patients as part of their practice was 67%, 63%, and 47%, respectively. All surgeons worked in the AYA age group whereas 82% of medical oncologists, 56% of radiation oncologists, and 43% of pediatric oncologists worked in this age group. The majority of clinicians saw fewer than or equal to 10 new cases of bone sarcoma per year (69%) with higher case load (defined as >10 new cases per year) seen by orthopedic surgeons (6/7, 86%) and medical oncologists (6/11, 55%) compared to other disciplines ($p = 0.009$).

4. Disease Surveillance

4.1. Assessing Radiologic Response to Treatment. Preferences regarding end of treatment disease restaging investigations for localized limb bone sarcoma divided by discipline are shown in Table 3. With regard to assessment at the primary site, there were no differences identified in the use of CT, MRI, FDG-PET, and bone scan for assessing local disease. However, POs were more likely than NPs to use X-ray imaging alone or as part of pulmonary DS ($p < 0.001$). Regarding metastatic site response assessment, 100% of POs ($n = 23$, $N = 23$) and 93% of NPs ($n = 24$, $N = 26$) conducted CT chest; however, 10/26 NPs compared to 1/23 POs chose this as part of a CT chest/abdomen/pelvis study ($p = 0.006$). POs were more likely than NPs to use CXR in addition to CT chest ($p = 0.02$) and were more likely

Table 1: Differences in RS protocols between COG, NCCN, and ESMO.

	COG [8]		NCCN [9]		ESMO [10]	
	OS	ES	OS	ES	OS and ES	For ES only
Frequency	(i) Primary site: every 3 months × 8 (yr 0–2) and then every 6 mo × 6 (yr 3–5) and then every 12 months × 5 (yr 6–10) (ii) Chest: CT chest every 3 mo × 8 (yr 0–2) and then every 6 mo × 2 (yr 3) and then every 12 months × 2 (yr 4-5). CXR, every 12 months × 5 (starting after last scheduled CT, yr 6–10)	(i) Primary site: every 3 months × 8 (yr 0–2) and then every 6 mo × 6 (yr 3–5) and then every 12 months × 5 (yr 6–10) (ii) Chest: CXR every 3 mo × 8 (yr 0–2) and then every 6 mo × 6 (yr 3–5) and then every 12 months × 5 (yr 6–10)	(i) Every 3 mo (yr 0–2) (ii) Every 4 mo (yr 3) (iii) Every 6 months (yr 4-5) (iv) Every year (>yr 5)	Every 2-3 months for 2 years and then increasing intervals up to 5 years and then annually indefinitely	(i) Every 2-3 mo (yr 0–2) (ii) Every 2–4 mo (yr 3-4) (iii) Every 6 mo (yr 5–10) (iv) Every 6–12 mo (>yr 10)	
Modality	(i) Primary site: AP and lateral X-ray (ii) Chest: CT chest and CXR (iii) Bone scan if symptoms or abnormal imaging (iv) FDG-PET if symptoms or abnormal imaging (v) MRI or CT primary if symptoms or abnormal imaging	(i) Primary site: AP and lateral X-ray (ii) Chest: AP and lateral (iii) Bone scan if symptoms or abnormal imaging (iv) FDG PET if symptoms or abnormal imaging (v) Chest CT if abnormal CXR (vi) MRI or CT primary if symptoms or abnormal imaging	(i) Physical exam (ii) Laboratory studies (iii) Chest imaging (iv) Imaging of primary site (v) Consider FDG/PET or bone scan (vi) Functional assessment at every visit	(i) Physical exam (ii) Laboratory studies (iii) Cross-sectional imaging (MRI with or without CT) and X-ray of primary site (iv) Chest CT (v) Consider PET/CT or bone scan	(i) Physical exam (ii) Laboratory studies (iii) Functional assessment (iv) Imaging of primary site (v) CXR/CT chest	Bone scan can be added

TABLE 2: Baseline demographics.

		Number (%)
Discipline	Pediatric medical oncology	23 (45%)
	Adult medical oncology	11 (22%)
	Radiation	9 (18%)
	Orthopaedics	7 (14%)
	Other	1 (2%)
Age demographic	Exclusively pediatric*	15 (29%)
	Exclusively adult*	4 (8%)
	Exclusively AYA	2 (4%)
	Pediatric as part of practice	34 (67%)
	Adult as part of practice	24 (47%)
	AYA as part of practice	32 (63%)
Institutional location	Private practice	2 (4%)
	Private general hospital	2 (4%)
	Public general hospital	36 (71%)
	Oncology specific hospital	11 (22%)
Volume of new patients per year	0–10	35 (69%)
	11–20	12 (24%)
	20–30	1 (2%)
	30–50	2 (4%)
	>50	1 (2%)

*Including Adolescent and Young Adult (AYA), defined as 15–25 years old.

TABLE 3: Approach to end of treatment radiological assessment.

	PO	Med Onc	Radiation	Ortho	p value**	OR	OR 95% CI
Number of responses	23	10	9	7			
End of treatment response assessment							
Local disease							
X-ray	20 (87%)	3 (30%)	2 (22%)	2 (29%)	<0.001	14.78	[3.15, 99.95]
CT	5 (22%)	2 (20%)	1 (11%)	2 (29%)	1.00	0.97	[0.20, 4.57]
MRI	18 (78%)	7 (70%)	9 (100%)	6 (86%)	0.72	0.63	[0.11, 3.42]
FDG-PET	16 (70%)	5 (50%)	7 (78%)	3 (43%)	0.56	1.56	[0.42, 6.07]
Bone scan	6 (26%)	0 (0%)	0 (0%)	1 (14%)	0.12	4.28	[0.66, 48.30]
Metastatic disease							
CXR	7 (30%)	0 (0%)	0 (0%)	0 (0%)	0.02	10.87	[1.22, 530.27]
CT chest	23 (100%)	5 (50%)	5 (56%)	4 (57%)	<0.001	*	[3.47, *]
CT chest/abdomen/pelvis	1 (4%)	4 (40%)	3 (33%)	3 (43%)	0.006	0.07	[0.00, 0.56]
FDG-PET	15 (65%)	8 (80%)	7 (78%)	4 (57%)	0.55	0.66	[0.16, 2.62]
Whole body scintigraphy	5 (22%)	0 (0%)	0 (0%)	1 (14%)	0.23	3.39	[0.49, 39.36]
Whole body MRI	0 (0%)	0 (0%)	0 (0%)	0 (0%)	1.00	*	[0.00, 45.75]
Bone marrow aspirate	6 (26%)	0 (0%)	0 (0%)	0 (0%)	0.006	*	[1.60, *]

*Inestimable due to insufficient data.
** p value represents comparison between PO and NP.

to include bone marrow aspirate ($p = 0.006$) (presumed with reference to Ewing sarcoma patients with bone marrow involvement at diagnosis; data not collected). There were no differences identified in the use of FDG-PET for assessing metastatic disease at the end of treatment ($p = 0.55$).

4.2. Radiologic Surveillance (RS) after Treatment. The relationship between posttreatment RS and discipline is shown in Table 4. There were no differences identified in the use of X-ray, MRI, CT, or FDG-PET for assessment of local recurrence when using either radiotherapy or surgery as the treatment

TABLE 4: Approach to radiological surveillance.

	PO	Med Onc	Radiation	Ortho	p value**	OR	OR 95% CI
Number of responses	17	10	9	7			
Radiologic surveillance after treatment							
Local disease (after surgery)							
X-ray	12 (71%)	4 (40%)	2 (22%)	5 (71%)	0.12	2.97	[0.70, 14.29]
CT	6 (35%)	3 (30%)	1 (11%)	1 (14%)	0.31	2.14	[0.43, 11.20]
MRI	13 (76%)	8 (80%)	8 (89%)	6 (86%)	0.41	0.45	[0.06, 3.14]
FDG-PET	7 (41%)	2 (20%)	2 (22%)	3 (43%)	0.51	1.77	[0.40, 8.00]
Local disease (after radiation)							
X-ray	5 (29%)	3 (30%)	1 (11%)	1 (14%)	0.48	1.73	[0.32, 9.28]
CT	4 (24%)	3 (30%)	1 (11%)	0 (0%)	0.69	1.67	[0.26, 10.68]
MRI	16 (94%)	8 (80%)	9 (100%)	5 (71%)	0.63	2.85	[0.25, 151.94]
FDG-PET	7 (41%)	1 (10%)	4 (44%)	3 (43%)	0.53	1.56	[0.36, 6.73]
Metastatic disease							
CXR	9 (53%)	2 (20%)	1 (12%)	0 (0%)	0.006	7.77	[1.47, 56.24]
CT chest	13 (76%)	7 (70%)	6 (75%)	2 (29%)	0.33	2.13	[0.47, 11.61]
Alternating CXR and CT	7 (41%)	2 (20%)	1 (12%)	3 (43%)	0.31	2.17	[0.48, 10.34]
CT C/A/P	0 (0%)	0 (0%)	1 (12%)	2 (29%)	0.26	*	[*, 3.52]
FDG-PET	6 (35%)	5 (50%)	4 (50%)	4 (57%)	0.35	0.51	[0.12, 2.10]
Bone scan	0 (0%)	0 (0%)	1 (12%)	1 (14%)	0.51	*	[*, 7.84]

*Inestimable due to insufficient data.
**p value represents comparison between PO and NP.

TABLE 5: Late effects monitoring.

	PO	Med Onc	Radiation	Ortho	p value*	OR	OR 95% CI
Number of responses	17	10	9	7			
Late effects clinic for complex patients	16 (94%)	4 (40%)	8 (89%)	4 (57%)	0.03	9.56	[1.12, 459.37]
Referral to GP/relevant subspecialists	11 (65%)	8 (80%)	8 (89%)	0 (0%)	1.00	1.14	[0.27, 5.04]
Give written information about health maintenance/lifestyle to patient	8 (47%)	1 (10%)	3 (33%)	0 (0%)	0.04	4.69	[0.97, 27.15]
Give verbal information about health maintenance/lifestyle	9 (53%)	6 (60%)	5 (56%)	1 (14%)	0.76	1.3	[0.33, 5.32]

*p value represents comparison between PO and NP.

modality. Several participants described that the type of surgical intervention was relevant to the disease surveillance strategy (e.g., in the setting of an amputation or the presence of a prosthetic implant (less likely to do MRI)). Additionally, some respondents commented that patients with cutaneous and superficial ESFT could be monitored clinically without primary site imaging. Regarding RS for metastatic disease, POs were more likely than NPs to use CXR for pulmonary surveillance ($p = 0.006$). Some respondents described alternating CXR and CT chest. There were no significant differences identified in the use of FDG-PET scans for metastatic disease, but typically this modality was used as a secondary investigation (i.e., to further investigate suspicious findings on CT). In addition, cumulative radiation exposure factored into the decision process for the RS modality being utilized ($n = 31$, $N = 42$; 74%) (e.g., CXR replacing CTs; the presence of *TP53* mutation; risk stratification with radiation minimization in low risk patients).

4.3. Frequency of Review. Overall, clinicians undertook 3-month follow-up (median) in years 1 and 2 and 6-month follow-up in years 3, 4, and 5, with no differences identified between disciplines. Differences between osteosarcoma and ES were identified in the free text analysis with clinicians described closer monitoring and longer lag time for relapse in ES patients. Others additionally described protocol related differences such as those mandated by COG.

4.4. Treatment Summary. When comparing POs to NPs, written information was more likely to be given to patients for health maintenance (47% versus 11%, $p = 0.037$). POs were also more likely to refer to a late effects clinic for complex patients (94% versus 44%, $p = 0.03$) (Table 5).

4.5. Duration of Surveillance. POs were more likely than NPs to follow up bone sarcoma patients for shorter time periods

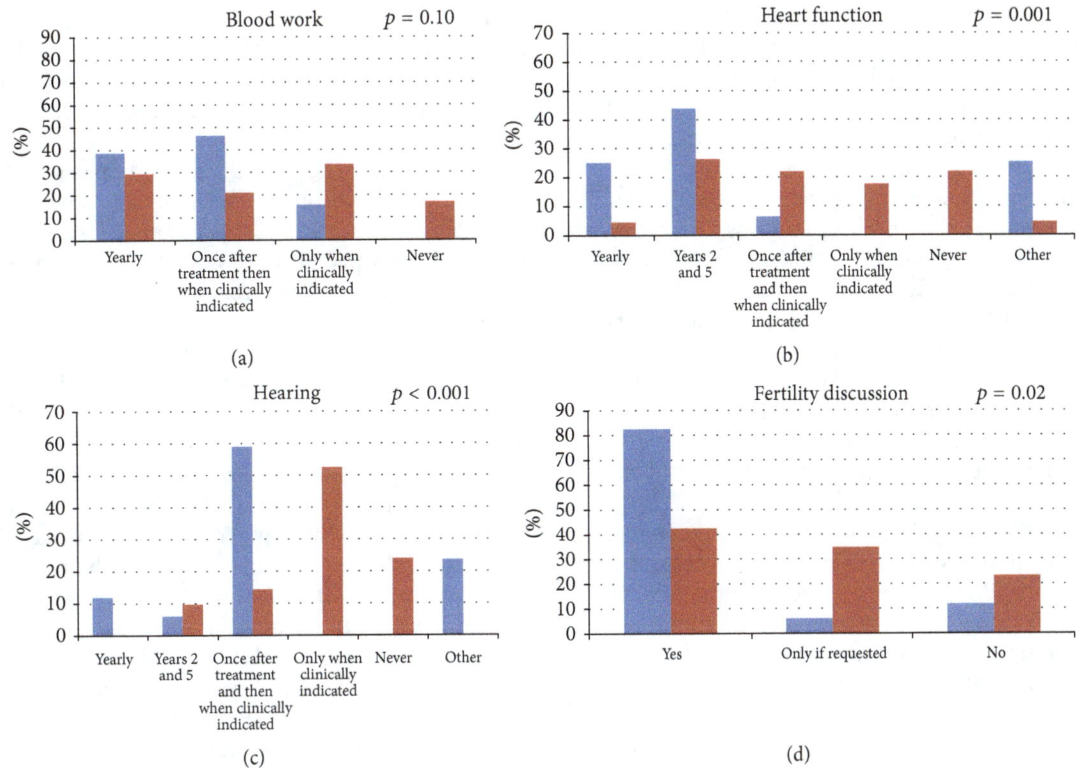

FIGURE 1: Timing of blood work (a), heart function assessment (b), hearing assessment (c), and fertility discussion (d). p values represent comparison between PO (blue) and NP disciplines (red).

(5 years' duration: PO 69%, NP 26%; 10 years' duration: PO 13%, NP 43%; no endpoint: PO 19%, NP 22%; $p = 0.04$).

5. Screening for Late Effects

5.1. Blood Work. No differences were identified in the utilization of blood work with 38% of POs ($n = 5$, $N = 13$) and 29% of NPs ($n = 7$, $N = 24$) drawing blood yearly and 46% of POs ($n = 6$, $N = 13$) and 21% of NPs ($n = 5$, $N = 24$) drawing blood once after treatment and then when clinically indicated (p = NS) (Figure 1(a)). 17% of NPs ($n = 4$, $N = 24$) did not undertake screening blood work. The role of screening blood work conducted by radiation oncologists was described in the context of checking biochemistry if the kidney and/or liver were within the radiotherapy field. Although not specifically asked, some clinicians described undertaking screening urinary cytology for those receiving alkylating agents.

5.2. Cardiotoxicity, Ototoxicity, and Fertility. POs were more likely to have more prescriptive intensity in assessing heart function with multiple heart function assessment occurring in 94% of POs compared with 32% in NPs ($p = 0.001$) (Figure 1(b)). In addition to standard evaluations, clinicians described other factors that influenced the timing of heart scans such as cumulative doxorubicin dose, previous chest irradiation, according to established guidelines (e.g., COG), and in the setting of pregnancy. Similarly, the assessment of ototoxicity was more intensive by POs with 77% assessing hearing function at least once after treatment compared to 24% of NPs ($p < 0.001$) (Figure 1(c)). Two respondents described that ototoxicity screening may occur through external programs and thus surveillance procedures occur outside of sarcoma clinics. Routine fertility discussions were more likely to be conducted by POs (82%) than NPs (42%) ($p = 0.02$) (Figure 1(d)).

5.3. Psychosocial Support. Although the overwhelming majority of respondents describe routinely enquiring about psychosocial aspects of health ($n = 33$, $N = 37$, 89%), a routine formal psychosocial screen was only used in 23% ($n = 6$, $N = 26$). The majority of respondents had the support of allied health (e.g., social worker, physiotherapy, and psychology) and nursing services to assess psychosocial support needs for patients off treatment and manage/refer accordingly ($n = 24$, $N = 31$, 77%).

6. Discussion

Posttreatment surveillance in patients with bone sarcoma aims to detect asymptomatic recurrences and to manage the chronic toxicities associated with primary treatment. However, the rarity of bone sarcoma and limited research in this area have led to significant practice variation amongst Australian clinicians involved in the follow-up of these patients.

Follow-up for bone sarcoma patients serves a number of purposes. The primary aim is to identify asymptomatic recurrences early enough to initiate treatment that will lead to improved outcomes. However, currently it is unclear whether RS is associated with improved outcomes [15–18], and opinion is divided, with only 67% of musculoskeletal tumor surgeons believing that early relapse detection led to improved survival [13]. It is currently unknown whether that belief holds true with nonsurgical clinicians. Nevertheless, in this survey there was wide consensus on the utility of RS and the timing of follow-up was consistent with intervals described by international guidelines [8–10]. Of note, POs were more likely than NPs to follow-up bone sarcoma patients for shorter time periods. However, this may be accounted for by transition of care to adult centers in AYA patients and more frequent referral to dedicated late effects service.

A major concern of intensive DS is the cumulative radiation exposure and corresponding concerns of secondary malignancy [7, 19, 20]. As a result, a general trend has been seen with the use of low dose protocol in children and improved scanning techniques that may result in reduced radiation exposure [8, 21]. Reflecting this, over 70% of respondents altered the timing or modality of RS on the basis of patient concerns, hereditary disposition syndromes, or based on risk stratification approaches. Not unexpectedly, POs were more likely to adopt an RS schedule cognisant of radiation exposure. They were thus more likely to alternate CT chest with CXR in RS for pulmonary metastasis ($p = 0.02$) and less likely to conduct full body CTs in end of treatment response assessments ($p = 0.003$). Given that pulmonary metastasis is the usual site of distant metastatic spread, there is arguably no role for routine whole body CTs. In addition, Australian PO's practice departs from established COG guidelines in that DS had variable inclusion of functional imaging which is recommended by COG. Of note, the only published trial comparing differing RS approaches in bone and soft tissue sarcoma did not demonstrate any differences in outcome with reduced intensity, either in the timing (3 versus 6 months) or in the modality (CXR versus CT) [18]. However, as this study included all extremity sarcomas (including low grade lesions with lower metastatic potential), it is unknown whether exchanging modalities and reducing radiation exposure are acceptable in high grade bone sarcoma where relapse rates are considerably higher. Although not specifically addressed in this survey (but reflected in COG guidelines [8]), the case for routine surveillance using CT chest in ESFT is less compelling. This is because relapses in ESFT are usually multifocal, compared to OS, where surgical salvage alone is likely to be appropriate, making early detection advantageous.

Regarding screening of local disease, previous reports demonstrated a high rate of patient detection of local relapse. In the TOSS trial [18], 90% of local recurrences were identified on the basis of symptoms. This is in keeping with other similar reports showing low rates of asymptomatic radiological detection [16, 17]. Although most clinicians in this survey described conducting RS of the local site without significant variation in modality, the timing/frequency of such undertaking were not explored. The question of whether these tests were conducted for assessing disease relapse or for other reasons such as prosthetic alignment was also not addressed.

In addition to DS, identifying and managing late effects of primary treatment are an important aspect of sarcoma surveillance care. Most of the literature assessing LTFU has stemmed from pediatric survivorship research. This is due to the many decades survivors of pediatric cancers live after intensive treatments and given that these treatments are delivered at an age where critical growth and maturation of organ systems are taking place [22–24]. It was consequently not unexpected to discover variations in practice identified with screening for late effects (with more prescriptive intensity in screening for ototoxicity, cardiotoxicity, and fertility discussions by POs). However, these variations in practice are important, as AYAs may be managed in adult based surveillance programs. They may therefore be treated according to lines of a more elderly cancer population, with limited thought given beyond cure. The potential for late effects is considerable with the Childhood Cancer Survivor Study showing that 62% of survivors of pediatric cancer had at least one chronic condition and 28% had a severe or life-threatening condition at a median of 17.5 years after diagnosis [22]. Thus a unifying late effect surveillance approach, aligned across pediatric, and adult institutions would allow early recognition and intervention thus minimizing the frequency of severe complications [25]. Variation in late effects surveillance may also exist because POs are supported by pediatric based international guidelines, which present exposure and risk-based guidelines for management of late effects [26]. Of note, adult based surveillance sarcoma guidelines such as those from NCCN [9] and ESMO [10] do not expand on specific surveillance in the timing or mechanisms for LTFU screening. This is an important underserved area as late effects are of considerable concern to those in survivorship (e.g., infertility risks [27]) and empowering patients with unified LTFU plans is important for self-care management. Risk stratification and arming low risk patients with treatment summaries/suggested late effects surveillance that can be enacted by local doctors may assist in overcoming practice variation and allow late effects resources to focus on high risk patients. However, even if adult based guidelines were developed targeting late effects screening, it is likely that practice variations would continue. This is due to the lack of uniformity in resource allocation, with subsequent effects on AYA service provision and availability of late effects clinics.

Although this survey identified that 89% of the respondents routinely enquired about psychosocial aspects of health, few undertook systemic psychosocial screening. Given the peak incidence of sarcoma in the AYA years [28], developing systems, such as screening tools, that proactively identify those at increased risk of psychological distress or those who need intervention/assistance is imperative. There are many aspects of a new cancer diagnosis that may be particularly confronting for AYAs. These include premature confrontation with mortality, disruption in the capacity to feel "normal," increased dependency on parents, social life interference, and fertility concerns. Developmentally appropriate targeted support for this age group is therefore required [29, 30]. However, assessing the specific overall quality of life (QOL) specifically in bone sarcoma patients is difficult with significant heterogeneity in patient populations (age, tumor type) and instrumentation used in established QOL literature [31]. Mechanisms for routine systematic screening of AYAs are currently in development [32]. However, with the increasing costs associated with implementing AYA programs and screening tools, it is unclear as to when to implement them, how they should be validated, and how to evaluate their cost-effectiveness.

We acknowledge several limitations in this survey. Firstly, although the number of participants is similar to previous sarcoma surveys [11–13], the corresponding overall response rate of 15% is low. This is driven by the large denominator of nonpracticing clinicians/general oncologists on the ASSG and ANZCHOG database who are likely not involved in sarcoma surveillance. Although we aimed to be overinclusive, the low response rate does raise the potential for nonresponse bias. Counteracting this weakness is that this survey focused exclusively on bone sarcoma clinicians with a focus on looking at variations in practice between POs and NP specialties. In addition, it is unclear as to whether this information is generalizable to clinicians at large, as current practices in Australia may not reflect global clinician practices. Similarly, survey amalgamation of RS questions for EFST/OS and site of disease (e.g., pelvic versus limb) does not allow for variations of practice in subtypes of bone sarcoma. Furthermore, clinicians were not enquired as to whether patients' insurance status had an effect on surveillance preferences. Lastly, given the small numbers of individual subspecialties, comparisons between individual groups and analysis of variation within groups could not be undertaken.

7. Conclusion

In conclusion, despite a relatively small and specialized field, this survey of Australian clinicians has identified significant variation in practice with regard to DS and LTFU for patients with bone sarcoma. A uniform holistic approach is important for patients treated with bone sarcoma as coherent pathways empower patients and families irrespective of age of diagnosis, place of care, or identified clinician. Lack of uniformity puts AYA patients undergoing transition at risk of disengaging. Therefore, confident transition plans are required between pediatric and adult centers. DS requires a sensible, radiation cognizant schedule adopted in line with current international guidelines and appropriate to local health system contexts. The impetus for its development should be generated from pediatric and adult multidisciplinary collaborative efforts and the development of such a standardized guideline should be mindful of the paucity of evidence base supporting practice. Efforts to harmonize DS and LTFU approach between pediatric and adult centers, factoring in available evidence, treatment protocols, cost, and radiation exposure, would allow early late effects recognition and intervention and facilitate improved patient care/transition, data collection, and research.

Disclosure

This work was presented as a poster presentation at Teenage Cancer Trust, December 2016, Edinburgh, Scotland.

Competing Interests

The authors declare that there is no conflict of interests regarding the publication of this paper.

Acknowledgments

The authors are grateful to the clinicians who responded to the survey and to the Australasian Sarcoma Study Group and Australasian and New Zealand Children Oncology Group for distributing the survey.

References

[1] J. Lewin, A. Puri, R. Quek et al., "Management of sarcoma in the asia-pacific region: resource-stratified guidelines," *The Lancet Oncology*, vol. 14, no. 12, pp. e562–e570, 2013.

[2] https://seer.cancer.gov/statfacts/html/bones.html.

[3] Cancer Council Australia Sarcoma Guidelines Working Party, *Clinical Practice Guidelines for the Management of Adult Onset Sarcoma*, Cancer Council Australia, Sydney, Australia, 2014, http://wiki.cancer.org.au/australia/Guidelines:Sarcoma, http://wiki.cancer.org.au/australiawiki/index.php?oldid=138276.

[4] Ø. S. Bruland, H. Høifødt, G. Sæter, S. Smeland, and Ø. Fodstad, "Hematogenous micrometastases in osteosarcoma patients," *Clinical Cancer Research*, vol. 11, no. 13, pp. 4666–4673, 2005.

[5] H. E. Grier, M. D. Krailo, N. J. Tarbell et al., "Addition of ifosfamide and etoposide to standard chemotherapy for Ewing's sarcoma and primitive neuroectodermal tumor of bone," *New England Journal of Medicine*, vol. 348, no. 8, pp. 694–701, 2003.

[6] A. Goel, M. E. L. Christy, K. S. Virgo, W. G. Kraybill, and F. E. Johnson, "Costs of follow-up after potentially curative treatment for extremity soft-tissue sarcoma," *International Journal of Oncology*, vol. 25, no. 2, pp. 429–436, 2004.

[7] A. B. de González, M. Mahesh, K.-P. Kim et al., "Projected cancer risks from computed tomographic scans performed in the United States in 2007," *Archives of Internal Medicine*, vol. 169, no. 22, pp. 2071–2077, 2009.

[8] J. S. Meyer, H. R. Nadel, N. Marina et al., "Imaging guidelines for children with Ewing sarcoma and osteosarcoma: a report from the Children's Oncology Group Bone Tumor Committee," *Pediatric Blood and Cancer*, vol. 51, no. 2, pp. 163–170, 2008.

[9] NCCN Guidelines, Cancer, https://www.nccn.org/professionals/physician_gls/pdf/bone.pdf.

[10] The ESMO/European Sarcoma Network Working Group, "Bone sarcomas: ESMO Clinical Practice Guidelines for diagnosis, treatment and follow-up," *Annals of Oncology*, vol. 25, supplement 3, pp. iii113–iii123, 2014.

[11] A. L. Beitier, K. S. Virgo, F. E. Johnson, J. F. Gibbs, and W. G. Kraybill, "Current follow-up strategies after potentially curative resection of extremity sarcomas: results of a survey of the members of the society of surgical oncology," *Cancer*, vol. 88, no. 4, pp. 777–785, 2000.

[12] C. H. Gerrand, L. J. Billingham, P. J. Woll, and R. J. Grimer, "Follow up after primary treatment of soft tissue sarcoma: A

Survey of Current Practice in The United Kingdom," *Sarcoma*, vol. 2007, Article ID 34128, 6 pages, 2007.

[13] D. D. Greenberg and B. Crawford, "Surveillance strategies for sarcoma: results of a survey of members of the musculoskeletal tumor society," *Sarcoma*, vol. 2016, Article ID 8289509, 5 pages, 2016.

[14] R Core Team, *R: A Language and Environment for Statistical Computing*, R Core Team, 2013.

[15] M. F. Brennan, "Follow-up is valuable and effective: true, true and unrelated?" *Annals of Surgical Oncology*, vol. 7, no. 1, pp. 2–3, 2000.

[16] D. Korholz, J. Verheyen, H. F. Kemperdick, and U. Gobel, "Evaluation of follow-up investigations in osteosarcoma patients: suggestions for an effective follow-up program," *Medical and Pediatric Oncology*, vol. 30, no. 1, pp. 52–58, 1997.

[17] S. Postovsky, M. Barzilai, I. Meller, Y. Kollander, B. Futerman, and M. W. Ben Arush, "Does regular follow-up influence the survival of patients with sarcoma after recurrence? The miri shitrit pediatric oncology department experience," *Journal of Pediatric Hematology/Oncology*, vol. 30, no. 3, pp. 189–195, 2008.

[18] A. Puri, A. Gulia, R. Hawaldar, P. Ranganathan, and R. A. Badwe, "Does intensity of surveillance affect survival after surgery for sarcomas? Results of a randomized noninferiority trial," *Clinical Orthopaedics and Related Research*, vol. 472, no. 5, pp. 1568–1575, 2014.

[19] D. J. Brenner, C. D. Elliston, E. J. Hall, and W. E. Berdon, "Estimated risks of radiation-induced fatal cancer from pediatric CT," *American Journal of Roentgenology*, vol. 176, no. 2, pp. 289–296, 2001.

[20] M. S. Pearce, J. A. Salotti, M. P. Little et al., "Radiation exposure from CT scans in childhood and subsequent risk of leukaemia and brain tumours: a retrospective cohort study," *The Lancet*, vol. 380, no. 9840, pp. 499–505, 2012.

[21] M. K. Kalra, N. Naz, S. M. R. Rizzo, and M. A. Blake, "Computed tomography radiation dose optimization: scanning protocols and clinical applications of automatic exposure control," *Current Problems in Diagnostic Radiology*, vol. 34, no. 5, pp. 171–181, 2005.

[22] K. C. Oeffinger, A. C. Mertens, C. A. Sklar et al., "Chronic health conditions in adult survivors of childhood cancer," *The New England Journal of Medicine*, vol. 355, no. 15, pp. 1572–1582, 2006.

[23] M. M. Hudson, A. C. Mertens, Y. Yasui et al., "Health status of adult long-term survivors of childhood cancer: a report from the childhood cancer survivor study," *Journal of the American Medical Association*, vol. 290, no. 12, pp. 1583–1592, 2003.

[24] K. C. Oeffinger and M. M. Hudson, "Long-term complications following childhood and adolescent cancer: foundations for providing risk-based health care for survivors," *Ca-A Cancer Journal for Clinicians*, vol. 54, no. 4, pp. 208–236, 2004.

[25] R. Skinner, W. H. B. Wallace, and G. A. Levitt, "Long-term follow-up of people who have survived cancer during childhood," *The Lancet Oncology*, vol. 7, pp. 489–498, 2006.

[26] W. Landier, S. Bhatia, D. A. Eshelman et al., "Development of risk-based guidelines for pediatric cancer survivors: the children's oncology group long-term follow-up guidelines from the children's oncology group late effects committee and nursing discipline," *Journal of Clinical Oncology*, vol. 22, no. 24, pp. 4979–4990, 2004.

[27] K. Saito, K. Suzuki, A. Iwasaki, Y. Yumura, and Y. Kubota, "Sperm cryopreservation before cancer chemotherapy helps in the emotional battle against cancer," *Cancer*, vol. 104, no. 3, pp. 521–524, 2005.

[28] K. H. Albritton, "Sarcomas in adolescents and young adults," *Hematology/Oncology Clinics of North America*, vol. 19, no. 3, pp. 527–546, 2005.

[29] B. Zebrack, M. A. Chesler, and S. Kaplan, "To foster healing among adolescents and young adults with cancer: what helps? what hurts?" *Supportive Care in Cancer*, vol. 18, pp. 131–135, 2010.

[30] C. J. Stava, A. Lopez, and R. Vassilopoulou-Sellin, "Health profiles of younger and older breast cancer survivors," *Cancer*, vol. 107, no. 8, pp. 1752–1759, 2006.

[31] J. Stokke, L. Sung, A. Gupta, A. Lindberg, and A. R. Rosenberg, "Systematic review and meta-analysis of objective and subjective quality of life among pediatric, adolescent, and young adult bone tumor survivors," *Pediatric Blood and Cancer*, vol. 62, no. 9, pp. 1616–1629, 2015.

[32] S. Palmer, P. Patterson, and K. Thompson, "A national approach to improving adolescent and young adult (AYA) oncology psychosocial care: the development of AYA-specific psychosocial assessment and care tools," *Palliative and Supportive Care*, vol. 12, no. 3, pp. 183–188, 2014.

28

Biomechanical Analysis of a Novel Acetabulum Reconstruction Technique with Acetabulum Reconstruction Cage and Threaded Rods after Type II Pelvic Resections

Vivek Ajit Singh,[1] Hassan Elbahri,[2] and Rukmanikanthan Shanmugam[1]

[1]*Department of Orthopaedic Surgery, University of Malaya Medical Centre, 59100 Kuala Lumpur, Malaysia*
[2]*Khartoum Teaching Hospital, 11111 Khartoum, Sudan*

Correspondence should be addressed to Vivek Ajit Singh; drvivek69@gmail.com

Academic Editor: Eugenie S. Kleinerman

Background. Periacetabular resections with reconstruction has high rates of complications due to the complexity of the reconstruction. We have improvised a novel technique of reconstruction for type II and type II + III pelvic resections with the use of a commercially available acetabulum reconstruction cage (gap II, Stryker) and threaded rods. *Objectives.* The aim of our study is to determine the biomechanical strength of our reconstruction compared to the traditional cemented total hip replacement (THR) designs in normal acetabulum and establish its mode of failure. *Methods.* Five sets of hemipelvises were biomechanically tested (Instron® 3848, MA, USA). These constructs were subjected to cyclic loading and load to failure. *Results.* The reconstructed acetabulum was stiffer and required a higher load to failure compared to the intact pelvis with a standard THR. The mean stiffness of the reconstructed pelvis was 1738.6 ± 200.3 Nmm^{-1} compared to the intact pelvis, which was 911.4 ± 172.7 Nmm^{-1} (P value = 0.01). The mean load to failure for the standard acetabular cup construct was 3297.3 ± 117.7 N while that of the reconstructed pelvis with the acetabulum cage and threaded rods was 4863.8 ± 7.0 N. *Conclusion.* Reconstruction of the pelvis with an acetabular reconstruction cage and threaded rods is a biomechanical viable option.

1. Introduction

Primary sarcomas of the pelvis account for 10% to 15% of primary bone tumours and pelvis is considered the third most common site for metastasis. Enneking and Dunham had classified pelvic resection depending on the site of the tumour. Tumour involving ilium is classified as type I, tumours involving the periacetabular area as type II, and pubis as type III [1]. Periacetabular bone tumours are considered the most challenging site of all pelvic tumours to treat as they involve the hip joint. Therefore, it is difficult to achieve a good oncological and functional outcome. Periacetabular resections are associated with a high incidence of complications, mainly infection and reconstruction failure [2–4]. This is usually due to the difficulty of reconstruction of the acetabulum cup and the local forces acting on this anatomical region. Type II pelvic resection with wide margin and reconstruction of the soft tissue and bony defect to restore weight bearing along anatomic axes is considered the goal standard management of periacetabular tumours [5, 6]. Many options are available for reconstruction of the bony defect after resections. These include autograft, allograft, allograft composite, and endoprosthesis [7–9]. Endoprostheses are developed to give the most durable and least complicated construct that can cope with the complex anatomy and biomechanical demands of the hip joint [10]. There are various custom-made endoprosthesis available but these are expensive and their long term results are not encouraging. They are associated with high rate of morbidity, infection, and failures [11]. Therefore, we have devised our own method of reconstruction for the acetabular defect using commercially available acetabular reconstruction cage (gap II acetabular cage; Stryker Howmedica), threaded rods, and cemented flanged acetabular cup. We believe that our method of reconstruction for periacetabular tumours might offer a cheaper and easily available alternative compared to other forms of endoprosthesis reconstruction.

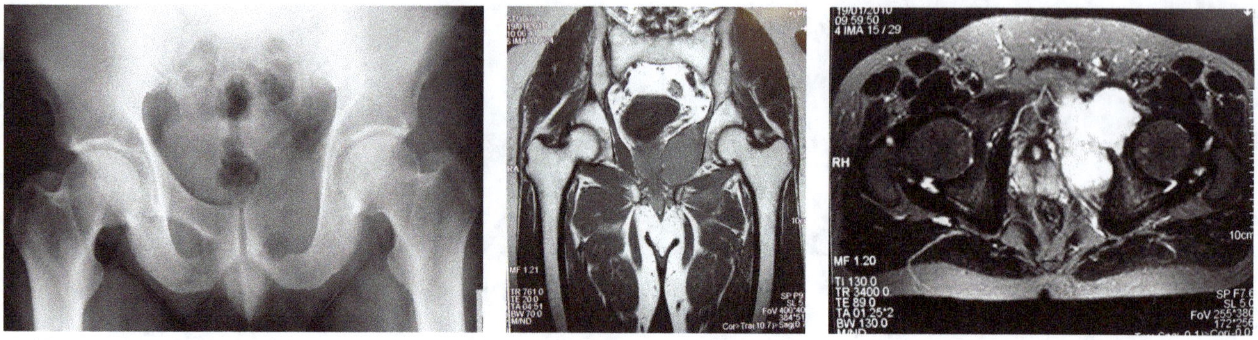

FIGURE 1: Grade 2 Chondrosarcoma arising from the left superior pubic rami extending into the medial wall of the acetabulum.

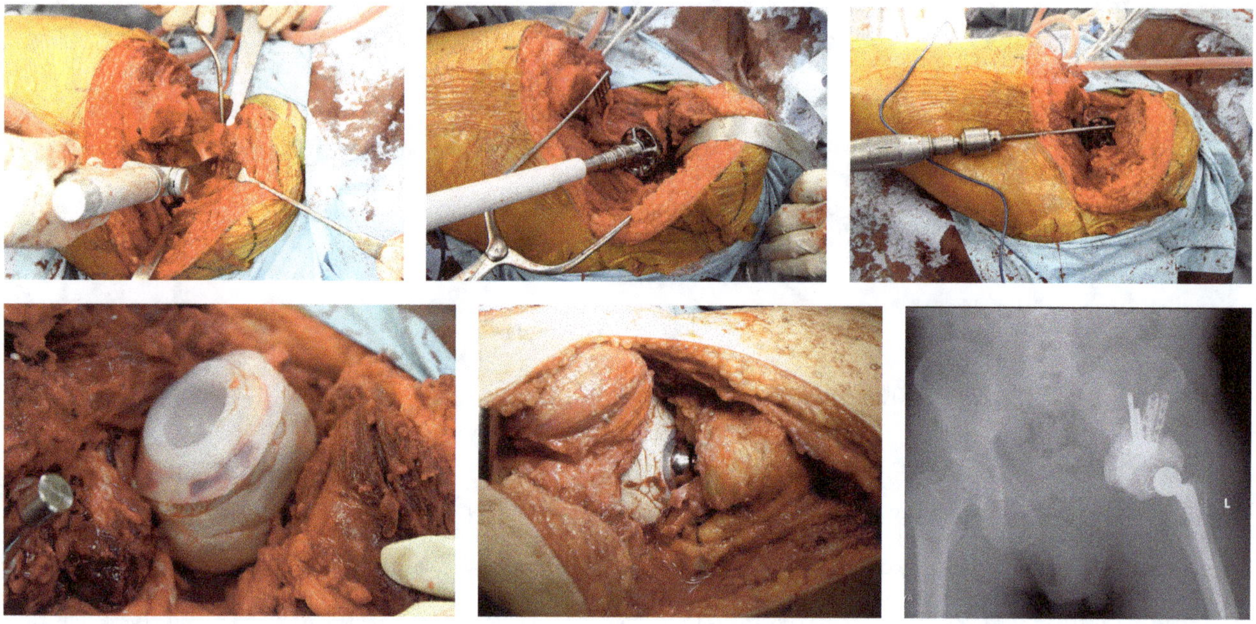

FIGURE 2: Showing the type II + III resection with acetabulum reconstruction with a acetabulum reconstruction cage and threaded rods.

The example of this form of reconstruction is shown in Figures 1 and 2. This is a 42-year-old gentleman who presented with Chondrosarcoma grade 2 of the left superior pubic rami extending to the medial wall of the acetabulum. He underwent a wide resection and reconstruction with an acetabulum reconstruction cage and threaded rods.

In order to determine the biomechanical strength of this construct, we compared the biomechanical properties of this construct to the standard cemented acetabular component of the total hip replacement.

2. Objective

The objective is as follows:

(i) To determine the biomechanical strength of acetabulum reconstruction cage and threaded rods reconstruction after a combined type II + III pelvic resection.

(ii) To compare the strength of the acetabular reconstruction using acetabulum reconstruction cage and threaded rods in type II and III pelvic resection against the traditional cemented cup in a normal acetabulum.

(iii) To determine the mode of failure of the acetabular reconstruction cage and threaded rods reconstruction designs.

3. Materials and Methods

Mechanical testing comparing intact pelvis implanted with the standard acetabular cup with those using the modified acetabular reconstruction cage and threaded rods was performed using solid foam bone models of large male full pelvis sourced from SAWBONES. This was to ensure a uniform material property to enable the fixation technique to be assessed with minimal bias. A total of five whole pelvises were used. Five hemipelvises were implanted with a standard acetabular cup (flanged cemented cup from Stryker Howmedica, Group A) according to the manufacturers recommended technique. And in the remaining five,

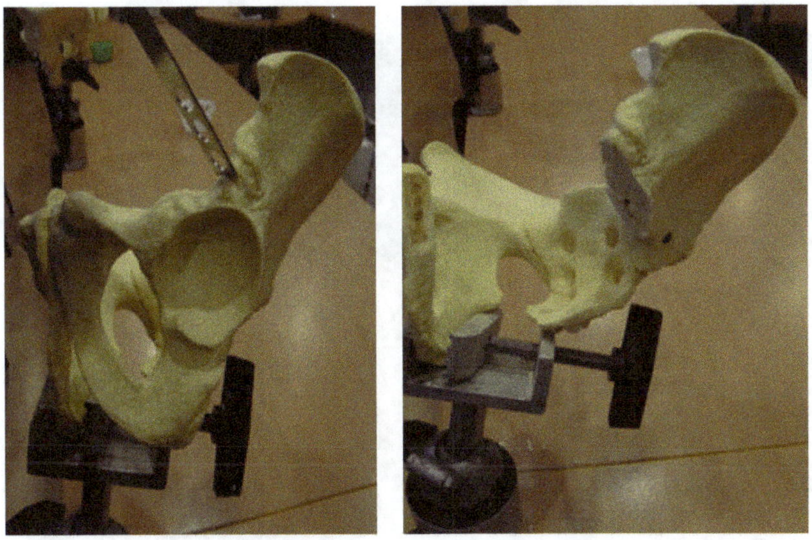

FIGURE 3: Resection of the pelvis at the level of the supra-acetabulum up to the symphysis pubis to mimic a type II + III pelvic resection.

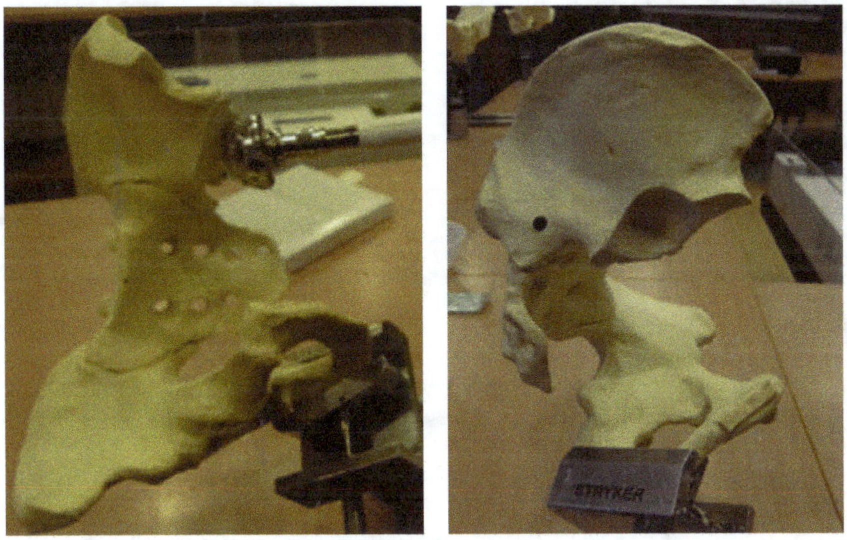

FIGURE 4: The reaming of the inferior border of the remnant iliac bone to create an indentation for better placement of the gap 2 acetabulum cage.

the acetabulum including the pubic bone was resected to simulate a combined type II + III pelvic resection (Figure 3). The inferior border of the remnant ilium is then reamed with the standard acetabulum reamers to create a curve indentation for better placement of the acetabular cage (Figure 4). A gap II acetabular reconstruction cage from Stryker Howmedica is then fitted to the remnant ilium and secured with long titanium screws (Figure 5) in the desired position (45 degrees' inclination and 15 degrees' anteversion) and construct is reinforced with 3 threaded rods. The rods are inserted in the thickest part of the pelvis, consisting of anterior and posterior borders of the ilium towards the anterior and posterior iliac spines and the centre in line with the iliac tubercle (Figure 6). This is known as Group B.

For the biomechanical testing, to ensure uniform loading conditions, the pelvis was positioned on a custom-made jig that would allow the acetabular cup to be placed in the same angle in relation to the femoral stem with a metal head. This was achieved by placing the Anterior Superior Iliac Spine (ASIS) and the anterior part of the pubic tubercle in the same plane and the posterior medial pubic tubercle and the sacroiliac joint surface on another plane which are at right angles to each other. By positioning it in this position, each intact pelvis was able to be placed within the jig and thus the femoral head component in the same position which represents the anatomical position in the natural hip.

The reconstructed specimens (Group B) were positioned in the similar position but since the pubic tubercle is absent,

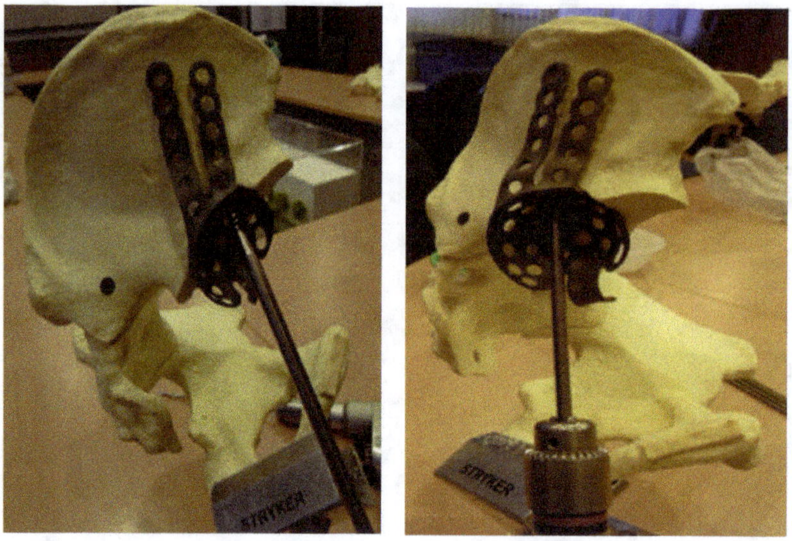

Figure 5: Insertion of long titanium screws and threaded rods to secure the construct.

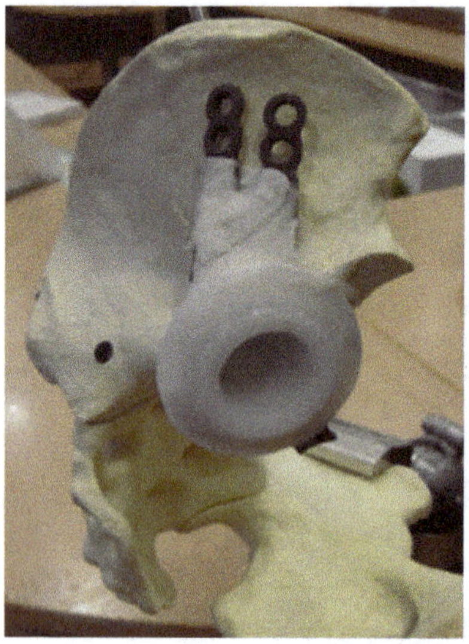

Figure 6: The end product of the reconstruction with a standard flanged cup cemented into the reconstructed acetabulum cage.

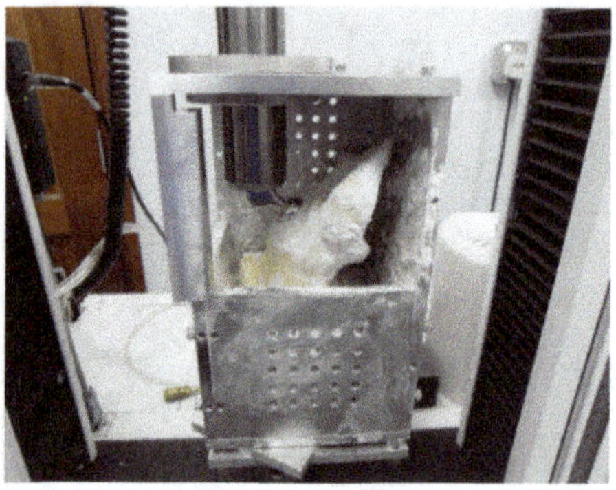

Figure 7: Placement of the test specimen in the test jig which is secured by plaster of Paris in an anatomical position.

the angle of the acetabular rim in relation to the horizontal and the two vertical planes was measured based on the standard (Group A) specimens thus ensuring a comparable positioning of the reconstructed specimens. This ensured that the force vectors acting on the acetabular cup are consistent for all specimens. The jig used is shown in Figure 7. The specimens were stabilised in the jig by using plaster of Paris.

Loading was done using a material testing machine (Instron® 3848, MA, USA) with a 5 kN load cell. A preload of 10 N was applied to take up the slack on the jigs and set the femoral head component well into the acetabulum. A fast ramp of 2000 N was applied with a ramp speed of 0.1 mm/sec. Once 2000 N was reached, load was cycled between 1800 N and 2000 N at a frequency of 1 Hz for 10 cycles. Following this, the 1800 N was held for 10 secs and the load subsequently increased by 100 N and cycled another 10 times. This cycle pattern was repeated until failure. A sample of the overall loading regime is as shown in Figure 8. And a full cycle pattern is shown in Figure 9. Loading was done till failure which was defined as either fracture of the acetabulum or the bony pelvis or displacement of the ramp by more than 20 mm.

The initial ramp was used to calculate the stiffness of the construct which was calculated from the slope of the linear portion of the load displacement curve. The maximum load to failure was also measured for each sample. Data analysis and statistical calculations were done using Microsoft Excel 2010. With the high degree of blocking that was done considering the use of standardised foam models with relatively consistent density and a standardised test setup, t-test was done to test for significance using the same software.

4. Results

A total of five full male pelvis sawbones were used. The acetabular reconstruction cage and threaded rods novel

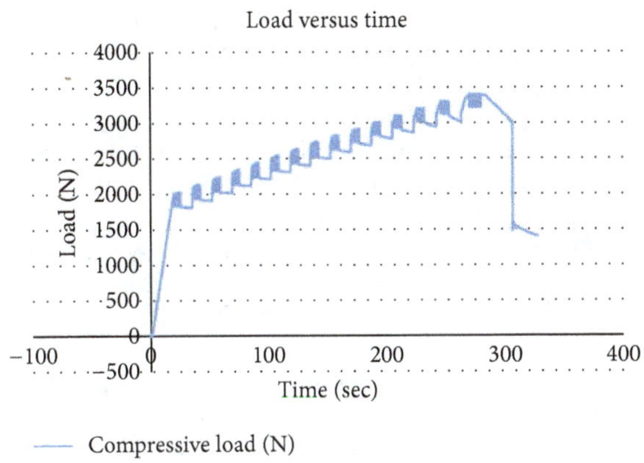

FIGURE 8: The loading regime for the test specimens.

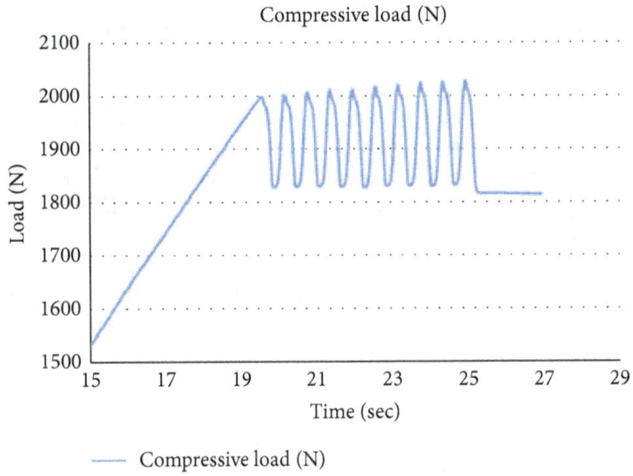

FIGURE 9: Full loading pattern of the test specimen.

reconstruction technique was carried out on half of five hemipelvises and a standard acetabular replacement was applied on the rest of the five hemipelvis sawbones. The reconstructed acetabulum (Group B) was generally stiffer and needed a higher load to failure compared to the intact pelvis with a standard total hip replacement. The mean stiffness of the reconstructed pelvis was 1738.6 ± 200.3 Nmm^{-1} compared to the intact pelvis (Group A) which was 911.4 ± 172.7 Nmm^{-1} (Figure 10). This was statistically significant with a P value of 0.01. The mean load to failure for the standard acetabular cup construct was 3297.3 ± 117.7 N while that of the reconstructed pelvis was 4863.8 ± 7.0 N.

All normal pelvis failed by fracture through the iliac bone just above the cemented acetabular cup. Due to the limitation of the testing machine used, none of the reconstructed pelvises could be loaded to failure as the maximum load that can be applied by the machine was reached before failure occurred (all operated specimens were loaded till about 4900 N without failure).

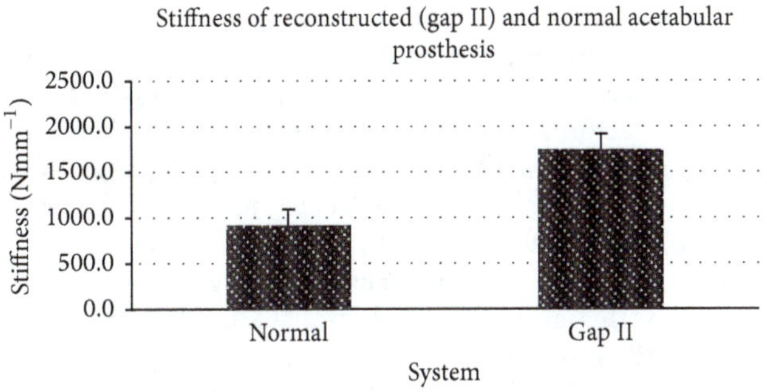

FIGURE 10: Bar graph showing the stiffness of the reconstructed pelvic and normal acetabular prosthesis.

5. Discussion

The common sarcomas involving the pelvis are Chondrosarcoma, Ewing's sarcoma, and osteosarcoma [12–14]. These tumours generally present late especially if they are located within the inner table of the pelvis and can grow up to a significant size before becoming clinically apparent [15].

The management of these tumours has always been challenging especially when it involves the pelvis. These surgeries are technically demanding due to the complex anatomy of the pelvis, in particular the acetabulum and hip joint (periacetabulum region) [2, 4, 16–18]. The goals of oncology surgery are the following: first is to get total clearance of the tumour with clear margins and second is to reconstruct the defect to enable best possible function with minimal functional deficit.

In the past decade, these tumours were managed with hindquarter amputations that gave good surgical clearance but poor functional outcome [4, 19, 20]. With advancements in imaging, adjuvant therapy, surgical planning using image fusion and navigation, better surgical techniques, and implant design, limb salvage surgery is possible in these cases [21–27].

Ennenking and Dunham [1] classified pelvic resections according to different regions centred around the acetabulum. In type II and type II + III resections, the acetabulum is removed, therefore, directly affecting the hip joint. Reconstruction options around the acetabulum generally involve fusion of the hip or recreating a new artificial hip joint. Reconstruction techniques without the use of prosthesis include iliofemoral arthrodesis or pseudarthrosis, ischiofemoral arthrodesis, massive allograft, and autoclaved autograft [27]. The common pelvic prosthesis used is the saddle prosthesis [2, 3, 25, 26] but it is associated with a high complication rate. There are numerous other prostheses that have been used and majority of them are custom-made [11, 16, 21, 23, 24, 27]. The Birmingham group recently also reported encouraging results with the use of an ice cream cone prosthesis [8]. Gou from China reported his experience with the use of their own version of a modular pelvic prosthesis that can be used off the shelf without customization [28, 29].

These prostheses are expensive and the majority are custom-made; therefore it takes time (a few weeks) for the product to be ordered, manufactured, shifted, and available for surgery. Sometimes during the wait, the preordered prosthesis is no longer suitable due to tumour progression. Furthermore, as they are custom-made, they are less forgiving to surgical errors made during tumour resections. Hence, we needed a cheaper and a surgical more forgiving alternative that suited our local needs. We decided to use an acetabular reconstruction cage, fortified by insertion of threaded rods into the remaining ilium bone and fixed together with bone cement. As this is a commercially available implant, the cost is much lower compared to a custom-made or a modular pelvic prosthesis. And it allowed us flexibility in terms of tumour progression and additional bone resection intraoperatively.

In order to determine the strength of this new construct, we decided to put it through some biomechanical testing. We compared the reconstructed pelvis to an acetabulum cup replacement in an intact pelvis. We found that the reconstructed pelvis with the acetabular cup was stiffer and required a bigger load to fail compared to a standard acetabulum cup replacement on an intact pelvis.

However, this is a cement bone construct and there is no avenue for bone in growth. Therefore, the long term survivorship of this construct is questionable as compared to other forms of implants that allow osteointegration. Furthermore, the increased stiffness of this construct might predispose this implant to long term fatigue failure especially at the bone cement interface.

Limitation of this study is that we used sawbones to compare the biomechanical strength of each construct. We will require a follow-up study using cadaveric pelvic bones which will give better representation of the biomechanical strength of the construct.

6. Conclusion

Acetabulum reconstruction with an acetabulum reconstruction cage and threaded rods after a type II or a type II + III resection is a biomechanically feasible option. The is a cheaper alternative and allows resection flexibility compared to other custom-made pelvic prostheses.

Competing Interests

The authors declare that there are no competing interests regarding the publication of this paper.

References

[1] W. F. Enneking and W. K. Dunham, "Resection and reconstruction for primary neoplasms involving the innominate bone," *The Journal of Bone & Joint Surgery—American Volume*, vol. 60, no. 6, pp. 731–746, 1978.

[2] A. J. Aboulafia, R. Buch, J. Mathews, W. Li, and M. M. Malawer, "Reconstruction using the saddle prosthesis following excision of primary and metastatic periacetabular tumors," *Clinical Orthopaedics and Related Research*, vol. 314, pp. 203–213, 1995.

[3] F. Aljassir, G. P. Beadel, R. E. Turcotte et al., "Outcome after pelvic sarcoma resection reconstructed with saddle prosthesis," *Clinical Orthopaedics and Related Research*, no. 438, pp. 36–41, 2005.

[4] M. Campanacci and R. Capanna, "Pelvic resections: the Rizzoli Institute experience," *Orthopedic Clinics of North America*, vol. 22, no. 1, pp. 65–86, 1991.

[5] L. A. Beck, M. J. Einertson, M. H. Winemiller, R. W. DePompolo, K. M. Hoppe, and F. F. Sim, "Functional outcomes and quality of life after tumor-related hemipelvectomy," *Physical Therapy*, vol. 88, no. 8, pp. 916–927, 2008.

[6] A. Hillmann, C. Hoffman, G. Gosheger, R. Rödl, W. Winkelmann, and T. Ozaki, "Tumors of the pelvis: complications after reconstruction," *Archives of Orthopaedic and Trauma Surgery*, vol. 123, no. 7, pp. 340–344, 2003.

[7] K. D. Harrington, "The use of hemipelvic allografts or autoclaved grafts for reconstruction after wide resections of malignant tumors of the pelvis," *The Journal of Bone & Joint Surgery—American Volume*, vol. 74, no. 3, pp. 331–341, 1992.

[8] N. E. Fisher, J. T. Patton, R. J. Grimer et al., "Ice-cream cone reconstruction of the pelvis: a new type of pelvic replacement. Early results," *The Journal of Bone & Joint Surgery—British Volume*, vol. 93, no. 5, pp. 684–688, 2011.

[9] E. Nieder, R. A. Elson, E. Engelbrecht, M. R. Kasselt, A. Keller, and K. Steinbrink, "The saddle prosthesis for salvage of the destroyed acetabulum," *Journal of Bone and Joint Surgery—Series B*, vol. 72, no. 6, pp. 1014–1022, 1990.

[10] A. J. S. Renard, R. P. H. Veth, H. W. B. Schreuder et al., "The saddle prosthesis in pelvic primary and secondary musculoskeletal tumors: functional results at several postoperative intervals," *Archives of Orthopaedic and Trauma Surgery*, vol. 120, no. 3-4, pp. 188–194, 2000.

[11] P. K. Jaiswal, W. J. S. Aston, R. J. Grimer et al., "Peri-acetabular resection and endoprosthetic reconstruction for tumours of the acetabulum," *The Journal of Bone & Joint Surgery—British Volume*, vol. 90, no. 9, pp. 1222–1227, 2008.

[12] A. J. Aboulafia and M. M. Malawer, "Surgical management of pelvic and extremity osteosarcoma," *Cancer*, vol. 71, no. 10, pp. 3358–3366, 1993.

[13] M. I. O'Connor, "Malignant pelvic tumors: limb-sparing resection and reconstruction," *Seminars in Surgical Oncology*, vol. 13, no. 1, pp. 49–54, 1997.

[14] K.-H. Shin, B. T. Rougraff, and M. A. Simon, "Oncologic outcomes of primary bone sarcomas of the pelvis," *Clinical Orthopaedics and Related Research*, no. 304, pp. 207–217, 1994.

[15] L. D. Wurtz, T. D. Peabody, and M. A. Simon, "Delay in the diagnosis and treatment of primary bone sarcoma of the pelvis," *The Journal of Bone & Joint Surgery—American Volume*, vol. 81, no. 3, pp. 317–325, 1999.

[16] A. Abudu, R. J. Grimer, S. R. Cannon, S. R. Carter, and R. S. Sneath, "Reconstruction of the hemipelvis after the excision of malignant tumours. Complications and functional outcome of prostheses," *The Journal of Bone & Joint Surgery—British Volume*, vol. 79, no. 5, pp. 773–779, 1997.

[17] F. R. Eilber, J. J. Eckardt, and T. G. Grant, "Resection of malignant bone tumors of the pelvis: evaluation of local recurrence, survival and function," in *Limb Salvage in Musculoskeletal Oncology*, W. F. Enneking, Ed., pp. 136–141, Churchill Livingstone, New York, NY, USA, 1987.

[18] I. Han, Y. M. Lee, H. S. Cho, J. H. Oh, S. H. Lee, and H.-S. Kim, "Outcome after surgical treatment of pelvic sarcomas," *Clinics in Orthopedic Surgery*, vol. 2, no. 3, pp. 160–166, 2010.

[19] S. R. Carter, D. M. Eastwood, R. J. Grimer, and R. S. Sneath, "Hindquarter amputation for tumours of the musculoskeletal system," *The Journal of Bone & Joint Surgery—British Volume*, vol. 72, no. 3, pp. 490–493, 1990.

[20] R. J. Grimer, C. R. Chandrasekar, S. R. Carter, A. Abudu, R. M. Tillman, and L. Jeys, "Hindquarter amputation: is it still needed and what are the outcomes?" *The Journal of Bone & Joint Surgery—British Volume*, vol. 95, no. 1, pp. 127–131, 2013.

[21] L. R. Menendez, E. R. Ahlmann, Y. Falkinstein, and D. C. Allison, "Periacetabular reconstruction with a new endoprosthesis," *Clinical Orthopaedics and Related Research*, vol. 467, no. 11, pp. 2831–2837, 2009.

[22] L. M. Jeys, A. Kulkarni, R. J. Grimer, S. R. Carter, R. M. Tillman, and A. Abudu, "Endoprosthetic reconstruction for the treatment of musculoskeletal tumors of the appendicular skeleton and pelvis," *The Journal of Bone & Joint Surgery—American Volume*, vol. 90, no. 6, pp. 1265–1271, 2008.

[23] Y. Falkinstein, E. R. Ahlmann, and L. R. Menendez, "Reconstruction of type II pelvic resection with a new peri-acetabular reconstruction endoprosthesis," *The Journal of Bone & Joint Surgery—British Volume*, vol. 90, no. 3, pp. 371–376, 2008.

[24] K.-C. Wong, S. M. Kumta, K.-H. Chiu et al., "Computer assisted pelvic tumor resection and reconstruction with a custom-made prosthesis using an innovative adaptation and its validation," *Computer Aided Surgery*, vol. 12, no. 4, pp. 225–232, 2007.

[25] Y. Kitagawa, E. T. Ek, and P. F. Choong, "Pelvic reconstruction using saddle prosthesis following limb salvage operation for periacetabular tumour," *Journal of Orthopaedic Surgery (Hong Kong)*, vol. 14, no. 2, pp. 155–162, 2006.

[26] R. Hugate Jr. and F. H. Sim, "Pelvic reconstruction techniques," *Orthopedic Clinics of North America*, vol. 37, no. 1, pp. 85–97, 2006.

[27] R. Hugate Jr. and F. H. Sim, "Pelvic reconstruction techniques," *Orthopedic Clinics of North America*, vol. 37, no. 1, pp. 85–97, 2006.

[28] W. Guo, D. Li, X. Tang, Y. Yang, and T. Ji, "Reconstruction with modular hemipelvic prostheses for periacetabular tumor," *Clinical Orthopaedics and Related Research*, no. 461, pp. 180–188, 2007.

[29] T. Ji, W. Guo, R. L. Yang, X. D. Tang, and Y. F. Wang, "Modular hemipelvic endoprosthesis reconstruction-experience in 100 patients with mid-term follow-up results," *European Journal of Surgical Oncology*, vol. 39, no. 1, pp. 53–60, 2013.

29

High-Dose Ifosfamide Chemotherapy in a Series of Patients Affected by Myxoid Liposarcoma

Vittoria Colia,[1] Elena Fumagalli,[1] Salvatore Provenzano,[1] Rossella Bertulli,[1] Silvia Stacchiotti,[1] Carlo Morosi,[2] Paola Collini,[3] Alessandro Gronchi,[4] Paolo G. Casali,[1,5] and Roberta Sanfilippo[1]

[1]*Medical Oncology Unit 2, Medical Oncology Department, Fondazione IRCCS Istituto Nazionale dei Tumori, Milan, Italy*
[2]*Department of Radiology, Fondazione IRCCS Istituto Nazionale dei Tumori, Milan, Italy*
[3]*Department of Diagnostic Pathology and Laboratory Medicine, Fondazione IRCCS Istituto Nazionale dei Tumori, Milan, Italy*
[4]*Department of Surgery, Fondazione IRCCS Istituto Nazionale dei Tumori, Milan, Italy*
[5]*Oncology and Haemato-Oncology Department, University of Milan, Milan, Italy*

Correspondence should be addressed to Vittoria Colia; vittoriacolia@outlook.com

Academic Editor: Quincy Chu

Background. To report on the activity of high-dose prolonged-infusion ifosfamide (HDIFX) chemotherapy in a retrospective series of patients affected by myxoid liposarcoma treated at Fondazione IRCCS Istituto Nazionale dei Tumori in Milan, Italy. *Patients and Methods.* Patients with an advanced myxoid liposarcoma treated with HDIFX (14 g/sqm, i.v., prolonged infusion of 14 days every 28 days) as a single agent between May 2002 and April 2017 were retrospectively reviewed. All pathologic diagnoses were centrally reviewed and molecularly confirmed. Response was evaluated by RECIST, and survival functions were computed by the Kaplan-Meier method. *Results.* Eleven patients with advanced myxoid liposarcoma were treated with HDIFX (male/female = 9/2, median age 33 years, range 31–75). Among these, 1/11 received HDIFX in first line, 5/11 in second line, 3/11 in third line, and 2/11 in fourth line for a median course number of 3 (range 2–7). No RECIST objective responses were observed. Overall median progression-free survival was 1,9 months. Median overall survival was 37 months. At a median follow-up of 115 months, 1 patient is alive. *Conclusions.* In this series of patients affected by advanced myxoid liposarcoma, chemotherapy with HDIFX was essentially inactive.

1. Introduction

Liposarcoma is the most common histological subtype among soft tissue sarcomas. Specifically, myxoid/round cell liposarcoma is the second of the three liposarcoma subtypes, accounting for 30% of liposarcoma cases. Myxoid/round cell liposarcoma typically occurs around the fifth decade (range 26–81 years) at any site of the body, mainly in the lower extremities [1–4].

The diagnosis is supported by the detection of the characteristic chromosomal recurrent translocation, namely, t(12; 16)(q13; p11), which results in the aberrant fusion gene FUS-CHOP/DDIT3 [5]. According to the most recent WHO classification, myxoid liposarcomas can be morphologically divided into high and low grade [3]. Standard treatment for localized disease is surgery alone or in combination with radiotherapy, while medical treatment may be offered in selected cases and is often the main choice in the advanced setting [6–9]. Myxoid liposarcomas are known as being particularly sensitive to chemotherapy compared with other soft tissue sarcomas [8–10], in particular to anthracycline-based combinations and trabectedin. In the whole group of advanced soft tissue sarcomas, first-line combination of anthracycline and ifosfamide provides response rates around 20–40%. It increases to 65% in myxoid liposarcoma [8, 11, 12]. On the other side, the expected response rate of myxoid liposarcoma to trabectedin is 50% [13–18], with a mechanism of action which is apparently specific inasmuch as implying an effect of the drug on the binding of the fusion transcript to target genes [16–18]. Recently, another marine-derived drug, eribulin, was shown to be effective in metastatic adipocytic sarcomas, with a significant improvement in overall survival which led to its approval by FDA and EMA [19–21]. However, its activity in myxoid liposarcoma compared to pleomorphic and well-differentiated/dedifferentiated liposarcoma is still not defined. No other agents commonly used for treatment of advanced soft tissue sarcoma (e.g., gemcitabine, dacarbazine, and pazopanib) have been demonstrated to be active in myxoid liposarcoma [2].

High-dose prolonged-infusion ifosfamide (HDIFX) is known to be active in soft tissue sarcoma patients, even in those previously treated with standard-dose ifosfamide [2, 22–24]. A peculiar activity has been demonstrated in dedifferentiated liposarcoma, especially with a high malignancy grade component [10]. By contrast, no data are reported so far on the activity of high-dose ifosfamide in myxoid liposarcoma and no prospective neither retrospective studies focusing on this drug in the disease are available.

The aim of this retrospective analysis was to review all patients affected by advanced myxoid liposarcoma treated with high-dose prolonged-infusion ifosfamide at our Institution.

2. Materials and Methods

All patients affected by advanced myxoid liposarcoma, consecutively treated with HDIFX chemotherapy between May 2002 and April 2017 at Fondazione IRCCS Istituto Nazionale dei Tumori, Milan, Italy, were retrospectively identified. Pathological diagnosis was centrally reviewed by expert pathologists in all the cases, following the most recent updated criteria. Data regarding clinical and histopathological characteristics, staging, surgical and systemic treatment, and survival were collected. The clinical records were reviewed and collected in one institutional database and a descriptive analysis was performed.

High-dose ifosfamide was administered as a single agent, at the daily dose of 1 g/sqm (total dose of 14 g/sqm per cycle), as a 14-day continuous infusion with the same dose of MESNA every 4 weeks, through external portable infusion devices (elastomeric pumps) each providing a 7-day infusion, so that 2 pumps were used in each cycle. The infusion was stopped with no additional MESNA after day 14. No additional hydration was foreseen and only oral hydration with 1.5 L/day was recommended. When required, antiemetic prophylaxis was based on oral ondansetron, or dexamethasone, or metoclopramide. No granulocyte growth factors were administered. The treatment was continued until disease progression, serious adverse events, medical decision, or patient refusal. Data on chemotherapy tolerability and adverse effects were reviewed.

Treatment follow-up investigations included a whole-body computed tomography scan (CT), a magnetic resonance (MRI), or a CT of the primary site at baseline and then were generally repeated after the first two courses of chemotherapy and then every 2-3 months. Response Evaluation Criteria in Solid Tumours (RECIST) were used to assess response to chemotherapy [25].

This retrospective analysis was approved by the Institutional Ethics Committee.

2.1. Statistical Analysis. Progression-free survival (PFS) and overall survival (OS) were estimated with Kaplan-Meier method [26]. Progression-free survival death and progressive disease according to RECIST were considered as failures, and death due to any cause was failure for OS. Patients alive were censored at the time of the last contact.

3. Results

Within the study period, 11 patients affected by advanced myxoid liposarcoma treated with HDIFX were identified.

Patient characteristics are summarized in Table 1. Male patients were prevalent (male/female 9/2); median age at the time of the treatment was 33 (range 31–75). Median number of ifosfamide cycles per patient was 3 (range 2–7). Among these, 1/11 received HDIFX in first line, 5/11 in second line, 3/11 in third line, and 2/11 in fourth line.

All patients had previously been treated with anthracycline ± ifosfamide in adjuvant or advanced setting. Among these, 7/11 patients were treated with epirubicin plus ifosfamide in the adjuvant setting and 4/11 as first-line treatment for advanced disease with 1/4 complete response (CR), 2/4 for partial response (PR), and 1/4 for stable disease (SD). In the latter, median progression-free survival was 16.5 months (range 6–21), with the only patient with SD experiencing a PFS shorter than 1 year. Three/11 patients were pretreated with trabectedin as well, with 2 PR and 1 SD. All patients had metastatic disease when starting HDIFX, with a median of 2 sites involved (range: 1–3); among these, the lung was the most common involved site (8/11, 73%), followed by the abdominal cavity (7/11, 64%), the bone (1/11, 9%), and the soft tissues (1/11, 9%). Four patients (36%) had, in addition, a local relapse.

All patients treated with HDIFX were evaluable for response. The best response was PD in 7/11 (36%) and SD in 4/11 (14%) with no PR or CR (Figure 1). Treatment was withdrawn because of progressive disease in all cases. No febrile neutropenia and renal failure were observed, as well as no toxic deaths or any other unexpected serious adverse events.

After a median follow-up of 115 months, OS was 37 months (Figure 2), with 10 patients dead and 1 patient alive at the time of this analysis. Median PFS was 1,9 months (Figure 3).

4. Discussion

In this small retrospective case-series of 11 patients with progressing advanced myxoid liposarcoma treated with chemotherapy on a 14-year span, no responses to continuous infusion high-dose ifosfamide were observed. Median PFS was 1,9 months, while median OS was 37 months.

Front-line ifosfamide combined with anthracyclines is clinically active in adult advanced soft tissue sarcomas, including liposarcomas [11, 12]. Following a histology-driven

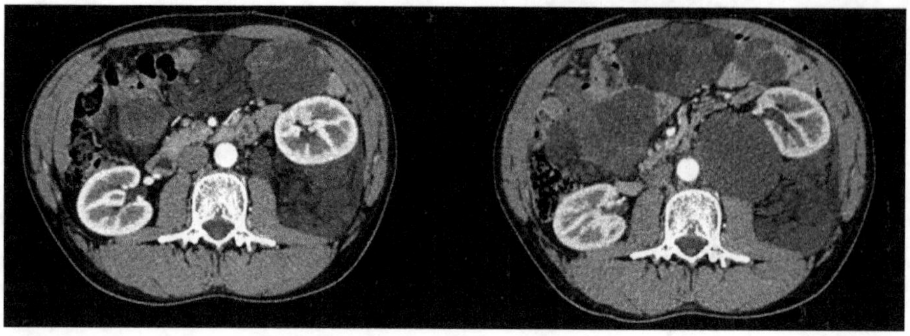

FIGURE 1: Multidetector computed tomography (MDCT) scan after contrast medium (arterial phase). Progression of abdominal metastasis from a myxoid liposarcoma after two cycles of high-dose prolonged-infusion ifosfamide.

TABLE 1: Patients characteristics at chemotherapy when starting ifosfamide.

Patients characteristics	
Age, years	
Median	33
Range	31–75
Histopathological diagnosis	
Round cell myxoid liposarcoma (high grade)	7 (63%)
Classical myxoid liposarcoma (low grade)	4 (37%)
Metastatic disease at diagnosis	2 (18%)
Localized disease at diagnosis	9 (82%)
Adjuvant chemotherapy	
Y	8 (73%)
N	3 (27%)
Adjuvant radiotherapy	
Y	7 (64%)
N	4 (36%)
Number of sites involved	
Median	2
Range	1–3
Local relapse	4 (36%)
Metastatic sites	
Lung	8 (73%)
Abdominal cavity	7 (64%)
Bone	1 (9%)
Soft Tissue	1 (9%)
Number of prior chemotherapy regimens	
0	1 (10%)
1	5 (45%)
2	3 (27%)
3	2 (18%)
Prior chemotherapy	
Anthracycline ± Ifosfamide	11 (100%)
Trabectedin	3 (27%)
Pemetrexed	1 (10%)
Liposomal doxorubicin	1 (9%)
Unknown	2 (18%)
High-dose ifosfamide infusion	
Elastomeric pump	11 (100%)
Number of ifosfamide courses	
Median	3
Range	(2–7)

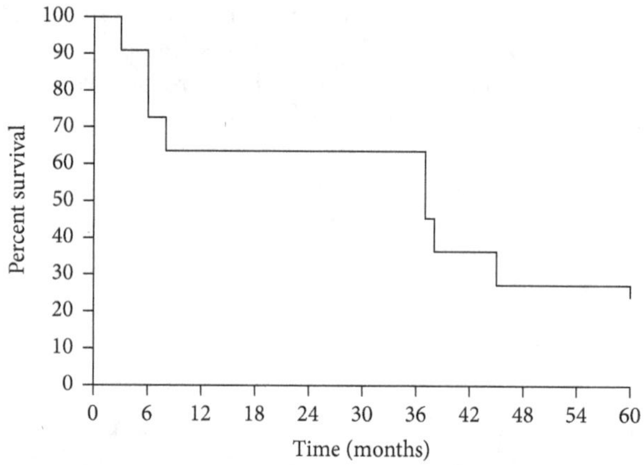

FIGURE 2: Overall survival (OS) of patients treated with high-dose prolonged-infusion ifosfamide chemotherapy (11 patients). Median OS was 37 months.

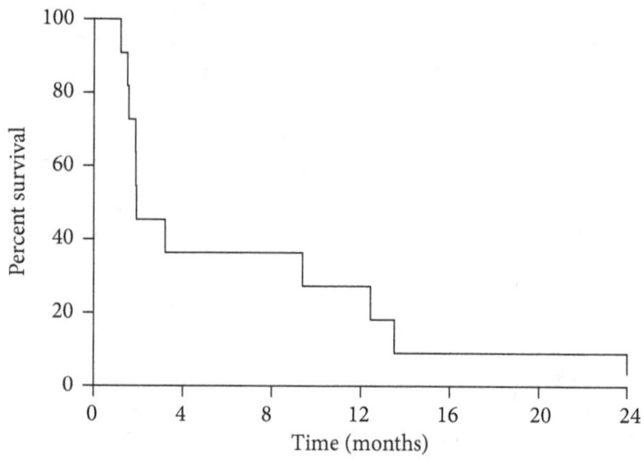

FIGURE 3: Overall progression-free survival (PFS) of patients treated with high-dose prolonged-infusion ifosfamide chemotherapy (11 patients). Median PFS was 1.9 months.

approach, high-dose ifosfamide as a single agent is often used as second-/further line treatment, even in patients previously treated with standard-dose ifosfamide.

HDIFX is known to be active in dedifferentiated liposarcoma and other histotypes [2, 10, 22–24, 27]. In our series, all patients had responded to anthracycline ± ifosfamide used as front-line treatment. These data are in line with studies pointing to a high sensitivity to cytotoxic chemotherapy of myxoid/round cell liposarcoma [8–10]. This is striking if compared to the apparent lack of activity of HDIFX in myxoid liposarcoma. Interestingly, there are no studies comparing the activity of anthracycline plus ifosfamide versus anthracycline alone in myxoid liposarcoma. On this basis, it is not known to which extent ifosfamide adds to anthracycline as a single agent in the first-line treatment of myxoid liposarcoma. The fact that in our series HDIFX did not show any antitumor activity raises doubts over its efficacy in myxoid liposarcomas. Clearly, all patients included in this series had been pretreated with doxorubicin plus ifosfamide, and we cannot rule out that this was an acquired resistance to the drug. However, the antitumor effect of ifosfamide as such may be better evaluated prospectively also in first line.

5. Conclusions

This was a retrospective analysis; the number of patients was limited and data refer to a 14-year span. However, it is difficult to extrapolate evidence pertaining to this subgroup of patients, let alone the lack of published retrospective and prospective studies on HDIFX selectively in myxoid liposarcoma. Thus, we believe that this series may stimulate collection of further cases. It is unfortunate that even if myxoid liposarcoma is considered chemosensitive among soft tissue sarcomas, only anthracyclines and trabectedin are active agents in this subtype at the moment. New medical treatments would be definitely needed.

Disclosure

This research did not receive any specific grant from funding agencies in the public, commercial, or not-for-profit sectors.

References

[1] C. A. Stiller, A. Trama, D. Serraino et al., "Descriptive epidemiology of sarcomas in Europe: report from the RARECARE project," *European Journal of Cancer*, vol. 49, no. 3, pp. 684–695, 2013.

[2] M. Saponara, S. Stacchiotti, and A. Gronchi, "Pharmacological therapies for Liposarcoma," *Expert Review of Clinical Pharmacology*, vol. 10, no. 4, pp. 361–377, 2017.

[3] C. D. M. Fletcher, J. A. Bridge, P. C. W. Hogendoorn et al., *WHO Classification of Tumours of Soft Tissue and Bone*, IARC Press, Lyon, France, 2013.

[4] M. Fiore, F. Grosso, S. Lo Vullo et al., "Myxoid/round cell and pleomorphic liposarcomas: prognostic factors and survival in a series of patients treated at a single institution," *Cancer*, vol. 109, no. 12, pp. 2522–2531, 2007.

[5] C. R. Antonescu, S. J. Tschernyavsky, R. Decuseara et al., "Prognostic impact of P53 status, TLS-CHOP fusion transcript structure, and histological grade in myxoid liposarcoma: a molecular and clinicopathologic study of 82 cases," *Clinical Cancer Research*, vol. 7, no. 12, pp. 3977–3987, 2001.

[6] The ESMO/European Sarcoma Network Working Group, "Soft tissue and visceral sarcomas: ESMO Clinical Practice Guidelines for diagnosis, treatment and follow-up," *Annals of Oncology*, vol. 25, supplement 3, pp. iii102–iii112, 2014.

[7] G. Pitson, P. Robinson, D. Wilke et al., "Radiation response: an additional unique signature of myxoid liposarcoma," *International Journal of Radiation Oncology Biology Physics*, vol. 60, no. 2, pp. 522–526, 2004.

[8] R. L. Jones, C. Fisher, O. Al-Muderis, and I. R. Judson, "Differential sensitivity of liposarcoma subtypes to chemotherapy," *European Journal of Cancer*, vol. 41, no. 18, pp. 2853–2860, 2005.

[9] F. Grosso, R. L. Jones, G. D. Demetri et al., "Efficacy of trabectedin (ecteinascidin-743) in advanced pretreated myxoid liposarcomas: a retrospective study," *The Lancet Oncology*, vol. 8, no. 7, pp. 595–602, 2007.

[10] R. Sanfilippo, R. Bertulli, A. Marrari et al., "High-dose continuous-infusion ifosfamide in advanced well-differentiated/dedifferentiated liposarcoma," *Clinical Sarcoma Research*, vol. 4, no. 1, p. 16, 2014.

[11] I. Judson, J. Verweij, H. Gelderblom et al., "Doxorubicin alone versus intensified doxorubicin plus ifosfamide for first-line treatment of advanced or metastatic soft-tissue sarcoma: a randomised controlled phase 3 trial," *The Lancet Oncology*, vol. 15, no. 4, pp. 415–423, 2014.

[12] R. Ratan and S. R. Patel, "Chemotherapy for soft tissue sarcoma," *Cancer*, vol. 122, no. 19, pp. 2952–2960, 2016.

[13] F. Grosso, R. Sanfilippo, E. Virdis et al., "Trabectedin in myxoid liposarcomas (MLS): a long-term analysis of a single-institution series," *Annals of Oncology*, vol. 20, no. 8, pp. 1439–1444, 2009.

[14] G. Germano, R. Frapolli, M. Simone et al., "Antitumor and anti-inflammatory effects of trabectedin on human myxoid liposarcoma cells," *Cancer Research*, vol. 70, no. 6, pp. 2235–2244, 2010.

[15] E. Charytonowicz, M. Terry, K. Coakley et al., "PPARγ agonists enhance ET-743 - Induced adipogenic differentiation in a transgenic mouse model of myxoid round cell liposarcoma," *Journal of Clinical Investigation*, vol. 122, no. 3, pp. 886–898, 2012.

[16] R. Dossi, R. Frapolli, S. Di Giandomenico et al., "Antiangiogenic activity of trabectedin in myxoid liposarcoma: involvement of host TIMP-1 and TIMP-2 and tumor thrombospondin-1," *International Journal of Cancer*, vol. 136, no. 3, pp. 721–729, 2015.

[17] C. Forni, M. Minuzzo, E. Virdis et al., "Trabectedin (ET-743) promotes differentiation in myxoid liposarcoma tumors," *Molecular Cancer Therapeutics*, vol. 8, no. 2, pp. 449–457, 2009.

[18] S. Di Giandomenico, R. Frapolli, E. Bello et al., "Mode of action of trabectedin in myxoid liposarcomas," *Oncogene*, vol. 33, no. 44, pp. 5201–5210, 2014.

[19] P. Schöffski, I. L. Ray-Coquard, A. Cioffi et al., "European Organisation for Research and Treatment of Cancer (EORTC) Soft Tissue and Bone Sarcoma Group (STBSG). Activity of eribulin mesylate in patients with soft-tissue sarcoma: a phase 2 study in four independent histological subtypes," *The Lancet Oncology*, vol. 12, no. 11, pp. 1045–1052, 2011.

[20] P. Schöffski, S. Chawla, R. G. Maki et al., "Eribulin versus dacarbazine in previously treated patients with advanced liposarcoma or leiomyosarcoma: a randomised, open-label, multicentre, phase 3 trial," *The Lancet*, vol. 387, no. 10028, pp. 1629–1637, 2016.

[21] S. P. Chawla, P. Schöffski, G. Grignani et al., "Subtype-specific activity in liposarcoma (LPS) patients (pts) from a phase 3, open-label, randomized study of eribulin (ERI) versus dacarbazine (DTIC) in patients with advanced LPS and leiomyosarcoma (LMS)," *Journal of Clinical Oncology*, vol. 34, no. suppl_6, 2016.

[22] A. Le Cesne, E. Antoine, M. Spielmann et al., "High-dose ifosfamide: circumvention of resistance to standard-dose ifosfamide in advanced soft tissue sarcomas," *Journal of Clinical Oncology*, vol. 13, no. 7, pp. 1600–1608, 1995.

[23] S. R. Patel, S. Vadhan-Raj, N. Papadopolous et al., "High-dose ifosfamide in bone and soft tissue sarcomas: results of phase II and pilot studies: sose-response and schedule dependence," *Journal of Clinical Oncology*, vol. 15, no. 6, pp. 2378–2384, 1997.

[24] R. Palumbo, S. Palmeri, M. Antimi et al., "Phase II study of continuous-infusion high-dose ifosfamide in advanced and/or metastatic pretreated soft tissue sarcomas," *Annals of Oncology*, vol. 8, no. 11, pp. 1159–1162, 1997.

[25] P. Therasse, S. G. Arbuck, E. A. Eisenhauer et al., "New guidelines to evaluate the response to treatment in solid tumors. European Organization for Research and Treatment of Cancer, National Cancer Institute of the United States, National Cancer Institute of Canada ," *Journal of the National Cancer Institute*, vol. 92, no. 3, pp. 205–216, 2000.

[26] E. L. Kaplan and P. Meier, "Nonparametric estimation from incomplete observations," *Journal of the American Statistical Association*, vol. 53, pp. 457–481, 1958.

[27] G. Rosen, C. Forscher, S. Lowenbraun et al., "Synovial sarcoma. Uniform response of metastases to high dose ifosfamide," *Cancer*, vol. 73, no. 10, pp. 2506–2511, 1994.

Permissions

All chapters in this book were first published in SARCOMA, by Hindawi Publishing Corporation; hereby published with permission under the Creative Commons Attribution License or equivalent. Every chapter published in this book has been scrutinized by our experts. Their significance has been extensively debated. The topics covered herein carry significant findings which will fuel the growth of the discipline. They may even be implemented as practical applications or may be referred to as a beginning point for another development.

The contributors of this book come from diverse backgrounds, making this book a truly international effort. This book will bring forth new frontiers with its revolutionizing research information and detailed analysis of the nascent developments around the world.

We would like to thank all the contributing authors for lending their expertise to make the book truly unique. They have played a crucial role in the development of this book. Without their invaluable contributions this book wouldn't have been possible. They have made vital efforts to compile up to date information on the varied aspects of this subject to make this book a valuable addition to the collection of many professionals and students.

This book was conceptualized with the vision of imparting up-to-date information and advanced data in this field. To ensure the same, a matchless editorial board was set up. Every individual on the board went through rigorous rounds of assessment to prove their worth. After which they invested a large part of their time researching and compiling the most relevant data for our readers.

The editorial board has been involved in producing this book since its inception. They have spent rigorous hours researching and exploring the diverse topics which have resulted in the successful publishing of this book. They have passed on their knowledge of decades through this book. To expedite this challenging task, the publisher supported the team at every step. A small team of assistant editors was also appointed to further simplify the editing procedure and attain best results for the readers.

Apart from the editorial board, the designing team has also invested a significant amount of their time in understanding the subject and creating the most relevant covers. They scrutinized every image to scout for the most suitable representation of the subject and create an appropriate cover for the book.

The publishing team has been an ardent support to the editorial, designing and production team. Their endless efforts to recruit the best for this project, has resulted in the accomplishment of this book. They are a veteran in the field of academics and their pool of knowledge is as vast as their experience in printing. Their expertise and guidance has proved useful at every step. Their uncompromising quality standards have made this book an exceptional effort. Their encouragement from time to time has been an inspiration for everyone.

The publisher and the editorial board hope that this book will prove to be a valuable piece of knowledge for researchers, students, practitioners and scholars across the globe.

List of Contributors

Robert J. Wilson, Jennifer L. Halpern, Herbert S. Schwartz and Ginger E. Holt
Department of Orthopaedics and Rehabilitation, Vanderbilt University Medical Center, Nashville, TN 37232, USA

Vignesh K. Alamanda
Department of Orthopaedics, Carolinas Medical Center, Charlotte, NC 28203, USA

Katherine G. Hartley
Department of Radiology and Radiological Sciences, Vanderbilt University Medical Center, Nashville, TN 37232, USA

Nathan W. Mesko
Department of Orthopaedics, Cleveland Clinic, Cleveland, OH 44195, USA

Xiaodong Mu and Johnny Huard
Department of Orthopaedic Surgery, University of Texas Health Science Center at Houston, Houston, TX 77030, USA

Stuti Patel, Adel Mahjoub and Kurt Weiss
Cancer Stem Cell Laboratory, Department of Orthopaedic Surgery, University of Pittsburgh, Pittsburgh, PA 15219, Kazakhstan

Damel Mektepbayeva
Laboratory of Cellular Technology, Nazarbayev University, Astana, Akmola 010000, USA

Tomohiro Fujiwara, Koichi Ogura, Eisuke Kobayashi, Yoshikazu Tanzawa, Fumihiko Nakatani, Hirokazu Chuman and Akira Kawai
Division of Musculoskeletal Oncology, National Cancer Center Hospital, 5-1-1 Tsukiji, Chuo-ku, Tokyo 104-0045, Japan

ShyamK. Tanguturi
Harvard Radiation Oncology Program, Boston, MA 02115, USA

Suzanne George and George D. Demetri
Center for Sarcoma and Bone Oncology, Dana-Farber Cancer Institute, Boston, MA 02115, USA
Department of Medical Oncology, Dana-Farber Cancer Institute, Boston, MA 02115, USA

Karen J. Marcus and Elizabeth H. Baldini
Center for Sarcoma and Bone Oncology, Dana-Farber Cancer Institute, Boston, MA 02115, USA
Department of Radiation Oncology, Dana-Farber Cancer Institute, Boston, MA 02115, USA
Department of Radiation Oncology, Brigham and Women's Hospital, Boston, MA 02115, USA
Department of Radiation Oncology, Boston's Children's Hospital, Boston, MA 02115, USA

Sjoerd P. F. T. Nota, Yvonne Braun and Joseph H. Schwab
Orthopaedic Oncology Service, Massachusetts General Hospital, Harvard Medical School, Boston, MA 02114, USA

C. Niek van Dijk and Jos A. M. Bramer
Department of Orthopaedic Surgery, Academic Medical Center, 1105 AZ Amsterdam, Netherlands

Winnie W. Lo and Irene L. Andrulis
Department of Molecular Genetics, University of Toronto, ON, Canada M5S 1A8
Lunenfeld-Tanenbaum Research Institute, Mount Sinai Hospital, 600 University Avenue, Toronto, ON, Canada M5G 1X5

Dushanthi Pinnaduwage and Nalan Gokgoz
Lunenfeld-Tanenbaum Research Institute, Mount Sinai Hospital, 600 University Avenue, Toronto, ON, Canada M5G 1X5

Jay S. Wunder
Lunenfeld-Tanenbaum Research Institute, Mount Sinai Hospital, 600 University Avenue, Toronto, ON, Canada M5G 1X5
University Musculoskeletal Oncology Unit, Mount Sinai Hospital, Toronto, ON, Canada M5G 1X5
Department of Surgery, University of Toronto, ON, Canada M5G 1L5

Koichi Ogura, Tomohiro Fujiwara, Hirokazu Chuman and Akira Kawai
Department of Musculoskeletal Oncology, National Cancer Center Hospital, 5-1-1 Tsukiji, Chuo-ku, Tokyo 104-0045, Japan

Shimpei Miyamoto and Minoru Sakuraba
Department of Plastic and Reconstruction Surgery, National Cancer Center Hospital, 5-1-1 Tsukiji, Chuo-ku, Tokyo 104-0045, Japan

Mohamad Farid, Linda Ahn, Andrew Brohl, Angela Cioffi and Robert G. Maki
Mount Sinai Medical Center, One Gustave L. Levy Place, New York, NY 10029-6574, USA

Juan Martin-Liberal, Salma Alam, Anastasia Constantinidou, Omar Al-Muderis, Aisha Miah, Mark Linch, Robin L. Jones, Michelle Scurr, Ian Judson and Charlotte Benson
Sarcoma Unit, The Royal Marsden Hospital, Fulham Road, London SW3 6JJ, UK

Cyril Fisher
Department of Histopathology, The Royal Marsden Hospital, Fulham Road, London SW3 6JJ, UK

Komel Khabra
Department of Statistics, The Royal Marsden Hospital, Downs Road, Sutton SM2 5PT, UK

Christina Messiou
Department of Radiodiagnostics, The Royal Marsden Hospital, Fulham Road, London SW3 6JJ, UK

David Olmos
Spanish National Cancer Research Centre (CNIO), Clinical Research Programme, 3 Melchor Fernandez Almagro, 28029 Madrid, Spain

Scott Mitchell
Department of Pharmacy, The Royal Marsden Hospital, Fulham Road, London SW3 6JJ, UK

Jordan Amdahl and Thomas E. Delea
Policy Analysis Inc. (PAI), Four Davis Court, Brookline, MA 02445, USA

Stephanie C. Manson, Robert Isbell and Jose Diaz
GlaxoSmithKline, Stockley Park West, Uxbridge, Middlesex UB11 1BT, UK

Ayman Chit
GlaxoSmithKline, 7333 Mississauga Road, Mississauga, ON, Canada L5N 6L4
University of Toronto, 144 College Street, Toronto, ON, Canada M5S 3M2

Lily Lewis
York Health Economics Consortium, Level 2, Market Square, University of York, Heslington, York YO10 5NH, UK

Tine Cuppens and Sandra Tuyaerts
Department of Oncology, Gynaecologic Oncology, KU Leuven (University of Leuven), 3000 Leuven, Belgium

Frédéric Amant
Department of Oncology, Gynaecologic Oncology, KU Leuven (University of Leuven), 3000 Leuven, Belgium
Department of Obstetrics and Gynaecology, University Hospitals Leuven, 3000 Leuven, Belgium
Center for Gynaecologic Oncology Amsterdam (CGOA), Antoni van Leeuwenhoek-Netherlands Cancer Institute, 1066 CX Amsterdam, Netherlands

Judith U. Cope
Office of Pediatric Therapeutics, Office of Special Medical Programs, Office of the Commissioner/Food and Drug Administration, Building 32, Room 5156, 10903 New Hampshire Avenue, Silver Spring, MD 20993, USA

Gregory H. Reaman
Office of Hematology and Oncology Products, OND, Center for Drug Evaluation and Research, U.S. Food and Drug Administration, White Oak Bldg. 22, Room2202, 10903 New Hampshire Avenue, Silver Spring, MD 20993, USA

Joseph M. Tonning
U.S. Public Health Service Commissioned Corps, Office of Translational Sciences, Center for Drug Evaluation and Research, U.S. Food and Drug Administration, White Oak Bldg. 22, Room3410, 10903 New Hampshire Avenue, Silver Spring, MD 20993,USA

Mark A. Dickson, Mary L. Keohan, Sandra P. D'Angelo, Mrinal M. Gounder, Olivia R. McKennon, Catherine M. Hirst and William D. Tap
Department of Medicine, Memorial Sloan-Kettering Cancer Center and Weill Cornell Medical College, New York, NY, USA

David R. D'Adamo
Eisai, Inc., Woodcliff Lake, NJ, USA

Richard D. Carvajal and Gary K. Schwartz
Department of Medicine, Columbia University, New York, NY, USA

Robert G. Maki
Departments of Medicine and Pediatrics, Mount Sinai School of Medicine, New York, NY, USA

Li-Xuan Qin
Department of Biostatistics, Memorial Sloan-Kettering Cancer Center and Weill Cornell Medical College, New York, NY, USA

Robert A. Lefkowitz
Department of Radiology, Memorial Sloan-Kettering Cancer Center and Weill Cornell Medical College, New York, NY, USA

Christopher J. Forlenza, Brian H. Kushner, Nancy Kernan, Farid Boulad, Heather Magnan, Leonard Wexler and Shakeel Modak
Department of Pediatrics, Memorial Sloan-Kettering Cancer Center, 1275 York Avenue, New York, NY 10065, USA

Suzanne L. Wolden
Department of Radiation Oncology, Memorial Sloan-Kettering Cancer Center, 1275 York Avenue, New York, NY 10065, USA

Michael P. LaQuaglia
Department of Pediatrics, Memorial Sloan-Kettering Cancer Center, 1275 York Avenue, New York, NY 10065, USA
Department of Surgery, Memorial Sloan-Kettering Cancer Center, 1275 York Avenue, New York, NY 10065, USA

Scott Evans, Michele Boffano, Samena Chaudhry, Lee Jeys and Robert Grimer
Royal Orthopaedic Hospital, Birmingham B31 2AP, UK

Henry J. Conter and Vancheswaran Gopalakrishnan
Division of Cancer Medicine, M.D. Anderson Cancer Center, 1400 Holcombe Boulevard, Unit 463, Houston, TX 77030, USA

Vinod Ravi, Shreyaskumar Patel and Dejka M. Araujo
Department of Sarcoma Medical Oncology, M.D. Anderson Cancer Center, 1400Holcombe Boulevard, Unit 463, Houston, TX 77030, USA

Joann L. Ater
Department of Pediatrics Patient Care, M.D. Anderson Cancer Center, 1400 Holcombe Boulevard, Unit 463, Houston, TX 77030, USA

Patrick W. O'Donnell
Department of Orthopaedic Surgery, Markey Cancer Center, University of Kentucky, 740 S. Limestone Avenue, Lexington, KY 40536, USA

Anthony M. Griffin, Amir Sternheim, Lawrence M. White, Jay S. Wunder and Peter C. Ferguson
Department of Orthopaedic Surgery, Mount Sinai Hospital, Toronto, ON, Canada M5G 1X5

William C. Eward
Department of Orthopaedic Surgery, Duke Cancer Center, Duke University, Durham, NC 27710, USA

Julie J. Willeumier, C. W. P. G. van der Wal, Robert J. P. van der Wal, P. D. S. Dijkstra, Thea P. M. Vliet Vlieland and Michiel A. J. van de Sande
Department of Orthopaedic Surgery, Leiden University Medical Center, Leiden, Netherlands

Thale M. Asp Strøm and Olga Zaikova
Department of Orthopedic Surgery, The Norwegian Radium Hospital, Oslo University Hospital, Oslo, Norway

Anette Torød Skeie
Department of Radiology, The Norwegian Radium Hospital, Oslo University Hospital, Oslo, Norway

Ingvild Koren Lobmaier
Department of Pathology, The Norwegian Radium Hospital, Oslo University Hospital, Oslo, Norway

Michael J. Nathenson
Dana–Farber Cancer Institute, 450 Brookline Ave., Boston, MA 02215, USA

Anthony P. Conley and Vinod Ravi
Department of Sarcoma Medical Oncology, The University of Texas MD Anderson Cancer Center, 1515 Holcombe Blvd Unit 450, Houston, TX 77030, USA

Heather Lin
Department of Biostatistics, The University of Texas MD Anderson Cancer Center, 1515 Holcombe Blvd Unit 450, Houston, TX 77030, USA

Nicole Fleming
Department of Gynecologic Oncology and Reproductive Medicine, The University of Texas MD Anderson Cancer Center, 1515 Holcombe Blvd Unit 450, Houston, TX 77030, USA

Johnathan R. Lex
University of Birmingham, Birmingham B15 2TT, UK

Ahmed Aoude, Nikolaos A. Stavropoulos, Krista Goulding and Robert E. Turcotte
McGill University Health Centre, Montreal, QC, Canada H4A 3J1

Jonathan D. Stevenson and Scott Evans
Royal Orthopaedic Hospital, Birmingham B31 2AP, UK

Jay S. Wunder and Peter C. Ferguson
University of Toronto Musculoskeletal Oncology Unit, Mount Sinai Hospital, Toronto, ON, Canada M5G 1X5

Lee Jeys
Royal Orthopaedic Hospital, Birmingham B31 2AP, UK
School of Life and Health Sciences, Aston University, Birmingham B4 7ET, UK

Kayleen Bailey
Division of Pediatric Hematology Oncology, Memorial Sloan Kettering Cancer Center, New York Presbyterian Hospital Cornell, New York, NY, USA

Michael Roth and Jonathan Gill
Division of Pediatrics, University of Texas MD Anderson Cancer Center, Houston, TX, USA

Daniel Weiser
Division of Pediatric Hematology, Oncology, Marrow and Blood Cell Transplantation, The Children's Hospital at Montefiore, Bronx, NY, USA

Heather Miller
Department of Obstetrics & Gynecology, Baylor College of Medicine, Houston, TX 77030, USA

Chiemeka Ike and Jennifer Parma
College of Pharmacy, University of Houston, Houston, TX 77030, USA

Claire M. Mach
Department of Obstetrics & Gynecology, Baylor College of Medicine, Houston, TX 77030, USA
College of Pharmacy, University of Houston, Houston, TX 77030, USA

Ramya P. Masand
Department of Pathology & Immunology, Baylor College of Medicine, Houston, TX 77030, USA

Matthew L. Anderson
Department of Obstetrics & Gynecology, Baylor College of Medicine, Houston, TX 77030, USA
Department of Pathology & Immunology, Baylor College of Medicine, Houston, TX 77030, USA
Dan L Duncan Cancer Center, Baylor College of Medicine, Houston, TX 77030, USA

Fabian Wolpert
Department of Neurology, University Hospital Zurich, Frauenklinikstrasse 26, 8091 Zurich, Switzerland
Department of Medical Oncology, University Hospital Zurich, Rämistrasse 100, 8091 Zurich, Switzerland

Michael A. Grotzer and Felix Niggli
Department of Pediatric Oncology, University Children's Hospital, Zurich, Steinwiesstrasse 75, 8032 Zurich, Switzerland

Dieter Zimmermann and Beata Bode-Lesniewska
Institute of Surgical Pathology, University Hospital Zurich, Schmelzbergstrasse 12, 8091 Zurich, Switzerland

Elisabeth Rushing
Department of Neuropathology, University Hospital Zurich, Schmelzbergstrasse 12, 8091 Zurich, Switzerland

David D. Greenberg and Brooke Crawford
Saint Louis University Hospital, 7th Floor, Desloge Towers, 3635 Vista Avenue, St. Louis, MO 63110, USA

A. Sanchez, B. Lala, N. Schmidt and C. Okoli
Sarcoma Oncology Service, Department of Medicine, Memorial Sloan Kettering Cancer Center, 1275 York Avenue, New York, NY 10065, USA

A. N. Shoushtari, P. Chi, M. A. Dickson, M. M. Gounder, M. L. Keohan, W. D. Tap and S. P. D'Angelo
Sarcoma Oncology Service, Department of Medicine, Memorial Sloan Kettering Cancer Center, 1275 York Avenue, New York, NY 10065, USA
Weill Cornell Medical College, 1300 York Avenue, New York, NY 10065, USA

J. Landa
Department of Radiology, Memorial Sloan Kettering Cancer Center, 1275 York Avenue, New York, NY 10065, USA

D. Kuk
Department of Epidemiology and Biostatistics, Memorial Sloan Kettering Cancer Center, 1275 York Avenue, New York, NY 10065, USA

A. M. Crago
Weill Cornell Medical College, 1300 York Avenue, New York, NY 10065, USA
Department of Surgery, Memorial Sloan Kettering Cancer Center, 1275 York Avenue, New York, NY 10065, USA

Kate Thompson and Deborah Howell
Victorian Adolescent & Young Adult Cancer Service, Peter MacCallum Cancer Centre, Melbourne, VIC, Australia

Jeremy Lewin
Victorian Adolescent & Young Adult Cancer Service, Peter MacCallum Cancer Centre, Melbourne, VIC, Australia
Adolescent and Young Adult Oncology, Princess Margaret Cancer Centre, Toronto, ON, Canada

Susie Bae, Jayesh Desai and Denise Caruso
Australasian Sarcoma Study Group, Melbourne, VIC, Australia

Robyn Strong
Australian and New Zealand Children's Hematology/ Oncology Group, Melbourne, VIC, Australia

Alan Herschtal
Centre for Biostatistics and Clinical Trials, Peter MacCallum Cancer Centre, Melbourne, VIC, Australia

Michael Sullivan
Children's Cancer Centre, Royal Children's Hospital, Melbourne, VIC, Australia
Department of Paediatrics, University of Melbourne, Melbourne, VIC, Australia

Lisa Orme
Victorian Adolescent & Young Adult Cancer Service, Peter MacCallum Cancer Centre, Melbourne, VIC, Australia
Children's Cancer Centre, Royal Children's Hospital, Melbourne, VIC, Australia

Vivek Ajit Singh and Rukmanikanthan Shanmugam
Department of Orthopaedic Surgery, University of Malaya Medical Centre, 59100 Kuala Lumpur, Malaysia

Hassan Elbahri
Khartoum Teaching Hospital, 11111 Khartoum, Sudan

Vittoria Colia, Elena Fumagalli, Salvatore Provenzano, Rossella Bertulli, Silvia Stacchiotti and Roberta Sanfilippo
Medical Oncology Unit 2, Medical Oncology Department, Fondazione IRCCS Istituto Nazionale dei Tumori, Milan, Italy

Carlo Morosi
Department of Radiology, Fondazione IRCCS Istituto Nazionale dei Tumori, Milan, Italy

Paola Collini
Department of Diagnostic Pathology and Laboratory Medicine, Fondazione IRCCS Istituto Nazionale dei Tumori, Milan, Italy

Alessandro Gronchi
Department of Surgery, Fondazione IRCCS Istituto Nazionale dei Tumori, Milan, Italy

Paolo G. Casali
Medical Oncology Unit 2, Medical Oncology Department, Fondazione IRCCS Istituto Nazionale dei Tumori, Milan, Italy
Oncology and Haemato-Oncology Department, University of Milan, Milan, Italy

Index

www.ingramcontent.com/pod-product-compliance
Lightning Source LLC
LaVergne TN
LVHW081030210926
848485LV00004B/992